D1594250

The Biosynthesis of Mycotoxins

A STUDY IN SECONDARY METABOLISM

Contributors

John A. Anderson

W. Breitenstein

J. D. Bu'Lock

Heinz G. Floss

Burchard Franck

Cedric W. Holzapfel

G. W. Kirby

D. J. Robins

U. Sankawa

Pieter S. Steyn

Ch. Tamm

Robert Vleggaar

Philippus L. Wessels

Mikio Yamazaki

Lolita O. Zamir

The Biosynthesis of Mycotoxins

A STUDY IN SECONDARY METABOLISM

Edited by

Pieter S. Steyn

National Chemical Research Laboratory
Council for Scientific and Industrial Research
Pretoria, South Africa

1980

ACADEMIC PRESS
A Subsidiary of Harcourt Brace Jovanovich, Publishers
New York   London   Toronto   Sydney   San Francisco

ACADEMIC PRESS, INC.
111 Fifth Avenue, New York, New York 10003

United Kingdom Edition published by
ACADEMIC PRESS, INC. (LONDON) LTD.
24/28 Oval Road, London NW1 7DX

Library of Congress Cataloging in Publication Data

Main entry under title:

The Biosynthesis of Mycotoxins.

Includes bibliographies and index.
1. Mycotoxins––Synthesis. 2. Metabolism,
Secondary. 3. Fungi––Physiology. I. Steyn,
Pieter S. [DNLM: 1. Mycotoxins––Biosynthesis.
QW630 B615]

QP632.M9B56   599.02'326   80–12013
ISBN 0–12–670650–6

PRINTED IN THE UNITED STATES OF AMERICA

80 81 82 83   9 8 7 6 5 4 3 2 1

Contents

11 The Biosynthesis of Anthraquinonoid Mycotoxins from Penicillium islandicum Sopp and Related Fungi
U. SANKAWA

12 The Biosynthesis of Some Miscellaneous Mycotoxins
ROBERT VLEGGAAR AND PIETER S. STEYN

List of Contributors

Numbers in parentheses indicate the pages on which the authors' contributions begin.

John A. Anderson (17), Department of Chemistry, Texas Tech University, Lubbock, Texas 79409

W. Breitenstein (69), Central Research Laboratories, Ciba-Geigy AG, 4002 Basel, Switzerland

J. D. Bu'Lock (1), Weizmann Microbial Chemistry Laboratory, Department of Chemistry, The University, Manchester M13 9PL, England

Heinz G. Floss (17), Department of Medicinal Chemistry and Pharmacognosy, School of Pharmacy and Pharmacal Sciences, Purdue University, West Lafayette, Indiana 47907

Burchard Franck (157), Institute for Organic Chemistry, University of Münster, D-4400 Münster, West Germany

Cedric W. Holzapfel (327), Department of Chemistry, Rand Afrikaans University, Johannesburg 2000, South Africa

G. W. Kirby (301), Chemistry Department, The University, Glasgow G12 8QQ, Scotland

D. J. Robins (301), Chemistry Department, The University, Glasgow G12 8QQ, Scotland

U. Sankawa (357), Faculty of Pharmaceutical Sciences, University of Tokyo, Bunkyo-ku, Tokyo, Japan

Pieter S. Steyn (105, 395), National Chemical Research Laboratory, Council for Scientific and Industrial Research, Pretoria 0001, South Africa

Ch. Tamm (69, 269), Institute of Organic Chemistry, University of Basel, 4056 Basel, Switzerland

Robert Vleggaar (105, 395), National Chemical Research Laboratory, Council for Scientific and Industrial Research, Pretoria 0001, South Africa

Philippus L. Wessels (105), National Chemical Research Laboratory, Council for Scientific and Industrial Research, Pretoria 0001, South Africa

Mikio Yamazaki (193), Research Institute for Chemobiodynamics, Chiba
    University, Chiba 280, Japan
Lolita O. Zamir (223), Department of Chemistry, Biology, and Center for
    Somatic Cell Genetics and Biochemistry, State University of New
    York at Binghamton, Binghamton, New York 13901

Foreword

Microorganisms have a marvelous capacity to produce secondary metabolites which show biological activity. Since these compounds frequently have complex and interesting structures, they have long been welcome to chemists as research challenges worthy of the most sophisticated effort.

The spectacular developments in antibiotic chemistry, which began in the 1940s and have continued with unabated effort and progress up to the present, are well appreciated. The importance of mycotoxins was perhaps less well known until in the early 1960s the extremely powerful and dangerous biological effects of the aflatoxins were discovered. Since that time the subject has developed enormously and the time is certainly ripe for an authoritative book.

Almost all secondary metabolites of microorganisms have structures that betray their biosynthetic origins. Indeed the biosynthetic analysis of these metabolites, frequently by the Birch hypothesis, is a powerful unifying principle.

This volume represents an excellent account of the biosynthesis of the mycotoxins. Dr. Steyn, himself an internationally accepted authority on the subject, has been able to persuade an outstanding group of authors to contribute chapters. This book will not only be the standard reference work for anyone concerned with mycotoxins, but it will also inspire a lot of challenging synthetic chemistry. Recent progress in the synthesis of the cytochalasans admirably illustrates this point.

Finally, this book would have given great pleasure to the outstanding microbial chemist of the first half of this century, the late Harold Raistrick.

Derek Barton
Institute for the Chemistry of
Natural Products
Gif-sur-Yvette, France

Preface

This volume is devoted to the biosynthesis of mycotoxins (from Greek, *mykes:* fungus).

The constituents of microorganisms such as fungi and bacteria may be classified formally as those molecules which are of primary metabolic concern and those which have no obvious utility for the organisms producing them. Primary metabolism is basically the same for most living systems and has been studied in great detail by biochemists as it provides the system with energy, synthetic intermediates, and key macromolecules. Secondary metabolites are produced from a few key intermediates of primary metabolism (e.g., acetate, propionate, pyruvate, malonate, mevalonate, and amino acids) by a consecutive series of enzyme-catalyzed reactions along pathways which branch from the primary network at a relatively small number of points.

Due to their structural complexity and unique biological properties, these highly specialized secondary microbial metabolites (e.g., antibiotics and mycotoxins), which are characteristic of the lower forms of life, are species-specific and often are strain-specific, and have long excited the curiosity of natural product chemists. Owing to their work, the dynamic relationship between primary metabolism and secondary pathways is now becoming clearer.

Mycotoxins are inherently a heterogeneous group of metabolites that are formed along the polyketide route (e.g., aflatoxins, patulin, penicillic acid, anthraquinones, and ergochromes) and the terpene route (e.g., trichothecanes), as well as from amino acids (e.g., ergot toxins and gliotoxins). An increasing number of newly discovered mycotoxins (e.g., ochratoxins, cyclopiazonic acids, and cytochalasans) are formed by an intriguing combination of some of the foregoing pathways.

We have attempted to include in this volume representative members of all the presently known mycotoxins as well as all the principal pathways involved in secondary fungal metabolism. However, the omission of the newest toxins and information which has accumulated on currently known toxins since the volume went to press is unavoidable, due to the rapidity with which this field is developing. The biogenesis of algal and mushroom toxins is not included in this volume.

Fungi are convenient organisms for the study of both primary and secondary metabolism and have been employed in the investigation of the details of many biosynthetic processes. The use of isotopically labeled precursors established the building units of several mycotoxins, the mechanisms involved in the linkage of the units and the transformations of intermediates. Experiments employing stereoselectively labeled (^{2}H and ^{3}H) precursors provided evidence for the subtle stereochemical control characteristic of enzymatically controlled processes.

Ergotism, certainly the first described form of a mycotoxicosis (a disease caused by the consumption of a mycotoxin), was recorded very early in history. More recently, molds (fungi) were also implicated in the etiology of diseases such as alimentary toxic aleukia and stachybotryotoxicosis in Russia, yellow rice toxicosis in Japan, and facial eczema in New Zealand.

Mycotoxins and mycotoxicoses were relatively obscure in scientific iterature until the dramatic discovery in the early 1960s of the aflatoxins, which are metabolites of the ubiquitous fungi *Aspergillus flavus* and *Aspergillus parasiticus*. The biochemical significance of aflatoxin B_1 was soon realized when Butler recognized it as the most potent hepatocellular carcinogen. Subsequent population-based studies in fact implicated aflatoxin contamination in the high incidence of human liver cancer occurring in various underdeveloped countries. This led to a reappraisal of the mycotoxin problem. Mycological surveys of foods and feeds revealed the international nature of the problem which only recently attracted much-needed attention from the scientific community. Research has also expanded greatly to other mycotoxins, particularly those from the genera *Aspergillus, Penicillium,* and *Fusarium*. Since the discovery of the aflatoxins, impressive progress has been made on the isolation of mycotoxins and the structure, synthesis, and biosynthesis of these compounds.

Research activities on mycotoxins are of necessity interdisciplinary. This volume will, therefore, be useful to biochemists and enzymologists who are interested in secondary metabolism, as well as to organic chemists, mycologists, plant pathologists, toxicologists, and graduate students.

I wish to express my sincere appreciation to the contributors to this book. The contributions of each of the eminent scientists demonstrate a high level of excellence. Each chapter contains introductory comments on the structure and biological significance of the mycotoxins involved. However, the selection and manner of description will inevitably reflect the authors' own interests and commitments in this field. I also acknowledge with gratitude the support of Dr. Robert Vleggaar whose interest and cooperation have been invaluable to me. A special word of thanks is also due the staff of Academic Press for their practical assistance and sympathetic cooperation.

Pieter S. Steyn

1

Mycotoxins as Secondary Metabolites

J. D. BU'LOCK

I. INTRODUCTION

In this introductory chapter the mycotoxins are considered as representative of wider range of fungal products which have come to be known as secondary metabolites (Bu'Lock, 1975). These have been defined in terms of several characteristics which do have some bearing on the problems of mycotoxin production. They include their problematic function, the combination of their structural diversity with their restricted biological occurrence, and the generally inverse relationship between their production and growth of the producing fungi. Each of these features is well exemplified within the mycotoxins, and this approach will be followed here, bearing in mind that these are a limited category within the range of secondary metabolites generally, and leaving until last the difficult question of function and its relevance, if any, to the mycotoxins *per se*.

II. DIVERSITY

However narrowly they are defined, the mycotoxins do not constitute a chemical category and they have no molecular features in common. All that

1

The Biosynthesis of Mycotoxins
Copyright © 1980 by Academic Press, Inc.
All rights of reproduction in any form reserved.
ISBN 0-12-670650-6.

can be found among their variety is a series of structurally related groups, which emerge most clearly and rationally when they are considered alongside other fungal products and classified in terms of biosynthetic pathways rather than structural features as such.

Both the diversity of the mycotoxins and their biogenetic relationships are of course fully covered in the ensuing chapters of this book, and here it is sufficient to indicate, as shown in Table I, hcw the principal mycotoxins are distributed between the main biosynthetic groups exemplified in fungal metabolism generally. This list is not intended as an exhaustive one, either for fungal metabolite categories or for mycotoxins, but simply to show how the smaller category is in fact fairly representative of the larger. This extends to aspects difficult to represent in tabular forms, for example to products whose biosynthesis involves combinations of two or more of the major pathways.

A further general feature which becomes apparent when the full range of secondary metabolites is analyzed in biosynthetic terms is the way in which variety within a group is generated by the multiple branching of biosynthetic

TABLE I

Mycotoxins as Representative of the Main Biosynthetic Categories of Secondary Metabolites

Biosynthetic category	Representative mycotoxins
Polyketides	
Tetra-	Patulin, penicillic acid, chlorflavonin
Penta-	Citrinin, ochratoxins
Hexa-	Maltoryzine
Hepta-	Viriditoxin, cytochalasins, rugulosin, etc.
Octa-	Ergochromes
Nona-	Zearalenone, viridicatumtoxin
Deca-	Aflatoxins, austocystins, erythroskyrine
Tetronic/tetramic acids	Tenuazonic acid, cyclopiazonic acid, cytochalasins
Diketopiperazines	
Simple	Aspergillic acid, echinulins
Modified	Brevianamides, sporidesmins, fumitremorgens, oxaline
Peptides	Tentoxin, ergotamine, tryptoquivaline
C_6C_3 Products	Chlorflavonin, xanthocillin, terphenyllin
Terpenes	
Mono-	Viridicatumtoxin
Sesqui-	Trichothecenes
Di-	Paspaline

pathways. This is an interesting feature of the pathway which leads to the ergot alkaloids (see Chapter 2), particularly when this is considered together with the wider range of products which can result from the introduction of dimethylallyl groups into tryptophan derivatives. This is outlined (not exhaustively) in Scheme 1, where the "ergoline branch" is not set out fully, from which the relationships among an interesting group of mycotoxins will be apparent. Such schemes, it should be noted, describe pathways which may or may not occur together. That is, branches lead on the one hand to metabolites produced by different organisms—for instance, roquefortine by *Penicillium roquefortii* and oxaline by *Penicillium oxalicum*—and on the other hand, through subsidiary branches which have been omitted in Scheme 1 for clarity, to the variety of metabolites produced in a single strain. An example is provided by the occurrence of different selections from the total range of compounds in the fumitremorgen series in cultures of *Aspergillus fumigatus, Aspergillus caespitosus*, and *Pencillium verruculosum* (Steyn, 1977). The situation is particularly well exemplified in the "ergot series" of compounds derived from 4-dimethylallyltryptophan, discussed in Chapter 2.

In another review (Bu'Lock, 1975) I discussed how even within a single isolate of a fungus, environmental effects on such branching reaction series can lead to considerable variations in the relative proportions of the different

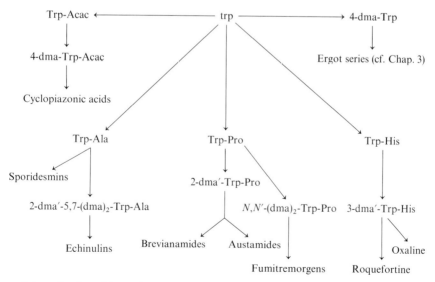

Scheme 1.   Branching pathways to mycotoxins involving dimethylallylation of tryptophan and its derivatives. Abbreviations: Trp, tryptophan; Acac, acetoacetyl; Ala, alanine; Pro, proline; His, histidine; dma, 3,3-dimethylallyl; dma', 1,1-dimethylallyl.

possible products, and commented on the parallels which thereby arise between such phenotypic variations and the genotypic differences among isolates of one or several species. A classic example of this situation exists with regard to the production of patulin, dealt with in Chapter 7, where the several products and intermediates in the overall complex of transformations of 6-methylsalicylic acid can either be found to predominate among the secondary metabolites of various different strains and species, or be made to predominate among the products of a given strain of *Penicillium urticae* by manipulating its nutritional and environmental history and state. The fact that within such a set of biosynthetically related products the predominant selection may be determined by both genotypic and phenotypic factors is a matter of some consequence in the field of mycotoxins.

One further comment on biogenetic diversity as it concerns the mycotoxins is offered rather tentatively. To some extent, it appears that the most potent individual mycotoxins tend to stand toward the end of quite long reaction sequences in which substances of much lower toxicity are intermediates. The particular case of the aflatoxins, detailed in Chapter 4, exemplifies this rather well. In approaching the difficult problem of assigning a function—or, in evolutionary terms, a selection advantage—to secondary metabolism in general, it can be argued that the great variety of secondary metabolites could only arise if they were nearly neutral in selection terms. However, it is also unlikely that they are absolutely so, and indeed there are many instances where they can be shown to be somehow "useful" though by no means essential to the organism. It appears that in this sense there has been some selection advantage, however minor, in evolving the high physiological activity which the true mycotoxins display; this is not to say that the particular aspects of that activity with which our own agrourban society is most concerned have been the relevant ones in evolution (see Section V).

III. OCCURRENCE

We have already seen that the sporadic occurrence of the mycotoxins as fungal metabolites is not unconnected with their biogenetic diversity. Here, however, we will consider the relationships between mycotoxin production and the accepted classification of fungal species. If in a diagram such as that in Scheme 1 we insert, in place of the various metabolic products, the names of the fungal species in which each product is found, then the branching tree denotes reactions (hence enzymes, and hence presumed genes) which they have in common, and others which are less widely shared; thus, for an admittedly short series of "characters" it constitutes a type of taxonomic classification. In higher plants such chemotaxonomic classifications usually correspond quite closely with, and indeed may sometimes usefully clarify, the normal taxonomic descriptions based on morphology; conversely, the conventional taxonomy is a useful and functional guide to the likely chemical constituents of a plant species. Unfortunately, this is only true to a very limited extent for fungi and fungal metabolites. The classification of fungi by predominantly morphological criteria into genera and species (and into higher and lower categories) is better founded than most microbial chemists would think. On the other hand, its correspondence with a "true" (phylogenetic) taxonomy based on gradations of relatedness, and ultimately on the molecular basis of transmitted genetic features, is very problematic. Nowhere is this more true than among the Fungi Imperfecti, which despite the devotion of many distinguished mycologists remains little more than a taxonomist's miscellany—unfortunately containing a high proportion of the mycotoxin-producing organisms.

We have every right to expect that a character such as aflatoxin production should have fairly high taxonomic value. If we consider the number of reaction steps specific to aflatoxin production, multiply this by (say) two for the number of specific enzymes involved and by two again to give the number of structural and regulatory genes directly connected with the aflatoxin sequence, we see that this character probably accounts for some 75–150 genes. The same is probably true for most other mycotoxins. Yet such characters are not given any agreed weight in accepted taxonomy, and there is no satisfactory correspondence between their incidence and the accepted morphological classifications.

The question is one of more than academic significance, yet it is not uncommon to find statements which ignore it. Even if we leave aside such obvious (but frequent) blunders of the type "this fungus is toxic," and consider only statements to the effect that such-and-such a species is known to be toxigenic, it may come as some surprise to find that when a series of isolates all assigned morphologically to that species has been carefully examined, in an adequate variety of culture conditions, only a proportion, and sometimes only a minority, has been found to produce the purportedly characteristic toxin. On the other hand, that same product may be (no more and no less) characteristic of several other isolates which, on classical grounds, are classed as belonging to different and even quite unrelated species. For example, the production of citrinin is recorded from, *inter alia*, *Aspergillus terreus*, *Aspergillus candidus*, *Penicillium viridicatum*, *Penicillium citrinum*, and *Penicillium citreoviride*—but it is only produced by a minority of strains of *A. terreus*.

Attitudes toward such problems vary. Morphologists have classed *Aspergillus flavus* and *Aspergillus oryzae* very close together, while those concerned with mycotoxins and (particularly) with the uses of fungi in the food industry regard them as sharply distinct, with no aflatoxin-producing strains then included in *A. oryzae*. In attempting to answer questions in this difficult area, it is important to know why a particular question is being asked, and to answer it in terms relevant to that context. For example, with regard to the possible presence of mycotoxins in a given foodstuff, we can say that the isolation from the sample of a fungus classified as belonging to a "toxigenic species" is an excellent guide to the type of mycotoxin whose presence might be suspected, but is of little value in establishing the presence of that product, which remains a matter for analytical chemistry.

As the technical uses of fungal cultures, and of preparations obtained from them, become more and more widespread, increasing importance attaches to questions of a rather different type. If citric acid produced by *Aspergillus niger* is acceptable in soft drinks, what safeguards would be needed for citric acid produced by *Aspergillus parasiticus* instead? (We leave on one side the question of health safeguards in the manufacturing process.) How do we regard the use of an enzyme preparation from *A. oryzae* or *A. flavus*? We are perhaps called to weigh a mycologist's conclusion that the production strain belongs to a species "known to be toxigenic" against a manufacturer's claim that mycotoxin production by that strain has never been detected. Can we be sure that in some part of the production process a particular combination of conditions might not lead, even occasionally, to mycotoxin production? Can we be sure that if the strain is improved for process use by mutation and selection, a hitherto unrealized potential for toxin production might not be uncovered?

It would be easier to answer such questions if the state of fungal taxonomy, and in particular its relevance to secondary metabolite production capabilities, were rather considerably advanced. A recent reviewer is hopeful of such advances, but meanwhile can only recount confusion in precisely those areas with which we are most concerned: by one of the newer criteria, "differences between strains of both *A. flavus* and *A. oryzae* appeared to be as great as differences between the two species," while "*A. parasiticus* showed a somewhat higher similarity to nine *Penicillium* spp. than to the other three species in the *A. flavus* group," etc. (Fennell, 1977).

However, the problems are not confined to questions of taxonomic evidence. If we are instead to rely wholly on analytical evidence (assuming our assay methods are adequately sensitive and also specific), we need to arrange sets of growth conditions such that any genotypic potential for mycotoxin production will be realized in at least some of our test cultures, because strains differ at least as much in the regulation mechanisms governing secondary metabolism, which are discussed in Section IV, as they do in their metabolic potential.

Consequently, we can only attempt to answer some of the practical problems raised by the sporadic occurrence of mycotoxin production in fungi by taking a balanced view, neither too rigidly stultifying nor too elastically permissive, of how much weight to attach to identification (either of a contaminant or of a commercially used strain) as belonging to, or being related to, a "toxigenic species," and equally of how much reliability to require from characterizations by chemically identifiable metabolites. Beyond these practical considerations, there remain unanswered fundamental questions about how the assembly of characteristics that we find in a fungal isolate has actually been brought together. We may suspect that there has been more to the process than the simple linear descent which the quest for a "true" taxonomy usually assumes. In that case, only a radically different approach to classifying the fungi will give us a system of real predictive value, capable of describing complex patterns of relatedness between different isolates.

IV. REGULATION

A. General Aspects

Fundamentally, the definition of secondary metabolism is a statement about the manner in which the biosynthesis of certain metabolites is regulated (Bu'Lock, 1975).

Very roughly, the biochemical processes in a living cell are of three kinds. First are the basal processes which provide energy and raw materials for all other cell functions, with respect to which (and to each other) they are normally controlled. Second are the synthetic processes involved in duplicating the cell substances, i.e., in growth (sometimes qualified as replicatory or vegetative growth to distinguish it from mere accretion). Replicatory growth involves the energy-dependent utilization of freely available substrates in a balanced manner. The biochemistry of both basal and replicatory processes is usually controlled by rather strict and very specific mechanisms, and it tends to be the same over very large taxonomic groups; this so-called "unity of biochemistry" indicates that within these types of processes there has been very little scope for the evolution of variety.

The third kind of process is secondary biosynthesis. This provides for the utilization of substrates (and energy) in modes which may be qualitatively similar to those in vegetative growth (e.g., accumulations of "normal" cell components like triglycerides or citric acid) or entirely different, in which case the variety of products is very great, but in either case the process is regulated more or less inversely to replicatory growth and the balance of nutrients that is required to sustain it is entirely different. Within secondary biosynthesis the unity of biochemistry breaks down, and it is here that the evolved individuality of microbial species is manifested at the molecular level (see Section III).

The mechanisms by which basal metabolism and replicatory growth are controlled have been one of the main topics of biochemical research for many years. A great deal is now known about them, particularly for bacteria but increasingly for the more complex eukaryotes, which include the fungi. Control is exerted at several levels, ranging from the simple mass action effects of substrate levels to subtle mechanisms controlling the expression of individual genes. Our knowledge of the corresponding control mechanism in secondary metabolism is considerably less in respect of molecular detail, partly because there are so many different systems to be studied, but the general outlines of their working are becoming clear (Bu'Lock, 1975; Demain, 1978), and they are at least consistent with types of regulatory mechanism known to control primary metabolism. Much of the effort in this field has been made in order to improve our understanding of industrial processes in which secondary metabolites such as antibiotics are the objective (Bu'Lock, 1965; Demain, 1968), but we shall be able to illustrate the general principles with examples from the field of mycotoxins (Sections IV,B–IV,D). However, a more general account is given as an introduction.

Particular attention has been given to the regulation of secondary biosynthesis in relation to replicatory growth. In controlling this balance, mechanisms which act at the level of gene expression, and govern *de novo* enzyme synthesis, seem to be particularly important (Bu'Lock, 1965, 1975; Luckner *et al.*, 1977). In effect, during secondary metabolism a microorganism expresses series of genes which are silenced under optimum growth conditions. A relevant type of mechanism is the one known as "catabolite repression," which in bacteria controls the initiation of gene transcription by means which act in the inverse sense to growth-linked metabolism and which provide common control for a multiplicity of unlinked gene sites. Each individual site can still be subject to more specific controls, such as substrate- or product-linked derepression or induction. To avoid an unwarrantedly precise implication that the controlling agents for secondary metabolism in general are the same as those for particular catabolite-repression systems in bacteria, the term "growth-linked repression" (or non-growth-linked derepression) is perhaps preferable for the general case.

This approach emphasizes what has been indicated in Section III, that the potential secondary metabolic activities of an organism are as much a part of its genetic complement as the coding for activities manifest during growth, but being less subject to the unity of biochemistry that the requirements for replicatory growth impose, it is in the "secondary genome" that related organisms are most capable of being different. A complication is that this scope for variety extends (to some extent) to the genes concerned with regulatory effects in secondary biosynthesis, so that two strains capable of producing the same pattern of secondary metabolites may well differ with regard to the circumstances under which their production is elicited and correspondingly in the quantitative pattern of products found under a given set of conditions. An instructive example is found in the classic studies of Taber and co-workers on alkaloid-producing strains of *Claviceps*. On a standard synthetic medium, most of the strains studied showed the typical pattern of a period of rapid growth, with little or no alkaloid synthesis (see below). One strain was markedly different in that it showed slow growth throughout the fermentation, accompanied by alkaloid production throughout; however, this one strain showed the normal pattern when grown on a richer complex medium (Taber *et al.*, 1968).

As in the above instance, there is a tendency in many laboratory (and industrial) fermentations for there to be an initial phase of proliferation in which replicatory growth predominates, followed by a differentiation phase in which secondary metabolism is most active. A similar succession may sometimes occur in the wild, but the phasing is most conspicuous in well-controlled laboratory systems, and the terms "trophophase" and "idiophase" have been coined to describe it. However, these are only short-hand descriptions, and the real situation is frequently more subtle. As in the example already cited, a small genetic difference may lead to super-ficially quite different phenomena. Moreover, an organism may have several different pathways of secondary metabolism (this is probably true in all fungi), and the precise conditions for the initiation of each can vary, so that the onset of idiophase is not a single event. Nor is it necessarily a simple one. For example, in studies with *Gibberella fujikuroi* (Bu'Lock *et al.*, 1974), which produces several distinct series of metabolites in response to slower growth, the fact that the substrate supply in ordinary batch cultures becomes kinetically limiting well before the limiting nutrient is actually "exhausted" could be directly linked to the observation that the different pathways of secondary biosynthesis become active at different degrees of nutrient limita-tion, and their products therefore appear in a corresponding succession. Here the restriction of growth, and the corresponding expressions of secondary metabolic potential, take place progressively and not in a simple on–off way.

Such observations are consistent with our understanding of a generalized growth-linked repression mechanism similar to catabolite repression in bacteria. Such a mechanism, in allowing for the interaction of a limited number of effectors with a larger number of genes, will allow different affinities at the interaction sites, i.e., for different sets of genes to have different sensitivities to the growth-linked controls.

Another practical complication arises from the fact that most fungi are able to build up internal reserves from surplus nutrients, so that a colony which has been grown on a very rich medium may well respond differently to one which has been only moderately well-nourished on transfer to minimal media; more generally, changes in an organism produced in response to one environment may well affect its response to another environment, and this can affect its secondary metabolic activities.

These general principles will now be illustrated from secondary metabolic pathways leading to acknowledged mycotoxins. We can summarize them in the statement that under conditions which are optimal for its growth a fungus will display little or none of its potential for secondary biosynthesis, but under suboptimal conditions (and with minor genetic changes that have the same effect) the precise pattern of secondary metabolism elicited will depend both on the prior history of the culture and on its current environmental conditions.

B. Patulin

The secondary biosynthesis of the mycotoxin patulin, as described in detail in Chapter 7, begins with the formation of 6-methylsalicylic acid, and the regulation of this first step is therefore rate-limiting overall. However, it is the control of further steps beyond 6-methylsalicylate that determines the extent to which patulin, or other products of the pathway, actually accumulate (Bu'Lock et al., 1965).

When fungi of the *Penicillium urticae/patulum* type are grown on a rich nutrient medium, no 6-methylsalicylate synthase activity is detectable, but if mycelium thus grown is transferred to Czapek–Dox medium (in which nitrogen is supplied as nitrate and is to that extent a limiting nutrient) a period of slower growth follows, during which the synthase is formed, becoming detectable after a delay period whose duration is strain dependent (Light, 1967a). It is not clear whether this delay is caused by carryover of reserves accumulated on the richer medium, or by a need to attain a more depleted nutrient state than the fresh nitrate medium provides, as either effect could vary from strain to strain in the manner described. There is, however, evidence that the component proteins of the synthase are actually formed during the slower growth on nitrate before any active synthase complex can be detected and before any 6-methylsalicylate synthesis begins, so that formation of the functioning synthase complex does seem to require the more severe nutrient limitation (Bu'Lock et al., 1969). As in several other systems which are usually controlled by progressive nutrient depletion, partial inhibition of protein synthesis (by inhibitors used at intermediate concentrations) also promotes appearance of the synthase complex (Light,

1967b), whereas higher levels, applied during the period when its component enzymes are being synthesized, prevent it.

Once the active 6-methylsalicylate synthase has been formed it is metabolically stable, and persists independent of new protein synthesis. In this it differs from some of the later enzymes on the route to patulin. These are only formed under even more stringent growth restriction. In addition, being metabolically labile (i.e., subject to turnover), they disappear quite quickly either when protein synthesis is stopped (with inhibitors) or when fresh nutrients are made available. As a result, such cultures accumulate 6-methylsalicylate. The regulation of these later enzymes is a clear instance of control by nutrient limitation, and some of them may also be controlled by specific induction mechanisms. In well-phased laboratory cultures they are formed in a regular succession (Bu'Lock *et al.*, 1969; Forrester and Gaucher, 1972; Murphy *et al.*, 1974).

Although nutrient restriction is also conducive to the formation of spores (conidia) in *P. urticae*, there is no direct connection with patulin synthesis (Sekiguchi and Gaucher, 1977). Equally, in other species where the patulin pathway exists alongside independent pathways to other secondary metabolites, such as byssochlamic acid, the optimum conditions for one pathway may be significantly different from those for the other (Escoula, 1975).

C. Ergot Alkaloids

Regulation mechanisms in the synthesis of ergot alkaloids by *Claviceps* fungi have been studied in several laboratories, often in connection with the biosynthetic studies described here in Chapter 3. Here we are concerned only with the earliest steps in the process, from tryptophan to the simple bases such as agroclavine.

The overall relationship between replicatory growth and alkaloid production, already alluded to in Section IV,A, was very thoroughly established by Taber and co-workers (Taber, 1964; Taber *et al.*, 1968). Laboratory cultures for alkaloid production are usually grown with phosphate as the limiting nutrient. In the growth phase, tryptophan synthesis (for proteins, etc.) is controlled by normal feedback mechanisms, but when the phosphate level becomes limiting there is a disproportionate increase in the tryptophan pool, suggesting that there is a change in the feedback control at this stage (Robbers *et al.*, 1972). The other alkaloid precursor, dimethylallyl pyrophosphate, is never limiting. Consequently, the rate of alkaloid synthesis is governed overall by the level of the first enzyme in the pathway, the 4-dimethylallyltryptophan synthase (Heinstein *et al.*, 1971).

This enzyme is metabolically labile and its level in the mycelium is controlled by modulating *de novo* synthesis against breakdown (Bu'Lock and

Barr, 1968). Synthesis of the enzyme is in turn controlled by at least two factors: while phosphate levels are high it is subject to the growth-linked repression mechanism, and it is derepressed by its substrate, tryptophan. It is also derepressed by nonsubstrate analogues such as thiotryptophan and 5-methyltryptophan (Floss et al., 1974), and the fact that these do not stop synthesis of tryptophan itself confirms that feedback regulation of trypto-phan synthesis is weakened during alkaloid synthesis.

Typically, then, alkaloid production does not begin until the initial phos-phate supply has been virtually used up, and thereafter it is controlled by the supply of tryptophan. More difficult to interpret is the repeated obser-vation that tryptophan and its analogues are most effective as inducers when added during the initial growth phase, in the presence of excess phosphate, i.e., under conditions when the synthetase is not detectable and no alkaloid synthesis actually occurs (Floss and Mothes, 1964; Bu'Lock and Barr, 1968; Floss et al., 1974). The inducer effect is therefore cumulative (and delayed) while growth-linked repression operates, yet it appears to be direct when the more general control is lifted. This effect is not explicable in terms of the classic mechanisms established for regulatory processes in bacteria, and perhaps it illustrates some of the additional complexities which more complex organisms can accommodate.

Other groups have compared the succession of changes in laboratory cultures, both of biochemistry and of morphology, with that in *Claviceps* growing parasitically on its natural hosts (Pazoutova et al., 1977; Rehacek, 1974; Mantle and Nisbet, 1976). In general, conditions favoring alkaloid production in laboratory cultures lead to a succession quite comparable to that in the wild. One biochemical feature common to both, for example, is the postgrowth accumulation of ricinoleyl lipids. However, these studies have not been extended to include other secondary products important in the overall mycotoxicosis, such as the secalonic acids (ergochromes) (Chapter 5) and paspaline.

D. Cyclopiazonic Acids

The biosynthesis of the cyclopiazonic acids in cultures of *Penicillium cyclopium*, detailed in Chapter 10, comprises relatively few steps, and its regulation has been particularly investigated in terms of effects at enzyme level (McGrath et al., 1976). An early step in the development of the system is the diversion of tryptophan from growth-linked protein synthesis into a pool of the precursor *cyclo*-acetoacetyltryptophan. However, the supply of this precursor is not subsequently rate-limiting. Apparently the synthesis of β-cyclopiazonic acid (by the introduction of a dimethylallyl group into this precursor) is then controlled by competition between the corresponding enzyme and dimethylallyltransferase (the "polymerase" of prenol synthesis) for dimethylallyl pyrophosphate, their common substrate. This competition is affected partly by the levels of the two enzymes but more markedly by inhibitory and stimulatory feedback exerted by the cyclopiazonic acids, and perhaps also by indirect effects caused by the strong metal-chelating properties of these tetramic acids. The system is perhaps especially interesting since it has been more thoroughly explored in terms of its enzymology. It would be interesting to know how widely the observed dependence on dimethylallyl pyrophosphate availability applies, in view of the importance of similar prenylation steps in so many other secondary biosynthetic pathways. As already noted, the effect is not seen in ergot alkaloid biosynthesis.

V. FUNCTION

The question of the function of secondary metabolism is one which has been inconclusively, though frequently, discussed. It is of course only legitimate when it is posed in a way which in biological terms is valid and meaningful; here it is helpful to confine our discussion to microbial metabolites. We can first ask whether secondary metabolism as a general phenomenon plays such a significant part in the natural life processes of a microorganism that we must necessarily conclude that it has a function, or in evolutionary terms that it has conferred any selection advantage. If we conclude that it does, can we then identify the nature of that advantage— remembering that having answered the first question on the basis of our understanding of secondary metabolism as a general phenomenon, we are precluded from answering the second in terms of any specific properties or effects in this or that particular instance? Only beyond this stage does it become legitimate to ask whether our general answer also permits (or requires, or precludes) specific answers concerning special advantages conferred by particular instances of secondary metabolism—and it is in this last context alone that the mycotoxins *per se* might play a role.

In the broadest sense, the ability to carry out metabolism disjoined from replicatory growth is essential for any microorganism, for none can multiply indefinitely. In this sense, the evolution of mechanisms for the operational segregation of the "nonvegetative genome" (in which are located the genetic determinants of secondary metabolism) has been wholly functional, because it is essential for the development of a complete life cycle. The partial (but very often incomplete) association of secondary metabolite biosynthesis with the formation of spores or other propagules is to that extent anticipated; conversely, such a genome can accommodate nonessential novelties more readily than the strictly regulated gene complement concerned with the precise replication of cell materials. It is probably true that all microorganisms are capable of producing secondary metabolites of some kind, and even if we exclude from consideration such man-made monsters as the strains used for industrial antibiotics production we can also find a great number of wild-type fungi which under certain circumstances will divert a substantial part of their total metabolic flow into secondary metabolite accumulation. Indeed, several are known to do so even in the wild, although the number of studies on this aspect has been limited. At the other end of the scale are those which produce their particular metabolites only in very small amounts—but in general, we only know about such cases because the product has very high activity in some humanly contrived test situation and has hence received our own disproportionate attention. All in all, most workers would agree that secondary metabolism in microorganism is a general activity sufficiently important to justify our inquiring into its selection advantage, or function.

Various suggestions regarding that general function have been raised (by some—and dismissed by others). One view is that they are simple waste products; against this, our picture of primary metabolism is that it is too finely adjusted to permit such an explanation, which in any case explains neither the elaboration nor the variety of secondary metabolite structures. Related to this is the view that they are produced as an overflow process to accommodate metabolic flows which have somehow overridden the normal regulatory mechanisms; the same objections (in my view) apply. Somewhat different is the proposal that secondary biosynthesis serves to maintain basic metabolism in circumstances when its products (high-energy phosphates, reduced coenzymes, and substrates for synthesis) cannot—through nutritional imbalances—be used for cell replication, and to do this in a way which can safely be turned off when environmental circumstances improve or when a new program of activity, such as propagule formation, can be fully activated. In all these views, it is the process of secondary biosynthesis which is seen as advantageous, and not, in the general case, its products, and in my opinion this is still the most likely type of general explanation.

Another type of view (e.g., Muller, 1974), at first appearing rather attractive, is that the general function of secondary biosynthesis is to provide a reservoir of nonfunctional variety out of which new functional processes can emerge at some future time by continuing natural selection. In this view, then, it is the products themselves which are functional (paradoxically, because they have no immediate function). This is either an extremely profound insight into the mechanism of evolution by natural selection at a molecular level, or it is a teleological fallacy; frankly, I am not sure which, but it is one of the few new ideas to have been introduced into this discussion in recent years.

If the variety of secondary metabolites is not directly functional (in the way just suggested), then it must be explained as a result of there being very little selection pressure on their identity; i.e., the products bring no great advantages nor disadvantages *per se*. As already indicated, however, this is a statement about secondary metabolism as a general phenomenon, and it in no way precludes the idea that particular organisms may derive an additional selection advantage from having evolved specific uses for specific secondary metabolites. We would even expect such uses to have evolved, given such a wide range of neutral possibilities for this kind of exploitation, just as organisms have evolved so as to take advantage of very specific features of their habitat and ecological context. Moreover, it is at precisely this level of evolution that the great variety of species has arisen, and we have already seen that the variety of secondary metabolism is to some extent an expression of this in molecular terms. Therefore, on this view the fact that some organisms demonstrably utilize some substances which we would class in general terms as secondary metabolites for a very considerable variety of needs (hormone action, interactions with other organisms, structural differentiation, physical protection, and so on), each of which we can find being met by quite different substances in other organisms, is *not* an argument against the view that the *general* function of secondary metabolism has little or nothing to do with the properties of the products.

Where they have evolved, the analyses of these specific functions can of course throw considerable light on the variety of microbial existence. In the present context, however, we must restrict outselves to the question of whether we can detect any such specific functions in the class of natural products now being considered—the mycotoxins. Now it would be churlish of me to suggest that this category, to which (after all) the rest of this book is devoted, is not a valid one. But it must be pointed out that for whatever purposes and needs this category has been constructed, it bears very little discernible relationship to the life of microorganisms in their natural state (whatever that may mean). The fact that an organism produces a substance toxic (in one of many different ways) to humans, or to our more favored domestic mammals, when it happens to grow on a substrate whose particular characteristics and interest are equally a creation of human culture, is of considerable interest to us, but corresponds to no clearly defined sector of the biological world at large. If we are to find specific functions—from the microbes' point of view—for the mycotoxins, we must try to establish their role in the microorganism's own interactions with its habitat, its survival and proliferation parameters, and its interaction with predators, hosts, and commensal species. So far as I am aware, this has hardly been attempted to date—a comment which would perhaps be better made in a postscript rather than in an introduction!

REFERENCES

Bu'Lock, J. D. (1965). *In* "Biogenesis of Antibiotic Substances" (Z. Vanek and Z. Hostalek, eds.), pp. 61–71. Academic Press, New York.

Bu'Lock, J. D. (1975). *In* "The Filamentous Fungi" (J. E. Smith and D. R. Berry, eds.), Vol. I, pp. 33–58. Arnold, London.

Bu'Lock, J. D., and Barr, J. G. (1968). *Lloydia* **31**, 342–354.

Bu'Lock, J. D., Hamilton, D., Hulme, M. A., Powell, A. J., Smalley, H. M., Shepherd, D., and Smith, G. N. (1965). *Can. J. Microbiol.* **11**, 765–778.

Bu'Lock. J. D., Shepherd, D., and Winstanley, D. J. (1969). *Can. J. Microbiol.* **15**, 279–285.

Bu'Lock, J. D., Detroy, R. W., Hostalek, Z., and Munim-Al-Shakarchi, A., (1974). *Trans. Br. Mycol. Soc.* **62**, 377–389.

Demain, A. L. (1968). *Lloydia* **31**, 395–418.

Demain, A. L. (1978). *In* "The Filamentous Fungi" (J. E. Smith and D. R. Berry, eds.), Vol. III, pp. 426–450. Arnold, London.

Escoula, L. (1975). *Ann. Rech. Vet.* **6**, 155–163 and 311–314.

Fennell, D. I. (1977). *In* "British Mycological Society Symposia No. 1: Genetics and Physiology of Aspergillus" (J. E. Smith and J. A. Pateman, eds.), pp. 1–22. Academic Press, New York.

Floss, H. G., and Mothes, V. (1964). *Arch. Mikrobiol.* **48**, 213–221.

Floss, H. G., Robbers, J. E., and Heinstein, P. F. (1974). *Recent Adv. Phytochem.* **8**, 141–178.

Forrester, P. I., and Gaucher, G. M. (1972). *Biochemistry* **11**, 1102–1107.

Heinstein, P. F., Lee, S. L., and Floss, H. G. (1971). *Biochem. Biophys. Res. Commun.* **44**, 1244–1251.

Light, R. J. (1967a). *J. Biol. Chem.* **242**, 1880–1886.

Light, R. J. (1967b). *Arch. Biochem. Biophys.* **122**, 494–500.

Luckner, M., Nover, L., and Bohm, H. (1977). "Secondary Metabolism and Cell Differentiation," Springer Verlag, Berlin and New York.

McGrath, R. M., Steyn, P. S., Ferreira, N. P., and Neethling, D. C. (1976). *Bioorg. Chem.* **4**, 11–23.

Mantle, P. G., and Nisbet, L. J. (1976). *J. Gen. Microbiol.* **93**, 321–331.

Muller, E. (1974). *In* "Secondary Metabolism and Coevolution" (M. Luckner, K. Mothes, and L. Nover, eds.), pp. 123–128. Dtsch Akad. Naturforscher Leopoldina Halle, Saale.

Murphy, G., Vogel, G., Krippahl, G., and Lynen, F. (1974). *Eur. J. Biochem.* **49**, 443–455.

Pazoutova, S., Pokorny, V., and Rehacek, Z. (1977). *Can. J. Microbiol.* **23**, 1182–1187.

Rehacek, Z. (1974). *Zentralbl. Bakteriol. Parasitenkd. Infektionskr. Hyg. Abt. 2*, **129**, 20–49.

Robbers, J. E., Robertson, L. W., Hornemann, K. M., Jindra, A., and Floss, H. G. (1972). *J. Bacteriol.* **112**, 791–796.

Sekiguchi, J., and Gaucher, G. M. (1977). *Appl. Env. Microbiol.*, **33**, 147–158.

Steyn, P. S. (1977). *Pure Appl. Chem.* **49**, 1771–1778.

Taber, W. A. (1964). *Appl. Microbiol.* **12**, 321–326.

Taber, W. A., Brar, S. S. and Giam, C. S. (1968). *Mycologia*, **60**, 806–826.

2

Biosynthesis of Ergot Toxins

HEINZ G. FLOSS AND JOHN A. ANDERSON

17

The Biosynthesis of Mycotoxins
Copyright © 1980 by Academic Press, Inc.

I. INTRODUCTION

A. Ergotism

General reviews of ergot have been published, including the classic work of Barger (1931) (Guggisberg, 1954; Hofmann, 1964; Bove, 1970; Gröger, 1972). Ergotism is the disease which results from consumption of the ergot body of sclerotium from rye or other grains infected by a parasitic fungus, genus *Claviceps*. The disease is due to the effects of the alkaloids produced by the fungus and contained in the ergot body.

There were two types of ergotism epidemics, convulsive and gangrenous. The epidemics of gangrenous ergotism occurred from the Middle Ages to the nineteenth century. Epidemics of convulsive ergotism arose between 1581 and the last large outbreak in Russia in 1928. Many deaths occurred in these epidemics: for example, 8000 people died in one district in France in the epidemic of 1770–1771.

In gangrenous ergotism the affected part (more often a foot than a hand) became swollen and inflamed. The patient experienced violent, burning pains (hence the Fire of St. Anthony). The affected part gradually became numb, turned black, shrank, and finally became mummified and dry. The gangrenous part often separated spontaneously at a joint.

An early symptom of convulsive ergotism was a tingling sensation such as experienced when one's foot "goes to sleep." Then the entire body was racked by spasms. In severe cases general convulsions caused the body to roll into a ball or to stretch out straight. Severe diarrhea followed the convulsions. On postmortem examination, patients who died of convulsive ergotism exhibited bleeding and softening of the brain and lesions of the posterior horn of the spinal column.

Very large quantities of ergot were consumed during the epidemics. It is estimated that the grain in the gangrenous epidemics in France was 25% ergot. A patient who died of gangrenous ergotism had consumed 100 gm of ergot over a few days. Death occurred when flour containing 7% ergot was ingested in the last Russian convulsive-type epidemics. A presence of 2% ergot is sufficient to cause epidemics. Since the Russian epidemics, most European countries have set limits of 0.1–0.2% ergot in flour.

The occurrence of ergotism has declined as the diet has become more varied. Use of clean seed, crop rotation, cutting of wild grasses near the fields, deep planting, and selection of varieties in which all plants flower at the same time are cultural practices which have reduced infection in the field. A flotation method can be used to remove ergot from grain before milling.

Early epidemics of gangrenous ergotism ("holy fire") were thought to be a sign of divine wrath. The later incidences of convulsive ergotism occurred at a time when belief in witchcraft was prevalent, and many believed that sufferers were possessed by demons. Ergot poisoning has been suggested as the reason for the behavior of the bewitched girls in the Salem village witch trials in New England (Caporael, 1976), although this proposal has been questioned (Spanos and Gottlieb, 1976). The death of poultry that had been fed ergot led to the recognition by Dodart in France in 1630 that ergot caused ergotism. However, the cause of ergotism was debated in Germany into the nineteenth century.

B. Life Cycle

Ergot was recognized as a fungus as early as 1711, but the complete life cycle was not described until 1853 by Tulasne. The ergot or ergot body is a hard, dark purple, sickel-shaped body in the seedhead of various grains. The ergot body or sclerotium falls to the ground and germinates the next spring. Short stalks terminated by a head (hence *Claviceps*) which contains the elongated ascospores grow from the sclerotium. The ascospores are produced in a sexual process which involves the fusion of two nuclei and subsequent formation of eight ascospores. The ascospores are released into the air, land on the moist stigmata of the flower, and germinate. The hyphae (sphacelia) grow around and then within the ovary of the flower. Asexual spores, or conidia, are produced and are spread to other flowers by honeydew produced by the host plant. In the final stage the hyphae become thicker and more closely packed to produce the hard sclerotium.

There are several species of ergot which differ in morphology and host plants. *Claviceps purpurea* readily infects rye but also infects barley, wheat, and more than 100 grasses. Other species infect rice, wheat, millet, and corn. The ergot of corn observed in the humid parts of Mexico is up to 8 cm long and 5 cm thick.

II. THE ALKALOIDS OF ERGOT

A. Lysergic Acid Derivatives

The ergot alkaloids are derivatives of the four-ring structure of ergoline (**1**). The pharmacologically most active components of ergot are amides of D-lysergic acid (**2**). The first crystalline alkaloid from ergot, which later was found to be a mixture of ergocornine, ergokryptine, and ergocristine was obtained in 1875 (Tanret, 1875). Another crystalline form of the same mixture of alkaloids, which was called ergotoxine, was reported in 1907 (Barger and Carr, 1907). Ergotamine, one of the most important alkaloids, was purified from ergot by Stoll (1918, 1945), and its structure was proved

TABLE I

Cyclol-Type Peptide Ergot Alkaloids

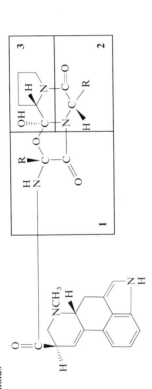

R	Amino Acid
CH_3	Alanine
$CH(CH_3)CH_3$	Valine
$CH_2CH(CH_3)CH_3$	Leucine
$CH(CH_3)CH_2CH_3$	Isoleucine
CH_2CH_3	α-Aminobutyric acid
$CH_2CH_2CH(CH_3)CH_3$	Homoleucine

Alkaloid	α-Hydroxy-L-amino acid **1**	L-amino acid **2**	Reference
Ergotamine	Alanine	Phenylalanine	Stoll (1918, 1945)
Ergosine	Alanine	Leucine	Smith and Timmis (1937)
Ergocristine	Valine	Phenylalanine	Stoll and Burckhardt (1937)
α-Ergokryptine	Valine	Leucine	Stoll and Hofmann (1943)
β-Ergokryptine	Valine	Isoleucine	Schlientz et al. (1968)
Ergocornine	Valine	Valine	Stoll and Hofmann (1943)
Ergostine	α-Aminobutyric acid	Phenylalanine	Schlientz et al. (1964)
Ergohexine	Alanine	Homoleucine[a]	Ohmomo and Abe (1976)
Ergoheptine	Valine	Homoleucine[a]	Ohmomo and Abe (1976)

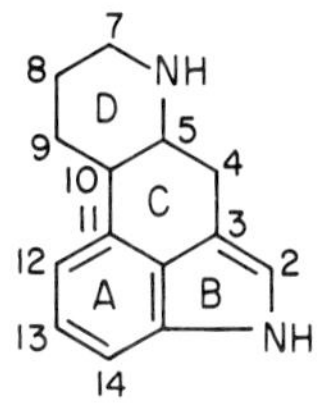

1 : Ergoline 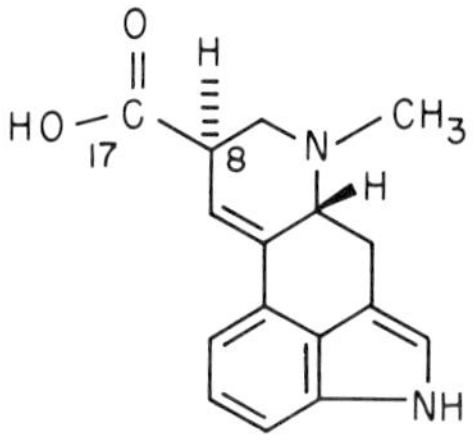   2 : D-Lysergic acid

by synthesis in 1961 (Hofmann et al., 1963). These compounds are representatives of the cyclol-type peptide alkaloids listed in Table I. Hydrolysis of the peptide alkaloids yields D-lysergic acid, proline, another L-amino acid, and an α-keto acid. The α-keto acid is produced from the amino acid moiety next to lysergic acid. The 9,10-dihydro derivative of ergosine has been isolated from *Sphacelia sorghi* (Mantle and Waight, 1968). Structure 3 has been proposed for ergosecaline, which contains only two amino acids (Abe et al., 1959). The structural proposal for ergohexine and ergoheptine was based in part on the isolation of L-homoleucyl-D-proline lactam (see Section III) from the cultures (Ohmoma and Abe, 1976).

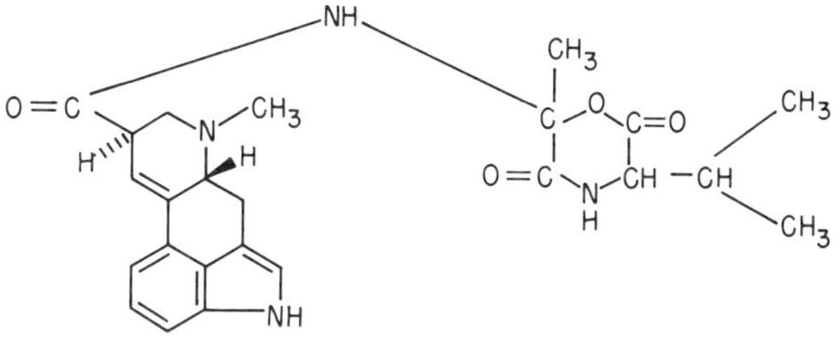

3 : Ergosecaline

Nonpeptide amides of lysergic acid found in ergot are ergonovine, lysergic acid α-hydroxyethylamide, and lysergic acid amide (ergine) (Table II). Ergonovine (ergobasine, ergometrine) was isolated simultaneously in several laboratories in 1935 (Dudley and Moir, 1935; Stoll and Burckhardt, 1935; Kharasch and Legault, 1935; Thompson, 1935). The α-hydroxyethylamide spontaneously decomposes to lysergic acid amide, and the naturally occurring amide may arise by this process. *Claviceps paspali* produces paspalic acid, which differs from lysergic acid in having a $\Delta^{8,9}$ double bond instead of the $\Delta^{9,10}$ double bond.

TABLE II

Naturally Occurring Lysergic Acid Derivatives Other Than Peptides

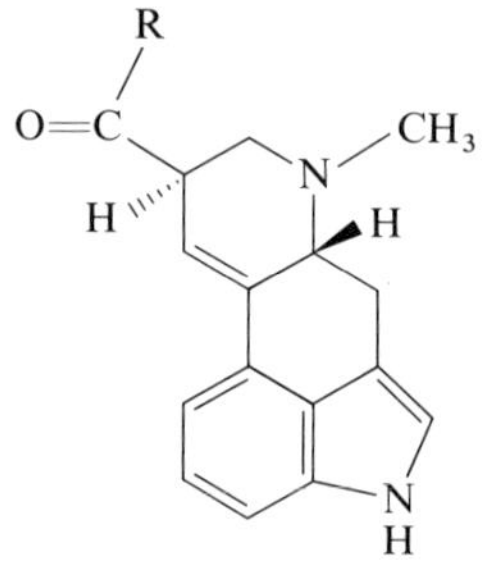

Name	R	Reference
Ergonovine (ergobasine, ergometrine)	$\begin{array}{c} CH_3 \\ \mid \\ -HN-C_{\prime\prime\prime}H \\ \mid \\ CH_2OH \end{array}$	Dudley and Moir (1935); Stoll and Burckhardt (1935); Kharasch and Legault (1935); Thompson (1935)
Lysergic acid α-hydroxyethylamide	$\begin{array}{c} CH_3 \\ \mid \\ -HN-CH-OH \end{array}$	Arcamone et al. (1961)
Lysergic acid amide	$-NH_2$	Arcamone et al. (1961)
Lysergic acid	$-OH$	Abou-Chaar et al. (1961)
$\Delta^{8,9}$-Lysergic acid (paspalic acid)	$-OH^a$	Kobel et al. (1964)

^{a} $\Delta^{9,10}$ double bond shifted to $\Delta^{8,9}$ position.

B. Clavine Alkaloids and Secoergolines

A new class of alkaloids, the clavine alkaloids (Table III), was isolated from saprophytic cultures of the ergot fungus. These alkaloids do contain not the carboxyl but a group of lower oxidation state at position 17, usually methyl or hydroxymethyl. Agroclavine, the first alkaloid of this series, was identified in saprophytic cultures by Abe (1951). Later, small amounts of clavine alkaloids were found accompanying the lysergic acid alkaloids in the ergot body (e.g., Voigt, 1962). Costaclavine is the only tetracyclic clavine alkaloid with a *cis* C/D ring junction.

A class of related structures is that of the 6,7-secoergolenes, or chano-clavines (Table III). Ring D is not closed in the chanoclavines. Chanoclavines I and II have hydrogens *trans* or *cis*, respectively, at positions 5 and 10. The *E* and *Z* isomers about the double bond are chanoclavine and isochano-clavine, respectively. *N*-Demethyl- or norchanoclavine I and chanoclavir

TABLE III

Clavine Alkaloids and Secoergolines

Ergolines	Alkaloid	R_1	R_2	R_3	R_4	References
$\Delta^{8,9}$-Ergolines 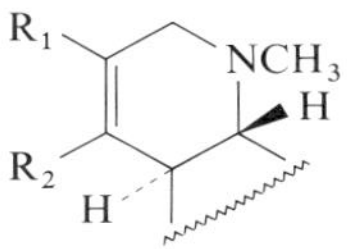	Agroclavine	CH_3	H			Abe (1951)
	Elymoclavine	CH_2OH	H			Abe et al. (1952)
	Molliclavine[a]	CH_2OH	OH			Abe and Yamatadoni (1955)
	Elymoclavine-O-β-D-fructoside	CH_2OH 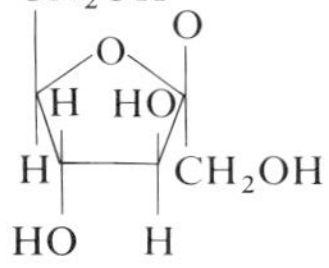 (fructoside)	H			Floss et al. (1967)
$\Delta^{9,10}$-Ergolenes 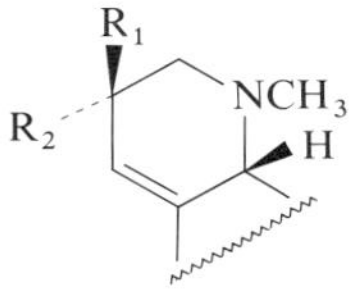	Lysergine	CH_3	H			Abe et al. (1961)
	Lysergol	CH_2OH	H			Abe et al. (1961)
	Isolysergol	H	CH_2OH			Hofmann (1961)
	Lysergene	CH_2				Agurell (1966a)
	Setoclavine	CH_3	OH			Abe et al. (1961)
	Isosetoclavine	OH	CH_3			Hofmann et al. (1957)
	Norsetoclavine (NH instead of NCH_3)	CH_3	OH			Hofmann et al. (1957)
						Ramstad et al. (1967)
	Penniclavine	CH_2OH	OH			Stoll et al. (1954)
	Isopenniclavine	OH	CH_2OH			Hofmann et al. (1957)
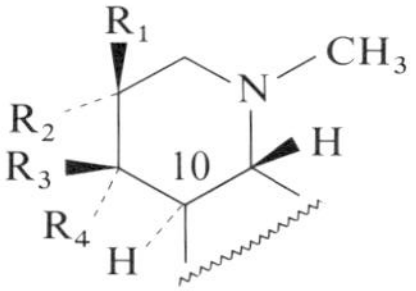	Festuclavine	CH_3	H	H	H	Abe and Yamatodani (1954)
	Costaclavine [epimeric at C(10)]	CH_3	H	H	H	Abe et al. (1956)
	Pyroclavine	H	CH_3	H	H	Abe et al. (1956)
	Dihydrolysergol I	CH_2OH	H	H	H	Agurell and Ramstad (1965)
	Dihydrosetoclavine	CH_3	OH	H	H	Tscherter and Hauth (1974)

(continued)

TABLE III (*continued*)

Ergolines	Alkaloid	R₁	R₂	R₃	R₄	References
	Fumigaclavine A	H	CH₃	CH₃COO	H	Spilsbury and Wilkinson (1961); Bach *et al.* (1974)
	Fumigaclavine B	H	CH₃	HO—	H	Spilsbury and Wilkinson (1961); Bach *et al.* (1974)
	Isofumigaclavine A (roquefortine A)	CH₃	H	H	CH₃COO	Ohmomo *et al.* (1975, 1977) Scott *et al.* (1976)
	Isofumigaclavine B (roquefortine B)	CH₃	H	H	OH	Ohmomo *et al.* (1975, 1977) Scott *et al.* (1976)
6,7-Secoergolenes	Chanoclavine I	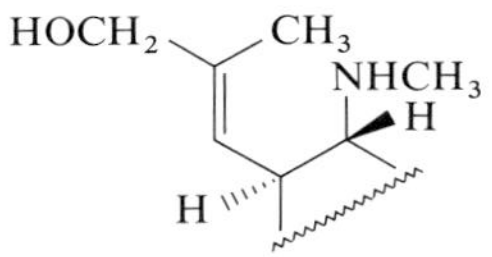				Abe *et al.* (1956) Hofmann *et al.* (1957)
	Chanoclavine II	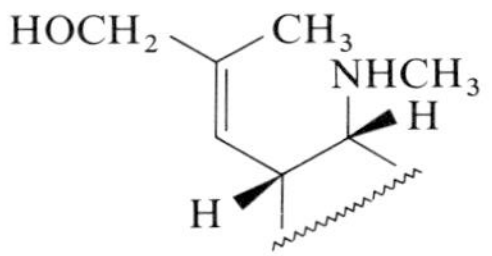 + enantiomer				Stauffacher and Tscherter (1964)
	Isochanoclavine I	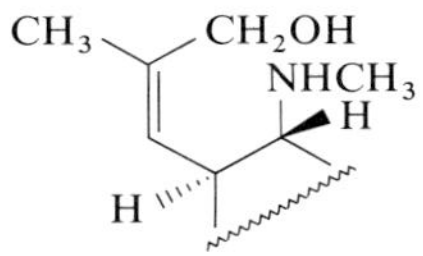				Stauffacher and Tscherter (1964)

Norchanoclavine I

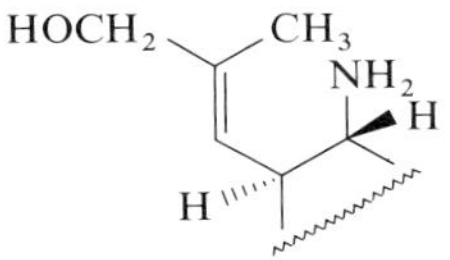

$HOCH_2$ CH_3 NH_2 H
H

Acklin (personal communication)

Norchanoclavine II

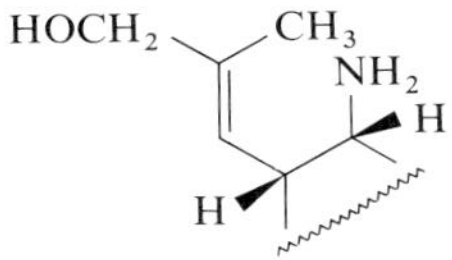

$HOCH_2$ CH_3 NH_2 H
H

and/or enantiomer

Cassady *et al.* (1973)
Acklin (personal communication)

Chanoclavine I acid

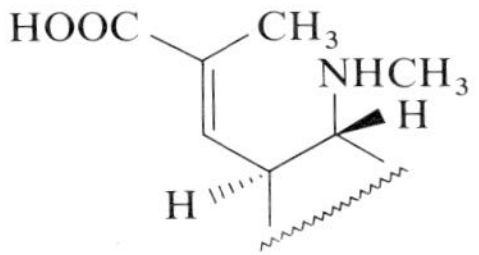

$HOOC$ CH_3 $NHCH_3$ H
H

Choong and Shough (1977)

Paliclavine

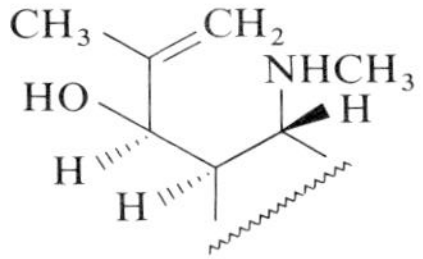

CH_3 CH_2 $NHCH_3$ H
HO H

Tscherter and Hauth (1974)

Paspaclavine

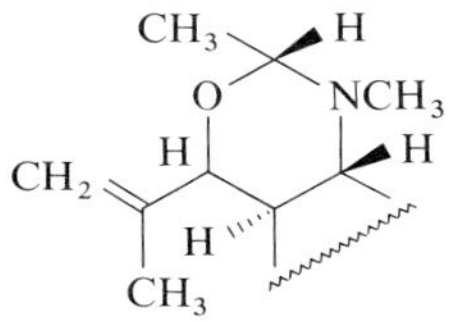

CH_3 H NCH_3 H
O
CH_2 CH_3

Tscherter and Hauth (1974)

(*continued*)

TABLE III (*continued*)

Ergolines	Alkaloid	R_1	R_2	R_3	R_4	References
	Rugulovasine A (R = H)	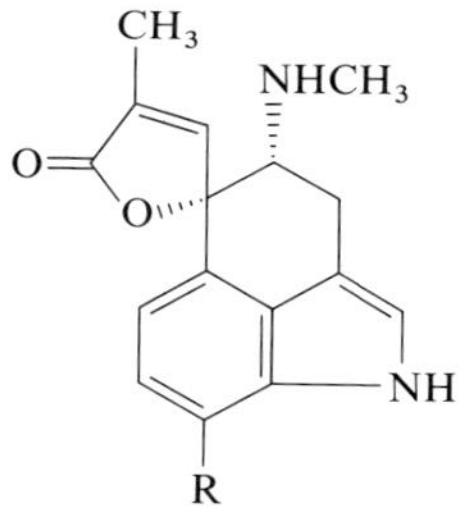				Yamatodani *et al.* (1970) Cole *et al.* (1976)
	8-Chlororugulovasine A (R = Cl)					Cole *et al.* (1976)
	Rugulovasine B (R = H)	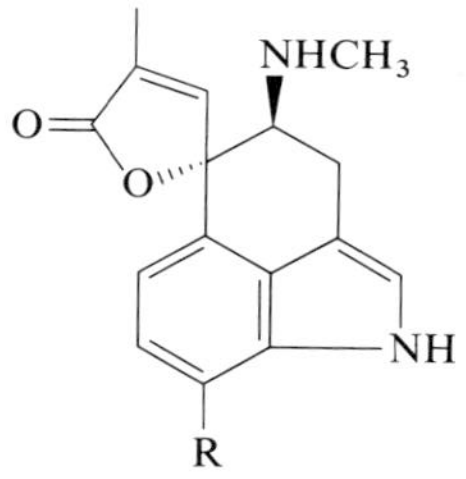				Yamatodani *et al.* (1970) Cole *et al.* (1976)
	8-Chlororugulovasine B (R = Cl)					Cole *et al.* (1976)
Other	Cycloclavine	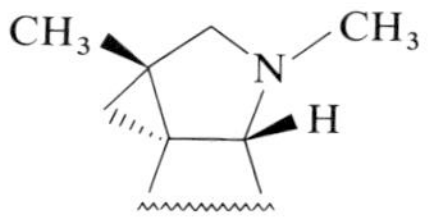				Stauffacher *et al.* (1976)

CH₃ NHCH₃ NH R + enantiomer O

NHCH₃ NH R + enantiomer O

CH₃ N—CH₃ H

Clavicipitic acid

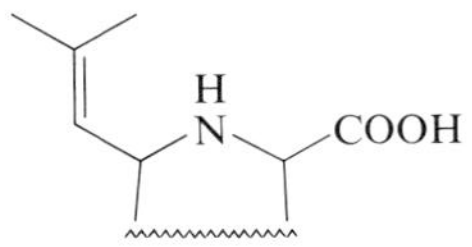

Robbers and Floss (1969)
King et al. (1977)

Dihydrochanoclavine I

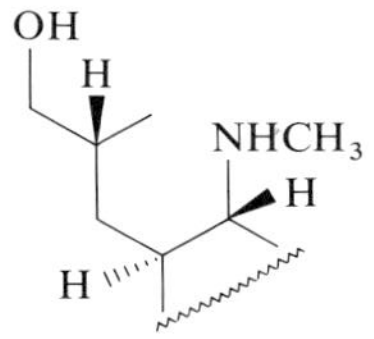

Voigt and Zier (1970)

Isodihydrochanoclavine I

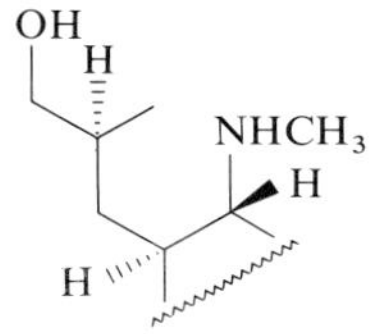

Voigt and Zier (1970)

[a] This structure should be considered tentative.

27

II occur in nature and appear to be formed by demethylation of the parent compounds (Ramstad *et al.*, 1967; Cassady *et al.*, 1973).

Interestingly, many of the clavine alkaloids have been found in other fungi. Festuclavine, agroclavine, elymoclavine, chanoclavine, and fumigaclavines A, B, and C were found in *Aspergillus fumigatus* (Spilsbury and Wilkinson, 1961; Yamano *et al.*, 1962). Costaclavine was isolated from *Penicillium chermesinum* (Agurell, 1964). Abe's group (Abe *et al.*, 1969; Yamatodani *et al.*, 1970) isolated chanoclavine I and two new alkaloids, rugulovasines A and B, from *Penicillium concavo-rugulovasum*. No lysergic acid derivatives have so far been found in fungi outside the genus *Claviceps*.

C. Ergolines in Higher Plants

The ergot alkaloids occur in a single family of higher plants, Convolvulaceae (Hofmann and Tscherter, 1960). The seeds of the two species *Ipomoea violaceae* L. (common morning glory) and *Rivea corymbosa* (L.) Hall f. were used for their hallucinogenic properties in a magic drug "ololiuqui" by Indians of Central America. Ergoline derivatives which have been isolated are lysergic acid amide, which is largely responsible for the hallucinogenic effects; isolysergic acid amide and chanoclavine (Hofmann and Tscherter, 1960); lysergic acid and isolysergic acid α-hydroxyethylamide (Gröger, 1963); elymoclavine and lysergol (Hofmann, 1961); ergonovine (Gröger, 1963; Taber *et al.*, 1963); ergosine and ergosinine (Stauffacher *et al.*, 1964); and a new clavine alkaloid, cycloclavine (Stauffacher *et al.*, 1969). Ergot alkaloids have not been found in any other plant family and are limited to a few genera in the Convolvulaceae.

D. Physiological Effects and Pharmacology

The various physiological activities of the ergot alkaloids can be divided into three types. The peripheral effects are the contraction of smooth muscle including the peripheral blood vessels and the muscle of the uterus.

The use of ergot to help contractions of the uterus at birth was reported in a German herbal in 1582. Methylergonovine (4), ergonovine, and ergotamine are now used to induce uterine contractions and reduce postpartal hemorrhage. The uterine muscle is only more sensitive than other smooth muscle at term. Ergot is therefore ineffective in causing abortions. Migraine headaches were first treated with extracts of ergot in 1883 and are currently treated with ergotamine and dihydroergotamine. The effectiveness of the ergot alkaloids is due primarily to the contraction of arteries in the brain.

The ergot alkaloids also block the action of the neurohormones serotonin and adrenalin. The antiserotonin effect contributes to the efficacy of the

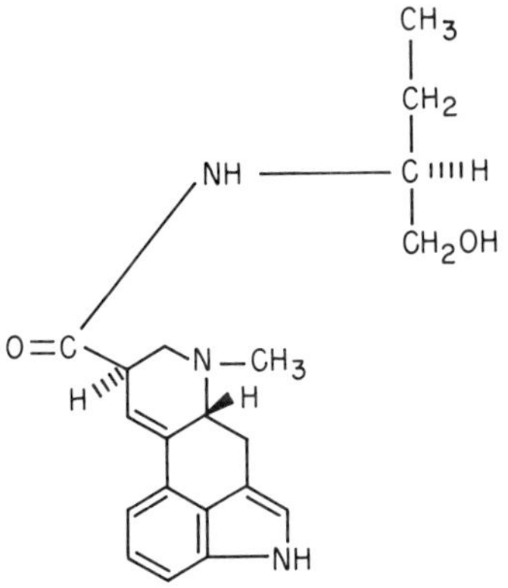

$$CH_3$$
$$|$$
$$CH_2$$
$$|$$
$$NH \longrightarrow C\ \text{IIII}\ H$$
$$|$$
$$CH_2OH$$

4

ergot alkaloids in relieving migraine headaches. Whereas the ergot alkaloids cause vasoconstriction, the dihydro derivative of ergotoxine, i.e., the 1:1:1 mixture of dihydroergocornine, dihydroergocristine, and dihydroergo-kryptine (Hydergine) causes vasodilation by blocking the action of adrenaline. Hydergine is used in the treatment of high blood pressure and cerebral circulatory disorders.

The ergot alkaloids also affect the central nervous system. Effects on the *medulla oblongata* cause decreased heart rate, vomiting, and reduction of vascular tone. Action on the midbrain causes hyperthermia, hyperglycemia, rapid breathing, dilation of the pupils of the eye, and exaggerated tendon reflexes. The derivative with the greatest effect on the midbrain is the diethyl-amide derivative of lysergic acid (LSD) (**5**). In addition to the above effects, LSD has the property of causing hallucinations in doses of 20–30 μg. For a time, illicit use of LSD was widespread. At present this use, as well as medical use in psychopharmacology, is limited. Ergoline derivatives act on the hypothalamic–pituitary system to inhibit the secretion of prolactin. The development of drugs for use in prolactin-dependent disorders is presently an active area of research (cf. Cassady and Floss, 1977).

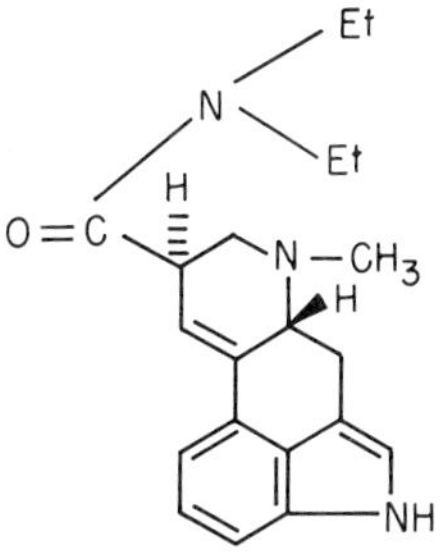

5 : LSD

E. Alkaloid Production in Laboratory Cultures

Abe (1951) obtained clavine alkaloid formation in surface cultures of several strains of *Claviceps*. However, high-yield production of lysergic acid derivatives in submerged cultures was not achieved until 1960, when Chain and co-workers reported the isolation of a strain of *C. paspali* which produced up to 2 gm/liter of lysergic acid α-hydroxyethylamide (Arcamone *et al.*, 1960; 1961). Kobel *et al.* (1964) isolated a strain which produced $\Delta^{8,9}$-lysergic acid (see Table II). Commercially, the products of these two high-producing strains are converted to lysergic acid, which then is used for the semisynthesis of ergonovine, methylergonovine, peptide alkaloids, and other commercially produced ergolines. More recently high-yielding fermentation methods have been developed for ergotamine and the ergo-tamine and the ergotoxine group of alkaloids (Arcamone *et al.*, 1970). Despite the recent development of fermentation methods for ergot alkaloid production, peptide ergot alkaloids are still obtained by field cultivation.

III. BIOSYNTHESIS OF THE ERGOLINE SYSTEM

A. Precursors of Ergot Alkaloids

Reviews have appeared throughout the course of studies on the bio-synthesis of the ergot alkaloids (e.g., Tyler, 1961; Winkler and Gröger, 1962; Weygand and Floss, 1963; Agurell, 1966b; Voigt, 1968; Ramstad, 1968; Gröger, 1969; Thomas and Bassett, 1972; Floss, 1971, 1976). Tryptophan was established as a precursor of the ergot alkaloids by Mothes *et al.* (1958), who showed that radioactivity from [^{14}C]tryptophan injected into plants infected with ergot was incorporated into ergonovine and the lysergic acid part of the peptide alkaloids. The specific incorporation into ergokryptine was 0.158% (Gröger *et al.*, 1959). (DL)-[β-^{14}C]Tryptophan was also shown to be incorporated into elymoclavine in saprophytic cultures of *Claviceps*, with specific incorporations of 10–39% (Gröger *et al.*, 1959). The use of saprophytic cultures of alkaloid-producing strains of *Claviceps*, most of which were isolated during the search for commercially useful strains, was subsequently also exploited by most other workers in the field for the study of ergot alkaloid biosynthesis. Mothes *et al.* (1958) and Birch *et al.* (1958) proposed that the ergoline ring structure is built up from tryptophan, a five-carbon isoprene unit, and a methyl group from C_1 donor. This proposal proved to be correct.

Incorporation of tryptophan labeled in different positions into the ergot alkaloids was consistent with the contribution of tryptophan to the ergoline

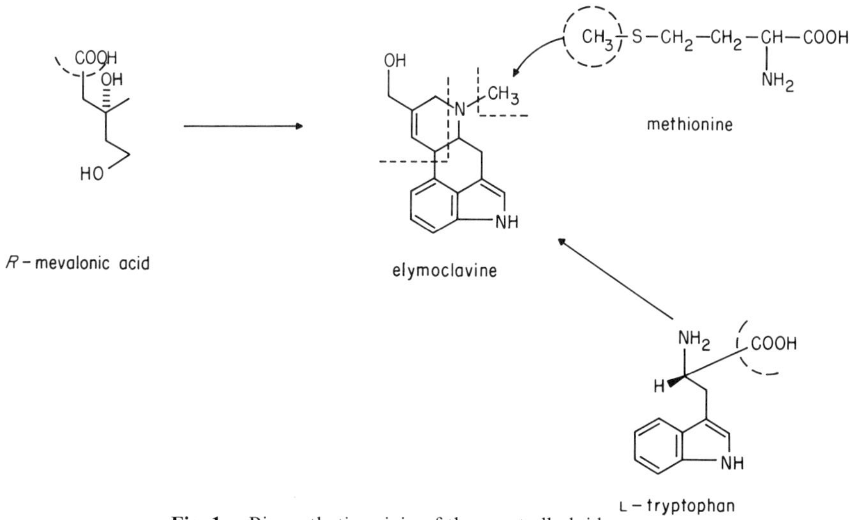

Fig. 1.   Biosynthetic origin of the ergot alkaloids.

skeleton shown in Fig. 1. The label from [1-^{14}C]tryptophan was not in-corporated (Gröger *et al.*, 1959, 1960). Incorporation studies also showed that hydrogens 5, 6 (Plieninger *et al.*, 1967; Bellati *et al.*, 1977), and 7 (Wil-son, 1970; Bellati *et al.*, 1977) and the amino nitrogen (Floss *et al.*, 1964), but not hydrogen 4 (Plieninger *et al.*, 1967; Bellatti *et al.*, 1977) of tryptophan were retained in the ergoline alkaloids. In a study where the position of the labeled hydrogen was established, the α hydrogen of tryptophan was shown to occupy position 5 of elymoclavine (Floss *et al.*, 1964). The conclusion from these studies is that tryptophan is incorporated intact into the ergoline ring structure, with the exception of the carboxy group and the hydrogen at position 4.

Both D- and L-tryptophan are incorporated into the ergoline alkaloids (Taber and Vining, 1959). Generally tritiated D-tryptophan was incorporated to the extent of 28% (Gröger *et al.*, 1960). The α hydrogen (98%) and amino nitrogen (90%) of D-tryptophan were lost during the incorporation into elymoclavine, compared to 47% and 56% loss with DL-tryptophan (Floss *et al.*, 1964). The results indicate that L-tryptophan is incorporated with almost complete retention of the α hydrogen and the amino nitrogen. L-Tryptophan is therefore the immediate precursor, and D-tryptophan is presumably incorporated via indole pyruvate and L-tryptophan. The configuration at position 5 in the ergoline ring is opposite to the configuration of L-tryptophan. The formation of ring C therefore involves an inversion of configuration of the α carbon of tryptophan with retention of the original hydrogen attached to this carbon (Floss et al., 1964).

Mevalonate is the precursor of terpenes, polyisoprenes, and steroids. In the biosynthesis of these compounds mevalonate is converted to dimethylallyl pyrophosphate and isopentenyl pyrophosphate, which provide the five-carbon isoprene unit. Three groups showed almost simultaneously the incorporation of mevalonate into the ergot alkaloids with efficiencies of 9–23% (Gröger et al., 1960; Birch et al., 1960; Taylor and Ramstad, 1960, 1961). The label from $[2-^{14}C]$mevalonate was shown to be specifically incorporated into C(17) by two different degradation procedures (Bhattacharji et al., 1962; Baxter et al., 1961, 1962a), but a fraction of the label is always found to be located at C(7). Baxter et al. (1961) established that the C(1) of mevalonate was not incorporated, and Plieninger's group reported the incorporation of isopentenyl pyrophosphate and dimethylallyl pyrophosphate (despite the usual impermeability of cell membranes to phosphate esters) (Plieninger et al., 1961, 1967).

$(R,S)-[2-^{14}C]$Mevalonate was incorporated 50 times better than $(3S)-[2-^{14}C]$mevalonate, indicating that $(3R)$-mevalonate is the precursor of the ergot alkaloids (Floss et al., 1968). This is the same isomer that is incorporated into squalene via dimethylallyl pyrophosphate in rat liver. In a related experiment, when a mixture of $(RS)-[2-^{14}C]$mevalonate and $(3R,5S)-[5-^{3}H]$mevalonate was fed, the $^{3}H:^{14}C$ ratio doubled owing to incorporation of half as much of the ^{14}C-labeled (R,S)-mevalonate as the ^{3}H-labeled (R)-mevalonate (Seiler et al., 1970a,b; Abou-Chaar et al., 1972).

Baxter's group (Baxter et al., 1964) found that the incorporation of (L)-$[methyl-^{14}C]$methionine was four times the incorporation of $[^{14}C]$formate into festuclavine. The label from methionine was shown by degradation experiments to be located exclusively in the N-methyl group of festuclavine. (L)-$[methyl-^{14}C,^{3}H]$Methionine was incorporated into the alkaloid without change in the $^{3}H:^{14}C$ ratio. The methyl goup of methionine is therefore transferred intact. Figure 1 summarizes the biogenetic origin of the ergoline ring system.

B. The First Step in Ergot Alkaloid Biosynthesis

During the biosynthesis of ergoline alkaloids, tryptophan is decarboxylated, isoprenylated at the 4 position, and methylated at the amino nitrogen. Neither tryptamine (Baxter et al., 1961; Floss and Gröger, 1963) nor N^{ω}-methyltryptamine (Floss and Gröger, 1963) was incorporated into the alkaloids. This ruled out decarboxylation as the first step. The tritium label from $N^{\alpha}-[side\ chain-^{14}C,methyl-^{3}H]$methyltryptophan was lost (Floss and Gröger, 1964). Only the tryptophan part was incorporated, the N-methyl

group apparently being added at a later stage. These results leave isoprenylation as the first step in the pathway. An early proposal was that tryptophan
was hydroxylated at the 4 position and that a "tail-to-tail" condensation
between dimethylallyl pyrophosphate and a phosphorylated 4-hydroxy-
indole derivative then occurred, analogous to the formation of squalene
from farnesyl pyrophosphate. However, the finding that 4-hydroxytryp-
tophan was not incorporated (Floss et al., 1965) ruled out this mechanism.

Direct isoprenylation remained as a likely first reaction. The initial point of
attachment could be either at the α position of the side chain or at the 4
position of the indole ring. Attachment at the α position could occur with
simultaneous decarboxylation to produce compound 6. γ,γ-Dimethylal-
lyltryptophan (DMAT), 7, was synthesized by Plieninger and Liede (1963),
and compound 6 by Weygand et al. (1964). Despite initial results suggesting
good incorporation of both compounds, direct comparisons showed that
DMAT was a much more efficient precursor of the alkaloids than compound
6 (Plieninger et al., 1964; Weygand et al., 1964), giving incorporation rates
up to 35%. DMAT labeled with tritium at the α-carbon of the alanine side
chain and with ^{14}C at $C(1)$ of the dimethylallyl group gave elymoclavine
without change in the $^{3}H:^{14}C$ ratio (Plieninger et al., 1967). DMAT was
isolated from ergot cultures incubated in the absence of oxygen (Robbers
and Floss, 1968) or with ethionine added (Agurell and Lindgren, 1968). The
final evidence that DMAT is the first intermediate was the isolation of the
enzyme from Claviceps mycelia which catalyzed the condensation of
tryptophan with dimethylallyl pyrophosphate (Heinstein et al., 1971; Lee
et al., 1976) to form DMAT.

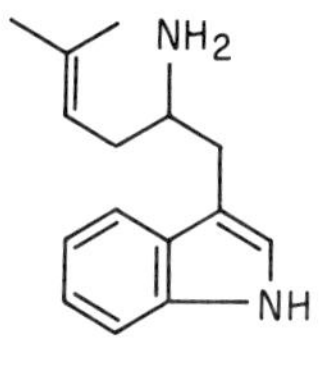

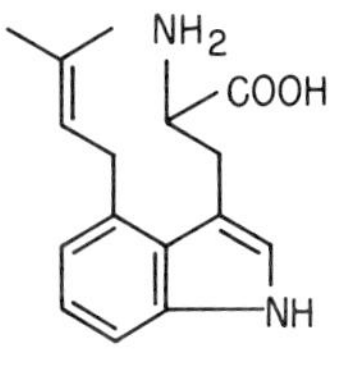

C. Interrelationships among the Clavine Alkaloids

In 1958 Rochelmeyer proposed the biosynthetic sequence chanoclavine →
agroclavine → elymoclavine → lysergic acid derivatives (Rochelmeyer, 1958).
Radioactive incorporation experiments in several laboratories have supported this route as the major pathway (Agurell, 1966b; Agurell and
Ramstad, 1961, 1962; Mothes et al., 1962; Baxter et al., 1962b). Early experiments showed that chanoclavine was not incorporated into agroclavine
(Agurell and Ramstad, 1962; Baxter et al., 1962b). However, it was later

found (see below) that a different isomer of chanoclavine is the intermediate in the biosynthetic pathway. Radioactive incorporation experiments by Agurell and Ramstad established the conversion of agroclavine to elymo-clavine and the failure of the reverse reaction (Agurell, 1966b; Agurell and Ramstad, 1962).

Agroclavine is a precursor of setoclavine and isosetoclavine, and elymo-clavine is a precursor of penniclavine and isopenniclavine (Agurell, 1966b; Agurell and Ramstad, 1962). The conversion involves a hydroxylation at the 8 position with an accompanying shift of the double bond from the 8,9 to the 9,10 position. Peroxidase catalyzes these conversions, and activity is widely distributed among fungal species (Ramstad, 1968; Taylor *et al.*, 1966;

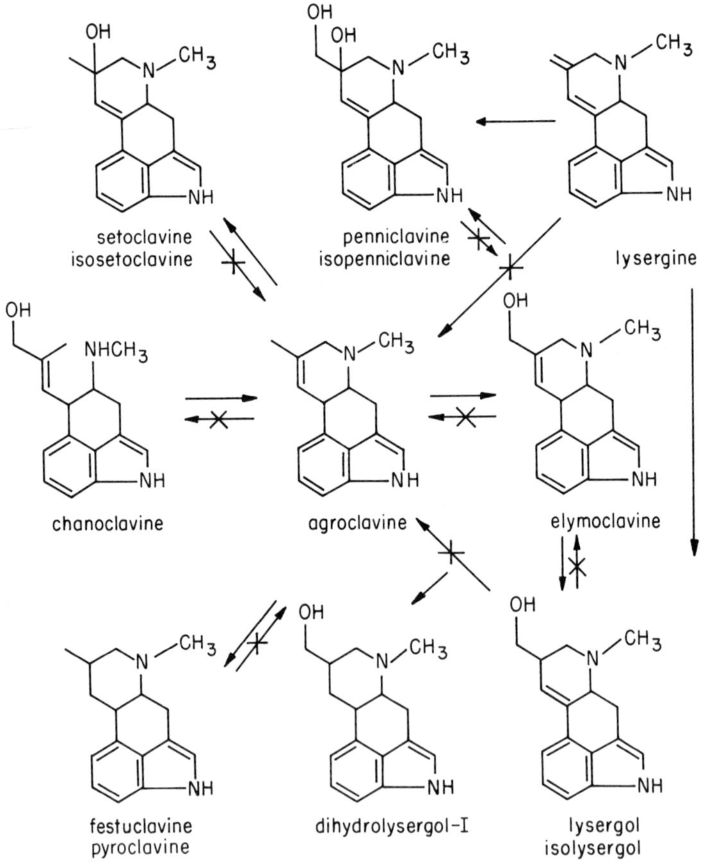

Fig. 2.   Relationships between clavine alkaloids.

Chan, 1967; Shough and Taylor, 1969; Lin *et al.*, 1967). A system consisting of thioglycolate, Fe^{2+}, and oxygen catalyzes the same conversion (Bajwa and Anderson, 1975), and the formation in strains where these alkaloids are not major products could be nonenzymatic. The dihydro derivatives are derived irreversibly from the corresponding $\Delta^{8,9}$-unsaturated clavines (Agurell and Ramstad, 1962; Baxter *et al.*, 1962b). The relationships among the clavine alkaloids determined by Agurell and Ramstad (1962), Agurell (1966b); and Baxter *et al.* (1962b) are summarized in Fig. 2.

In disagreement with the above sequence, Abe's group (Abe, 1963, 1966; Abe *et al.*, 1963) proposed, based on radioactive incorporation studies, that elymoclavine is a precursor of agroclavine. They proposed that lysergaldehyde is a precursor of both elymoclavine and the lysergic acid derivatives, and that elymoclavine is converted to lysergol, lysergene, and then to agroclavine. The retention of label in agroclavine (and also elymoclavine) observed when $[2\text{-}^{14}C,2\text{-}^{3}H]$- or $[2\text{-}^{14}C,5\text{-}^{3}H]$mevalonate was fed (Agurell, 1966; Baxter *et al.*, 1962b) is inconsistent with lysergaldehyde being a precursor of elymoclavine or lysergol and lysergene being precursors of agroclavine.

D. Role of the Chanoclavines

In the experiments of Agurell and Ramstad (1961, 1962) and of Baxter *et al.* (1962b), chanoclavine was not converted to agroclavine or elymoclavine. Furthermore, Mothes and Winkler (1962) reported the conversion of elymoclavine to chanoclavine. On the other hand, in feeding experiments with labeled tryptophan, the specific activity of chanoclavine was higher than that of the clavine alkaloids, a finding indicating that chanoclavine could not have been derived from the latter (Weygand and Floss, 1963). The apparent inconsistency was resolved with the isolation of chanoclavine I, ($-$)- and ($\pm$)-chanoclavine II, and isochanoclavine I (Stauffacher and Tscherter, 1964) (see Table III). The results of different investigators could be attributed to the metabolic properties of the isomers. Incorporation experiments showed that one of the isomers, chanoclavine I, was incorporated into the clavine alkaloids and lysergic acid derivatives (Gröger *et al.*, 1966; Fehr *et al.*, 1966; Floss *et al.*, 1968; Voigt *et al.*, 1967) with incorporation into elymoclavine as high as 40% (Gröger *et al.*, 1966) and dilution factors as low as 1.23 (Voigt *et al.*, 1967). Chanoclavine I was incorporated into elymoclavine with a higher dilution factor than into agroclavine, consistent with the sequence chanoclavine I → agroclavine → elymoclavine (Gröger *et al.*, 1966). Conversion of elymoclavine into chanoclavine I was reported by Abe (1971).

Neither chanoclavine II nor isochanoclavine I is converted to the tetra-cyclic clavine alkaloids or to chanoclavine I (Fehr *et al.*, 1966; Floss *et al.*, 1968). Chanoclavine II has the wrong stereochemistry at C(5) or C(10), but isochanoclavine I looks like a good potential precursor, because elimination of water to form the D ring would directly produce agroclavine.

E. *Cis–Trans* Isomerizations in Clavine Alkaloid Biosynthesis

The label from [2-^{14}C]mevalonic acid is incorporated predominantly into the methyl group of chanoclavine I and the other secoergolines, with some scrambling (7%) into the hydroxymethyl group (Fehr *et al.*, 1966). The finding that this label was incorporated into C(17) of the clavine alkaloids (Bhattacharji *et al.*, 1962; Baxter *et al.*, 1961, 1962a) suggested a *cis–trans* isomerization during the conversion of chanoclavine I to agroclavine. This was confirmed by feeding [17-^{14}C]- or [7-^{14}C]chanoclavine (Fehr *et al.*, 1966; Floss *et al.*, 1968) and degrading the isolated agroclavine and elymo-clavine. The labeling pattern showed that the hydroxymethyl group of chanoclavine I becomes C(7) of agroclavine, and that the methyl group becomes C(17).

The location of the label from C(2) of mevalonate in the methyl group of chanoclavine I (Fehr *et al.*, 1966) suggested a second *cis–trans* isomerization during the synthesis of chanoclavine I. In the conversion of isopentenyl pyrophosphate to dimethylallyl pyrophosphate, C(2) of mevalonate becomes the *trans*-methyl group of dimethylallyl pyrophosphate (Popjak and Corn-forth, 1966). Because the label is located in the *cis*-methyl group of chanoclavine I, a *cis–trans* isomerization apparently occurs in the formation of chanoclavine I from dimethylallyl pyrophosphate.

Loss of the *pro-S* hydrogen from C(4) of mevalonate occurs in the normal isomerization of isopentenyl pyrophosphate to dimethylallyl pyrophosphate, whereas the *pro-R* hydrogen is lost in the synthesis of rubber or dolichol, which results in the formation of *cis* double bonds. The *pro-4S* hydrogen of mevalonate was lost (Floss *et al.*, 1968) in forming elymoclavine, supporting the normal pathway for formation of dimethylallyl pyrophosphate and a *cis–trans* isomerization on the pathway to chanoclavine I.

Arigoni's group (Pachlatko *et al.*, 1975a,b) synthesized [Z-^{14}CH$_3$]-(**7**), fed it to *Claviceps* cultures, and showed that the label was located at C(7) (>98%) of agroclavine and elymoclavine, i.e., in the carbon occupying the *cis* position. As a *cis–trans* isomerization occurs between chanoclavine I and agroclavine, another *cis–trans* isomerization is unequivocally indi-cated between **7** and chanoclavine I. These isomerizations are shown in Fig. 3.

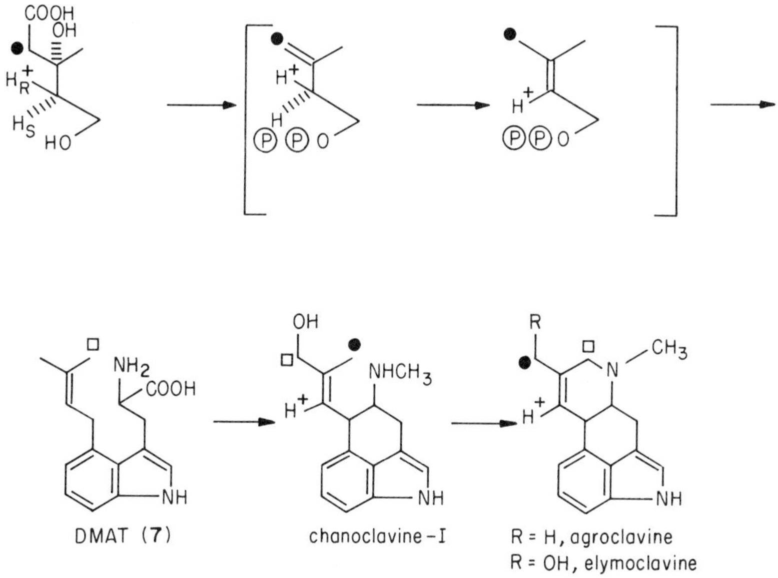

DMAT (7)   chanoclavine-I   R = H, agroclavine
                                          R = OH, elymoclavine

Fig. 3. Double bond isomerizations in ergoline biosynthesis.

F. Hydroxylation of 4-γ,γ-Dimethylallyltryptophan

Arigoni's group (Fehr, 1967) tested deoxychanoclavine I and nordeoxy-chanoclavine I and found that neither was a precursor of the clavine alkaloids. The hydroxylation at C(17) therefore precedes C-ring formation. Plieninger et al. (1971) synthesized 4-(4′-E-hydroxy-3′-methyl-2′-butenyl)-tryptophan (E-8) labeled with ^{14}C in the hydroxymethyl group and tested it for incorporation into agroclavine and elymoclavine. Incorporation was at first reported into both alkaloids, but it was later shown that only elymoclavine was labeled (Plieninger, personal communication and Pachlatko 1975). Pachlatko et al. (1975) then synthesized (Z)-[^{14}CH$_3$]-(8) from (E)-[^{14}CH$_3$]-(8) by a photoisomerization and found that the label from the Z

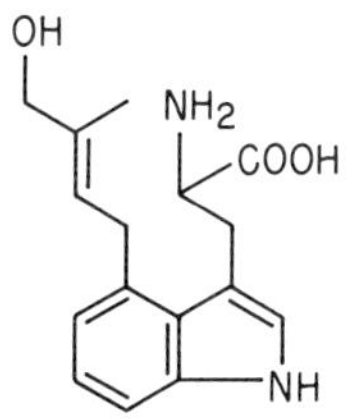

E-8

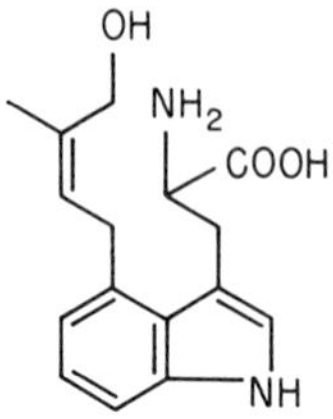

Z- **8**

isomer was also incorporated into elymoclavine but not into agroclavine. Compound **8**, therefore, cannot be an intermediate on the main pathway.

Anderson and Saini (1974) isolated **8** from *Claviceps*. The compound was found to be identical by mass spectroscopy and chromatography with reference to *E*-**8**. Cell-free conversion of **7** to **8** has been obtained by Petroski and Kelleher (1977) and by Saini and Anderson (in press). The above results indicate that there probably is a pathway in *Claviceps* **7** → **8** → elymoclavine independent of the main pathway via agroclavine. The contribution of this pathway to the total synthesis of elymoclavine is unknown.

In the radioactive incorporation experiments of Arigoni's group (Pachlatko, 1975; Pachlatko *et al.*, 1975), more than 97% of the label from (E)-$[^{14}CH_3]$-(**8**) and (Z)-$[^{14}CH_3]$-(**8**) was incorporated into C(7) of elymo-clavine. This labeling pattern would result if *E*-(**8**) went through the normal pathway with the two *cis–trans* isomerizations as though the hydroxyl was not there. The pathway for *Z*-(**8**) is difficult to explain unless it is assumed that *Z*-(**8**) is converted to *E*-(**8**) in the cell.

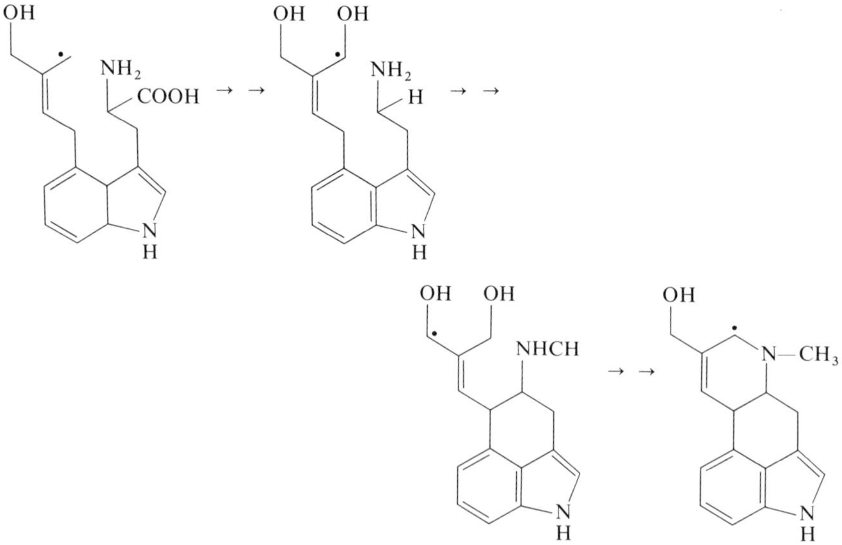

G. Clavicipitic Acid

Clavicipitic acid accumulates in cultures of *Claviceps* (Robbers and Floss, 1969; King *et al.*, 1977). Structure **9** was proposed (Robbers and Floss, 1969) based on the mass spectrum and biochemical evidence. Subsequently, King *et al.* (1973) deduced structure **10** from the spectra of derivatives of clavicipitic acid. The finding of 95.5% retention of the *pro*-(5*S*) hydrogen of mevalonate and 52.5% of the *pro*-(5*R*) hydrogen (Floss, 1976) is not easily reconciled with either structure. Clavicipitic acid is isolated as a pair of closely related compounds which are proposed by King *et al.* (1977) to be diastereomers, and study of the separate compounds may be necessary to resolve this discrepancy. The possibility exists that the biosynthesis of clavicipitic acid and clavine alkaloid biosynthesis, both of which require oxidation of the isoprene unit, involves a common enzymatic process, although no evidence to support such a relationship has so far been found.

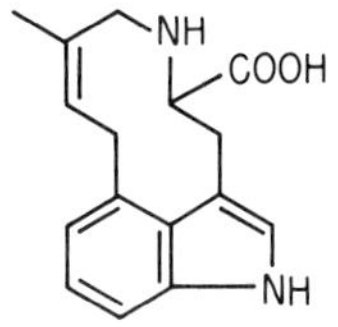

9

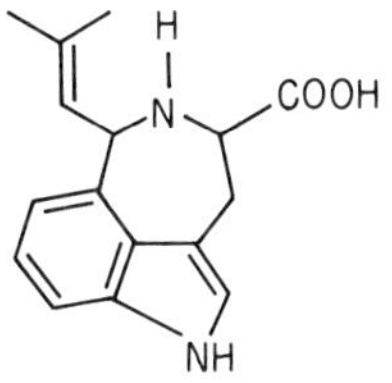

10

H. Possible Mechanisms for Closure of Ring C

The observations by Arigoni's group (Fehr, 1967; Pachlatko *et al.*, 1975) that deoxychanoclavine I, nordeoxychanoclavine I, and **8** are not intermediates in the biosynthesis of the ergot alkaloids require that (a) hydroxylation of either of the methyl groups in the isoprene unit cannot be the first step after formation of **7**, and (b) closure of ring C occurs after oxidation of the *cis*-methyl group of the isoprene unit unless ring C closes to form an as yet completely unsuspected product. A possible sequence is shown in Fig. 4. The initial hydroxylation could occur at C(1) of the isoprene unit, replacing the hydrogen originating from the *pro*-(5*R*) position of mevalonate (Seiler

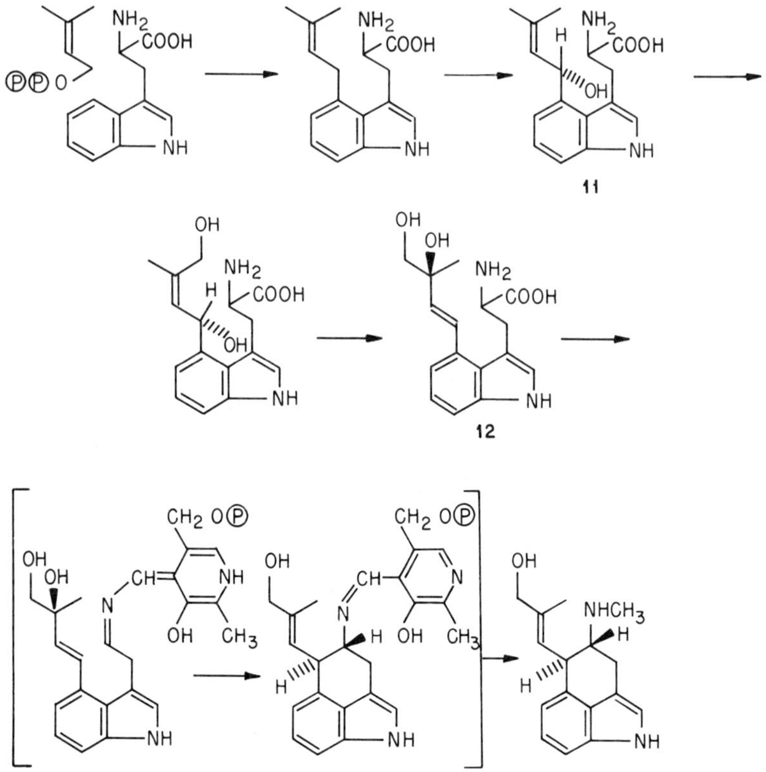

Fig. 4. Possible mechanism of C-ring formation in ergot alkaloid biosynthesis.

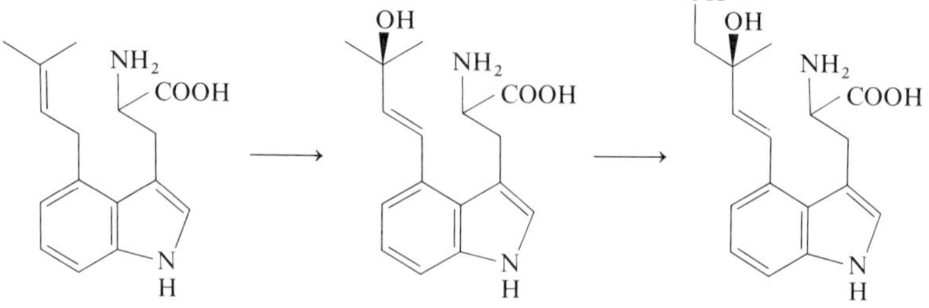

et al., 1970a,b; Abou-Chaar, *et al.*, 1972) to give **11**. After the hydroxylation of the methyl group, rearrangement takes place to give structure **12**. Alternatively, the initial hydroxylation could occur with simultaneous allylic rearrangement to give structure **13**, followed by hydroxylation of the methyl group to produce **12**. As another alternative, Pachlatko *et al.* (1975) proposed an epoxide intermediate that could be derived from a hydroperoxide:

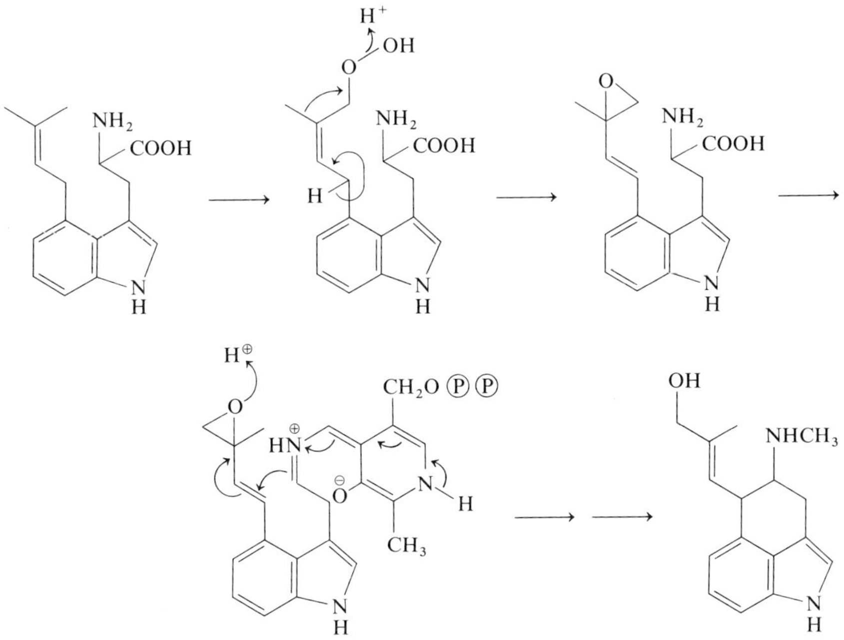

I. The *N*-Methylation Step

Methylation of the amino group must occur between **7** and chanoclavine I. Methylation after formation of ring C seems attractive because this would allow the involvement of pyridoxal 5′-phosphate in the ring closure reaction (see Fig. 4). Norchanoclavines I and II were detected in cultures of *Claviceps* (Acklin, personal communication; Cassady *et al.*, 1973), but feeding experiments with both labeled compounds showed no incorporation into agroclavine and elymoclavine (Cassady *et al.*, 1973). Consistent with this result, Acklin (personal communication) found that norchanoclavine I is derived from chanoclavine I. Because norchanoclavine I is not an intermediate in alkaloid biosynthesis, the methylation step must occur before or simultaneously with closure of ring C (unless the product of ring C formation is a completely unsuspected product). Acklin (personal communication) considers a mechanism in which methylation occurs simultaneously with ring closure. If the intermediate is a pyridoxal 5′-phosphate Schiff's base, CH_3^+ from *S*-adenosylmethionine adds to the Schiff's base double bond in place of H^+ in the final cleavage of pyridoxal 5′-phosphate. This mechanism, although chemically reasonable, requires a very complicated enzyme-active site:

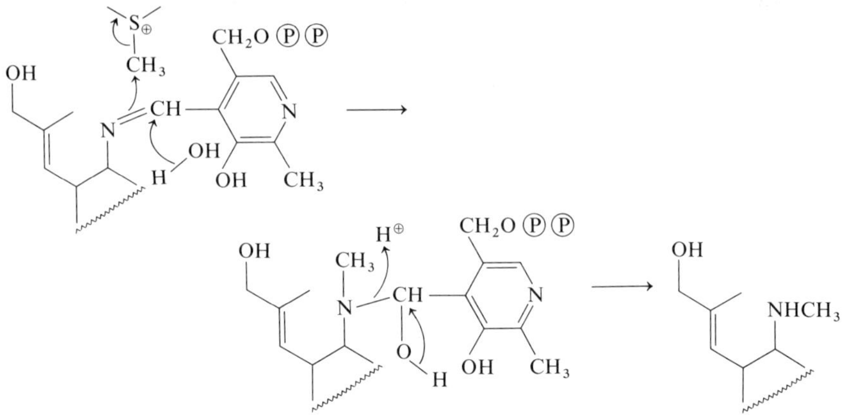

Methylation of an earlier stage has not been considered likely, because it would preclude participation of pyridoxal phosphate in the ring closure reaction. However, N^{α}-methyl-4-γ,γ-dimethylallyltryptophan (14) has been isolated from *Claviceps* cultures incubated under anaerobic conditions (Barrow and Quigley, 1975). The structure was established by spectroscopy. $[N\text{-}^{14}CH_3]$-(14) was produced by anaerobic incubation of *Claviceps fusiformis* with $[^{14}CH_3]$methionine. Refeeding of the $[N\text{-}^{14}CH_3]$-(14) then gave low (1.4%) incorporation into the clavine alkaloids. Further experimentation should be done to establish whether the methyl group remains with the rest of the molecule during conversion into the alkaloids. It is evident that the exact location of the methylation step has not yet been found, and early or late steps between 7 and chanoclavine I are possible.

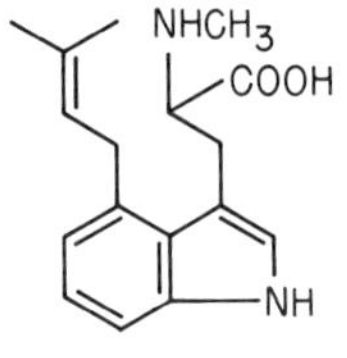

14

It has since been shown that $[^{15}N\text{-}CD_3]$-(14) is converted into elymoclavine with efficiencies of up to 50% and without cleavage of the N—CH_3 bond (Otsuka *et al.*, 1979). The corresponding decarboxylation product was not incorporated. Furthermore, an enzyme has been isolated from *Claviceps* which catalyzes the transfer of the methyl group of S-adenosylmethionine to 7 as substrate (F. Quigley, D. Gröger, and H. G. Floss, unpublished work). These results strongly suggest that N-methylation of 7 is the second step in the pathway of ergoline biosynthesis, followed by a reaction in the isoprenoid side chain. They also imply that the decarboxylation and the closure of ring C do not involve pyridoxal phosphate catalysis, but must proceed by a different mechanism.

J. Formation of Ring D

Fehr (1967) proposed a mechanism for the conversion of chanoclavine I into agroclavine in which the C(9) epimer of paliclavine (see Table III) is an intermediate:

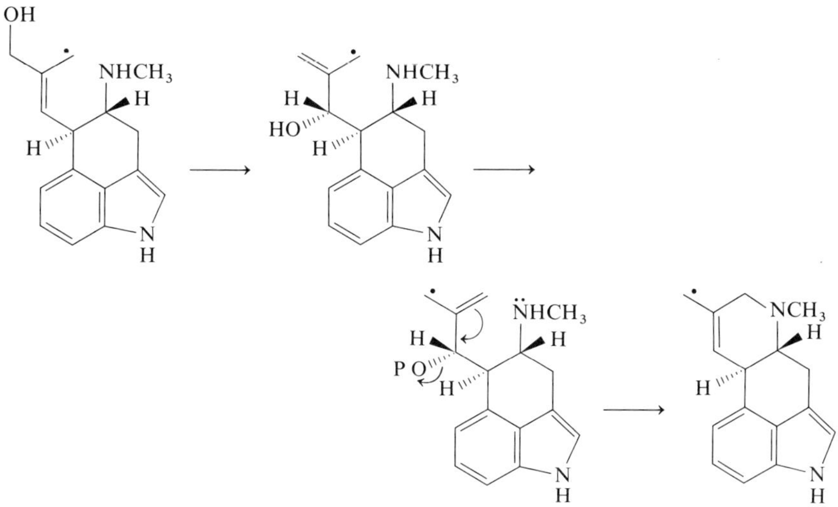

The isolation of paliclavine from *Claviceps* cultures (Tscherter and Hauth, 1974) lent support to this proposal. Acklin *et al.* (1975) synthesized [N-^{14}CH$_3$]chanoclavine I and [N-^{14}CH$_3$]paliclavine and tested them for incorporation into the ergot alkaloids in a *C. paspali* and in a clavine-producing strain. Paliclavine was not a precursor of paspalic acid, agro-clavine, elymoclavine, chanoclavine I, or isochanoclavine I. This rules out a mechanism for closure of ring D involving paliclavine. The results also show that paliclavine is formed by a route that does not involve chanoclavine I as an intermediate.

K. Chanoclavine I Aldehyde

[17-^{3}H,4-^{14}C]Chanoclavine was fed to *Claviceps* strain SD 58. The elymoclavine isolated from this culture showed a tritium retention of 53%, demonstrating the loss of one of the labeled hydrogens from C(17) of chanoclavine I (Floss *et al.*, 1974a). The results suggested that chanoclavine I aldehyde is formed as an intermediate in D-ring closure. [17-^{3}H,4-^{14}C]- Chanoclavine I aldehyde was prepared from chanoclavine I and tested for incorporation into elymoclavine. The incorporation of tritium was 40% into elymoclavine compared to 9.9% for chanoclavine I. The retention of the C(17) hydrogen of chanoclavine I aldehyde was 90%. Consistent with these results, elymoclavine isolated after feeding [3'-D_3]mevalonate contained one atom of deuterium at C(7), and chanoclavine I contained two deuterium atoms in the hydroxymethyl group. NMR analysis indicated that the deuterium at C(7) of elymoclavine was in the *pro-S* position. The newly introduced hydrogen was therefore the *pro-(7R)* hydrogen (Floss *et al.*, 1974a).

These results support a mode of ring closure shown in Fig. 5. So far, it has not been possible to synthesize the proposed intermediate isochanoclavine I aldehyde. Chanoclavine I aldehyde is converted to chanoclavine I in cultures of *Claviceps*, but the conversion of chanoclavine I to chanoclavine I aldehyde could not be demonstrated because chanoclavine I aldehyde could not be recovered from the cultures (Floss *et al.*, 1974a). Nevertheless, the evidence strongly suggests that chanoclavine I aldehyde is an intermediate between chanoclavine I and the clavine alkaloids.

L. Intermolecular Transfer of the C(9) Hydrogen

[7-^{14}C,9-^{3}H]Chanoclavine I was converted to elymoclavine with 70% tritium retention. (4R)-[2-^{14}C,4-^{3}H]Mevalonate also gave elymoclavine and lysergic acid α-hydroxyethylamide with 70% tritium retention (Floss *et al.*, 1968). The percent tritium retention varied in the range 40–80% with the rate of alkaloid biosynthesis (Floss *et al.*, 1974a). Low rates of alkaloid production correlated with low tritium retention at C(9). A mechanism was proposed to account for the loss of tritium (Fig. 6). The mechanism involves (a) transfer of H from a group on the enzyme to C(9) of chanoclavine I; (b) rotation around the 8,9 bond and formation of ring D; (c) removal of the original H (H*) at C(9) by Enz-X to form product and Enz-XH*; (d) partial exchange of Enz-XH* with solvent protons; and (e) transfer of H* from Enz-XH* to a second molecule of substrate.

To test this mechanism, a 1:1 mixture of [2-^{13}C]mevalonate (86% ^{13}C) and [4-^{2}H$_2$]mevalonate was fed to *Claviceps* strain SD 58, and the mass spectra of chanoclavine I and elymoclavine were analyzed for the percentage excess of M + 1 and M + 2 species (Floss *et al.*, 1974a). Chanoclavine I contained only M + 1 (monodeuterio or ^{13}C) species. However, elymoclavine contained 7% M + 2 species because of intermolecular transfer of deuterium from [9-^{2}H]chanoclavine I to a [^{13}C]chanoclavine I molecule. NMR analysis of elymoclavine biosynthesized from [4-^{2}H$_2$]mevalonate showed that all the deuterium was located at C(9), establishing that the hydrogen is transferred back to the 9 position.

When (4R)-[2-^{14}C,4-^{3}H]mevalonate was fed to *Claviceps* cultures (Floss *et al.*, 1974a; Tabacik *et al.*, unpublished results), tritium retention was

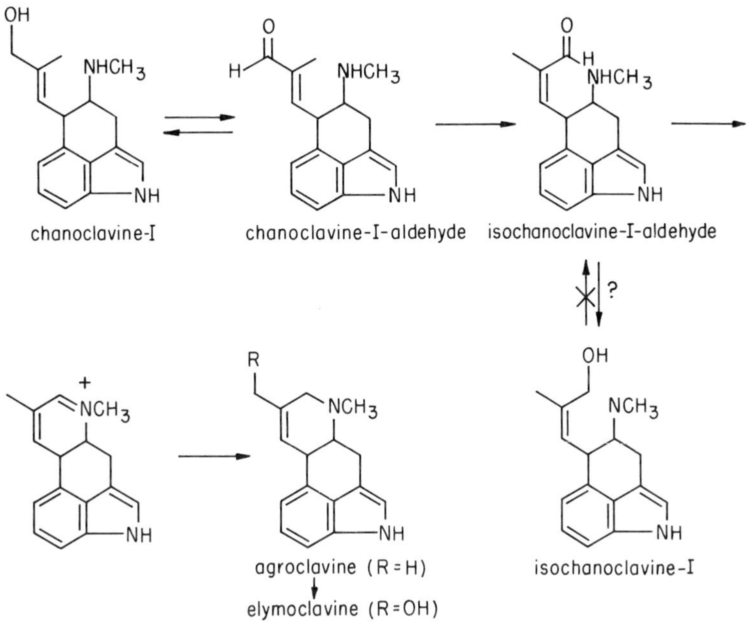

Fig. 5.   Conversion of chanoclavine I into tetracylic ergolines.

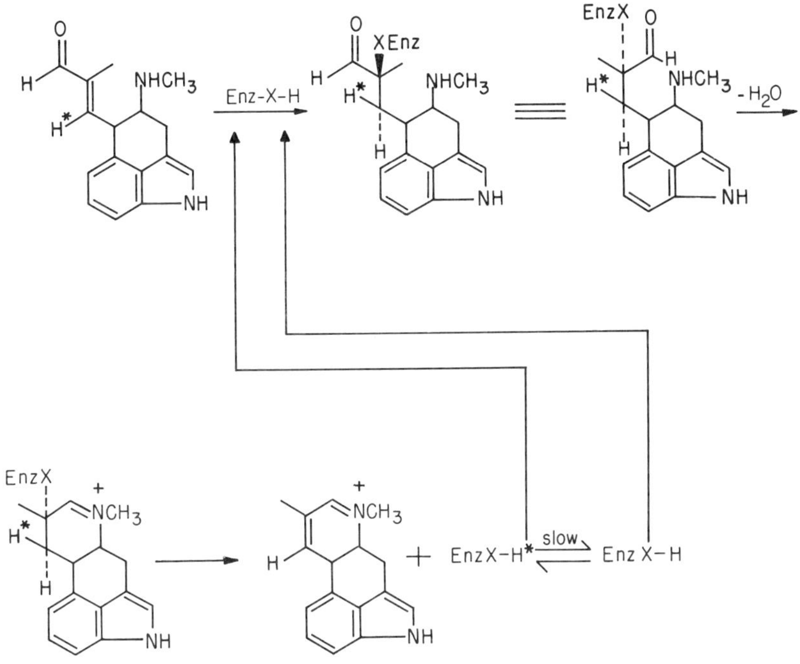

Fig. 6.   Mechanism of double bond isomerization and hydrogen recycling in ring D closure.

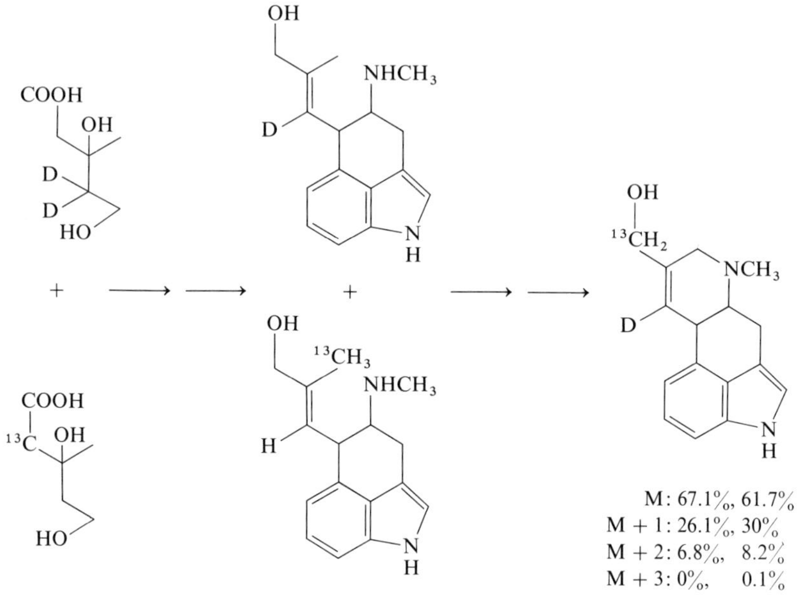

OH

COOH
OH

D
D
HO

NHCH₃
D

+   ⟶ ⟶   +   ⟶ ⟶

OH

COOH
^{13}C OH

HO

OH
^{13}CH₃
NHCH₃
H

M: 58%, 50.2%
M + 1: 42%, 49.8%
M + 2: 0%, 0%
M + 3: 0%, 0%

OH
^{13}CH₂
NCH₃
D

M: 67.1%, 61.7%
M + 1: 26.1%, 30%
M + 2: 6.8%, 8.2%
M + 3: 0%, 0.1%

nearly complete for isochanoclavine I and (−)-chanoclavine II, 63% for agroclavine, and 52% for elymoclavine, but it was 146% for chanoclavine I. This tritium enrichment of chanoclavine I must be due to an isotope effect and can be explained by the addition of a second hydrogen at C(9) followed by competition between removal of the original C(9) hydrogen (tritium) in a rate-determining irreversible reaction and back-reaction with removal of the newly introduced hydrogen. The reactions from chanoclavine I up to the elimination step must be reversible. The scheme shown in Fig. 6 is consistent with these observations. This explanation was supported by observations of the effect of carrying out the incorporation of (4R)-[2-^{14}C,4-^{3}H]mevalonate into elymoclavine in the presence of a large excess of [4-^{2}H]mevalonate. Under these conditions, elimination of tritium would compete primarily with the elimination of deuterium, because most of the molecules would contain deuterium at C(9), and the tritium enrichment in unreacted chanoclavine I would be less. As predicted, the tritium retention in chanoclavine I was reduced to 114–117% (Floss et al., 1974a).

A mechanism incorporating the formation of chanoclavine I aldehyde and the intermolecular transfer of the hydrogen at C(9) is shown in Fig. 7. The carbinolamine is the product in path a, and isochanoclavine I aldehyde

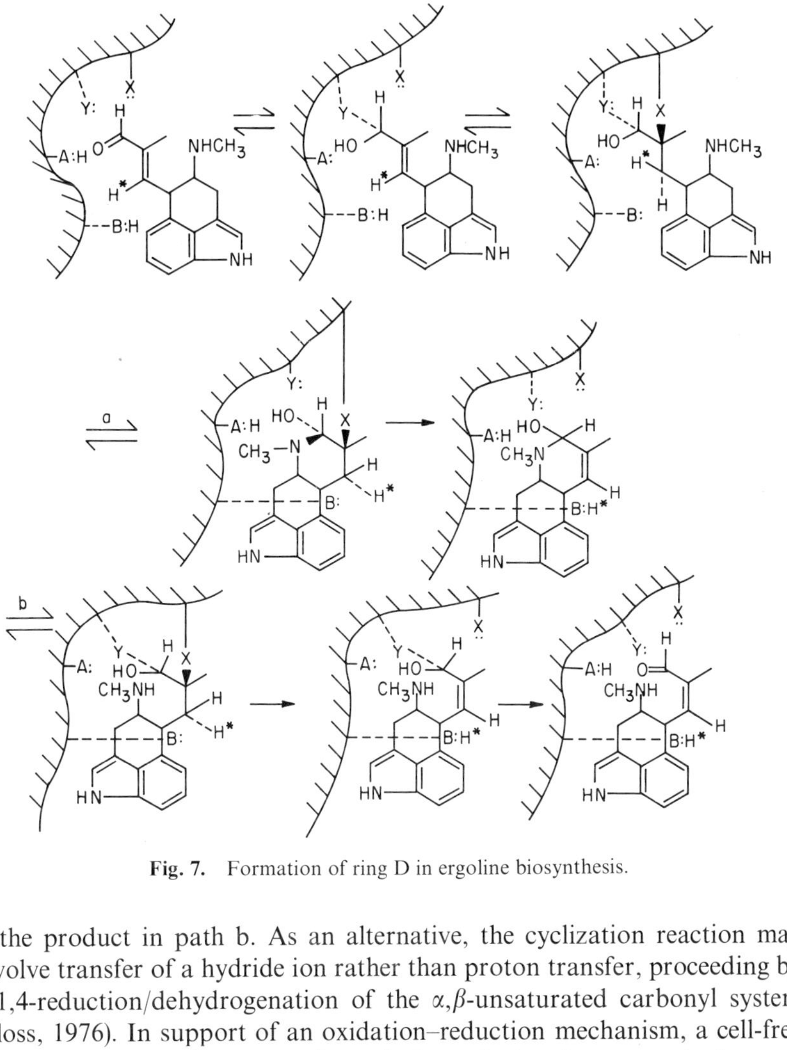

Fig. 7. Formation of ring D in ergoline biosynthesis.

is the product in path b. As an alternative, the cyclization reaction may involve transfer of a hydride ion rather than proton transfer, proceeding by a 1,4-reduction/dehydrogenation of the α,β-unsaturated carbonyl system (Floss, 1976). In support of an oxidation–reduction mechanism, a cell-free system catalyzing the conversion of chanoclavine I to agroclavine and elymoclavine was found to be flavin-dependent (Heinstein *et al.*, unpublished results).

M. Other Proposals

Voigt and Zier (1970, 1971) proposed that the biosynthesis of ergot alkaloids could occur by the pathway dihydrochanoclavine I → dihydro-agroclavine → agroclavine → elymoclavine. In experiments with ripening sclerotia of ergot, tritiated dihydrochanoclavines were incorporated into dihydroagroclavine, but there was little or no incorporation into agroclavine and the peptide alkaloids (Voigt *et al.*, 1972). In saprophytic cultures [G-³H]dihydrochanoclavines were not incorporated into dihydroagroclavine (Johne *et al.*, 1972). Chanoclavine I, agroclavine, and elymoclavine were labeled slightly (0.005–0.01%). Chanoclavine I had a higher specific activity than agroclavine or elymoclavine suggesting that dihydrochanoclavines were converted to chanoclavine I, which then was converted to agroclavine and elymoclavine. The results do not support a reductive pathway for ergoline biosynthesis.

The closing of the D ring could involve loss of a hydrogen from the methyl group of chanoclavine I:

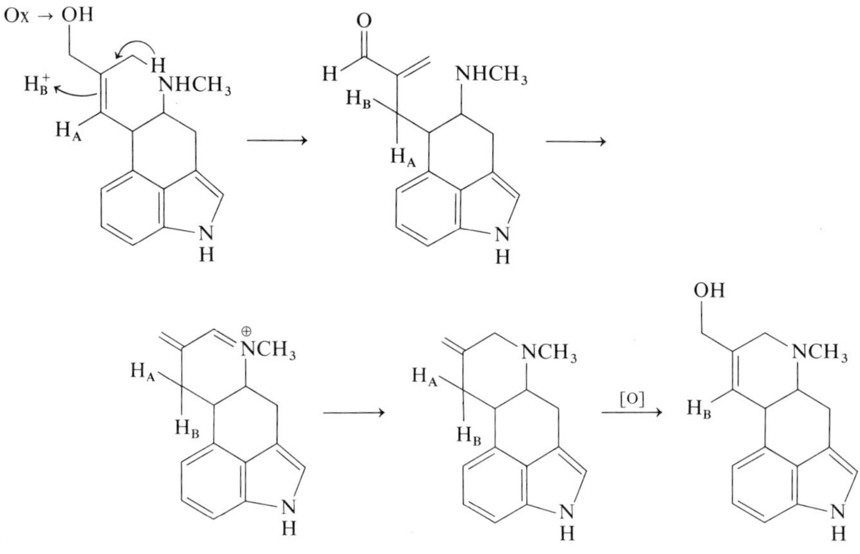

$\Delta^{8,17}$-agroclavine

The intermediate $\Delta^{8,17}$-agroclavine could either be oxidized to elymoclavine or isomerize to agroclavine. The tritium retentions from [2-¹⁴C,2-³H]-mevalonate in chanoclavine-I, agroclavine, and elymoclavine, were 92%, 69%, and 62%, respectively, suggesting that one hydrogen of the chanoclavine I methyl group is lost, in agreement with the above mechanism. Ogunlana *et al.*, (1970) also observed conversion of chanoclavine I to elymoclavine, but not agroclavine in a cell-free system, suggesting a pathway from chanoclavine I to elymoclavine independent of agroclavine. However, different activities were found by other investigators in cell-free systems with chanoclavine I as substrate (see Section V). Pachlatko (1975) synthesized tritium-labeled $\Delta^{8,17}$-agroclavine and tested it as a precursor of elymoclavine. There was no conversion of $\Delta^{8,17}$-agroclavine to elymoclavine, a finding that disproves the above mechanism. As another alternative, conversion of chanoclavine I to elymoclavine could involve hydroxylation of the other methyl group of chanoclavine I as the first step. Further reactions would occur as in Fig. 7 as though the methyl of chanoclavine I had not been oxidized [see discussion of possible mechanism for conversion of E-(8) to elymoclavine in Section III,F]. No experimental evidence on this possible route is presently available.

IV. BIOSYNTHESIS OF LYSERGIC ACID DERIVATIVES

A. Origin of the Lysergyl Moiety

As mentioned previously, elymoclavine is a precursor of the lysergic acid amides (Mothes et al., 1962). Gröger et al. (1963) showed by chemical degradation that the elymoclavine was incorporated specifically into the lysergic acid moiety of the lysergic acid amide. The sequence of steps involved in this pathway has not been elucidated. Penniclavine and lysergol are not intermediates in the conversion (Agurell and Johanson, 1964; Floss et al., 1966). The finding that lysergol is not an intermediate rules out double-bond isomerization at the stage of the alcohol. Labeled paspalic acid ($\Delta^{8,9}$-lysergic acid) is incorporated into the lysergic acid amides with an efficiency close to that of elymoclavine (Agurell, 1966c; Ohashi et al., 1970). This suggests that paspalic acid may be an intermediate in the biosynthesis of the amide alkaloids:

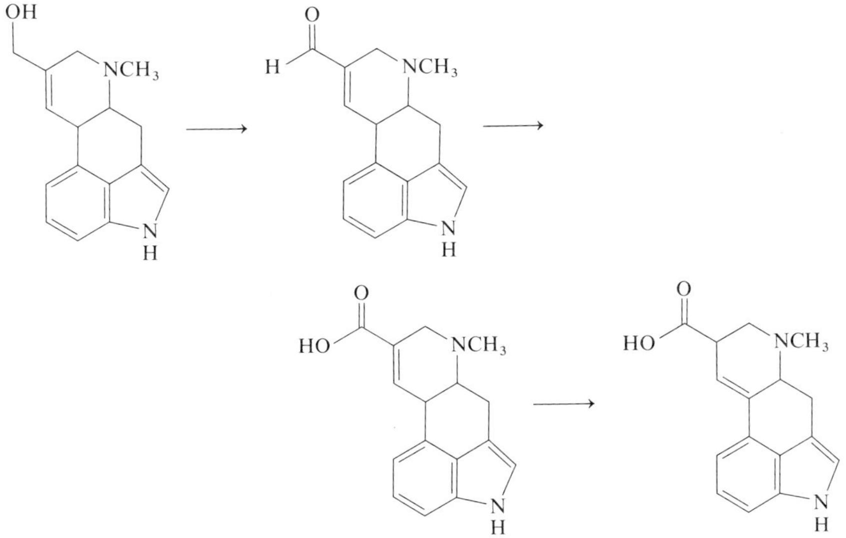

However, the incorporation of paspalic acid into the alkaloids does not necessarily prove that the biosynthesis proceeds by this pathway, because paspalic acid can isomerize in aqueous solution to lysergic acid and the labeled paspalic acid could have been converted nonenzymatically to lysergic acid before incorporation. The isomerization of the double bond from the $\Delta^{8,9}$ to the $\Delta^{9,10}$ position at the aldehyde stage therefore remains a possibility, particularly because lysergylaldehydes would be expected to exist almost exclusively in the enol form. Attempts to synthesize lysergaldehyde were unsuccessful, but the enol acetate **15** was synthesized and was found to be incorporated into the lysergic acid amide alkaloids (Lin *et al.*, 1973) with an efficiency similar to that of elymoclavine *O*-acetate. While these results are not conclusive concerning the involvement of $\Delta^{9,10}$-lysergaldehyde, they do indicate that the question of the sequence of double-bond isomerization and oxidation to the carboxyl is not yet settled.

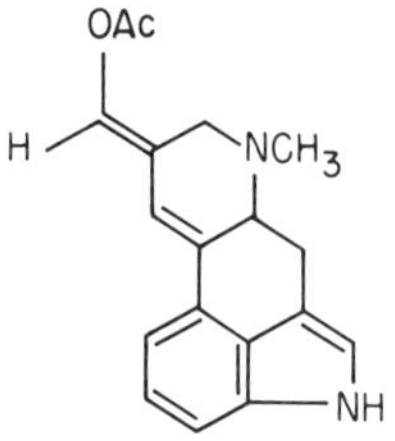

15

Labeled lysergic acid is incorporated into the amide alkaloids (Agurell, 1966d). This process presumably requires the activation of lysergic acid, and a likely activated form is lysergyl-CoA. Maier *et al.* (1972) demonstrated the formation of lysergyl-CoA in a cell-free system from *Claviceps*. However, activity was not correlated with alkaloid production, and nonproducing and clavine alkaloid-producing strains were able to form lysergyl-CoA. There is, therefore, some question whether the enzyme which catalyzes the formation of lysergyl-CoA is specific. Because of the uncertainty about the significance of the cell-free formation of lysergyl-CoA, the possibility remains that formation of a coenzyme A derivative takes place at the level of lysergaldehyde as proposed by Floss *et al.* (1966):

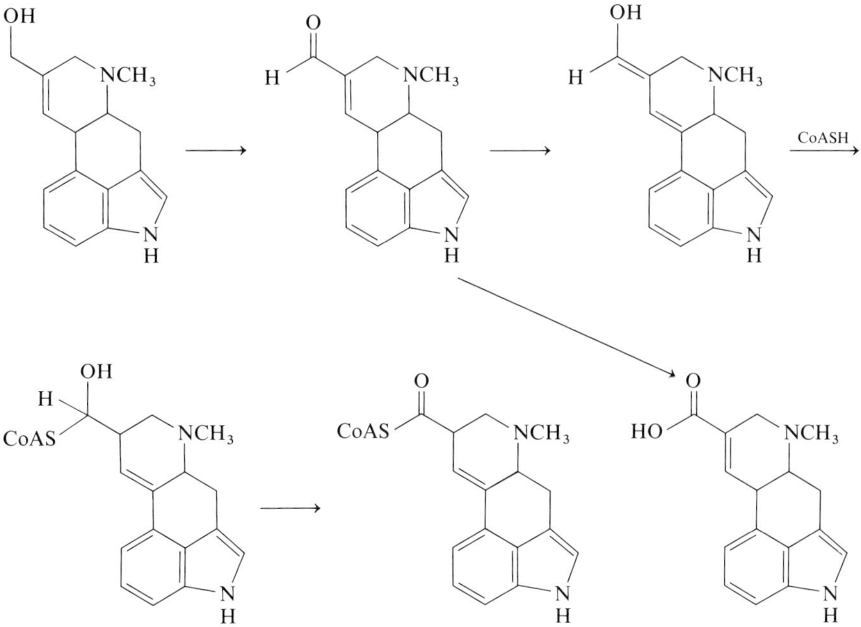

In this scheme, the enol form of $\Delta^{9,10}$-lysergaldehyde is converted to the coenzyme A hemiacetal. Paspalic acid is an end product formed in a side reaction from $\Delta^{8,9}$-lysergaldehyde. The scheme, which is admittedly speculative, explains the observations that no $\Delta^{8,9}$-amide alkaloids are found in nature and that paspalic acid but not lysergic acid accumulates in cultures.

Dihydroergosine, a dihydrolysergic acid peptide alkaloid, is formed in *Sphacelia sorghi* (Barrow *et al.*, 1974). One of the C(5) hydrogens of [2-^{14}C,5-^{3}H]mevalonate was retained in dihydroergosine. This rules out $\Delta^{9,10}$-lysergic acid derivatives as precursors of dihydroergosine. Festuclavine, dihydroelymoclavine, and dihydrolysergic acid were incorporated efficiently, but agroclavine was not. This indicates that the double bond is reduced before agroclavine in the biosynthetic sequence, possibly at the level of chanoclavine I. Dihydrochanoclavines were not found in the cultures (Barrow *et al.*, 1974) but were not tested as precursors of dihydroergosine. Dihydrolysergic acid added to the culture medium of an ergotamine-producing strain was converted to dihydroergotamine (Anderson and Floss, unpublished results). This finding suggests that the activating enzyme and the enzymes that catalyze synthesis of the peptide moiety can tolerate some change in the lysergic acid structure.

B. Biosynthesis of the Simple Lysergic Acid Amides

The biosynthesis of ergonovine and lysergic acid α-hydroxyethylamide has been studied extensively, but the biosynthetic process is still not well understood. Radioactive incorporation experiments (Agurell, 1966e) demonstrated that lysergic acid amide and isolysergic acid amide are not precursors of lysergic acid α-hydroxyethylamide. Consistent with this observation was the finding (Kleinerova and Kybal, 1973) that lysergic acid amide and isolysergic acid amide are formed from lysergic acid α-hydroxyethylamide. [1-^{14}C]Ethylamine (Agurell, 1966e) and [1-^{14}C]acetamide (Agurell, 1966b) were not incorporated into the α-hydroxyethylamide, but [U-^{14}C]alanine (Agurell, 1966b) was incorporated. The incorporation of radioactivity from [2-^{14}C]alanine occurred primarily in the carbinolamide carbon (Gröger et al., 1968; Castagnoli et al., 1970). The ^{15}N from (L)-[U-^{14}C,^{15}N]alanine was incorporated into the amide nitrogen (Gröger et al., 1968; Castagnoli et al., 1970).

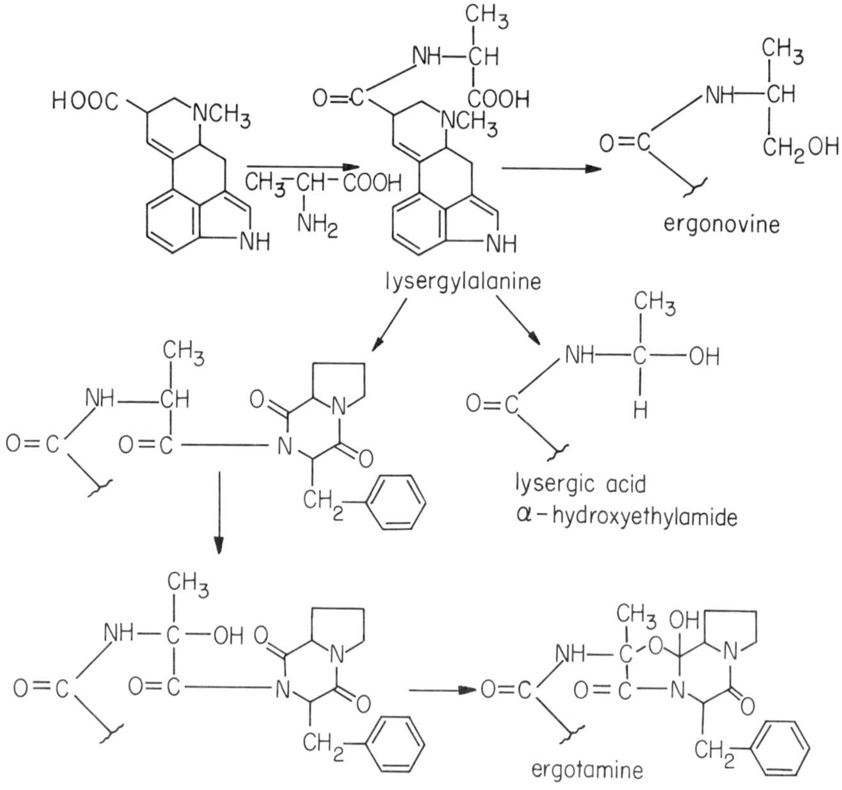

Fig. 8.   Biosynthesis of lysergic acid amide derivatives as proposed by Agurell.

Radioactive L-alanine was also incorporated into the L-alaninol moiety of ergonovine (Minghetti and Arcamone, 1969; Nelson and Agurell, 1969). Methylserine was not a precursor of ergonovine (Nelson and Agurell, 1969). The role of L-alaninol is unclear. Nelson and Agurell (1969) and Majer *et al.* (1967) found no incorporation of radioactive L-alaninol into ergonovine, whereas Minghetti and Arcamone (1969) found higher incorporation of L-alaninol than L-alanine into ergonovine.

Based on some of the above results and other evidence, Agurell (1966b) proposed a general scheme for the biosynthesis of lysergic acid derivatives in which lysergylalanine is the precursor of those compounds in which the amide is derived from alanine (Fig. 8). When lysergyl-(L)-$[2\text{-}^{14}C]$alanine was fed to *C. paspali* there was insignificant incorporation into lysergic acid α-hydroxyethylamide but a small (1.77%) incorporation of radioactivity into the C(2) + C(3) carbons of the alaninol moiety of ergonovine (Basmadjian *et al.*, 1969). The low incorporation and failure to demonstrate formation of lysergylalanine in *C. paspali* leaves questionable the role of lysergyl-L-alanine in ergonovine biosynthesis (Floss *et al.*, 1971a).

C. Biosynthesis of the Peptide Alkaloids

As expected, lysergic acid (Minghetti and Arcamone, 1969; Maier *et al.*, 1971) and the amino acids phenylalanine (Vining and Taber, 1963; Bassett *et al.*, 1973), proline (Gröger and Erge, 1970; Bassett *et al.*, 1973), valine (Maier *et al.*, 1971; Floss *et al.*, 1971b), and leucine (Maier *et al.*, 1971) are incorporated into the corresponding amino acid and/or hydroxyamino acid positions in the peptide alkaloids. (DL)-$[1\text{-}^{14}C]$Valine was incorporated into the α-hydroxyvaline moiety (59%) and into the valine moiety (37%) of ergocornine (Floss *et al.*, 1971b). Most of the radioactivity (92%) of the α-hydroxyvaline moiety was located at C(1) (Floss *et al.*, 1971b). $[^{15}N]$Valine labeled the lysergamide nitrogen of ergocornine (Maier *et al.*, 1971), whereas [*amide*-^{15}N]lysergic acid did not. This suggests that the lysergic acid amide nitrogen comes from valine. The radioactivity from (L)-$[U\text{-}^{14}C]$alanine was incorporated into the α-hydroxyalanine moiety of ergotamine but was also scrambled into the rest of the molecule (Minghetti and Arcamone, 1969; Majer *et al.*, 1967; Bassett *et al.*, 1973; Floss *et al.*, 1971c). However, with $[1\text{-}^{14}C]$alanine as precursor, 90% of the label in ergotamine was found in the α-hydroxyalanine moiety (Floss *et al.*, 1971c).

Several proposals for the mode of assembly of the peptide alkaloids have been made. Voigt and Bornschein (1964), observing that addition of ergonovine increased the levels of peptide alkaloids, proposed that ergonovine was a precursor of the peptide alkaloids. However, ergonovine labeled in the lysergic acid (Vicario *et al.*, 1967) or the L-alaninol moiety (Floss *et al.*

1971c) gave insignificant incorporation into ergotamine. Agurell (1966b) proposed that lysergyl-L-alanine was a precursor of the peptide alkaloids containing the α-hydroxylalanine moiety, ergotamine, and ergosine (see Fig. 8).

Abe (1971) proposed that lysergyl-L-valine was the precursor of the ergotoxines. The isolation of lysergylvaline methyl ester from ergot (Schlientz et al., 1963) apparently supported this proposal. However, lysergyl-(L)-[U-14C]alanine, (L)-[U-14C]alanine, and isolysergyl-(L)-[U-14C]alanine were incorporated into ergotamine to about the same extent and with similar labeling patterns. The results suggest that lysergyl- and isolysergylalanine were hydrolyzed before incorporation into ergotamine (Floss et al., 1971c). Similar results were obtained when the incorporation of lysergyl-L-valine into ergocornine and ergokryptine was determined (Floss et al., 1971b). Incorporation of lysergyl- and isolysergyl-L-valine labeled in the valine portion, and of L-valine were about equal, and the isotope distributions were similar in the products from all three compounds. The similarity of labeling in the α-hydroxyvaline and valine moieties of the alkaloids with lysergyl-L-valine (59%/37%) and L-valine (51%/33%) as substrates shows that lysergyl-L-valine was incorporated only after hydrolysis to lysergic acid and L-valine, because direct incorporation of lysergyl-L-valine should label only the α-hydroxyvaline moiety. Abe's group (Ohashi et al., 1972a) observed 1.2% incorporation of lysergyl-(L)-[G-3H]valine methyl ester in a cell-free system from an ergokryptine-producing strain. Addition of the unlabeled compound reduced radioactivity incorporation from [14C]elymoclavine by a factor of three. However, no degradations were carried out, and the incorporation could have occurred after hydrolysis. Maier et al. (1974) found that lysergyl-L-alanine methyl ester and lysergyl-L-valine methyl ester were readily hydrolyzed by intact cells and cell-free extracts from C. purpurea. In trapping experiments, no lysergylalanine or lysergylvaline could be detected in peptide alkaloid-producing strains. The results indicate that the lysergyl amino acids are incorporated only after hydrolysis to lysergic acid and amino acids.

Abe's group (Abe, 1971; Abe et al., 1970) isolated L-leucyl-D-proline lactam and L-phenylalanyl-D- and L-proline lactam from cultures in which ergokryptine and ergotamine, respectively, were the major peptide alkaloids. The time course of production of the lactams was consistent with their involvement in peptide alkaloid biosynthesis (Abe et al., 1970). The role of the lactams as precursors of the peptide alkaloids was tested by carrying out incubations with the tritium-labeled lactams. Incorporation of L-leucyl-D- and -L-proline lactam into ergokryptine plus ergokryptinine was 0.06–1.45%, and incorporation of L-phenylalanine-D- and -L-proline lactam into ergotamine plus ergotaminine was 0.04–0.3%. The nearly equal incorporation of the D- and L-proline lactams and of L-proline into the peptide alkaloids suggests that the lactams were hydrolyzed prior to incorporation. Various other incorporation experiments with di- and tripeptides and the proline lactams have supported the interpretation that incorporation occurs only after hydrolysis (cf. Gröger, 1975). The distribution of radioactivity from [1-^{14}C]valine in the hydroxyvaline and valine moieties of ergocornine was not changed by the addition of unlabeled L-valyl-L-proline (Floss et al., 1971b). Gröger and Johne (1972) showed that L-valyl-(L)-[U-^{14}C]proline lactam was incorporated equally into ergocornine, which contains the L-valyl-L-proline moiety, and into ergokryptine, which contains hydroxyvaline and L-leucyl-L-proline as the terminal two amino acids. To account for the equal labeling of both peptides it must be assumed that the L-valyl-L-proline lactam had been hydrolyzed. Labeled L-valyl-L-leucine, L-leucyl-L-proline lactam, L-valyl-L-proline lactam (Gröger and Johne, 1972), L-valyl-(L)-[1-^{14}C]valyl-L-proline (Floss et al., 1974b), L-prolyl-(L)-[U-^{14}C]alanine, L-prolyl-[U-^{14}C]glycine, and L-valyl-L-leucyl-(L)-[U-^{14}C]proline (Gröger et al., 1974) were incorporated into the alkaloids regardless of whether they contained the right sequence. The lack of dependence of incorporation on amino acid sequence further indicates that incorporation occurs after hydrolysis to the amino acids. The latter work by Gröger et al. (1974) also demonstrated that washed mycelia of Claviceps hydrolyzed the added peptides, e.g., leucylproline lactam. Most recently, Gröger's group (Baumert et al., 1977) has synthesized a lysergyl tripeptide corresponding in sequence to ergocornine. This compound was not incorporated into the corresponding alkaloid, and it could be shown that it was not taken up by the fungal mycelium.

Thus far, no amide intermediate tested has been incorporated specifically into the peptide alkaloids. Floss et al. (1974b) have suggested that the structure is built up on a multienzyme complex similar to the enzyme systems which catalyze the synthesis of peptide antibiotics, e.g., gramicidin S and tyrocidin (Lipmann, 1973). By analogy with these systems, peptide bond formation would take place on an enzyme sulfhydryl group. Chain growth could begin either at the C-terminal L-proline, as suggested by the higher specific activity in the α-hydroxyvaline moiety compared to the valine moiety of ergocornine (Floss et al., 1971b; Maier et al., 1971) or at the N-terminal lysergic acid by analogy with tyrocidin and gramicidin S biosynthesis.

Assuming that synthesis begins at the C-terminal end of the peptide, L-proline would be activated and attached to the sulfhydryl group of the enzyme. Taking ergocristine synthesis as an example (Fig. 9), successive

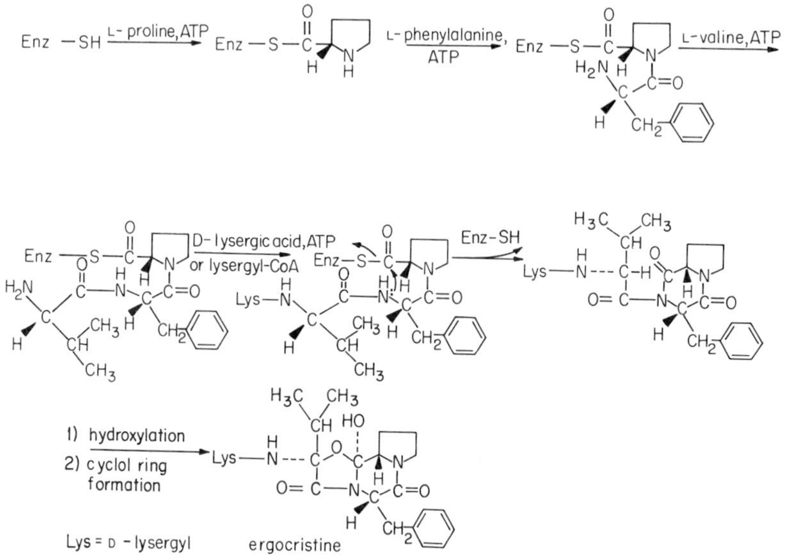

Fig. 9. Proposed formation of peptide ergot alkaloids on a multienzyme complex.

activation, thioester formation, and transfer reactions (cf. Lipmann, 1973) would form the enzyme-bound intermediate lysergyl-L-valyl-L-phenylalanyl-L-proline-S-E. Internal displacement of the sulfur would lead to release of this intermediate with simultaneous lactam formation. Hydroxylation of the α-carbon of the alanine moiety followed by enzymatic or spontaneous cyclol formation would complete the synthesis of the peptide alkaloids. The proposed pathway is supported by the isolation, from an ergocristine-producing strain, of N-[N-(lysergyl)-L-valyl]-L-phenylalanyl-D-proline lactam (**16**) (Stütz et al., 1973). Compound (**16**) could be formed from the lysergyl tripeptide lactam (**17**) (Fig. 9) by the readily occurring nonenzymatic epi-

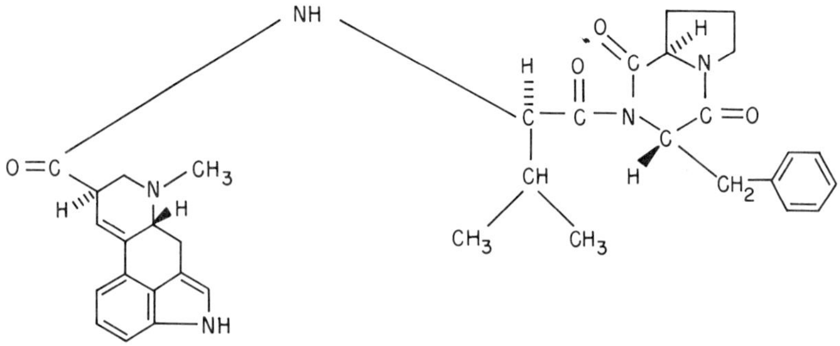

16

merization of the proline to the D isomer. Compound **16** underwent rapid methanolysis to lysergyl-L-valine methyl ester and L-phenylalanyl-D-proline lactam (Stütz *et al.*, 1973). The earlier isolation of lysergyl-L-valine methyl ester by the Sandoz group (Sschlientz *et al.*, 1963) was attributed to methanolysis of compound **16** during isolation. The isolation of lactams by Abe's group (Abe, 1971; Abe *et al.*, 1970) could also be due to the presence of compounds corresponding to **16** and **17** in those strains of *Claviceps* and their decomposition in the cultures or during work-up.

The mechanism of peptide bond formation remains an area of interest for future studies. A cell-free system for biosynthesis of the peptide alkaloids would greatly facilitate these studies, but attempts to carry out the cell-free synthesis have so far been unsuccessful (e.g., Maier *et al.*, 1972).

V. ENZYMOLOGY AND PHYSIOLOGY OF ERGOT ALKALOID BIOSYNTHESIS

A. Ergoline Biosynthesis in Cell-Free Extracts

Cell-free conversion of the precursors into the tetracyclic clavines and chanoclavine I and II was obtained by Cavender and Anderson (1970). Incubation of [^{14}C]tryptophan, isopentenyl pyrophosphate, methionine, ATP, and liver concentrate (mixture of cofactors) with the 60–80% ammonium sulfate fraction from *C. purpurea* PRL 1970 for 12 hr gave radioactive chanoclavine I and II, agroclavine, and elymoclavine. Conversion was 0.15% for chanoclavine I and II.

Abe's group (Abe, 1971; Ohashi *et al.*, 1972b) obtained cell-free biosynthesis of setoclavine from [^{14}C]tryptophan, mevalonate, and methionine in crude extracts from two *Claviceps* strains. Their system was considerably more efficient with 4.4% conversion in 3 hr. The product was identified by cocrystallization with authentic material. The system also converted (**7**), but not (**6**) into setoclavine. Abe's group also studied several other conversions in cell-free systems (Abe, 1971; Ohashi and Abe, 1970; Ohashi *et al.*, 1970a,b, 1972a).

B. Dimethylallyltryptophan Synthetase

Dimethylallyltryptophan synthetase (systematic name dimethylallylpyrophosphate:L-tryptophan dimethylallyltransferase) was isolated by Heinstein *et al.* (1971). The enzyme was purified to homogeneity from mycelia of *Claviceps* strain SD 58 (Lee *et al.*, 1976). The enzyme is a single polypeptide chain with molecular weight 73,000. It is activated by

Fe^{2+}, Mg^{2+}, and particularly Ca^{2+}. The K_m values for L-tryptophan and dimethylallyl pyrophosphate were determined as 0.067 and 0.2 M, respectively. Steady-state kinetics were consistent with either a random or an ordered mechanism. The enzyme is specific for dimethylallyl pyrophosphate. Analogues of tryptophan carrying methyl groups in the benzene ring showed decreased substrate activity; the closer the methyl group was to the reactive 4 position, the lower the activity. The enzyme is inhibited by the end products of the pathway in *Claviceps* species SD 58, agroclavine, and elymoclavine (Heinstein and Floss, 1976; Lee, 1974). The inhibition is not competitive with either substrate. The concentrations of agroclavine and elymoclavine which inhibit the enzyme are in the range of the concentrations in the cultures. Therefore, a process of feedback inhibition may operate in alkaloid biosynthesis, in which the rate of alkaloid production is regulated by the concentration of the alkaloids in the cells. The enzyme is not synthesized until the period of rapid growth is over. Enzyme synthesis immediately precedes biosynthesis of the alkaloids. The enzyme was also isolated from two other alkaloid-producing *Claviceps* strains, and it was characterized (Maier and Gröger, 1976). The enzyme from a peptide alkaloid-producing strain was not inhibited by clavine alkaloids.

C. Chanoclavine Cyclase

Three groups have obtained cell-free synthesis of agroclavine and/or elymoclavine from chanoclavine I. The three groups found activity in the soluble fraction and demonstrated a requirement for NADP or NADPH, but other properties were found to differ. Ogunlana *et al.* (1970) obtained 20% conversion of chanoclavine I to elymoclavine. Besides NADPH, molecular oxygen and ATP were required. Agroclavine was not produced and was poorly converted into elymoclavine. Based on these properties, the investigators proposed a pathway from chanoclavine I to elymoclavine without the intermediacy of agroclavine (see conversion of **8** to elymoclavine, discussed in Section III, F). Gröger's laboratory (Gröger and Sajdl, 1972; Erge *et al.*, 1973) obtained a cell-free system which produced agroclavine but not elymoclavine in 10–30% yield. The cell-free system of Heinstein *et al.* (unpublished results) required NADP but not ATP, and catalyzed the formation of both agroclavine and elymoclavine. Addition of FAD to column-fractionated preparations stimulated activity. The requirement for FAD and NADP(H) indicated that an oxidation–reduction reaction is involved in the conversion of chanoclavine I to agroclavine. Formation of chanoclavine I aldehyde (see Fig. 5) and/or hydride ion transfer in the isomerization reaction are oxidation–reduction reactions that have been proposed as part of the chanoclavine I cyclase mechanism.

D. Agroclavine Hydroxylase

Hsu and Anderson (1970, 1971) obtained conversion of agroclavine to elymoclavine with the 60–80% ammonium sulfate fraction from *C. purpurea* PRL 1980. NADPH or liver concentrate (mixture of cofactors) was required for activity. The reaction could be followed spectrophotometrically by following the oxidation of NADPH in the presence of agroclavine. Although few microorganisms can hydroxylate the C(17)-methyl (Beliveau and Ramstad, 1966), a microsomal system from liver can convert agroclavine to elymoclavine and noragroclavine (Wilson *et al.*, 1971) This system involves cytochrome *P*-450.

E. Cell-Free Conversion of Dimethylallyltryptophan to Clavicipitic Acid

A cell-free system for the conversion of **7** to clavicipitic acid was obtained by Anderson's group (Bajwa *et al.*, 1975; Saini *et al.*, 1976). Activity was in the particulate cell fraction and could be solubilized with Triton X-100. Hydrogen peroxide was shown to be the product of oxygen reduction by coupling with peroxidase. The activity was independent of pH in the range 6–8 and increased to a maximum at pH 10.5, with a pK_{app} of 9.4. Enzyme-specific activity increased during the growth phase and then remained constant during the stationary phase.

An intermediate compound could be envisioned which could either react further to close the C ring and form chanoclavine I or produce clavicipitic acid in a side reaction. The synthesis of the enzyme throughout the growth phase, with no enzyme synthesis during the stationary phase, does not correlate with the observation that alkaloid production starts after growth stops. This suggests that the enzyme which catalyzes the conversion of **7** to clavicipitic acid is not in the pathway of alkaloid biosynthesis, although direct evidence for or against involvement in the pathway is lacking.

F. Other Enzymatic Transformations

Saini and Anderson (unpublished results) have obtained a small (0.1–0.3%) conversion of **7** to **8** with the 60–80% ammonium sulfate fraction from *C. purpurea* PRL 1980. Activity was stimulated four-fold by NADPH. Petroski and Kelleher (1977) have also reported the conversion of **7** to **8** in cell-free extracts from *C. paspali*.

Ramstad and Taylor (Ramstad, 1968; Taylor *et al.*, 1966; Shough and Taylor, 1969) showed that horseradish peroxidase catalyzes the conversion of agroclavine and elymoclavine to their 8-hydroxy-$\Delta^{9,10}$ analogues seto-clavine/isosetoclavine and penniclavine/isopenniclavine, respectively. In addition, the 10-hydroxy-$\Delta^{8,9}$ product was formed. The 10-hydroxy compound rearranges nonenzymatically to the 8-hydroxy product and can be considered an intermediate in the reaction.

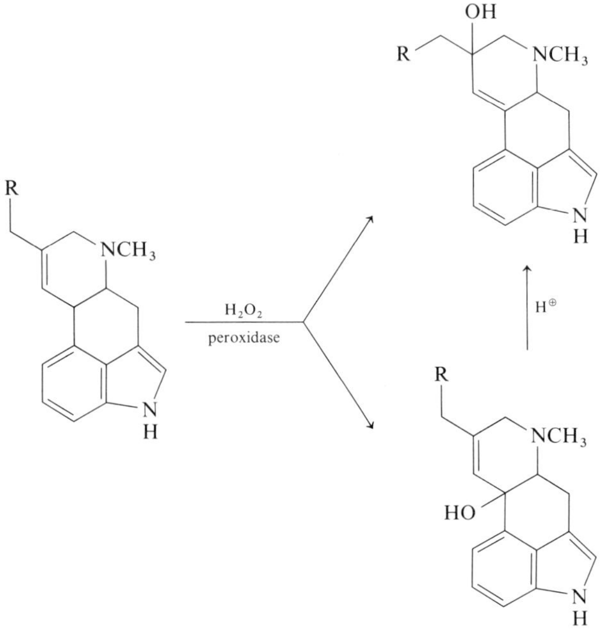

The involvement of peroxidase in the formation of the 8-hydroxy-$\Delta^{9,10}$-clavine alkaloids in *Claviceps* has not been established. Crude extracts can catalyze the nonenzymatic formation of the 8-hydroxy-$\Delta^{9,10}$-clavine alkaloids (Bajwa and Anderson, 1975).

With slant cultures of an Elymus-type *Claviceps* strain, Ohashi and Abe (1970) obtained cell-free conversion of agroclavine and elymoclavine to peptide alkaloids. There have been no reports so far of cell-free peptide alkaloid synthesis with shake cultures. Gröger's laboratory (Maier *et al.*, 1972) studied the activation reactions that could be involved in peptide alkaloid biosynthesis. They observed cell-free synthesis of lysergyl-CoA and activation of valine, serine, leucine, and proline. Activation was found in nonproducing, clavine alkaloid-producing, and peptide alkaloid-producing strains. The connection between these activities and peptide alkaloid synthesis is therefore uncertain.

Both L-tryptophan and 7 bound to cytochrome *P*-450 in a particulate preparation from *Claviceps* (Ambike and Baxter, 1970). However, the enzymatic activity associated with this binding is not known.

G. Physiology and Regulation of Ergot Alkaloid Biosynthesis

Alkaloid production begins after the stationary phase has been reached in *Claviceps* sp. SD 58 and in several other alkaloid-producing strains (Taber, 1964; Amici *et al.*, 1967; Kaplan *et al.*, 1969). As mentioned earlier, the production of two of the enzymes involved in alkaloid biosynthesis, DMAT synthetase and chanoclavine cyclase, occurs at the beginning of the stationary phase just prior to the onset of alkaloid biosynthesis. L-Tryptophan addition increased alkaloid production (cf. Tyler, 1961), but only when added early in the growth phase (Floss and Mothes, 1964; Vining, 1970). Bu'Lock and Barr (1968) showed cyclic variations in both intracellular tryptophan concentration and alkaloid production, with the increase in alkaloid production lagging behind the increase in tryptophan concentration. Krupinski *et al.* (1976) showed that thiotryptophan, which is inactive as a precursor of the alkaloids, was as effective as L-tryptophan in increasing alkaloid production. L-Tryptophan, therefore, acts as an inducer of alkaloid biosynthesis. L-Tryptophan and thiotryptophan increased the level of dimethylallyltryptophan synthetase, suggesting that L-tryptophan induces the production of this enzyme and possibly that of other enzymes in the pathway.

The enzymes involved in L-tryptophan synthesis have been studied in order to establish possible correlations between the rapid rate of tryptophan biosynthesis during the alkaloid production phase (Kaplan *et al.*, 1969) and the properties of the enzymes. Lingens *et al.* (1967) found that anthranilate synthetase from *C. paspali* was not inhibited by tryptophan. This unusual property suggested that the enzymes involved in tryptophan synthesis in *Claviceps* may not be subject to regulation by the endproduct. Mann and Floss (1977) isolated a three-enzyme complex from *Claviceps* strain SD 58 which contained anthranilate synthetase, phosphoribosylanthranilate isomerase, and indole-3-glycerolphosphate synthetase. Anthranilate synthetase from *Claviceps* strain SD 58 (Mann and Floss, 1977) and from two *C. purpurea* strains (Schmauder and Gröger, 1976) exhibited inhibition by L-tryptophan, in contrast to the enzyme from *C. paspali*. No unusual properties of the enzyme were observed that would relate to high tryptophan production during alkaloid biosynthesis, but the anthranilate synthetase activity was inhibited by elymoclavine. This may represent a second point of feedback control of alkaloid biosynthesis in addition to the inhibition of dimethylallyltryptophan synthetase by elymoclavine (Heinstein and Floss, 1976).

L-Tryptophan in the culture medium is actively taken up by the mycelium (Teuscher, 1965; Robertson *et al.*, 1973), although the maximum activity was seen during the early growth phase before initiation of alkaloid production. The level of intracellular free tryptophan increases two- to threefold early in the transition from growth to stationary phase (Robbers *et al.*, 1972). Whether this increase in tryptophan level is related to induction of alkaloid synthesis is, of course, an open question.

Our knowledge of the mechanism involved in maintaining the high flux of tryptophan from precursors to alkaloid is far from complete. This partially reflects the present paucity of knowledge about regulatory mechanisms in eukaryotic cells. Much more work has been done on various aspects of the physiology and regulation of ergot alkaloid synthesis, but lack of space prohibits us from discussing the subject in more depth. The reader is referred to an earlier review (Floss *et al.*, 1974c).

VI. CONCLUSION

It is clear from the above discussion that much has been learned about the biosynthesis of the toxic ergot alkaloids. What at one time appeared to be a very simple biosynthetic pathway, requiring perhaps only a few specific enzymes and some general oxidases, has turned out to be a highly complex sequence of rather specific reactions. Despite the very detailed knowledge of many aspects of this biosynthesis, there are still a number of major blank spots which need to be filled in before we have a complete picture of the pathway. The most important aspects which still have to be worked out are the mechanism and enzymology of C-ring formation and the enzymology of formation of ring D and of the peptide moiety. Some other interesting problems which should be examined are (a) the regulatory mechanisms which allow such a high flow of intermediary metabolites into alkaloid biosynthesis, (b) the reason why most *Claviceps* strains produce alkaloids parasitically but only very few do so under saprophytic culture conditions, and (c) the biosynthesis of these compounds in higher plants and its evolutionary relationship to alkaloid formation in the fungus. These unanswered questions, together with the continuing concern about potential ergot poisoning and the sustained promise for new drug development, should keep interest in the ergot alkaloids alive for years to come.

REFERENCES

Abe, M. (1963). *Abh. Dtsch. Akad. Wiss. Berlin Kl. Chem. Geol. Biol.*, No. 4, pp. 309–322.
Abe, M. (1966). *Abh. Dtsch. Akad. Wiss. Berlin Kl. Chem. Geol. Biol.*, No. 3, pp. 393–403.
Abe, M. (1971). *Abh. Dtsch. Akad. Wiss. Berlin Kl. Chem. Geol. Biol.*, pp. 411–422.
Abe, M., and Yamatodani, S. (1954). *J. Agric. Chem. Soc. Jpn*, **28**, 501.
Abe, M., and Yamatodani, S. (1955). *Bull. Agric. Chem. Soc., Jpn.* **19**, 161–162.
Abe, M., Yamano, T., Kozu, Y., and Kusumoto, M. (1952). *J. Agric. Chem. Soc. Jpn.* **25**, 458.

Abe, M., Yamatodani, S., Yamano, T., and Kusumoto, M. (1956). *Bull. Agric. Chem. Soc. Jpn.* **20**, 59–60.

Abe, M., Yamano, T., Yamatodani, S., Kozu, Y., Kusumoto, M., Komatsu, H., and Yamada, S. (1959). *Bull. Agric. Chem. Soc. Jpn.* **23**, 246–248.

Abe, M., Yamatodani, S., Yamano, T., and Kusumoto, M. (1961). *Agric. Biol. Chem.* **25**, 594–595.

Abe, M., Yamatodani, S., Yamano, T., Kozu, Y., and Yamada, S. (1963). *Agric. Biol. Chem.* **27**, 659–662.

Abe, M., Ohmomo, S., Ohashi, T., and Tabuchi, T. (1969). *Agric. Biol. Chem.* **33**, 469–471.

Abe, M., Fukuhara, T., Ohmomo, S., Hori, M., and Tabuchi, T. (1970). *J. Agric. Chem. Soc.* **44**, 573–579.

Abou-Chaar, C. I., Brady, L. R., and Tyler, V. E. (1961). *Lloydia* **24**, 89–93.

Abou-Chaar, C. I., Günther, H. F., Manuel, M. F., Robbers, J. E., and Floss, H. G. (1972). *Lloydia* **35**, 272–279.

Acklin, W., Fehr, T., and Stadler, P. (1975). *Helv. Chim. Acta.* **58**, 2492–2500.

Agurell, S. (1964). *Experientia* **20**, 25.

Agurell, S. (1966a). *Acta Pharm. Suec.* **3**, 7–10.

Agurell, S. (1966b). *Acta Pharm. Suec.* **3**, 71–100.

Agurell, S. (1966c). *Acta Pharm. Suec.* **3**, 65–70.

Agurell, S. (1966d). *Acta Pharm. Suec.* **3**, 23–32.

Agurell, S. (1966e). *Acta Pharm. Suec.* **3**, 33–36.

Agurell, S., and Johansson, M. (1964). *Acta Chem. Scand.* **18**, 2285–2293.

Agurell, S., and Lindgren, J.-E. (1968). *Tetrahedron Lett.*, pp. 5127–5128.

Agurell, S., and Ramstad, E. (1961). *Tetrahedron Lett.*, pp. 501–505.

Agurell, S., and Ramstad, E. (1962). *Arch. Biochem. Biophys.* **98**, 457–470.

Agurell, S., and Ramstad, E. (1965). *Acta Pharm. Suec.* **2**, 231–238.

Ambike, S. H., and Baxter, R. M. (1970). *J. Pharm. Sci.* **59**, 1149–1152.

Amici, A. M., Minghetti, A., Scotti, T., Spalla, C., and Tognoli, L. (1967). *Appl. Microbiol.* **15**, 597–610.

Anderson, J. A., and Saini, M. S. (1974). *Tetrahedron Lett.*, pp. 2107–2108.

Arcamone, F., Bonino, C., Chain, E. B., Ferretti, A., Pennella, P., Tonolo, A., and Vero, L. (1960). *Nature (London)* **187**, 238–239.

Arcamone, F., Chain, E. B., Ferretti, A., Minghetti, A., Pennella, P., Tonolo, A., and Vero, L. (1961). *Proc. Roy. Soc. London, Ser. B* **155**, 26–54.

Arcamone, F., Casinelli, G., Ferni, G., Penco, S., Pennella P., and Pol, C. (1970). *Can. J. Microbiol.* **16**, 923–931.

Bach, N. J., Boaz, H. E., Kornfeld, E. C., Chang, C.-j., Floss, H. G., Hagaman, E. W., and Wenkert, E. (1974). *J. Org. Chem.* **39**, 1272–1276.

Bajwa, R. S., and Anderson, J. A. (1975). *J. Pharm. Sci.* **64**, 343–344.

Bajwa, R. S., Kohler, R. D., Saini, M. S., Cheng, M., and Anderson, J. A. (1975). *Phytochemistry* **14**, 735–737.

Barger, G. (1931). "Ergot and Ergotism." Gurney and Jackson, London.

Barger, G., and Carr, F. H. (1907). *J. Chem. Soc.* **91**, 337–353.

Barrow, K. D., and Quigley, F. R. (1975). *Tetrahedron Lett.*, pp. 4269–4270.

Barrow, K. D., Mantle, P. G., and Quigley, F. R. (1974). *Tetrahedron Lett.*, pp. 1557–1560.

Basmadjian, G., Floss, H. G., Gröger, D., and Erge, D. (1969). *Chem. Commun.*, pp. 418–419.

Bassett, R. A., Chain, E. B., and Corbett, K. (1973). *Biochem. J.* **134**, 1–10.

Baumert, A., Gröger, D., and Maier, W. (1977). *Experientia* **33**, 881–882.

Baxter, R. M., Kandel, S. I., and Okany, A. (1961). *Tetrahedron Lett.*, pp. 596–600.

Baxter, R. M., Kandel, S. I., and Okany, A. (1962a). *J. Am. Chem. Soc.* **84**, 2997–2999.

64   Heinz G. Floss and John A. Anderson

Baxter, R. M., Kandel, S. I., Okany, A., and Tam, K. L. (1962b). *J. Am. Chem. Soc.* **84**, 4350–4352.
Baxter, R. M., Kandel, S. I., Okany, A., and Pyke, R. G. (1964). *Can. J. Chem.* **42**, 2936–2938.
Beliveau, J., and Ramstad, E. (1966). *Lloydia* **29**, 234–238.
Bellatti, M., Casnati, G., Palla, G., and Minghetti, A. (1977). *Tetrahedron* **33**, 1821–1822.
Bhattacharji, S., Birch, A. J., Brack, A., Hofmann, A., Kobel, H., Smith, D. C. C., Smith, H., and Winter, J. (1962). *J. Chem. Soc.*, pp. 421–425.
Birch, A. J. (1958). *In* "Ciba Foundation Symposium on Amino Acids and Peptides with Antimetabolic Activity" (G. E. W. Westenholme and C. M. O'Connor, eds.), p. 247. Churchill, London.
Birch, A. J., McLoughlin, B. J., and Smith, H. (1960). *Tetrahedron Lett.*, pp. 1–3.
Bové, F. J. (1970). "The Story of Ergot." Karger, Basel.
Bu'Lock, J. D., and Barr, J. G. (1968). *Lloydia* **31**, 342–354.
Caporael, L. R. (1976). *Science* **192**, 21–26.
Cassady, J. M., and Floss, H. G. (1977). *Lloydia* **40**, 90–106.
Cassady, J. M., Abou-Chaar, C. I., and Floss, H. G. (1973). *Lloydia* **36**, 390–396.
Castagnoli, N., Corbett, K., Chain, E. B., and Thomas, R. (1970). *Biochem. J.* **117**, 451–455.
Cavender, F. L., and Anderson, J. A. (1970). *Biochem. Biophys. Acta.* **208**, 345–348.
Choong, T.-C., and Shough, H. R. (1977). *Tetrahedron Lett.*, pp. 3137–3138.
Cole, R. J., Kirksey, J. W., Clardy, J., Eickman, N., Weinreb, S. M., Singh, P., and Kim, D. (1976). *Tetrahedron Lett.*, pp. 3849–3852.
Erge, D., Maier, W., and Gröger, D. (1973). *Biochem. Physiol. Pflanzen* **164**, 234–247.
Fehr, T. (1967). Ph.D thesis, ETH Zürich, Switzerland.
Fehr, T., Acklin, W., and Arigoni, D. (1966). *Chem. Commun.*, pp. 801–802.
Floss, H. G. (1971). *Abh. Dtsch. Akad. Wiss. Berlin Kl. Chem. Geol. Biol.* pp. 395–407.
Floss, H. G. (1976). *Tetrahedron* **32**, 873–912.
Floss, H. G. and Gröger, D. (1963). *Z. Naturforsch. Teil B.* **18**, 519–522.
Floss, H. G., and Gröger, D. (1964). *Z. Naturforsch. Teil B.* **19**, 393–395.
Floss, H. G., and Mothes, U. (1964). *Arch. Mikrobiol.*, **48**, 213–221.
Floss, H. G., Mothes, U., and Günther, H. (1964). *Z. Naturforsch. Teil B.* **19**, 784–788.
Floss, H. G., Mothes, U., Onderka, D., and Hornemann, U. (1965). *Z. Naturforsch. Teil B.* **20**, 133–136.
Floss, H. G., Günther, H., Gröger, D., and Erge, D. (1966). *Z. Naturforsch. Teil B.* **21**, 128–131.
Floss, H. G., Günther, H., Mothes, U., and Becker, I. (1967). *Z. Naturforsch. Teil B.* **22**, 399–402.
Floss, H. G., Hornemann, U., Schilling, N., Kelley, K., Gröger, D., and Erge, D. (1968). *J. Am. Chem. Soc.* **90**, 6500–6507.
Floss, H. G., Basmadjian, G. P., Gröger, D., and Erge, D. (1971a). *Lloydia*, **34**, 499–450.
Floss, H. G., Basmadjian, G. P., Tcheng, M., Gröger, D., and Erge, D. (1971b). *Lloydia* **34**, 446–448.
Floss, H. G., Basmadjian, G. P., Tcheng, M., Spalla, C., and Minghetti, A. (1971c). *Lloydia* **34**, 442–445.
Floss, H. G., Tcheng-Lin, M., Chang, C.-j., Naidoo, B., Blair, G. E., Abou-Chaar, C., and Cassady, J. M. (1974a). *J. Am. Chem. Soc.* **96**, 1898–1909.
Floss, H. G., Tcheng-Lin, M., Kobel, H., and Stadler, P. (1974b). *Experientia* **30**, 1369–1370.
Floss, H. G., Robbers, J. E., and Heinstein, P. F. (1974c). *Recent Adv. Phytochem.* **8**, 141–178.
Gröger, D. (1963). *Flora* **153**, 373–382.
Gröger, D. (1969). *In* "Biosynthese der Alkaloide" (K. Mothes and H. R. Schütte, eds.), pp. 486–509. Deut. Verlag Wissensch., Berlin.

Gröger, D. (1972). In "Microbial Toxins" (S. J. Ajl, S. Kadis, and T. C. Montie, eds.), Vol. 8, pp. 321–373. Academic Press, New York.

Gröger, D. (1975). Planta Med. 28, 37–51.

Gröger, D., and Erge, D. (1970). Z. Naturforsch. Teil B. 25, 196–199.

Gröger, D., and Johne, S. (1972). Experientia 28, 241–242.

Gröger, D., and Sajdl, P. (1972). Pharmazie 27, 188.

Gröger, D., Wendt, H. J., Mothes, K., and Weygand, F. (1959). Z. Naturforsch. Teil B. 14, 355–358.

Gröger, D., Mothes, K., Simon, H., Floss, H. G. and Weygand, F. (1960). Z. Naturforsch. Teil B. 15, 141–143.

Gröger, D., Schütte, H. R., and Stolle, K. (1963). Z. Naturforsch. Teil B. 18, 850.

Gröger, D., Erge, D., and Floss, H. G. (1966). Z. Naturforsch. Teil B. 21, 827–832.

Gröger, D., Erge, D., and Floss, H. G. (1968). Z. Naturforsch. Teil B. 23, 177–180.

Gröger, D., John, S., and Härtling, S. (1974). Biocehm. Physiol. Pflanzen 166, 33–43.

Guggisberg, H. (1954). "Mutterkorn, Vom Gift Zum Heilstoff." Karger, Basel.

Heinstein, P., and Floss, H. G. (1976). Nova Acta Leopold., Suppl. No. 7, 299–310.

Heinstein, P. F., Lee, S.-L., and Floss, H. G. (1971). Biochem. Biophys. Res. Commun., 44, 1244–1251.

Hofmann, A. (1961). Planta Med. 9, 354–367.

Hofmann, A. (1964). "Die Mutterkornalkaloide." Enke, Stuttgart.

Hofmann, A., and Tscherter, H. (1960). Experientia 16, 414.

Hofmann, A., Brunner, R., Kobel, H., and Brack, A. (1957). Helv. Chim. Acta, 40, 1358–1373.

Hofmann, A., Ott, H., Griot, R., Stadler, P. A., and Frey, A. J. (1963). Helv. Chim. Acta, 46, 2306–2328.

Hsu, J. C., and Anderson, J. A. (1970). Chem. Commun., pp. 1318.

Hsu, J. C., and Anderson, J. A. (1971). Biochem. Biophys. Acta. 230, 518–525.

Johne, S., Gröger, D., Zier, P., and Voigt, R. (1972). Pharmazie 27, 801–802.

Kaplan, H., Hornemann, U., Kelley, K. M., and Floss, H. G. (1969). Lloydia 32, 489–497.

Kharasch, M. S., and Legault, R. R. (1935). Science (Lancaster) 81, 388, 614–615.

King, G. S., Waight, E. S., Mantle, P. G., and Szczyrbak, C. A. (1977). J. Chem. Soc., Perkin Trans. 1, 2099–2103.

Kleinerova, E., and Kybal, J. (1973). Folia Microbiol. 18, 390–392.

Kobel, H., Schreier, E., and Rutschmann, J. (1964). Helv. Chim. Acta. 47, 1052–1064.

Krupinski, V. M., Robbers, J. E., Floss, H. G. (1976). J. Bacteriol. 125, 158–165.

Lee, S. L. (1974). Ph. D. thesis, Purdue University, West Lafayette, Indiana.

Lee, S. L., Floss, H. G., and Heinstein, P. F. (1976). Arch. Biochem. Biophys. 177, 84–94.

Lin, C. C. L., Blair, G. E., Cassady, J. M., Gröger, D., Maier, W., and Floss, H. G., (1973). J. Org. Chem. 38, 2249–2251.

Lin, W.-n. C., Ramstad, E., and Taylor, E. H. (1967). Lloydia 30, 202–208.

Lingens, F., Goebel, W., and Uesseler, H. (1967). Eur. J. Biochem. 2, 442–447.

Lipmann, F. (1973). Accts. Chem. Res. 6, 361–367.

Maier, W., and Gröger, D. (1976). Biochem. Physiol. Pflanzen (BBP), 170, 9–15.

Maier, W., Erge, D., and Gröger, D. (1971). Biochem. Physiol. Pflanzen 161, 559–569.

Maier, W., Erge, D., and Gröger, D. (1972). Biochem. Physiol. Pflanzen 163, 432–442.

Maier, W., Erge, D., and Gröger, D. (1974). Biochem. Physiol. Pflanzen 165, 479–485.

Majer, J., Kybal, J., and Komersova, I. (1967). Folia Microbiol. 12, 489–491.

Mann, D. F., and Floss, H. G. (1977). Lloydia 40, 136–145.

Mantel, P. G., and Waight, E. S. (1968). Nature (London) 218 581–582.

Minghetti, A., and Arcamone, F. (1969). Experientia 25, 926–927.

Mothes, K., and Winkler, K. (1962). *Tetrahedron Lett.*, pp. 1243–1248.
Mothes, K., Weygand, F., Gröger, D., and Grisebach, H. (1958). *Z. Naturforsch. Teil B.* **13**, 41–44.
Mothes, K., Winkler, K., Gröger, D., Floss, H. G., Mothes, U., and Weygand, F. (1962). *Tetrahedron Lett.*, pp. 933–937.
Nelson, U., and Agurell, S. (1969). *Acta Chem. Scand.* **23**, 3393–3397.
Ogunlana, E. O., Wilson, B. J., Tyler, V. E., and Ramstad, E. (1970). *Chem. Commun.*, pp. 775–776.
Ohashi, T., and Abe, M. (1970). *J. Agric. Chem. Soc.* **44**, 519–526.
Ohashi, T., Aoki, S., Abe, M. (1970a). *J. Agric. Chem. Soc.* **44**, 527–531.
Ohashi, T., Iimura, Y., and Abe, M. (1970b). *J. Agric. Chem. Soc.* **44**, 567–572.
Ohashi, T., Takahashi, H., and Abe, M. (1972a). *J. Agric. Chem. Soc.* **46**, 533–540.
Ohashi, T., Shibuya, N., and Abe, M. (1972b). *J. Agric. Chem. Soc.* **46**, 207–213.
Ohmomo, S., and Abe, M. (1976). *J. Agric. Chem. Soc. Jpn.* **50**, 543–546.
Ohmomo, S., Sato, T., Utagawa, T., and Abe, M. (1975). *Agric. Biol. Chem.* **39**, 1333–1334.
Ohmomo, S., Utagawa, T., and Abe, M. (1977). *Agric. Biol. Chem.* **41**, 2097–2098.
Pachlatko, P. (1975). Ph. D. thesis, No. 5481, ETH Zürich, Switzerland.
Pachlatko, P., Tabacik, C., Acklin, W., and Arigoni, D. (1975). *Chimia* **29**, 526–527.
Petroski, R. J., and Kelleher, W. J. (1977). *FEBS Lett.* **82**, 55–57.
Plieninger, H., Fischer, R., Keilich, G., and Orth, H. D. (1961). *Justus Liebig's Ann. Chem.* **642**, 214–224.
Plieninger, H., Höbel, M., and Liede, V. (1963). *Chem. Ber.* **96**, 1618–1629.
Plieninger, H., Fischer, R., and Liede, V. (1964). *Justus Liebig's Ann Chem.* **672**, 223–231.
Plieninger, H., Immel, H., and Völkl, A. (1967). *Justus Liebig's Ann. Chem.* **706**, 223–229.
Plieninger, H., Wagner, C., and Immel, H. (1971). *Justus Liebig's Ann. Chem.* **743**, 95–111.
Popjak, G., and Cornforth, J. W. (1966). *Biochem. J.* **101**, 553–568.
Ramstad, E. (1968). *Lloydia* **31**, 327–341.
Ramstad, E., Lin, W. N. Chan, Shough, R., Goldner, K. J., Parikh, R. P., and Taylor, E. H. (1967). *Lloydia* **30**, 441–444.
Robbers, J. E., and Floss, H. G. (1968). *Arch. Biochem. Biophys.* **126**, 967–969.
Robbers, J. E., and Floss, H. G. (1969). *Tetrahedron Lett.*, pp. 1857–1858.
Robbers, J. E., Robertson, L. W., Hornemann, K. M., Jindra, A., and Floss, H. G. (1972). *J. Bact.* **112**, 791–796.
Robertson, L. W., Robbers, J. E., and Floss, H. G. (1973). *J. Bact.* **114**, 208–219.
Rochelmeyer, H. (1958). *Pharm. Ztg.* **103**, 1269–1275.
Saini, M. S., Cheng, M., and Anderson, J. A. (1976). *Phytochemistry* **15**, 1497–1500.
Schlientz, W., Brunner, R., and Hofmann, A. (1963). *Experientia* **19**, 397.
Schlientz, W., Brunner, R., Stadler, P. A., Frey, A. J., Ott, H., and Hofmann, A. (1964). *Helv. Chim. Acta.* **47**, 1921–1933.
Schlientz, W., Brunner, R., Rüegger, A., Berde, B., Stürmer, E., and Hofmann, A. (1968). *Pharm. Acta Helv.* **43**, 497–509.
Schmauder, H.-P., and Gröger, D. (1976). *Biochem. Physiol. Pflanzen* **169**, 471–486.
Scott, P. M., Merrien, M.-A., and Polonsky, J. (1976). *Experientia* **32**, 140–142.
Seiler, M., Acklin, W., and Arigoni, D. (1970a). *Chem. Commun.*, pp. 1394–1395.
Seiler, M., Acklin, W., and Arigoni, D. (1970b). *Chimia* **24**, 449–450.
Shough, H. R., and Taylor, E. H. (1969). *Lloydia* **32**, 315–326.
Smith, S., and Timmis, G. M. (1937). *J. Chem. Soc.*, pp. 396–401.
Spanos, N. P., and Gottlieb, J. (1976). *Science* **194**, 1390–1394.
Spilsbury, J. F., and Wilkinson, S. (1961). *J. Chem. Soc.*, pp. 2085–2091.
Stauffacher, D., and Tscherter, H. (1964). *Helv. Chim. Acta* **47**, 2186–2194.

Stauffacher, D., Tscherter, H., and Hofmann, A. (1965). *Helv. Chim. Acta* **48**, 1379–1380.

Stauffacher, D., Niklaus, P., Tscherter, H., Weber, H. P., and Hofmann, A. (1969). *Tetrahedron* **25**, 5879–5887.

Stoll, A. (1918). Swiss Patent No. 79879.

Stoll, A. (1945). *Helv. Chim. Acta.* **28**, 1283–1308.

Stoll, A., Burckhardt, E. (1935). *Compt. Rend. Acad. Sci.* (*Paris*), **200**, 1680–1682; (1935). *Bull. Sci. Pharm.* **42**, 257–266.

Stoll, A., and Burckhardt, E. (1937). *Hoppe-Seyler's Z. Physiol. Chem.* **250**, 1–6.

Stoll, A., and Hofmann, A. (1943). *Helv. Chim. Acta.* **26**, 1570–1601.

Stoll, A., Brack, A., Kobel, H., Hofmann, A., and Brunner, R. (1954). *Helv. Chim. Acta.* **37**, 1815–1825.

Stutz, P., Brunner, R., and Stadler, P. A. (1973). *Experientia* **29**, 936–937.

Taber, W. A. (1964). *Appl. Microbiol.* **12**, 321 326.

Taber, W. A., and Vining, L. C. (1959). *Chem. Ind. N.Y.*, pp. 1218–1219.

Taber, W. A., Vining, L. C., and Heacock, R. A. (1963). *Phytochemistry* **2**, 65–70.

Tanret, C. (1875). *Compt. Rend. Acad. Sci., Paris* **81/82**, 896.

Taylor, E. H., and Ramstad, E. (1960). *Nature* (*London*) **188**, 494–495; (1961). *J. Pharm Sci.* **50**, 681–683.

Taylor, E. H., Goldner, K. J., Pong, S. F., and Shough, H. R. (1966). *Lloydia* **29**, 239–244.

Teuscher, E. (1965). *Pharmazie* **20**, 778–784.

Thomas, R., and Bassett, R. A. (1972). *Progr. Phytochem.* **3**, 47–111.

Thompson, M. R. (1935). *Science* **81**, 636–639.

Tscherter, H., and Hauth, H. (1974). *Helv. Chim. Acta* **57**, 113–121.

Tyler, V. E. (1961). *J. Pharm. Sci.* **50**, 629–640.

Vicario, G. P., Dubini, M., Minghetti, A., and Arcamone, F. (1967). *J. Labelled Compd.* **3**, 492–493.

Vining, L. C. (1970). *Can. J. Microbiol.* **16**, 473–480.

Vining, L. C., and Taber, W. A. (1963). *Can. J. Microbiol.* **9**, 291–302.

Voigt, R. (1962). *Pharmazie* **17**, 101–106.

Voigt, R. (1968). *Pharmazie* **23**, 285–296, 353–359, 419–436.

Voigt, R., and Bornschein, M. (1964). *Pharmazie* **19**, 772–775.

Voigt, R., and Zier, P. (1970). *Pharmazie* **25**, 272.

Voigt, R., and Zier, P. (1971). *Pharmazie* **26**, 494–503.

Voigt, R., Bornschein, M., and Rabitzsch, G. (1967). *Pharmazie* **22**, 326–329.

Voigt, R., Zier, P., and Rabitzsch, G. (1972). *Pharmazie* **27**, 175–178.

Weygand, F., and Floss, H. G. (1963). *Angew. Chem. Int. Ed. Eng.* **2**, 243–247.

Weygand, F., Floss, H. G., Mothes, U., Gröger, D., and Mothes, K. (1964). *Z. Naturforschg. Teil B.* **19**, 202–210.

Wilson, B. J. (1970). Ph.D. thesis, Purdue University, West Lafayette, Indiana.

Wilson, B. J., Ramstad, E., Jansson, I., and Orrenius, S. (1971). *Biochem. Biophys. Acta.* **252**, 348–356.

Winkler, K., and Gröger, D. (1962). *Pharmazie* **17**, 658–670.

Yamano, T., Kishino, K., Yamatodani, S., and Abe, M. (1962). *Ann. Rep. Takeda Res. Lab.* **21**, 95–101.

Yamatodani, S., Asahi, Y., Matsukura, A., Ohmomo, S., and Abe, M. (1970). *Agric. Biol. Chem.* **34**, 485–487.

3

The Biosynthesis
of Trichothecene Mycotoxins

CH. TAMM AND W. BREITENSTEIN

I. INTRODUCTION

The trichothecenes belong to a class of structurally closely related secondary metabolites produced by various species of Fungi Imperfecti and, as exemplified in one case, by higher plants. They are sesquiterpene alcohols or esters derived from a common tricyclic skeleton named trichothecane (**1**) (Godtfredsen *et al.*, 1967). The corresponding rearranged system is called apotrichothecane (**2**) (Fig. 1). Nearly all the naturally occurring compounds of this family, with known structures, possess an olefinic double bond between C(9) and C(10). In addition, most of the metabolites—there is only one known exception—contain an epoxy group at C(12) and C(13). Therefore, the name

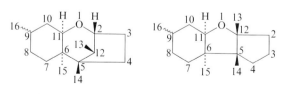

1 Trichothecane   **2** Apotrichothecane

Fig. 1. Structure, stereochemistry, and numbering system of the trichothecane and apotrichothecane skeletons.

The Biosynthesis of Mycotoxins
Copyright © 1980 by Academic Press, Inc.
ISBN 0-12-670650-6.

TABLE I

Trichothecene Derivatives: Simple Alcohols and Esters

Structure number	Trivial name	Systematic name	Molecular formula	References
5	—	12,13-Epoxytrichothec-9-ene	$C_{15}H_{22}O_2$	Machida and Nozoe (1972b)
6	Trichodermol (Roridin C)	4β-Hydroxy-12,13-epoxytrichothec-9-ene	$C_{15}H_{22}O_3$	Abrahamsson and Nilsson (1964, 1966); Härri et al. (1962)
7	Trichodermin	4β-Acetoxy-12,13-epoxytrichothec-9-ene	$C_{17}H_{24}O_4$	Godtfredsen and Vangedal (1964, 1965)
8	15-Deacetylcalonectrin	3α-Acetoxy-15-hydroxy-12,13-epoxytrichothec-9-ene	$C_{17}H_{24}O_5$	Gardner et al. (1972)
9	Calonectrin	3α,15-Diacetoxy-12,13-epoxytrichothec-9-ene	$C_{19}H_{26}O_6$	Gardner et al. (1972)
10	Di-O-acetylverrucarol	4β,15-Diacetoxy-12,13-epoxy-trichothec-9-ene	$C_{19}H_{26}O_6$	Okuchi et al. (1968)
11	Scirpentriol	3α,4β,15-Trihydroxy-12,13-epoxytrichothec-9-ene	$C_{15}H_{22}O_5$	Pathre et al. (1976)
12	Monoacetoxyscirpenol	15-Acetoxy-3α,4β-dihydroxy-12,13-epoxytrichothec-9-ene	$C_{17}H_{24}O_6$	Pathre et al. (1976)
13	Diacetoxyscirpenol	4β,15-Diacetoxy-3α-hydroxy-12,13-epoxytrichothec-9-ene	$C_{19}H_{26}O_7$	Brian et al. (1961); Dawkins (1966); Sigg et al. (1965)
14	7-Hydroxydiacetoxyscirpenol	4β,15-Diacetoxy-3α,7α-dihydroxy-12,13-epoxytrichothec-9-ene	$C_{19}H_{26}O_8$	Ishii (1975)
15	—	4β,8α-Dihydroxy-12,13-epoxytrichothec-9-ene	$C_{15}H_{22}O_4$	Machida and Nozoe (1972b)
16	T-2-Tetraol	3α,4β,8α,15-Tetrahydroxy-12,13-epoxytrichothec-9-ene	$C_{15}H_{22}O_6$	Mirocha and Pathre (1973)
17	HT-2-Toxin	15-Acetoxy-8α-(3-methylbutyryloxy)-3α,4β-dihydroxy-12,13-epoxytrichothec-9-ene	$C_{22}H_{32}O_8$	Bamburg and Strong (1969); Wei et al. (1971)
18	T-2-Toxin (fusariotoxin T2)	4β,15-Diacetoxy-8α-(3-methylbutyryloxy)-3α-hydroxy-12,13-epoxytrichothec-9-ene	$C_{24}H_{34}O_9$	Bamburg et al. (1968); Yates et al. (1968)
19	Acetyl-T-2-toxin	3α,4β,15-Triacetoxy-8α-(3-methylbutyryloxy)-12,13-epoxytrichothec-9-ene	$C_{26}H_{36}O_{10}$	Kotsonis et al. (1975)
20	Solaniol (neosolaniol)	4β,15-Diacetoxy-3α,8α-dihydroxy-12,13-	$C_{19}H_{26}O_8$	Ishii et al. (1971); Ueno

	Name	Systematic name	Formula	Reference
21	7,8-Dihydroxydiacetoxyscirpenol	$4\beta,15$-Diacetoxy-$3\alpha,7\alpha,8\alpha$-trihydroxy-12,13-epoxytrichothec-9-ene	$C_{19}H_{26}O_9$	Ishii (1975)
22	—	$4\beta,8\alpha,15$-Triacetoxy-$3\alpha,7\alpha$-dihydroxy-12,13-epoxytrichothec-9-ene	$C_{21}H_{28}O_{10}$	Brian et al. (1961); Grove (1970b)
23	—	$4\beta,8\alpha$-Diacetoxy-$3\alpha,15$-dihydroxy-12,13-epoxytrichothec-9-ene	$C_{19}H_{26}O_8$	Ilus et al. (1977)
24	Crotocin	4β-Isocrotonoyloxy-$7\beta,8\beta,12,13$-diepoxytrichothec-9-ene	$C_{19}H_{24}O_5$	Gläz et al. (1959, 1966); Gyimesi and Melera (1967)
25	Trichothecolone	4β-Hydroxy-12,13-epoxytrichothec-9-en-8-one	$C_{15}H_{20}O_4$	Achilladelis and Hanson (1969)
26	Trichothecin	4β-Isocrotonoyloxy-12,13-epoxytrichothec-9-en-8-one	$C_{19}H_{24}O_5$	Freeman and Morrison (1948); Freeman et al. (1959); Fishman et al. (1960); Godtfredsen and Vangedal (1964)
27	Vomitoxin (deoxynivalenol)	$3\alpha,7\alpha,15$-Trihydroxy-12,13-epoxytrichothec-9-en-8-one	$C_{15}H_{20}O_6$	Vesonder et al. (1973, 1976); Yoshizawa and Morooka (1973)
28	Deoxynivalenol monoacetate	3α-Acetoxy-$7\alpha,15$-dihydroxy-12,13-epoxytrichothec-9-en-8-one	$C_{17}H_{22}O_7$	Blight and Grove (1974); Yoshizawa and Morooka (1973)
29	Nivalenol	$3\alpha,4\beta,7\alpha,15$-Tetrahydroxy-12,13-epoxytrichothec-9-en-8-one	$C_{15}H_{20}O_7$	Tatsuno et al. (1968, 1969)
30	Fusarenon (fusarenon-X)	4β-Acetoxy-$3\alpha,7\alpha,15$-trihydroxy-12,13-epoxytrichothec-9-en-8-one	$C_{17}H_{22}O_8$	Tatsuno et al. (1969); Ueno et al. (1969, 1971)
31	Nivalenol diacetate	$4\beta,15$-Diacetoxy-$3\alpha,7\alpha$-dihydroxy-12,13-epoxytrichothec-9-en-8-one	$C_{19}H_{24}O_9$	Brian et al. (1961); Grove (1969, 1970a); Tatsuno et al. (1970); Tidd (1967)

TABLE II

Trichothecene Derivatives: Macrocyclic Di- and Triesters

Structure number	Trivial name	Origin	Molecular formula	References
32	Verrucarin A	*Myrothecium* species	$C_{27}H_{34}O_9$	Gutzwiller and Tamm (1965a); Tamm and Gutzwiller (1962)
33	Roridin A	*Myrothecium* species	$C_{29}H_{40}O_9$	Böhner and Tamm (1966a)
34	Verrucarin B	*Myrothecium* species	$C_{27}H_{32}O_9$	Gutzwiller and Tamm (1965b)
35	Roridin D	*Myrothecium* species	$C_{29}H_{38}O_9$	Böhner and Tamm (1966b)
36	Verrucarin J	*Myrothecium* species	$C_{27}H_{32}O_8$	Fetz *et al.* (1965)
37	Roridin E	*Myrothecium* species	$C_{29}H_{38}O_8$	Traxler *et al.* (1970)
38	2'-Dehydroverrucarin A	*Myrothecium roridum*	$C_{27}H_{32}O_9$	Zürcher and Tamm (1966)
39	Roridin H	*Myrothecium verrucaria*	$C_{29}H_{36}O_8$	Traxler and Tamm (1970)
40	Satratoxin H	*Stachybotrys atra*	$C_{29}H_{36}O_9$	Eppley and Bailey (1973); Eppley *et al.* (1977)
41	7β,8β-Epoxyroridin H	*Cylindrocarpon* species	$C_{29}H_{34}O_9$	Matsumoto *et al.* (1977a,b)
42	Vertisporin	*Verticimonosporium diffractum*	$C_{29}H_{36}O_{10}$	Minato *et al.* (1975)
43	7β,8β,2',3'-Diepoxyroridin H	*Cylindrocarpon* species	$C_{29}H_{34}O_{10}$	Matsumoto *et al.* (1977a,b)
44	Isororidin E	*Cylindrocarpon* species	$C_{29}H_{38}O_8$	Matsumoto *et al.* (1977a,b)
45	7β,8β-Epoxyisororidin E	*Cylindrocarpon* species	$C_{29}H_{36}O_9$	Matsumoto *et al.* (1977a,b)
46	Verrucarin K	*Myrothecium verrucaria*	$C_{27}H_{34}O_8$	Breitenstein and Tamm (1977)
47	Baccharin	*Baccharis megapotamica*	$C_{29}H_{38}O_{11}$	Kupchan *et al.* (1976)

trichothecene or 12,13-epoxytrichothec-9-ene is often used in connection with these substances. For recent reviews in this field see, e.g., Bamburg (1976) and Smalley and Strong (1974).

Two types of trichothecenes may be distinguished on the basis of structural characteristics: the alcohols and simple esters (Table I, Figs. 3–6), and the more complex macrocyclic di- and triesters (Table II, Figs. 7 and 8).

The first member belonging to the first group, trichothecin, was isolated from *Trichothecium roseum* by Freeman and Morrison (1948). It was shown to be an isocrotonic ester of a ketonic alcohol which was named trichothecolone. Structure **3** (Fig. 2) was proposed for the latter compound (Freeman *et al.*, 1959; Fishman *et al.*, 1960). Verrucarol, another sesquiterpenoid alcohol belonging to the same group, was obtained as a hydrolysis product of the cytostatic antibiotic verrucarin A (**32**) (Tamm and Gutzwiller, 1962). On the basis of chemical and spectroscopic evidence, structure **4** (Fig. 2) was assigned to the new compound (Gutzwiller and Tamm, 1963). In the following year, Godtfredsen and Vangedal (1964) isolated a new member of the trichothecene family, named trichodermin, from a strain of *Trichoderma viride*. The anti-fungal metabolite was recognized as an acetyl derivative of a sesquiterpene alcohol, called trichodermol. The latter was shown (Godtfredsen and Vangedal, 1964, 1965; Gutzwiller *et al.*, 1964) to be identical to roridin C, a metabolite of *Myrothecium roridum* (Härri *et al.*, 1962).

In view of the similarity of the chemical and spectroscopic properties, a relationship between trichodermin and trichothecin was suggested that subsequently was confirmed by the oxidative conversion of trichodermin into trichothecolone acetate (Godtfredsen and Vangedal, 1964, 1965). However, the structure of trichodermin, based on the proposed formula **3** of trichothecolone, was in conflict with the results of several chemical conversions. Therefore, a *p*-bromobenzoate derivative of trichodermol was prepared and subjected to X-ray analysis. Using this method, structure **6** was established for trichodermol (Abrahamsson and Nilsson, 1964, 1966). Because of the interrelation of trichodermin (**7**) with trichothecolone acetate, a revision of the old formula **3** for trichothecolone and trichothecin was required. The correct structures, **25** and **26**, are shown in Fig. 6.

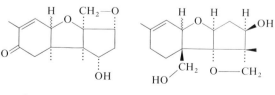

3 Trichothecolone   4 Verrucarol

Fig. 2.   Old formulas of trichothecolone and verrucarol.

In addition to these findings, Godtfredsen and Vangedal (1964) suggested that verrucarol should possess the same skeleton as trichodermol (**6**) and trichothecolone (**25**). This suggestion was proven unambiguously by chemical degradations and by the correlation of verrucarol with trichodermin (**7**) and trichothecolone (**25**) (Gutzwiller *et al.*, 1964). The revised formula (**49**) of verrucarol is represented in Fig. 9. The ring structure of diacetoxyscirpenol (**13**), a metabolite from *Fusarium equiseti* (Brian *et al.*, 1961), *Fusarium diversisporum*, and *Fusarium sambucinum* (Flury *et al.*, 1965; Sigg *et al.*, 1965), was also established by the interrelation with verrucarol (**49**) (Dawkins, 1966; Dawkins *et al.*, 1965; Flury *et al.*, 1965; Sigg *et al.*, 1965).

The systematic investigation of biologically active substances produced by molds has led during the last few years to the discovery of a number of new trichothecene derivatives. The structures of these compounds are summarized in Figs. 3–8.

The macrocyclic ester derivatives of trichothecene alcohols (Figs. 7 and 8) possess remarkable biological properties. Verrucarin A (**32**) was the first member of this group whose structure was established by the extensive use of chemical and spectroscopic methods (Gutzwiller and Tamm, 1965a; Tamm and Gutzwiller, 1962). The structure was then confirmed by an X-ray analysis

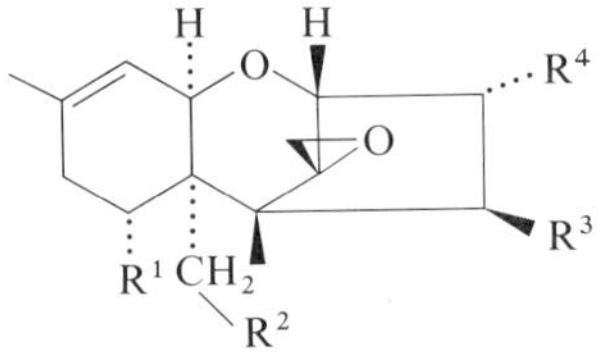

	R^1	R^2	R^3	R^4	
5	H	H	H	H	—
6	H	H	OH	H	Trichodermol (Roridin C)
7	H	H	OAc	H	Trichodermin
8	H	OH	H	OAc	15-Deacetylcalonectrin
9	H	OAc	H	OAc	Calonectrin
10	H	OAc	OAc	H	Di-*O*-acetylverrucarol
11	H	OH	OH	OH	Scirpentriol
12	H	OAc	OH	OH	Monoacetoxyscirpenol
13	H	OAc	OAc	OH	Diacetoxyscirpenol
14	OH	OAc	OAc	OH	7-Hydroxydiacetoxyscirpenol

Fig. 3. Structural types of naturally occurring trichothecene derivatives. I.

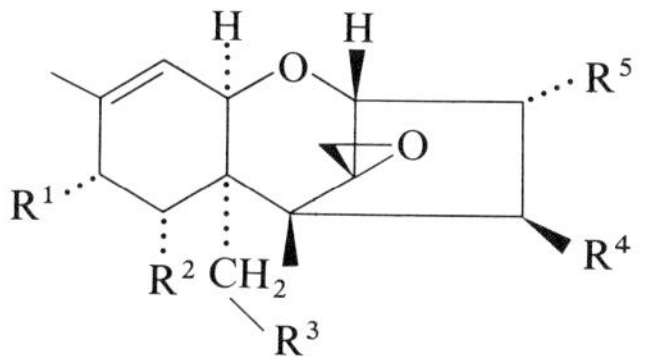

	R¹	R²	R³	R⁴	R⁵	
15	OH	H	H	OH	H	—
16	OH	H	OH	OH	OH	T-2-Tetraol
17	$O-C(=O)-CH_2-CH(CH_3)_2$	H	OAc	OH	OH	HT-2-Toxin
18	$O-C(=O)-CH_2-CH(CH_3)_2$	H	OAc	OAc	OH	T-2-Toxin (Fusariotoxin T2)
19	$O-C(=O)-CH_2-CH(CH_3)_2$	H	OAc	OAc	OAc	Acetyl-T-2-toxin
20	OH	H	OAc	OAc	OH	Solaniol (Neosolaniol)
21	OH	OH	OAc	OAc	OH	7,8-Dihydroxy-diacetoxyscirpenol
22	OAc	OH	OAc	OAc	OH	—
23	OAc	H	OH	OAc	OH	—

Fig. 4. Structural types of naturally occurring trichothecene derivatives. II.

Fig. 5. Structure of crotocin.

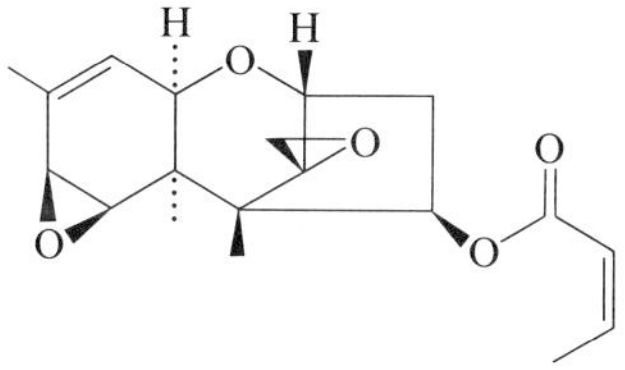

24

of the *p*-iodobenzene sulfonate of the antibiotic (McPhail and Sim, 1966). Besides verrucarin A (**32**), several other macrocyclic trichothecene derivatives were isolated from cultures of *Myrothecium verrucaria* and *M. roridum* (Böhner *et al.*, 1965; Härri *et al.*, 1962; Zürcher and Tamm, 1966). These include verrucarin B (**34**), verrucarin J (**36**), and 2′-dehydroverrucarin A (**38**) as well as the roridins A (**33**), D (**35**), E (**37**), and H (**39**) (Fig. 7) (Tamm, 1966,

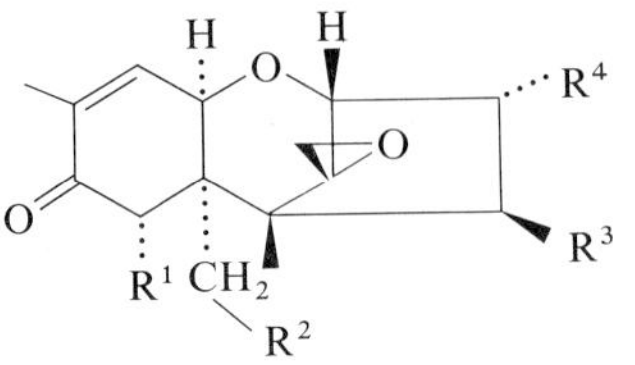

	R^1	R^2	R^3	R^4	
25	H	H	OH	H	Trichothecolone
26	H	H	O—C(=O)—CH=CH—CH₃	H	Trichothecin
27	OH	OH	H	OH	Vomitoxin (deoxynivalenol)
28	OH	OH	H	OAc	Deoxynivalenol monoacetate
29	OH	OH	OH	OH	Nivalenol
30	OH	OH	OAc	OH	Fusarenon (fusarenon-X)
31	OH	OAc	OAc	OH	Nivalenol diacetate

Fig. 6. Structural types of naturally occurring trichothecene derivatives. III.

1974). They are colorless, crystalline, optically active solids possessing high cytostatic activity. Base-catalyzed hydrolysis of the verrucarins and roridins yields the same sesquiterpene alcohol, verrucarol (49). However, whereas the roridins yield only two hydrolysis products, three moieties are formed by the hydrolysis of the verrucarins.

The physical and chemical properties of the verrucarins B (34) and J (36) and of 2′-dehydroverrucarin A (38) are very similar to those of verrucarin A (32). Therefore, it is difficult to separate the four closely related metabolites from each other. The structure elucidation of verrucarin B (34) (Gutzwiller and Tamm, 1965b) and verrucarin J (36) (Fetz et al., 1965) is based on chemical and spectroscopic evidence, whereas the structure of 2′-dehydroverrucarin A (38) was established by direct comparison with the product resulting from the oxidation of verrucarin A (32) (Zürcher and Tamm, 1966). The absolute configuration of verrucarin B (34) has been determined very recently by a single crystal X-ray diffraction analysis (Breitenstein et al., 1979). The structures of roridin A (33), the major metabolite of M. roridum, and of roridin D (35), a minor compound, were elucidated by Böhner and Tamm (1966a, 1966b).

A total hydrolysis of verrucarin J (36) yielded as one of three products the lactone of 5-hydroxy-3-methyl-cis-2-pentenoic acid. Therefore, it was antici- pated that a cis double bond would be present between the centers C(2′) and C(3′) in the side chain of verrucarin J (36) (Fetz et al., 1965). This conclusion

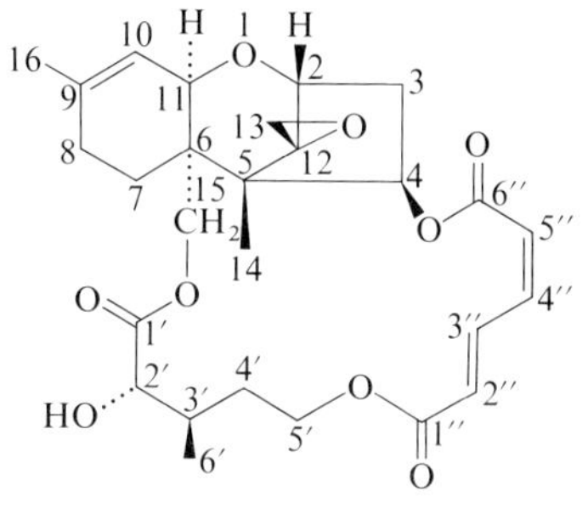

32 Verrucarin A 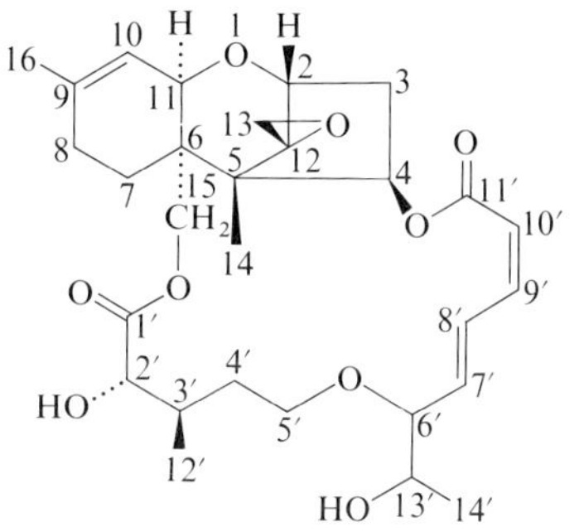   33 Roridin A

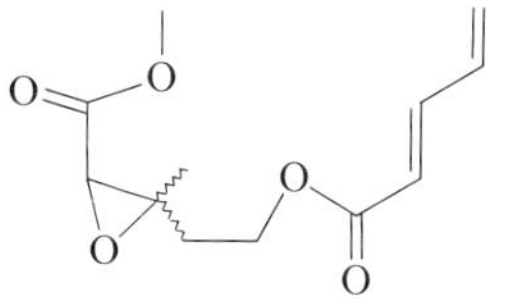

34 Verrucarin B 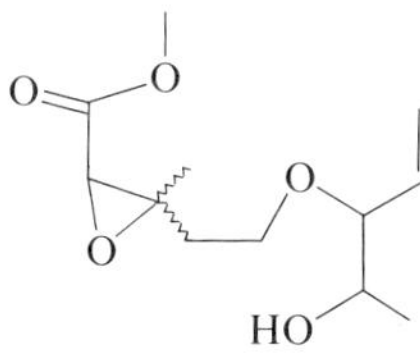   35 Roridin D

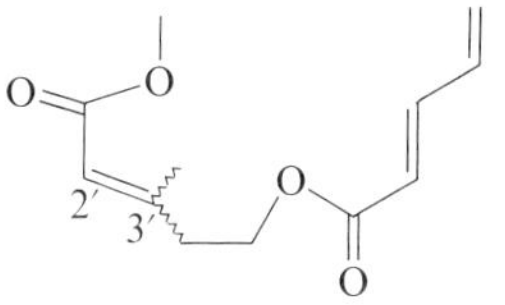

36 Verrucarin J 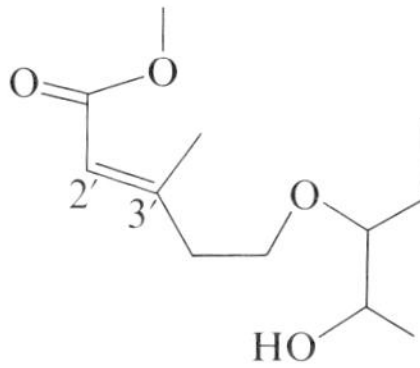   37 Roridin E

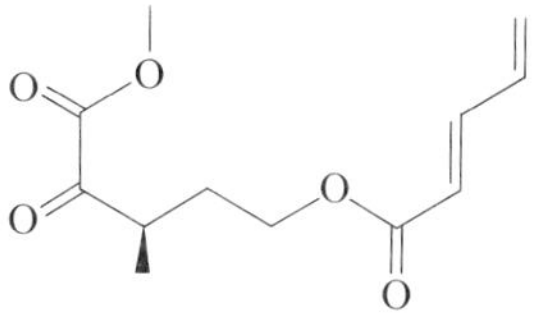

38 2′-Dehydroverrucarin A 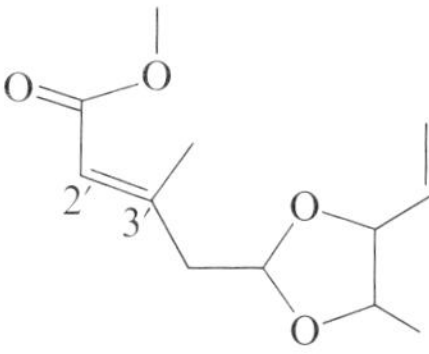   39 Roridin H

Fig. 7.   Macrocyclic di- and triesters of verrucarol.

was however, inconsistent with results obtained in the course of further spectroscopic investigations, and the *trans* configuration of this double bond was
suggested (Breitenstein, 1975). The same problem occurred in the structure
elucidations of roridin E (37) (Traxler *et al.*, 1970) and roridin H (39) (Traxler
and Tamm, 1970). In both these cases a *cis* relationship between the proton

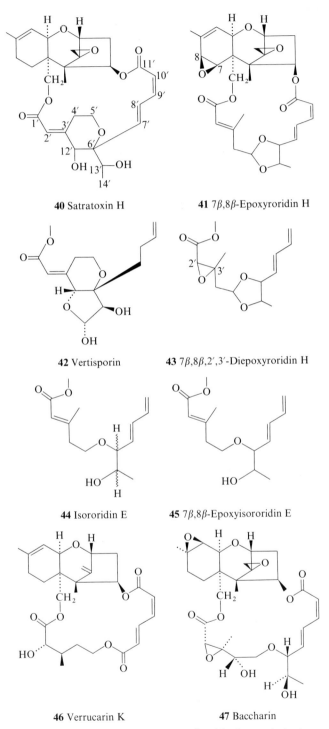

40 Satratoxin H

41 7β,8β-Epoxyroridin H

42 Vertisporin

43 7β,8β,2′,3′-Diepoxyroridin H

44 Isororidin E

45 7β,8β-Epoxyisororidin E

46 Verrucarin K

47 Baccharin

Fig. 8. Naturally occurring macrocyclic trichothecene derivatives.

at C(2') and the methyl group at C(3') was reported. The results of some recently performed NOE experiments, however, indicate that the C(2'),C(3') double bonds of roridin E (**37**) and roridin H (**39**) possess the *trans* configuration (Matsumoto *et al.*, 1977a,b).

Several new compounds belonging to the roridin group have been isolated recently from a species of *Cylindrocarpon*. The structures of four of these metabolites, namely, 7β,8β-epoxyroridin H (**41**), 7β,8β,2',3'-diepoxyroridin H (**43**), isororidin E (**44**), and 7β,8β-epoxyisororidin E (**45**) were elucidated (Matsumoto *et al.*, 1977a,b) (Fig. 8). Other compounds, representing diesters of verrucarol, are vertisporin (**42**) (Minato *et al.*, 1975) and satratoxin H (**40**) (Eppley and Bailey, 1973; Eppley *et al.*, 1977) (Fig. 8).

Very recently, the isolation and structure elucidation of baccharin (**47**), an antileukemic trichothecene triepoxide, from *Baccharis megapotamica* Spreng (Asteraceae) was reported (Kupchan *et al.*, 1976). This constitutes the first known case of a trichothecene derivative in higher plants. The full structure and stereochemistry of baccharin (**47**) were established by X-ray analysis.

The first naturally occurring trichothecene derivative without the 12,13-epoxy group has recently been isolated from a strain of *M. verrucaria* (Breitenstein and Tamm, 1977). The structure of this compound, named verrucarin K (**46**), is shown in Fig. 8.

II. BIOSYNTHESIS OF TRICHOTHECENES

The number of carbon atoms in the basic skeleton of the trichothecenes suggests that they belong to the class of sesquiterpenes. The biosynthetic formation of this type of compound has been the subject of several reports within the last few years. For a general review in this field see, e.g., Cordell (1976).

The sesquiterpenoid origin of the trichothecenes was first recognized by Fishman *et al.* (1959) and by Jones and Lowe (1960), who observed the incorporation of three molecules of [2-^{14}C]mevalonate into the trichothecane nucleus of trichothecin (**26**). The positions of the labeled carbon atoms were determined by extensive degradations. The results indicated that a double 1,2-methyl group migration had occurred during the biosynthetic formation of the skeleton. The trichothecin obtained after the incorporation of [1-^{14}C]acetate contained 95% of the activity in the isocrotonate moiety. The structure of trichothecolone which Fishman *et al.* (1959) and Jones and Lowe (1960) were using for their investigations proved later to be incorrect. A reinterpretation of their results on the basis of the revised formula led to the conclusion that the radioactivity from [2-^{14}C]mevalonate is distributed between C(4), C(10), and C(14) of trichothecolone (**25**) (Godtfredsen and Vangedal, 1965).

The results obtained from the incorporation of $[2\text{-}^{14}C]$mevalonate into diacetoxyscirpenol (13) (Dawkins, 1966) were in accord with the double 1,2-methyl shift, proposed by Fishman *et al.* (1959) and Jones and Lowe (1960). A similar kind of migration was also observed in the course of investigations on the biosynthesis of verrucarol (49) (Kocor and Siewinski, 1966). A γ-bisabolene derivative such as 58 (see Fig. 10) was postulated to be a key intermediate in the biosynthesis of the trichothecenes (Godtfredsen and Vangedal, 1965; Parker *et al.*, 1967; Ruzicka, 1963; Sigg *et al.*, 1965). Hanson and Achilladelis (1967) and Achilladelis and Hanson (1968) demonstrated that farnesyl pyrophosphate acts as a precursor of the trichothecenes.

When $[1\text{-}^{14}C]$farnesyl pyrophosphate prepared chemically as a mixture of the C(2)–C(3) double bond isomers was administered to a growing culture of *Trichothecium roseum*, an incorporation of 1.5% into trichothecin (26) was observed. Hydrolysis to trichothecolone (25) established that the radioactivity was confined to the terpenoid portion of the molecule. It is known that in the formation of *trans,trans*-farnesol from mevalonate it is the *pro*-4S mevalonoid hydrogen atom which is lost, whereas the corresponding *pro*-4R hydrogen atom is retained (see, e.g., Cordell, 1976). When $(4R)\text{-}[4\text{-}^{3}H,2\text{-}^{14}C]$ mevalonic acid was used as a precursor of trichothecin (26) in *Trichothecium roseum*, two of the three possible tritium labels were incorporated (Achilladelis *et al.*, 1970, 1972). One of them was located at C(2). $(4R)\text{-}[4\text{-}^{3}H,2\text{-}^{14}C]$ Mevalonic acid was also fed to *Trichoderma sporulosum* (Achilladelis *et al.*, 1970, 1972). Again, two of the three tritium labels were retained in the isolated trichodermol (6). Degradative conversions established the presence of one of the *pro*-4R mevalonoid hydrogen atoms at C(10), a result which apparently differs from the observations of Jones and Lowe (1960). The findings of Achilladelis *et al.* (1970, 1972) were confirmed by the work of Machida and Nozoe (1972b). $(4R)\text{-}[4\text{-}^{3}H,2\text{-}^{14}C]$Mevalonic acid was fed to a culture of *Trichothecium roseum*. Trichodiol A (68) and trichothecolone (25), obtained after hydrolysis of the extract, retained two of the three tritium labels. The trichothecolone (25) was then subjected to a series of degradations, permitting the selective removal of C(8) as radioactive carbon dioxide, which was isolated as $BaCO_3$. Thus, further evidence was provided that C(8) of trichothecolone corresponds to C(2) of mevalonate and that C(10) is derived from C(4) of the precursor.

Additional proof of this distribution came from experiments with verrucarol (Achini *et al.*, 1971; Müller *et al.*, 1975b). $[2\text{-}^{3}H_2,2\text{-}^{14}C]$Mevalonate was administered to growing cultures of *Myrothecium species* and the isolated metabolites were hydrolyzed to yield verrucarol (49). The oxidation of di-O-acetylverrucarol (10) via 52 to the corresponding 8-oxo compound (55) (Fig. 9) resulted in the loss of two tritium atoms from C(8). The second product of this oxidation, aldehyde 51, was characterized by a significant increase

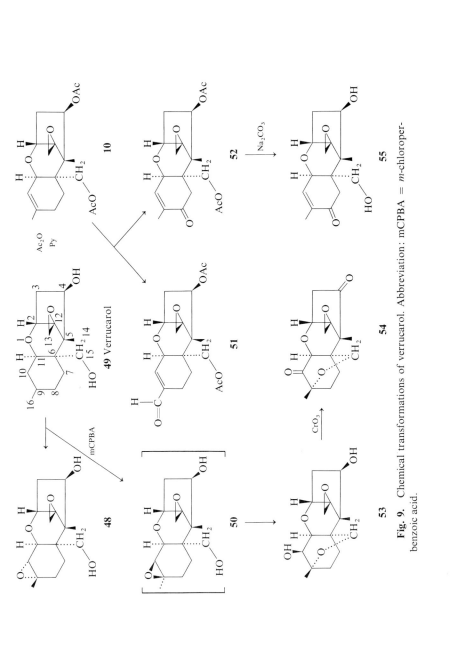

Fig. 9. Chemical transformations of verrucarol. Abbreviation: mCPBA = *m*-chloroperbenzoic acid.

in the tritium content caused by the kinetic isotope effect of tritium. Because C(8) contains tritium, this carbon atom is oxidized approximately 20 times more slowly than the competitive carbon atom C(16). This observation supports the labeling of C(8). To confirm that tritium was absent at C(10), verrucarol (**49**) was epoxidized. The resulting 9β,10β-epoxide **50** could not be isolated owing to isomerization to hydroxy ether **53**. On oxidation of **53** to diketo ether **54**, only the tritium atom at C(4) was lost (Fig. 9).

The location of a C(2) mevalonate hydrogen atom at C(8) in calonectrin (**9**) was also established by oxidation to the corresponding 8-oxo compound (Evans *et al.*, 1974).

The identity of C(8) of trichothecenes with C(2) of mevalonate was also proven directly, i.e., without the necessity of troublesome degradations and chemical conversions, by using $[^{13}C]$mevalonate (Hanson *et al.*, 1974). The only centers showing any enrichment in the ^{13}C-NMR spectrum after the incorporation of $[2-^{13}C]$mevalonic acid into trichothecolone (**25**) were C(4), C(8), and C(14). That C(8)—and not C(10), as reported by Jones and Lowe (1960)—is derived from C(2) of mevalonate gives rise to the suggestion that the farnesyl pyrophosphate precursor of the trichothecenes is coiled as shown in structure **56**, not as in structure **57** (Fig. 10) (Achilladelis *et al.*, 1970, 1972).

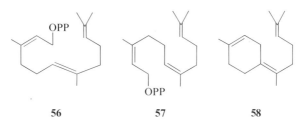

56   **57**   **58**

Fig. 10.   Folding of farnesyl pyrophosphate.

In order to distinguish conclusively between the two possibilities of folding the chain, $[1-^3H_2,2-^{14}C]$- and $[2-^3H,2-^{14}C]$farnesyl pyrophosphates were used as precursors of trichothecin (**26**) in *Trichothecium roseum* (Achilladelis *et al.*, 1970, 1972). The incorporation of $[1-^3H_2,2-^{14}C]$farnesyl pyrophosphate was accompanied by the elimination of one tritium label. No tritium was lost from $[2-^3H,2-^{14}C]$farnesyl pyrophosphate. In a similar experiment, $[1-^3H_2,2-^{14}C]$farnesyl pyrophosphate was fed to *Trichoderma sporulosum* to afford trichodermol (**6**). Again, only one of the two tritium labels was retained.

These results provide further support for the suggestion that 6,7-*trans*-farnesyl pyrophosphate (**56**) acts as an intermediate in the biosynthesis of the trichothecene skeleton. That the two methyl groups of the starter prenyl unit of this farnesyl pyrophosphate retain their individuality during the subsequent biosynthetic transformations was shown by Jones and Lowe (1960) and confirmed by Adams and Hanson (1970) and Achilladelis *et al.* (1972). Trichothecolone (**25**), obtained after incorporation of $[2-{}^3H_2,2-{}^{14}C]$mevalonate, was oxidized to trichothecodione (**59**). The latter was rearranged to yield **60** (Fig. 11). On further oxidation to the carboxylic acid **61**, no loss of activity was observed, confirming that tritium was absent from the epoxide group. Thus, of the two starter methyl groups of farnesyl pyrophosphate, only the group derived from C(2) of mevalonate is involved in the migration step.

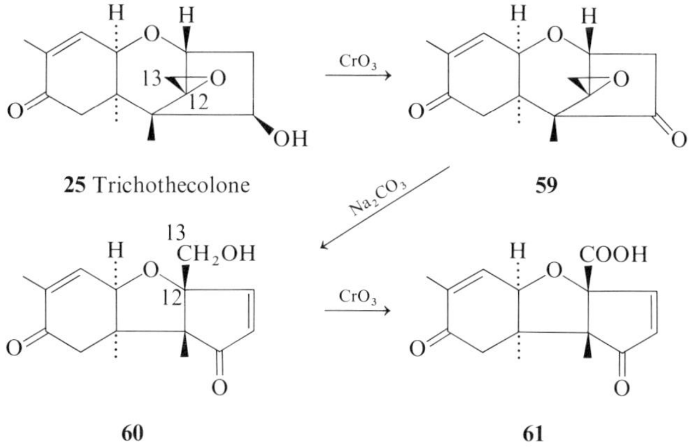

Fig. 11.   Rearrangement of trichothecolone.

In order to cast additional light on the mechanism of the transformation of the farnesyl precursor **56** to the trichothecene skeleton, several feeding experiments with ${}^3H$- and ${}^{14}C$-labeled geranyl and farnesyl pyrophosphates were carried out. When $[2-{}^3H,2-{}^{14}C]$geranyl pyrophosphate was administered to *Trichothecium roseum*, *Trichoderma polysporum*, and *Trichoderma sporulosum*, respectively, the isolated metabolites, trichothecin (**26**) and trichodermol (**6**), both retained the $[2-{}^3H]$geranyl label and hence the (4R)-$[4-{}^3H]$mevalonate hydrogen atom from the central prenyl unit of farnesyl pyrophosphate as well (Adams and Hanson, 1971; Achilladelis *et al.*, 1972).

The observation that only the two hydrogen atoms at C(2) and C(10) of trichodermol (**6**) and trichothecolone (**25**), respectively, are identical with a *pro*-4R-mevalonate hydrogen atom, implies a hydrogen shift. It is known (Achilladelis *et al.*, 1970, 1972) that the hydrogen at C(10) of the trichothecene skeleton originates from the terminal prenyl fragment of farnesyl pyrophosphate. This result indicates that the central *pro*-4R-mevalonate hydrogen atom is transferred to C(2) of trichodermol (**6**) and trichothecolone (**25**) in the course of the biosynthetic transformations. These findings clearly preclude the intermediacy of a bisabolene derivative (**58**) in the biosynthesis.

A similar type of intramolecular hydride shift was also shown by Arigoni *et al.* (1973) to occur during the biosynthetic formation of verrucarol (**49**). All-*trans*-[6-^{3}H,12,13-^{14}C$_2$]farnesyl pyrophosphate was administered to a culture of *M. roridum*, and the isolated roridin A (**33**) was hydrolyzed to give verrucarol (**49**). Acetylation followed by acid-catalyzed rearrangement gave the apotrichothecane derivative, **62** (Fig. 12). The latter was oxidized to the α,β-unsaturated ketone **63** which on hydrolysis yielded compound **64**. The almost complete loss of tritium associated with the conversion of diacetoxy-diol **62** into the keto ether **64** served to locate the tritium label at C(2) or, less likely, at C(3) in verrucarol (**49**). This result extended the findings on the biosynthesis of trichodermol (**6**) and trichothecolone (**25**) and confirmed that farnesyl pyrophosphate cyclizes directly, and not via the bisabolene inter-mediate **58**. This conclusion was further supported both by the low and non-specific incorporation of labeled α-bisabolol, β- and γ-bisabolenes, and monocyclofarnesol, respectively, into trichothecin (**26**) (Forrester and Money, 1972) and by the observation that α-bisabolol is not incorporated into verrucarol (**49**) after administration to cultures of *M. roridum* (Knöll and Tamm, 1975).

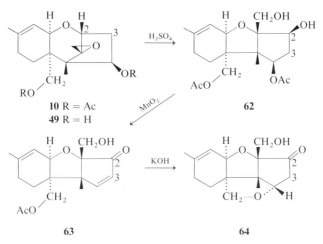

Fig. 12. Rearrangement of verrucarol. I.

On the basis of the observed hydride shift and of other evidence, Adams and Hanson (1971) and Achilladelis *et al.* (1972) proposed a concerted cycli-zation sequence initiated by the attack of an enzyme at C(10) of farnesyl pyrophosphate (**56**) (Fig. 13). This double addition to the central double bond (**56 → 65**) was stated to occur in an overall *cis* fashion (Arigoni *et al.*, 1973). Trichodiene (**66**) was postulated to be formed by a subsequent hydro-

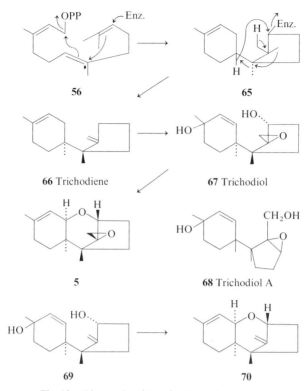

Fig. 13. Biogenetic scheme for the trichothecenes.

gen transfer from C(6) to C(10) of the precursor, followed by two methyl group rearrangements and abstraction of a proton. Trichodiene (**66**), which had already been suggested to be a precursor of trichothecin by Bu'Lock (1965), was later isolated from a strain of *Trichothecium roseum* (Nozoe and Machida, 1970b, 1972).

Other compounds of biogenetic significance were found in the same fungus; among them were trichodiol (**67**) and 12,13-epoxytrichothec-9-ene (**5**) (Machida and Nozoe, 1972b; Nozoe and Machida, 1972). In order to confirm the suggested relationship between these compounds and trichothecin (**26**), tritium-labeled trichodiene was prepared and administered to a culture of *Trichothecium roseum* (Machida and Nozoe, 1972a). An incorporation of 3.2% into trichothecolone (**25**) or trichothecin (**26**) was observed. The two minor metabolites isolated in this experiment, 12,13-epoxytrichothec-9-ene (**5**) and trichodiol A (**68**), were also shown to be labeled. Trichodiol A (**68**), first isolated by Nozoe and Machida (1970a), later proved to be an artefact produced from trichodiol (**67**) on treatment with base (Machida and Nozoe,

1972a; Nozoe and Machida, 1972). Therefore, trichodiene (66) may be considered a precursor of trichodiol (67), 12,13-epoxytrichothec-9-ene (5), and trichothecolone (25) or trichothecin (26). This biogenetic relationship was confirmed by Evans and Hanson (1976). Labeled trichodiene, prepared from [2-^{14}C]mevalonic acid, was fed to a growing culture of *Trichothecium roseum*. A 5.3% incorporation of the precursor into trichothecin (26) was observed.

The intermediacy of trichodiol (67) in the biosynthetic scheme has not yet been established conclusively. As stated by Machida and Nozoe (1972b), trichodiol (67) might be a metabolite of 12,13-epoxytrichothec-9-ene (5). In this connection, the recent isolation of verrucarin K (46) (Breitenstein and Tamm, 1977) is noteworthy. As stated earlier, this compound is the first naturally occurring trichothecene derivative lacking the 12,13-epoxy group. In view of this isolation, an alternative pathway may be postulated consisting of the direct cyclization of an intermediate of type 69 to the trichotheca-9,12-diene system 70 (Fig. 13).

Evans and Hanson (1976) and Evans *et al.* (1973) recognized that all-*trans*-farnesyl pyrophosphate acts as a precursor of trichodiene (66), although the cyclization step requires the 2-*cis* isomer, 56. Therefore, a *trans–cis* isomerization must take place. The experiments mentioned earlier using (4R)-[4-^{3}H,2-^{14}C]mevalonic acid had demonstrated that the *pro*-4R-mevalonate hydrogen atom, which was attached to C(2) of the double bond of farnesyl pyrophosphate, was retained through the biosynthesis of the trichothecene skeleton and hence in the isomerization step. Further details on the mechanism of the *trans–cis* isomerization and the subsequent cyclization were obtained via the incubation of some likely labeled farnesyl pyrophosphates with a cell-free system, prepared from *Trichothecium roseum* (Evans and Hanson, 1975, 1976; Evans *et al.*, 1973). In the presence of magnesium and manganese chlorides and reduced pyridine nucleotides, this cell-free preparation converted all-*trans*-[4,8,12-^{14}C$_3$]farnesyl pyrophosphate into trichodiene (66) within 2 hr in 50% yield. The specimen of trichodiene, obtained after incubation of all-*trans*-[2,6,10-^{3}H$_3$,4,8,12-^{14}C$_3$]farnesyl pyrophosphate was shown to retain all three tritium labels, thus confirming the above-mentioned result from (4R)-[4-^{3}H,2-^{14}C]mevalonic acid incorporation.

In a similar experiment, all-*trans*-[1,5,9-^{3}H$_6$,4,8,12-^{14}C$_3$]farnesyl pyrophosphate prepared enzymatically from [5-^{3}H$_2$,2-^{14}C]mevalonic acid was incubated with the cell-free preparation. From three isolated products, all-*trans*-farnesol retained all six tritium atoms, whereas only five labels were present in 2-*cis*-6-*trans*-farnesol as well as in trichodiene (66). Thus, the isomerization and cyclization of all-*trans*-farnesyl pyrophosphate takes place with the loss of one hydrogen atom. Bearing in mind the earlier results from the mevalonate incorporations, this hydrogen loss must occur at C(1) of the farnesyl pyrophosphate precursor.

In order to cast additional light on the stereochemistry of this elimination, all-*trans*-(1R)-[1,5,9-^{3}H$_3$,4,8,12-^{14}C$_3$]farnesyl pyrophosphate prepared enzymatically from (5R)-[5-^{3}H,2-^{14}C]mevalonic acid was incubated with the cell-free system. Trichodiene (**66**), isolated from this experiment, retained all three *pro*-5R-mevalonate hydrogen atoms. Therefore, the conversion of all-*trans*-farnesyl pyrophosphate into trichodiene (**66**) is accompanied by the loss of a *pro*-5S-mevalonate hydrogen atom which corresponds to the *pro*-1S hydrogen atom of farnesyl pyrophosphate. It was demonstrated that the lost hydrogen atom was replaced by a hydrogen from NADPH. Furthermore, it was established that, as in squalene biosynthesis (Cornforth *et al.*, 1966), it is the *pro*-4S hydrogen atom of NADPH which is transferred (Evans and Hanson, 1975, 1976).

Within the last few years, several cases pointing to the loss of the hydrogen atom at C(1) in the isomerization of farnesol have been reported implicating farnesals as intermediates (Overton and Roberts, 1973, 1974c; Suzuki and Marumo, 1972). The *trans–cis* reaction of farnesol in a cell-free system from *Andrographis paniculata* tissue cultures was demonstrated to proceed with the elimination of the *pro*-1S hydrogen atom (Overton and Roberts, 1974a, 1974b). Conversely, the *pro*-1R hydrogen atom was abstracted in the *trans–cis* isomerization of free farnesol when intact cultures of *Helminthosporium sativum* were used (Imai and Marumo, 1974). Chayet *et al.* (1973) investigated the biosynthesis of the farnesols from geranyl pyrophosphate and isopentenyl pyrophosphate in a cell-free preparation from orange flavedo. The order of appearance of the products was: *trans,trans*-farnesol; *trans,trans*-farnesal; *cis,trans*-farnesal; and *cis,trans*-farnesol. The cell-free system from *Trichothecium roseum*, however, could not utilize free farnesol as a substrate. Moreover, no significant radioactivity associated with farnesal was detected, and, in contrast to common redox systems, the introduced hydrogen atom originated from the "B" face of NADPH. Therefore, Evans and Hanson (1975) suggested that a different mechanism, not implicating farnesals as intermediates, might be involved in the *Trichothecium roseum* system. As outlined in Fig. 14, *trans,trans*-farnesyl pyrophosphate (**71**) was proposed to form first a cyclopropene intermediate **73** which on opening in the opposite stereochemical sense would yield, via carbenium ion **74** trichodiene (**66**).

In order to establish the fate of the retained *pro*-5R mevalonoid hydrogen atoms in farnesyl pyrophosphate during the later stages of the biosynthesis, several experiments were carried out with specifically tritiated precursors. Incorporation of (5R)-[5-^{3}H,2-^{14}C]mevalonate into trichothecolone (**25**)

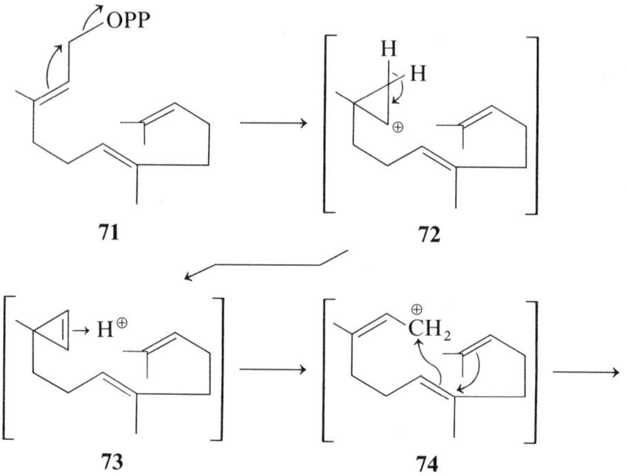

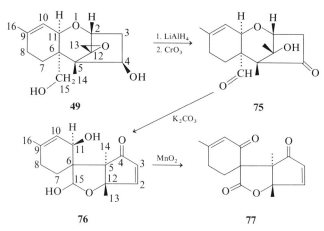

Fig. 14. Alternative mechanism for the cyclization of all-*trans*-farnesyl pyrophosphate.

(Evans *et al.*, 1974) and verrucarol (**49**) (Müller and Tamm, 1975) revealed that all three *pro-5R* mevalonate hydrogen atoms were retained during the formation of the metabolites. For the location of the labels, trichothecolone (**25**) from the $(5R)$-$[5$-$^3H,2$-$^{14}C]$mevalonate feeding was treated with aqueous sodium hydroxide. One label was lost, thus indicating the presence of a *pro-5R* mevalonate hydrogen atom at C(7) of trichothecolone (**25**). The distribution of the tritium labels in verrucarol (**49**) was determined by a series of degradations (Fig. 15) (Müller and Tamm, 1975). Reductive cleavage of the expoxy group of verrucarol (**49**) with lithium aluminum hydride yielded a triol which was oxidized with CrO_3 to the keto aldehyde **75**.

Fig. 15. Rearrangement of verrucarol. II.

Rearrangement of the oxidation product **75** to spirolactol **76** was accomplished by treatment with K_2CO_3 in aqueous methanol. During the conversion the tritium attached to C(3), i.e., in the α-position to the carbonyl group, was exchanged. Subsequent oxidation of compound **76** with MnO_2 to the spirolactone **77** resulted in the loss of a second tritium label, thus proving the identity of the hydrogen at C(11) of the trichothecene skeleton with a *pro-5R*-mevalonate hydrogen atom. This result indicates that the hydrogen atom which is introduced during the isomerization of *trans,trans*-farnesyl pyrophosphate is eliminated again during the subsequent steps.

In the last stage of the biosynthetic sequence, the 12,13-epoxytrichothec-9-ene system (**5**) formed is modified by various hydroxylations. The mechanism of these steps was studied by incorporation experiments with a number of mevalonates labeled at C(2) and C(5). $[2\text{-}^3H_2,2\text{-}^{14}C]$Mevalonate was administered to a culture of *Trichoderma sporulosum* (Adams and Hanson, 1970; Achilladelis *et al.*, 1972). Hydrolysis of the resulting trichodermin (**7**) afforded trichodermol (**6**), which showed the presence of 4.90 tritium atoms. Oxidation of trichodermol (**6**) to trichodermone (**78**) (Fig. 16) resulted in the loss of one tritium label from C(4). $[2\text{-}^3H_2,2\text{-}^{14}C]$Mevalonate was also fed to growing cultures of *Myrothecium species*. The isolated roridin A (**33**) was hydrolyzed to verrucarol (**49**), which contained 4.61 tritium atoms. On oxidation to the keto aldehyde **79**, verrucarol lost about one-fifth of its tritium activity, consistent with the attachment of one tritium at C(4) (Achini *et al.*, 1971; Müller *et al.*, 1975b).

In order to determine the stereochemistry of the C(4) hydroxylation of verrucarol (**49**), two separate feeding experiments with $(3R)\text{-}[(2S)\text{-}2\text{-}^3H]/$ $(3S)\text{-}[(2R)\text{-}2\text{-}^3H]$- and $(3R)\text{-}[(2R)\text{-}2\text{-}^3H]/(3S)\text{-}[(2S)\text{-}2\text{-}^3H]$mevalonate were carried out. From the incorporation of $(3R)\text{-}[5\text{-}^{14}C]$mevalonate into **49** it

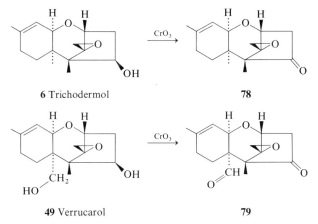

6 Trichodermol   **78**

49 Verrucarol   **79**

Fig. 16. Oxidation of trichodermol and verrucarol.

was already known that the natural $(3R)$ enantiomer of mevalonate is the biogenetic active unit. Oxidation of the verrucarol **(49)** from the $(3R)$-$[(2R)$-2-^{3}H$]/(3S)$-$[(2S)$-$[(2S)$-2-^{3}H$]$-$[2$-^{3}H$]$mevalonate experiment to the keto aldehyde **79** produced no change in the specific activity, whereas the same oxidative conversion of the verrucarol **(49)** from the $(3R)$-$[(2S)$-2-^{3}H$]/(3S)$-$[(2R)$-2-^{3}H$]$mevalonate incorporation was accompanied by the loss of about one-third the original tritium content (Achini et al., 1971; Müller et al., 1975b). When $(2R)$-$[2$-^{3}H,2-^{14}C$]$mevalonate was used as a precursor of trichodermol **(6)** in Trichoderma sporulosum (Adams and Hanson, 1970; Evans et al., 1974), 1.81 out of the three tritium labels were retained. Oxidation yielded trichodermone **(78)**, which showed the presence of 1.57 tritium atoms. (The departure from whole numbers in these experiments with $[2$-^{3}H$]$-labeled mevalonates was attributed to the reversible activity of prenyl isomerase.)

Incorporation of $(2R)$-$[2$-^{3}H,2-^{14}C$]$- and $(2S)$-$[2$-^{3}H,2-^{14}C$]$mevalonates into trichothecolone **(25)** gave similar results (Evans et al., 1974). Conversion of trichothecolone **(25)** from the $(2S)$-$[2$-^{3}H,2-^{14}C$]$mevalonate feeding to trichothecodione **(59)** resulted in the loss of half the activity, whereas the trichothecolone **(25)** from the $(2R)$-$[2$-^{3}H,2-^{14}C$]$mevalonate incorporation showed only a slight drop in activity on oxidation. Thus, in trichodermol **(6)**, trichothecolone **(25)**, and verrucarol **(49)**, respecitvely, the hydroxy group at C(4) replaces a pro-2R-mevalonate hydrogen atom. The assumption that the formation of the farnesyl pyrophosphate precursor takes place in the same manner as observed for the precursor of the steroids implies that hydroxylation at C(4) occurs with an overall retention of configuration (Adams and Hanson, 1970).

In order to establish the stereochemistry of the mevalonate labels at C(3) of the trichothecenes, Evans et al. (1974) used $(5R)$-$[5$-^{3}H,2-^{14}C$]$mevalonic acid as a precursor of calonectrin **(9)** in Fusarium culmorum. The isolated metabolite **9** which showed the presence of two out of three possible tritium labels was subjected to a partial hydrolysis, yielding 3-deacetylcalonectrin **(80)** (Fig. 17). Oxidation of **80** with the silver carbonate/celite reagent to ketone **81** resulted in only a slight drop in activity, thus indicating that hydroxylation at C(3) had replaced a pro-5R mevalonate hydrogen atom.

Further experiments were performed for the determination of the stereochemistry of the mevalonate labels at C(4) in calonectrin **(9)**. First it was demonstrated that the β-hydrogen atom at C(4) of ketone **81** exchanged with deuterium in the presence of sodium hydroxide in deuterium oxide and $[^2$H$_6]$acetone. $(2R)$-$[2$-^{3}H,2-^{14}C$]$- and $(2S)$-$[2$-^{3}H,2-^{14}C$]$Mevalonic acids were then administered in separate experiments to cultures of F. culmorum, and the isolated calonectrin **(9)** was converted into the ketone **81**. Subsequent hydrogen exchange with the ketone derived from the $(2R)$-

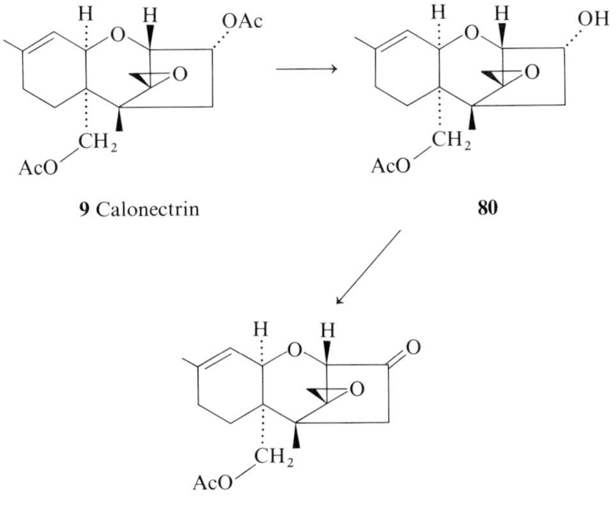

9 Calonectrin   **80**

81

Fig. 17.   Oxidative transformation of calonectrin.

$[2\text{-}^3\text{H},2\text{-}^{14}\text{C}]$mevalonate feeding was accompanied by the loss of nearly one tritium label, whereas when the ketone from the $(2S)\text{-}[2\text{-}^3\text{H},2\text{-}^{14}\text{C}]$-mevalonate incorporation was subjected to the same reaction no characteristic change in the tritium content was observed. It is concluded that a *pro-2R*-mevalonate hydrogen atom is located at the β-position of C(4). The labeling pattern at the centers C(3) and C(4) in the trichothecenes, resulting from a simple folding of farnesyl pyrophosphate as shown in Fig. 18, is in agreement with the results from calonectrin (**9**). Hydroxylations at C(3) and C(4) occur with retention of configuration (Evans *et al.*, 1974).

   Further feeding experiments with C(2)- and C(5)-labeled mevalonates were carried out to establish the origin of the C(8) carbonyl group in trichothecolone (**25**) and trichothecin (**26**), respectively. After the incorporation of $[2\text{-}^3\text{H}_2,2\text{-}^{14}\text{C}]$mevalonate trichothecolone retained four tritium atoms

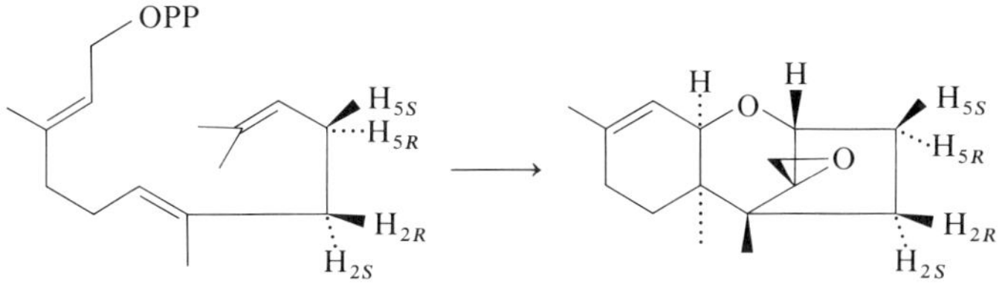

71   **5**

Fig. 18.   Labeling pattern at C(3) and C(4) of trichothecenes.

(Adams and Hanson, 1970; Achilladelis *et al.*, 1972). One of them, probably attached to C(7), was readily lost in an exchange reaction. If the C(8) carbonyl group was the result of a simple oxidation, trichothecolone (**25**) should contain only three tritium labels in this experiment. When $[5\text{-}^3H_2,2\text{-}^{14}C]$-mevalonate was used as a precursor, the isolated trichothecin (**26**) retained only four of the expected five labels. Therefore, Adams and Hanson (1970) and Achilladelis *et al.* (1972) suggested crotocin (**24**), which is also present in the same fungus, or a similar epoxide as a precursor of trichothecin (**26**). Rearrangement of the epoxide to the ketone would be accompanied by a hydrogen shift from C(8) to C(7). When, however, $(2R)\text{-}[2\text{-}^3H,2\text{-}^{14}C]$-mevalonate was used as a precursor, the isolated trichothecolone (**25**) retained one tritium atom, whereas the trichothecolone (**25**) derived from $(2S)\text{-}[2\text{-}^3H,2\text{-}^{14}C]$mevalonate showed the presence of two tritium labels, one of them at C(4) (Evans *et al.*, 1974). These results were not compatible with the suggested hydrogen transfer.

On repeating the feeding experiments with $[2\text{-}^3H_2,2\text{-}^{14}C]$- and $[5\text{-}^3H_2,2\text{-}^{14}C]$mevalonates, Evans *et al.* (1976) obtained results which differed from the earlier findings. Trichothecin (**26**) derived from $[2\text{-}^3H_2,2\text{-}^{14}C]$mevalonate contained three tritium atoms, whereas five labels were retained after incorporation of $[5\text{-}^3H_2,2\text{-}^{14}C]$mevalonate. Both preparations were subjected to an exchange reaction with concomitant hydrolysis in methan-$[^2H]$ol containing sodium deuteroxide. On this treatment, the trichothecin derived from $[5\text{-}^3H_2,2\text{-}^{14}C]$mevalonate lost two tritium atoms from C(7). On the other hand, no loss of label was observed when trichothecin derived from the $[2\text{-}^3H_2,2\text{-}^{14}C]$mevalonate incorporation was subjected to the same exchange. These results clearly precluded the intermediacy of a 7,8-epoxide, such as crotocin, in the biosynthesis of trichothecolone.

Further investigations directed toward establishing the origin of the C(8) carbonyl group of trichothecolone (**25**) were carried out. It was demonstrated that trichodermol (**6**), a trichothecene metabolite lacking the C(8)-carbonyl group, co-occurs with trichothecin (**26**) in *Trichothecium roseum* (Evans *et al.*, 1976). $[2,10\text{-}^3H_2,4,8,14\text{-}^{14}C_3]$Trichodermol was prepared by administering $(4R)\text{-}[4\text{-}^3H,2\text{-}^{14}C]$mevalonate to a growing culture of *Trichoderma sporulosum* followed by hydrolysis of the isolated trichodermin. The labeled trichodermol was incorporated with a 3.4% yield into trichothecin by *Trichothecium roseum* (Evans *et al.*, 1976). A possible biogenetic intermediate in this conversion from trichodermol (**6**) to trichothecin (**26**) is the diol **15**, which had already been isolated from *Trichothecium roseum* by Machida and Nozoe (1972b). In order to establish this biogenetic relationship, the two epimeric diols $[8\beta\text{-}^3H,4,8,14\text{-}^{14}C_3]-4\beta$,8$\alpha$-dihydroxy-12,13-epoxytrichothec-9-ene and $[8\alpha\text{-}^3H,4,8,14\text{-}^{14}C_3]-4\beta$, 8$\beta$-dihydroxy-12, 13-epoxytrichothec-9-ene were prepared and administered to a growing culture of *Trichothecium* *roseum.* Both preparations were incorporated into trichothecin (**26**) with a 6.6% and 5.6% yield, respectively, (Evans *et al.*, 1976). Only 4β,8α-dihydroxy-12,13-epoxytrichothec-9-ene (**15**) has so far been isolated from *Trichothecium roseum* (Machida and Nozoe, 1972b). Therefore, this is the likely intermediate.

The esterification of trichothecolone (**25**), which co-occurs with trichothecin (**26**) in *Trichothecium roseum*, is probably one of the last steps in the biosynthesis of trichothecin (**26**). The intermediacy of trichothecolone was demonstrated by the successful conversion of a suitably labeled trichothecolone preparation into trichothecin (**26**) by *Trichothecium roseum* (Evans *et al.*, 1976). The sequence of the last stages in the biosynthetic formation of trichothecin (**26**) in *Trichothecium roseum* is outlined in Fig. 19 (Evans *et al.*, 1976; Machida and Nozoe, 1972b).

6 Trichodermol   15

25 Trichothecolone   26 Trichothecin

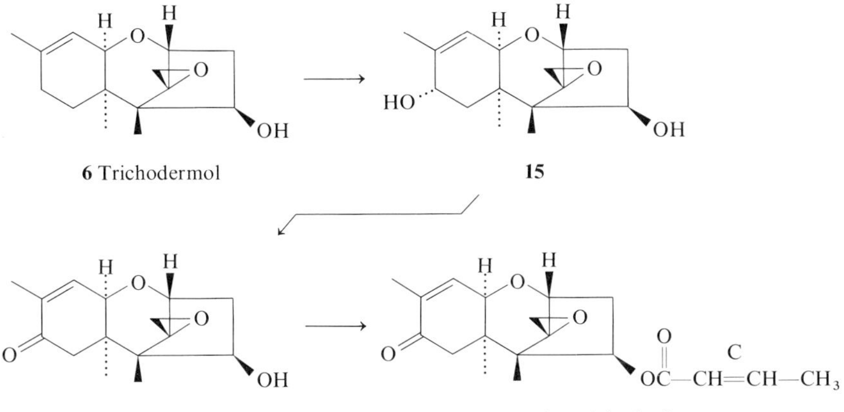

Fig. 19.   Last stages in the biosynthetic formation of trichothecin.

III. BIOSYNTHESIS OF THE RORIDINS AND VERRUCARINS

For the elucidation of the biosynthesis of the macrocyclic part of the verrucarins and roridins, a number of feeding experiments were carried out by adding likely [14]C- and ^{3}H-labeled precursors to cultures of *Myrothecium species*. In order to determine the distribution of the radioactivity, the isolated metabolites were subjected to several degradation reactions (Achini *et al.*, 1974; Müller *et al.*, 1975a; Tamm, 1968).

Verrucarin A (**32**) obtained after the incorporation of [1-^{14}C]acetate was hydrolyzed with K_2CO_3 in aqueous methanol to afford, after acidification, verrucarol (**49**), *cis,trans*-muconic acid (**83**), and verrucarinic acid (**86**), isolated as a lactone (**87**) (Fig. 20). The measurement of the radioactivities of the three products (**49**, **84**, and **87**) suggested that of the 12 acetate units of verrucarin A (**32**), six were located in verrucarol (**49**) and three each in *cis,trans*-muconic acid (**83**) and verrucarinolactone (**87**). Radioactivity was located by converting *cis,trans*-muconic acid (**83**) into adipic acid (**89**). Schmidt degradation of the latter afforded 1,4-diaminobutane (**90**) along with two equivalents of CO_2, isolated as $BaCO_3$ (Fig. 21). 1,4-Diaminobutane (**90**) contained two-thirds the total radioactivity of the starting material. Only one of the two carboxy groups of *cis,trans*-muconic acid (**83**) was labeled.

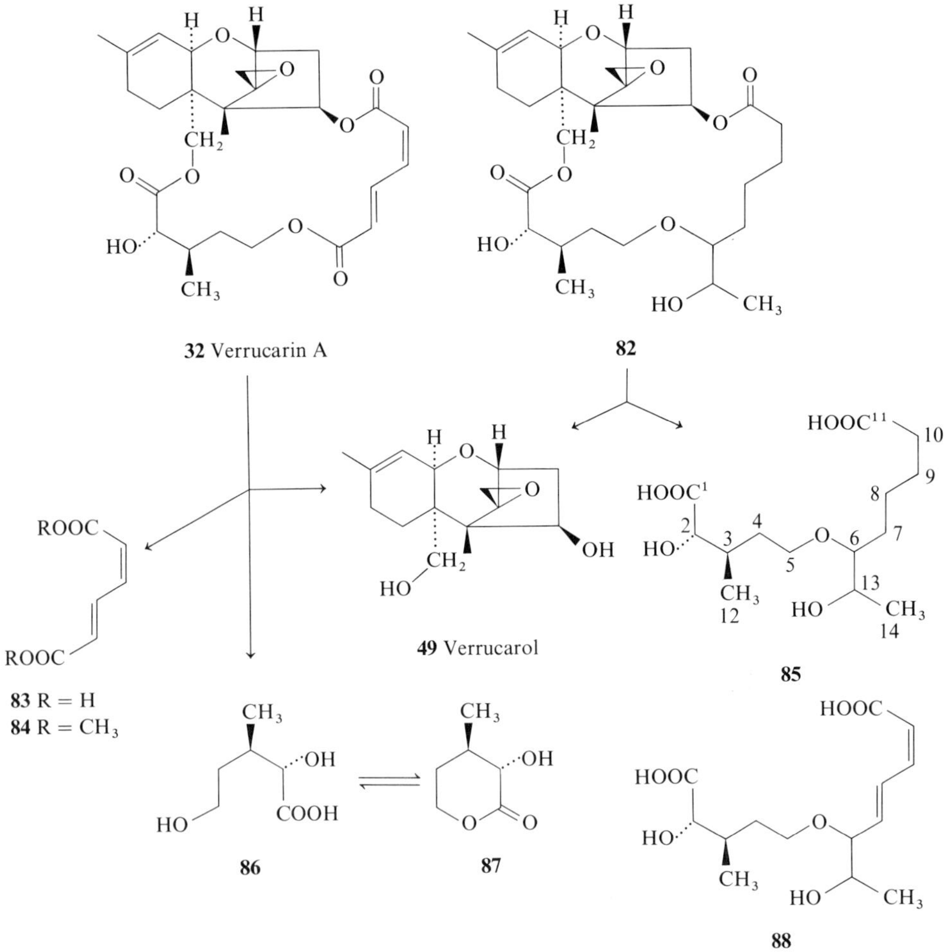

Fig. 20.   Hydrolysis of verrucarin A and tetrahydrororidin A.

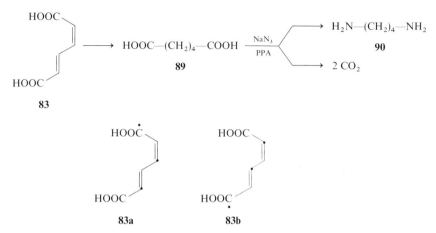

Fig. 21. Degradation of muconic acid. PPA = polyphosphoric acid.

On the basis of these results, two different labeling patterns (**83a** and **83b**) were proposed for muconic acid (Fig. 21) (Müller *et al.*, 1975a). However, the possibility that these two distributions could arise at the same time was not precluded by the experimental data available.

For the location of the labeled centers in the macrocyclic part of roridin A (**33**), the latter was converted into the corresponding tetrahydro derivative **82** and then hydrolyzed with KOH in aqueous methanol to afford verrucarol (**49**) and tetrahydrororidinic acid (**85**). Careful oxidation of the isolated acid **85** with $KMnO_4$ yielded CO_2, which contained 13.8% of the total ^{14}C-activity, suggesting that seven acetate units are involved in the biosynthetic formation of roridinic acid (**88**). Further oxidation of the nonvolatile residue of the oxidative cleavage led to the nor-acid **92**, which was subjected to a Schmidt degradation (Fig. 22). The CO_2 derived from C(2) and C(11) was collected as $BaCO_3$ and the radioactivity was measured. The results indicated that C(11) originated from the carboxyl group of acetic acid. By analogy, it was concluded that the *cis*-carboxy group of muconic acid (**83**) is also derived from C(1) of acetate. Thus, the alternating labeling shown in formula **83a** is probably realized in *cis,trans*-muconic acid. By subjecting tetrahydrororidinic acid (**85**) from the incorporation of $[2\text{-}^{14}C]$mevalonate to the same sequence of degradative conversions, the label of mevalonate could be located in the carboxy group of the nor-acid **92**. Consequently, roridinic acid (**88**) is probably built up from an isoprenoid unit and a polyketide or its biogenetic equivalent.

A heterocyclic fragmentation reaction was elaborated, permitting the separation of these two suggested biogenetic moieties (Müller *et al.*, 1975a). Dimethyl tetrahydrororidinate (**91**), derived from the incorporation of

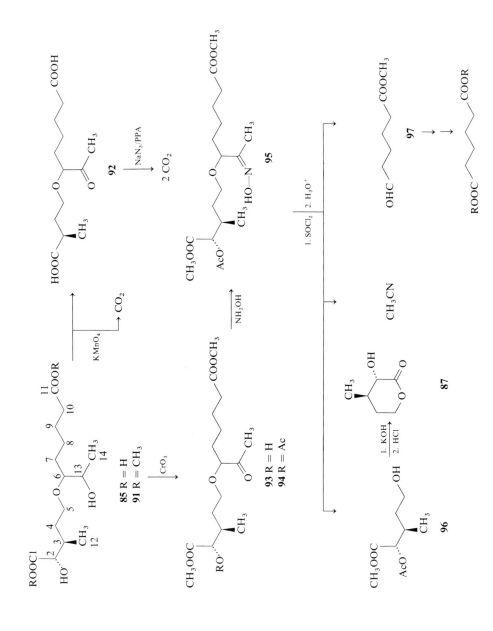

[2-^{14}C,2-^{3}H$_2$]mevalonate, was oxidized to the corresponding 13-dehydro derivative **93**. Acetylation of the free hydroxy group yielded the acetyl derivative **94**, which was transformed into oxime **95**. Subsequent Beckmann fragmentation, induced by treatment of the oxime **95** with SOCl$_2$, gave three products. One of them, the methyl ester **96**, was hydrolyzed to yield verruca-rinolactone (**87**). The aldehyde **97** was converted into the *p*-bromophenacyl ester of adipic acid (**98**). The results of the measurements of the ^{3}H- and ^{14}C-activity of the cleavage products **87** and **98** indicated that the radioactivity was confined to the verrucarinic acid portion of roridinic acid (**88**). On the basis of these findings, a hypothetical scheme for the biogenetic formation of muconic acid and roridinic acid was proposed to be as outlined in Fig. 23 (Müller *et al.*, 1975a).

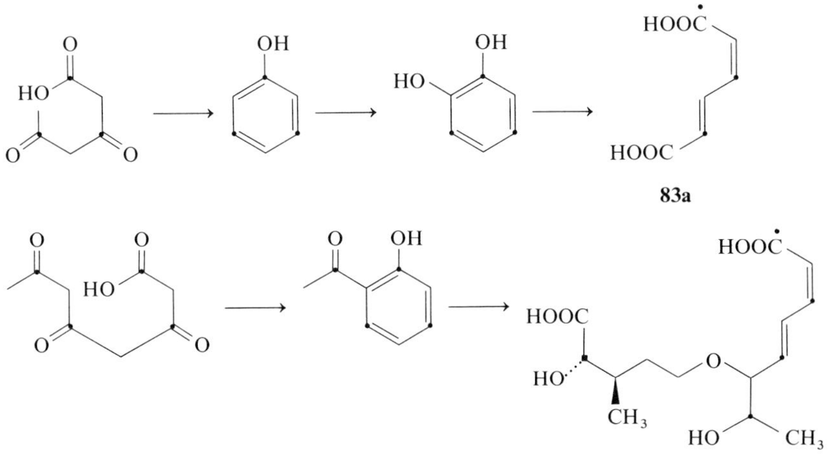

83a

88a

Fig. 23. Biogenetic scheme for the formation of muconic acid and roridinic acid. Filled circles = C(1) of acetate; filled squares = C(2) of mevalonate.

Further feeding experiments were necessary for investigations on the origin of verrucarinic acid (**86**) and on the mechanism of its formation. Upon hydrolysis, verrucarin A (**32**) that was obtained after incorporation of [2-^{14}C]mevalonate yielded radioactive verrucarol (**49**) and verrucarino-lactone (**87**) as well as inactive muconic acid (**83**). The measured activity suggested that one mevalonate unit participates in the formation of verru-carinic acid (**86**). For the location of the labeled centers, the verrucarino-lactone from the [2-^{14}C]mevalonate experiment was reduced to the triol **99**. Cleavage of the latter with HIO$_4$ yielded 2-methyl-4-hydroxybutanal

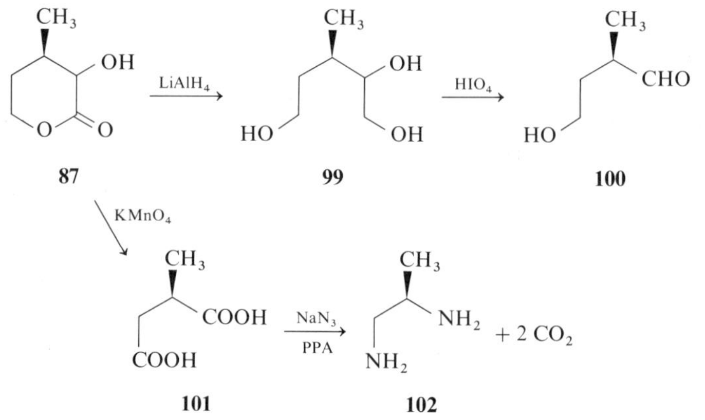

Fig. 24. Degradation of verrucarinolactone. I. PPA = polyphosphoric acid.

(100) along with practically inactive formaldehyde (Fig. 24) (Achini et al., 1974).

In a second degradation sequence, verrucarinolactone (87) was oxidized to (R)-(+)-methylsuccinic acid (101). Schmidt degradation of this acid afforded radioinactive 1,2-diaminopropane (102) and two equivalents of active CO_2, isolated as $BaCO_3$. From these results it was concluded that the carbon skeleton of mevalonate had undergone neither a rearrangement nor an exchange of the state of oxidation of C(1) and C(5), respectively.

In order to study the mechanism of the conversion of mevalonic acid into verrucarinic acid (86), feeding experiments with doubly labeled mevalonates were carried out. Verrucarinolactone obtained from the incorporation of [2-$^3H_2$,2-^{14}C]mevalonate into verrucarin A (32) was reduced with lithium aluminum hydride (Fig. 25). Subsequent cleavage with $NaIO_4$ and oxidation of the formed hydroxyaldehyde with bromine in water gave, after acidification, 2-methylbutyrolactone (103), which was treated with phenylmagnesium bromide in ether to yield the carbinol 104. Selective esterification of the primary hydroxy group of compound 104 led to the 3,5-dinitrobenzoyl derivative 105, which showed an unchanged $^3H:^{14}C$ ratio in comparison with verrucarinolactone (87).

Dehydration of compound 105 with $SOCl_2$ resulted in the complete loss of ^3H-activity. Oxidative cleavage of the double bond of 106 with OsO_4 and $NaIO_4$ yielded the 3,5-dinitrobenzoyl derivative of 4-hydroxybutan-2-one (107), which was radioinactive, and benzophenone (108), containing 99.5% of the original ^{14}C-activity. Therefore, C(2) of verrucarinic acid (86) is biogenetically identical with C(2) of mevalonic acid. Furthermore, the results of the degradation studies provide strong evidence that the biogenetic

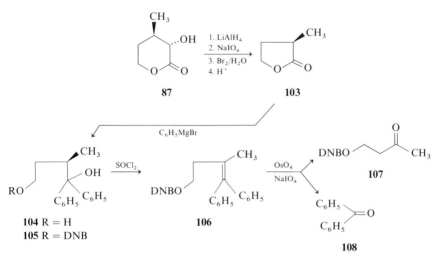

Fig. 25. Degradation of verrucarinolactone. II. DNB = 3,5-dinitrobenzoyl.

transformation of mevalonic acid into verrucarinic acid is accompanied by a hydrogen transfer from C(2) of mevalonate to C(3) of verrucarinate.

In order to cast additional light on the stereochemical aspects of this migration, feeding experiments with stereospecifically tritiated mevalonates were performed. The separate administration of $(3R)$-$[(2S)$-2-^{3}H$]$/(3S)-$[(2R)$-2-^{3}H$]$- and $(3R)$-$[(2R)$-2-^{3}H$]$/(3S)-$[(2S)$-2-^{3}H$]$mevalonates to cultures of *Myrothecium* species gave radio-inactive verrucarinolactone (**87**) from the first and active verrucarinolactone from the second incorporation. Because it is the natural $(3R)$ enantiomer of mevalonate that is incorporated into verrucarinate, these results indicate that the *pro*-2S-mevalonate hydrogen atom is lost during formation of verrucarinic acid (**86**). The *pro*-2R hydrogen atom is retained and transferred to C(3) of verrucarinate.

A possible mechanism for the formation of verrucarinate was proposed by Achini *et al.* (1974) and is outlined in Fig. 26. It is anticipated that the first step is a *trans*- or *cis*-elimination of H$_2$O from mevalonate (**109**) leading to *cis*- or *trans*-anhydromevalonate (**110a** or **110b**). On epoxidation of the olefinic double bond, two pairs of enantiomeric glycidic acids (**111** and **112**) are formed. Cleavage of the C(3) oxygen bond of the protonated "*β*-epoxide" **113** followed by a 1,2-shift of the *pro*-2R hydrogen atom H$_A$ of mevalonate (**109**) yields 2-dehydroverrucarinate (**115**) with concurrent inversion of the center C(3). In the last step, ketone **115** is stereospecifically reduced to yield verrucarinate (**117**). As shown in Fig. 26, formation of verrucarinate (**117**) from the "*α*-epoxide" **112** is also possible. Nevertheless the *β*-epoxide **111** was assumed to be the real intermediate (Achini *et al.*,

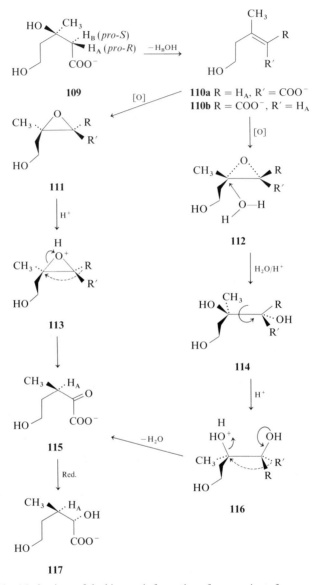

Fig. 26. Mechanisms of the biogenetic formation of verrucarinate from mevalonate.

1974). According to the X-ray analysis of verrucarin B (34) the 2,3-epoxy-anhydromevalonic acid moiety possesses the 2S,3R-configuration. On this basis Breitenstein *et al.* (1979) have proposed very recently that the biogenetic transformation of mevalonate to verrucarinate (117) proceeds via *cis*-elimination of water to yield *trans*-anhydromevalonate (110b). The latter is epoxidized to the glycidic acid 111 and transformed to verrucarinate (117) via the intermediates 113 and 115.

According to the proposed mechanism for the transformation of meva-lonate (109) into verrucarinate (117), a biogenetic sequence of the macrocyclic metabolites of *Myrothecium species* may be formulated, starting with verrucarin J (36), followed by verrucarin B (34) and 2'-dehydroverrucarin A (38), and ending with the major metabolite verrucarin A (32). For the roridins the corresponding order would be roridin E (37) and roridin H (39), roridin D (35), and roridin A (33). However, numerous problems remain unresolved. Thus, it is not yet known if the trichothecene portion and the acids are built up separately, simultaneously, or in subsequent steps before they are combined. Furthermore, it is not yet clear at which stage the ester linkages are formed.

REFERENCES

Abrahamsson, S., and Nilsson, B. (1964). *Proc. Chem. Soc. London*, 188.
Abrahamsson, S., and Nilsson, B. (1966). *Acta Chem. Scand.* 20, 1044–1052.
Achilladelis, B., and Hanson, J. R. (1968). *Phytochemistry* 7, 589–594.
Achilladelis, B., and Hanson, J. R. (1969). *Phytochemistry* 8, 765–767.
Achilladelis, B., Adams, P. M., and Hanson, J. R. (1970). *Chem. Commun.*, pp. 511.
Achilladelis, B. A., Adams, P. M., and Hanson, J. R. (1972). *J. Chem. Soc. Perkin Trans. 1*, 1425–1428.
Achini, R., Müller, B., and Tamm, Ch. (1971). *Chem. Commun.*, pp. 404–405.
Achini, R., Müller, B., and Tamm, Ch. (1974). *Helv. Chim. Acta.* 57, 1442–1459.
Adams, P. M., and Hanson, J. R. (1970). *Chem. Commun.*, pp. 1569–1570.
Adams, P. M., and Hanson, J. R. (1971). *Chem. Commun.*, pp. 1414–1415.
Arigoni, D., Cane, D. E., Müller, B., and Tamm, Ch. (1973). *Helv. Chim. Acta.* 56, 2946–2949.
Bamburg, J. R. (1976). *Adv. Chem. Ser.* 149, 144–162.
Bamburg, J. R., and Strong, F. M. (1969). *Phytochemistry*, 8, 2405–2410.
Bamburg, J. R., Riggs, N. V., and Strong, F. M. (1968). *Tetrahedron* 24, 3329–3336.
Blight, M. M., and Grove, J. F. (1974). *J. Chem. Soc. Perkin Trans. 1*, pp. 1691–1693.
Böhner, B., and Tamm, Ch. (1966a). *Helv. Chim. Acta.* 49, 2527–2546.
Böhner, B., and Tamm, Ch. (1966b). *Helv. Chim. Acta.* 49, 2547–2554.
Böhner, B., Fetz, E., Härri, E., Sigg, H. P., Stoll, Ch., and Tamm, Ch. (1965). *Helv. Chim. Acta.* 48, 1079–1087.
Breitenstein, W. (1975). Ph.D. thesis, University of Basel, Basel, Switzerland.
Breitenstein, W., and Tamm, Ch. (1977). *Helv. Chim. Acta.* 60, 1522–1527.
Breitenstein, W., Tamm, Ch., Arnold, E. V., and Clardy, J. (1979). *Helv. Chim. Acta.* 62, 2699–2705.

Brian, P. W., Dawkins, A. W., Grove, J. F., Hemming, H. G., Lowe, D., and Norris, G. L. F. (1961). *J. Exp. Bot.* **12**, 1–12.

Bu'Lock, J. D. (1965). "The Biosynthesis of Natural Products." McGraw-Hill, New York.

Chayet, L., Pont-Lezica, R., George-Nascimento, C., and Cori, O. (1973). *Phytochemistry* **12**, 95–101.

Cordell, G. A. (1976). *Chem. Rev.* **76**, 425–460.

Cornforth, J. W., Cornforth, R. H., Donninger, C., Popjak, G., Ryback, G., and Schroepfer, G. J. (1966). *Proc. Roy. Soc. London, Ser. B* **163**, 436–464.

Dawkins, A. W. (1966). *J. Chem. Soc. C.*, pp. 116–123.

Dawkins, A. W., Grove, J. F., and Tidd, B. K. (1965). *Chem. Commun.*, pp. 27–28.

Eppley, R. M., and Bailey, W. J. (1973). *Science* **181**, 758–760.

Eppley, R. M., Mazzola, E. P., Highet, R. J., and Bailey, W. J. (1977). *J. Org. Chem.* **42**, 240–243.

Evans, R., and Hanson, J. R. (1975). *J. Chem. Soc. Chem. Commun.*, pp. 231–232.

Evans, R., and Hanson, J. R. (1976). *J. Chem. Soc. Perkin Trans. 1*, pp. 326–329.

Evans, R., Holtom, A. M., and Hanson, J. R. (1973). *J. Chem. Soc., Chem. Commun.*, p. 465.

Evans, R., Hanson, J. R., and Marten, T. (1974). *J. Chem. Soc. Perkin Trans. 1*, pp. 857–860.

Evans, R., Hanson, J. R., and Marten, T. (1976). *J. Chem. Soc. Perkin Trans. 1*, pp. 1212–1214.

Fetz, E., Böhner, B., and Tamm, Ch. (1965). *Helv. Chim. Acta* **48**, 1669–1679.

Fishman, J., Jones, E. R. H., Lowe, G., and Whiting, M. C. (1959). *Proc. Chem. Soc. London*, 127–128.

Fishman, J., Jones, E. R. H., Lowe, G., and Whiting, M. C. (1960). *J. Chem. Soc.*, pp. 3948–3959.

Flury, E., Mauli, R., and Sigg, H. P. (1965). *Chem. Commun.* pp. 26–27.

Forrester, J. M., and Money, T. (1972). *Can. J. Chem.* **50**, 3310–3314.

Freeman, G. G., and Morrison, R. I. (1948). *Nature (London)*, **162**, 30.

Freeman, G. G., Gill, J. E., and Waring, W. S. (1959). *J. Chem. Soc.*, pp. 1105–1132.

Gardner, D., Glen, A. T., and Turner, W. B. (1972). *J. Chem. Soc. Perkin Trans. 1*, pp. 2576–2578.

Gláz, E. T., Scheiber, E., Gyimesi, J., Horvath, I., Steczek, K., Szëntirmai, A., and Bohus, G. (1959). *Nature (London)* **184**, 908.

Gláz, E. T., Csányi, E., and Gyimesi, J. (1966). *Nature (London)* **212**, 617–618.

Godtfredsen, W. O., and Vangedal, S. (1964). *Proc. Chem. Soc. London*, 188–189.

Godtfredsen, W. O., and Vangedal, S. (1965). *Acta Chem. Scand.* **19**, 1088–1102.

Godtfredsen, W. O., Grove, J. F., and Tamm, Ch. (1967). *Helv. Chim. Acta.* **50**, 1666–1668.

Grove, J. F. (1969). *Chem. Commun.*, pp. 1266–1267.

Grove, J. F. (1970a). *J. Chem. Soc. C*, pp. 375–378.

Grove, J. F. (1970b). *J. Chem. Soc. C*, pp. 378–379.

Gutzwiller, J., and Tamm, Ch. (1963). *Helv. Chim. Acta* **46**, 1786–1790.

Gutzwiller, J., and Tamm, Ch. (1965a). *Helv. Chim. Acta* **48**, 157–176.

Gutzwiller, J., and Tamm, Ch. (1965b). *Helv. Chim. Acta* **48**, 177–182.

Gutzwiller, J., Mauli, R., Sigg, H. P., and Tamm, Ch. (1964). *Helv. Chim. Acta* **47**, 2234–2262.

Gyimesi, J., and Melera, A. (1967). *Tetrahedron Lett.* pp. 1665–1673.

Hanson, J. R., and Achilladelis, B. (1967). *Chem. Ind. (London)*, 1643–1644.

Hanson, J. R., Marten, T., and Siverns, M. (1974). *J. Chem. Soc. Perkin Trans. 1*, pp. 1033–1036.

Härri, E., Loeffler, W., Sigg, H. P., Stähelin, H., Stoll, Ch., Tamm, Ch., and Wiesinger, D. (1962). *Helv. Chim. Acta* **45**, 839–853.

Ilus, T., Ward, P. J., Nummi, M., Adlercreutz, H., and Gripenberg, J. (1977). *Phytochemistry* **16**, 1839–1840.

Imai, K., and Marumo, S. (1974). *Tetrahedron Lett.*, pp. 4401–4404.

Ishii, K. (1975). *Phytochemistry* **14**, 2469–2471.

Ishii, K., Sakai, K., Ueno, Y., Tsunoda, H., and Enomoto, M. (1971). *Appl. Microbiol.* **22**, 718–720.

Jones, E. R. H., and Lowe, G. (1960). *J. Chem. Soc.*, pp. 3959–3962.

Knöll, W., and Tamm, Ch. (1975). *Helv. Chim. Acta.* **58**, 1162–1171.

Kocor, M., and Siewinski, A. (1966). *Acad. Polon. Sci. Ser. Sci. Chim.* **14**, 341–345.

Kotsonis, F. N., Ellison, R. A., and Smalley, E. B. (1975). *Appl. Microbiol.* **30**, 493–495.

Kupchan, S. M., Jarvis, B. B., Dailey, R. G. Jr., Bright, W., Bryan, R. F., and Shizuri, Y. (1976). *J. Am. Chem. Soc.* **98**, 7092–7093.

Machida, Y., and Nozoe, S. (1972a). *Tetrahedron Lett.*, pp. 1969–1971.

Machida, Y., and Nozeo, S. (1972b). *Tetrahedron* **28**, 5113–5117.

McPhail, A. T., and Sim, G. A. (1966). *J. Chem. Soc. C*, pp. 1394–1406.

Matsumoto, M., Minato, H., Uotani, N., Matsumoto, K., Kondo, E. (1977a). *J. Antibiot.* **30**, 681–682.

Matsumoto, M., Minato, H., Tori, K., and Ueyama, M. (1977b). *Tetrahedron Lett.*, pp. 4093–4096.

Minato, H., Katayama, T., and Tori, K. (1975). *Tetrahedron Lett.*, pp. 2579–2582.

Mirocha, C. J., and Pathre, S. (1973). *Appl. Microbiol.* **26**, 719–724.

Müller, B., and Tamm, Ch. (1975). *Helv. Chim. Acta* **58**, 483–488.

Müller, B., Achini, R., and Tamm, Ch. (1975a). *Helv. Chim. Acta* **58**, 453–470.

Müller, B., Achini, R., and Tamm, Ch. (1975b). *Helv. Chim. Acta* **58**, 471–482.

Nozoe, S., and Machida, Y. (1970a). *Tetrahedron Lett.*, pp. 1177–1179.

Nozoe, S., and Machida, Y. (1970b). *Tetrahedron Lett.*, pp. 2671–2674.

Nozoe, S., and Machida, Y. (1972). *Tetrahedron* **28**, 5105–5111.

Okuchi, M., Itoh, M., Kaneko, Y., and Doi, S. (1968). *Agr. Biol. Chem. (Tokyo)* **32**, 394–395.

Overton, K. H., and Roberts, F. M. (1973). *J. Chem. Soc., Chem. Commun.*, pp. 378–379.

Overton, K. H., and Roberts, F. M. (1974a). *J. Chem. Soc., Chem. Commun.*, pp. 385–386.

Overton, K. H., and Roberts, F. M. (1974b). *Biochem. J.* **144**, 585–592.

Overton, K. H., and Roberts, F. M. (1974c). *Phytochemistry* **13**, 2741–2743.

Parker, W., Roberts, J. S., and Ramage, R. (1967). *Quart. Rev. Chem. Soc.* **21**, 331–363.

Pathre, S. V., Mirocha, C. J., Christensen, C. M., and Behrens, J. (1976). *J. Agric. Food Chem.* **24**, 97–103.

Ruzicka, L. (1963). *Pure Appl. Chem.* **6**, 493–522.

Sigg, H. P., Mauli, R., Flury, E., and Hauser, D. (1965). *Helv. Chim. Acta* **48**, 962–988.

Smalley, E. B., and Strong, F. M. (1974). *In* "Mycotoxins" (I. F. H. Purchase, ed.), pp. 199–228. Elsevier, Amsterdam.

Suzuki, Y., and Marumo, S. (1972). *Tetrahedron Lett.*, pp. 5101–5104.

Tamm, Ch. (1966). *Angew. Chemie* **78**, 496–497.

Tamm, Ch. (1968). *Chimia* **22**, 315–316.

Tamm, Ch. (1974). *Progr. Chem. Org. Nat. Prod.* **31**, 64–117.

Tamm, Ch., and Gutzwiller, J. (1962). *Helv. Chim. Acta* **45**, 1726–1731.

Tatsuno, T., Saito, M., Enomoto, M., and Tsunoda, H. (1968). *Chem. Pharm. Bull.* **16**, 2519–2520.

Tatsuno, T., Fujimoto, Y., and Morita, Y. (1969). *Tetrahedron Lett.*, pp. 2823–2826.

Tatsuno, T., Morita, Y., Tsunoda, H., and Umeda, M. (1970). *Chem. Pharm. Bull.* **18**, 1485–1487.

Tidd, B. K. (1967). *J. Chem. Soc. C*, pp. 218–220.

Traxler, P., and Tamm, Ch. (1970). *Helv. Chim. Acta* **53**, 1846–1869.

Traxler, P., Zürcher, W., and Tamm, Ch. (1970). *Helv. Chim. Acta* **53**, 2071–2085.

Ueno, Y., Ueno, I., Tatsuno, T., Ohokubo, K., and Tsunoda, H. (1969). *Experientia* **25**, 1062.

Ueno, Y., Ueno, I., Amakai, K., Ishikawa, Y., Tsunoda, H., Okubo, K., Saito, M., and Enomoto, M. (1971). *Jpn. J. Exp. Med.* **41**, 507–519.

Ueno, Y., Ishii, K., Sakai, K., Kanaeda, S., Tsunoda, H., Tanaka, T., and Enomoto, M. (1972). *Jpn. J. Exp. Med.* **42**, 187–203.

Vesonder, R. F., Ciegler, A., and Jensen, A. H. (1973). *Appl. Microbiol.* **26**, 1008–1010.
Vesonder, R. F., Ciegler, A., Jensen, A. H., Rohwedder, W. K., and Weisleder, D. (1976). *Appl. Environ. Microbiol.* **31**, 280–285.
Wei, R. D., Strong, F. M., Smalley, E. B., and Schnoes, H. K. (1971). *Biochem. Biophys. Res. Commun.* **45**, 396–401.
Yates, S. G., Tookey, H. L., Ellis, J. J., and Burkhardt, H. J. (1968). *Phytochemistry* **7**, 139–146.
Yoshizawa, T., and Morooka, N. (1973). *Agric. Biol. Chem.* **37**, 2933–2934.
Zürcher, W., and Tamm, Ch. (1966). *Helv. Chim. Acta* **49**, 2594–2597.

4

The Biosynthesis of Aflatoxin and Its Congeners

PIETER S. STEYN, ROBERT VLEGGAAR,
AND PHILIPPUS L. WESSELS

I. INTRODUCTION

The discovery in 1960 of the Turkey-X disease in England initiated the present tremendous resurgence of interest in mycotoxins among scientists of many disciplines. The etiological agent was found to be Brazilian peanut meal, contaminated with toxins produced by the ubiquitous mold, *Aspergillus flavus*. The characterization of the toxic components (Asao *et al.*, 1965), given the generic name of aflatoxins, is one of the notable accomplishments in the chemistry of natural products in recent times. The aflatoxins constitute a number of structurally related metabolites which differ considerably in their biological effects. All these toxins, however, contain a

The Biosynthesis of Mycotoxins

coumarin ring fused to a bisdihydrofurano moiety and additionally either a cyclopentenone ring (B series) or a six-membered lactone (G series). The coumarins (**1–7**) (see Fig. 1) are formed by the cultivation of *A. flavus* both on solid and in liquid media.

Aflatoxin B_1 occurs most widely and has the greatest biological activity of this group of toxins. It is carcinogenic in several animal species and is the most potent hepatocarcinogen known for the rat and the rainbow trout (Wogan *et al.*, 1974). Data from several population-based studies indicated that elevated aflatoxin intake is associated with an increased incidence of human liver cancer, e.g., in Mozambique (Van Rensburg *et al.*, 1974); it may also be related to Reye's syndrome in Thailand (Shank, 1976). Aflatoxins can contaminate many commodities, e.g., peanuts, Brazil nuts,

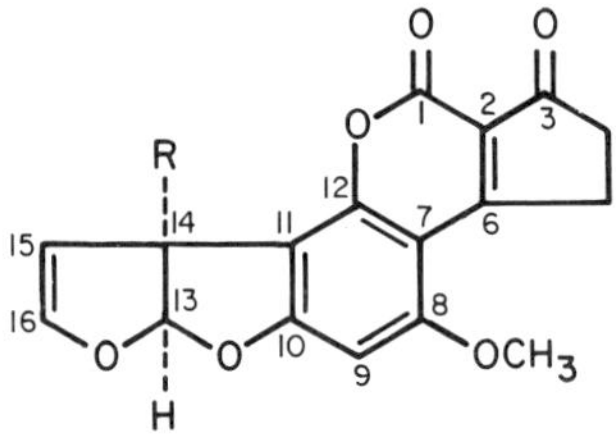

1 R = H : AFLATOXIN B_1
2 R = OH : AFLATOXIN M_1

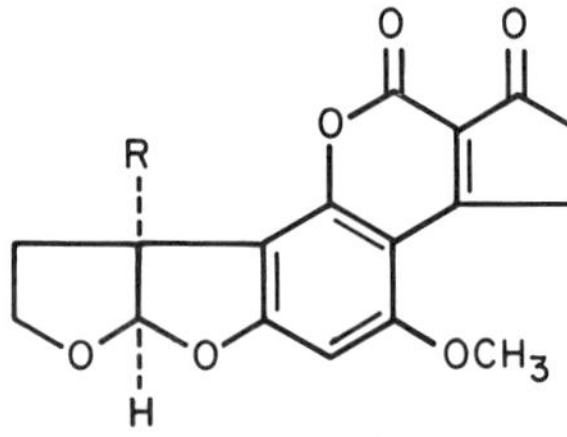

3 R = H : AFLATOXIN B_2
4 R = OH : AFLATOXIN M_2

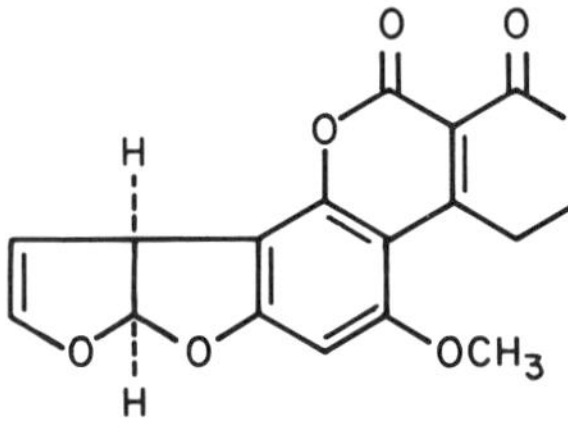

5 AFLATOXIN G_1

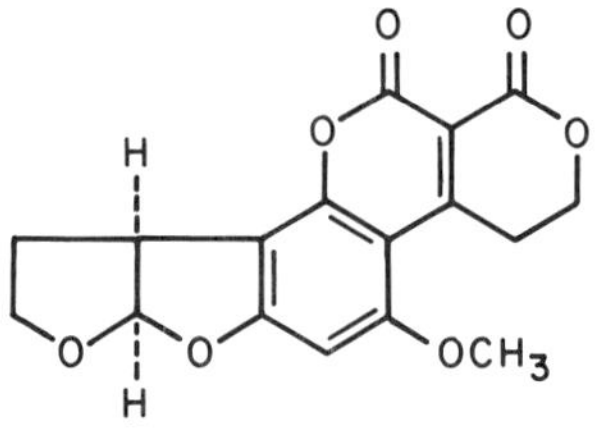

6 AFLATOXIN G_2

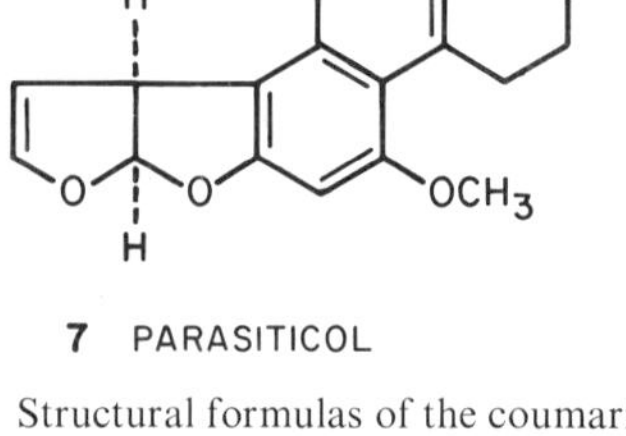

7 PARASITICOL

Fig. 1. Structural formulas of the coumarins.

pistachio nuts, cottonseed meal, and corn and grain sorghum during growth, harvesting, processing, storage and shipment, thereby causing a serious economic and health problem. The three most important factors controlling aflatoxin formation in field crops are relative humidity, moisture, and temperature.

The production of the aflatoxins is confined to certain strains of *A. flavus* Link ex Fries and *Aspergillus parasiticus* Speare (Wilson *et al.*, 1968), two closely related species of the *A. flavus* group which are commonly encountered as agents of decomposition in soil and foodstuffs. Members of this group are broadly identified by the production of yellowish-green conidia. *Aspergillus flavus* and *A. parasiticus* are differentiated from each other primarily by the color of their colonies and the morphology of their conidial structures. The sterigmata of *A. flavus* are typically biseriate, whereas those of *A. parasiticus* are uniseriate.

Toxicologically, the aflatoxins may be regarded as a multiple threat; e.g., aflatoxin B_1 can function as a potent toxin, a carcinogen, a teratogen, and a mutagen (Ciegler, 1975), and it can impair the immune system in animals (Thaxton *et al.*, 1974). *In vivo* aflatoxin B_1 is metabolized by different animal species to derivatives of lower toxicity. Its metabolism in relation to its biological activity has been studied, and convincing evidence indicates that aflatoxin B_1 requires metabolic activation to exert its carcinogenic and mutagenic effects (Campbell and Hayes, 1976; Roebuck and Wogan, 1977; Swenson *et al.*, 1977). Structure–activity as well as chemical studies indicate that the major route for activation proceeds through attack by liver mixed-function oxygenases, which yield the very toxic but short-lived 15,16-oxide as the ultimate carcinogen. Essigman *et al.* (1977) and Lin *et al.* (1977) established that 15,16-dihydro-16-[N^7-*guanyl*]15-hydroxyaflatoxin B_1 is the major acid hydrolysis product of aflatoxin B_1–DNA or aflatoxin B_1–ribosomal RNA adducts formed in hepatic microsome-mediated reactions and in rat liver *in vivo*. The covalent binding of aflatoxin B_1 with the guanine residue of informational molecules is then likely to induce frame-shift mutations, caused by intercalation of aflatoxin B_1, together with base-substitution mutations as a result of misrepair (Martin and Garner, 1977).

Only related bisdihydrofuran-containing substances [sterigmatocystin (**32**), austocystins (**42–50**), and versicolorin A (**21**)] with proven *in vivo* or *in vitro* toxicity will be discussed in this introduction. Sterigmatocystin (**32**), a xanthone which contains an angularly fused bisdihydrofuran system, was originally isolated from the mycelium of *Aspergillus versicolor* (Vuillemin) Tiraboschi by a Japanese group (Hatsuda and Kuyama, 1954). The marked similarity in structure between sterigmatocystin and the aflatoxins became apparent when the structures of the latter became known. This led to renewed interest in the production, natural occurrence, and chemical and biological properties of sterigmatocystin (Rabie *et al.*, 1977; Van der Watt, 1974; Roberts, 1974; Hamasaki and Hatsuda, 1977). In rats, the hepatocarcinogenicity of sterigmatocystin is approximately one-tenth of that of aflatoxin B_1. The activity of sterigmatocystin is furthermore attested to by its ability to induce neoplastic skin lesions, whereas for aflatoxin B_1 there is an absence of percutaneous absorption (Purchase and Steyn, 1973). Rodricks *et al.* (1968) reported the isolation of aspertoxin (**37**), a toxin which is closely related to sterigmatocystin (**32**), from *A. flavus*.

Steyn and Vleggaar (1974, 1975) characterized nine austocystins (**42**–**50**) from *Aspergillus ustus* (Bainier) Thom. and Church. The xanthone and bisdihydrofuran moieties of the austocystins are linearly fused and frequently contain either an isopentyl side chain or a chlorine atom. The cytotoxicity of the austocystins was determined in primary kidney epithelial cells of *Cercopithecus aethiops pygerythrus*; austocystins A–D (**42**–**45**) are more toxic than sterigmatocystin in this system (Steyn *et al.*, 1977). The most toxic compounds caused severe lesions in cells (nucleolar segregation), an indication of disturbed nucleic acid metabolism.

Versicolorin A (**21**), a yellow-orange polyhydroxyanthraquinone, is elaborated by *A. versicolor* (Hamasaki *et al.*, 1965a, 1967a) and by *A. parasiticus* (Lee *et al.*, 1975). Wong *et al.* (1977) employed *Salmonella typhimurium* T_{98} for testing the mutagenicity of versicolorin A, sterigmatocystin, and aflatoxin B_1; the compounds had a relative mutagenic potency of 5.83, 10.66, and 100, respectively. The mutagenicity and carcinogenicity of these compounds are associated with the bisdihydrofuran moiety.

Reviews covering facets of the aflatoxins and their attendant problems have been compiled by Wogan (1966), Goldblatt (1969), Detroy *et al.* (1971), Butler (1974), Roberts (1974), Ciegler (1975), Jammali (1976), Venkitasubramanian (1977), Stoloff (1977), and Maggon *et al.* (1977). The novel structural and biological features of the aflatoxins and sterigmatocystin soon stimulated investigations on their biogenesis and *in vitro* production. The biosyntheses of the aflatoxins and biosynthetically related compounds will be reviewed in this chapter.

II. STRUCTURAL TYPES BIOGENETICALLY RELATED TO THE AFLATOXINS

A number of secondary metabolites are biogenetically related to the aflatoxins in apparently having a common C_{20} poly-β-ketide precursor. Although these metabolites do not belong to a single class of compounds, they can be conveniently subdivided into the following structural types relative to the postulated sequence of the aflatoxin biosynthesis: (acetate–

polymalonate) → polyhydroxyanthraquinones (see Figs. 2–4) → xanthones (see Figs. 5,6) → coumarins (see Fig. 1). The reported numbering of the basic skeletons of these compounds differed. The numbering used for each group of compounds in this chapter is shown in Figs. 1–6.

In the final biosynthetic analysis of the foregoing compounds, an example from each group will be discussed (Section V); the biosynthetic implications will pertain to all compounds in that group.

A. Polyhydroxyanthraquinones

Most of these compounds are orange-red 1,3,6,8-tetraoxygenated-2-alkylanthraquinones.

1. *Anthraquinones Containing an Unbranched C_6 Side Chain*

This group of pigments is mainly produced by genotypically similar *Aspergillus* species namely, *A. versicolor, A. nidulans,* and *A. ustus.* None of these species produces aflatoxins, hence indicating a metabolic block in aflatoxin biosynthesis.

Averufin (**8**) is the first characterized natural product containing a 1,3-benzodioxane system. Holker *et al.* (1966) proposed the correct structure (**8**) from data obtained from an acid-catalyzed deuteriation of the open-chain hydrate which resulted in exchange of five hydrogens alpha to the ketone group. Synthetic and mass spectral information (Roffey *et al.*, 1967), ^{13}C nuclear magnetic resonance (NMR) data (Gorst-Allman *et al.*, 1977), and X-ray crystallography (Katsube *et al.*, 1972) confirmed structure **8** for averufin. Berger *et al.* (1976) characterized the related deoxyaverufinone (**13**) and dehydroaverufin (**11**) from *A. versicolor*. The additional nonaromatic hydroxy group in nidurufin (**9**), isolated from *A. nidulans* (Aucamp and Holzapfel, 1970), was located by methylation and oxidation reactions. Kingston *et al.* (1976) isolated 6,8-*O,O*-dimethylnidurufin (**10**) from *A. versicolor* and proposed it as an intermediate in aflatoxin biosynthesis. Holker *et al.* (1966) obtained averufanin (**12**) and its 8-*O*-methyl- and 6,8-*O,O*-dimethyl derivatives from a mutated strain of *A. versicolor*. Averufanin was obtained by Aucamp and Holzapfel (1970) from *A. versicolor* as well as from a *Bipolaris* sp.

Solorinic acid (**15**) from *Solorina crocea* was characterized by Koller and Russ (1937). The demethyl compound, norsolorinic acid (**14**), was produced by *A. versicolor* (Hamasaki *et al.*, 1967b) and *S. crocea* L. (Anderson *et al.*, 1966). *Aspergillus versicolor* furthermore yielded both averantin (**16**) (Birkinshaw *et al.*, 1966) and 1′-*O*-methylaverantin (**17**) (Aucamp and Holzapfel, 1970). Drastic acid treatment converted these two compounds into averythrin (**18**), a metabolite of *A. versicolor* (Roberts and Roffey, 1965).

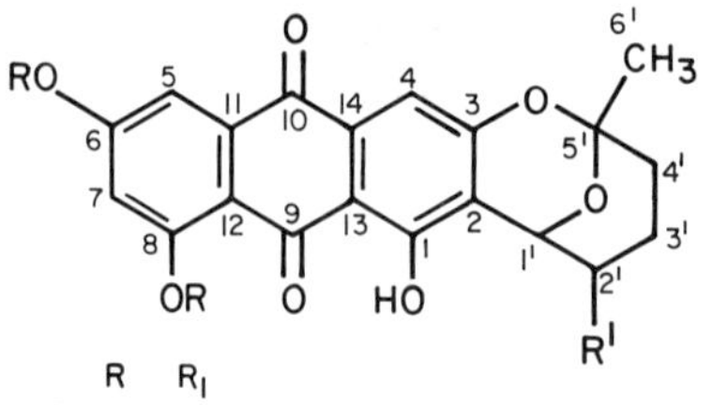

R R_1
8   H   H: AVERUFIN
9   H   OH: NIDURUFIN
10 CH_3 OH: 6,8-O,O-DIMETHYLNIDURUFIN

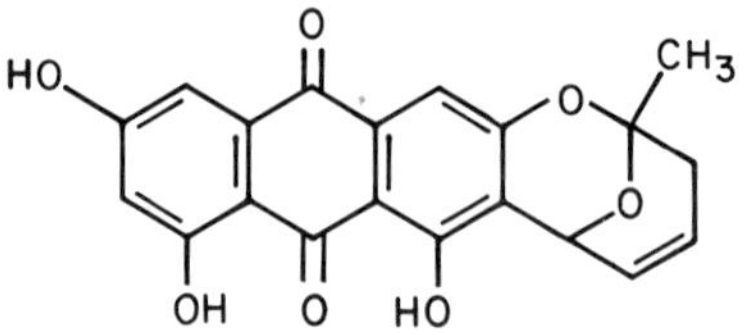

11 DEHYDROAVERUFIN

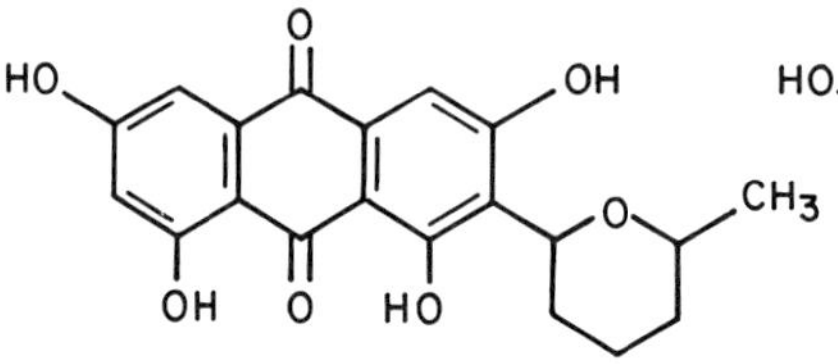

12 AVERUFANIN

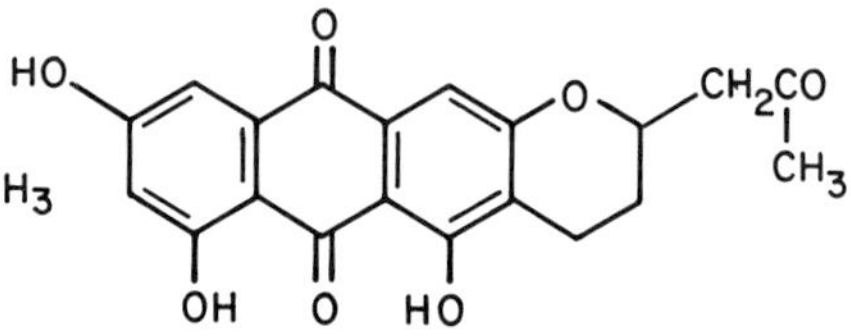

13 DEOXYAVERUFINONE

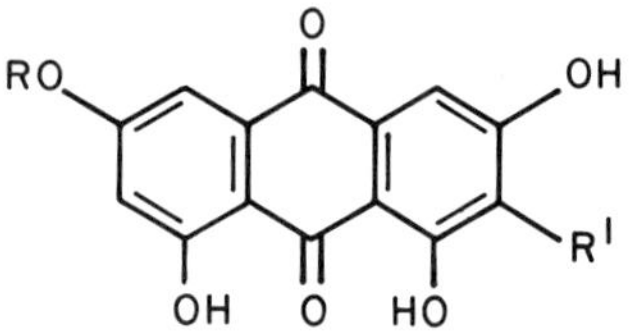

R R_1
14 H $CO(CH_2)_4CH_3$: NORSOLORINIC ACID
15 CH_3 $CO(CH_2)_4CH_3$: SOLORINIC ACID
16 H $CH(OH)(CH_2)_4CH_3$: AVERANTIN
17 H $CH(OCH_3)(CH_2)_4CH_3$: $1'-O$-METHYLAVERANTIN
18 H $CH=CH-(CH_2)CH_3$: AVERYTHRIN

Fig. 2.   Structural formulas of the C_{20}-hydroxyanthraquinones.

Although a number of the above compounds are elaborated by *A. versicolor*, the sequence of biosynthetic events remains speculative. Dehydroaverufin and norsolorinic acid were suggested as precursors of averufin by Berger *et al.* (1976) and Hsieh *et al.* (1976a), respectively.

2. Anthraquinones Containing a Branched C_6 Side Chain

Yao and Hsieh (1974) observed that treatment of *A. parasiticus* with dichlorvos[O,O-dimethyl-O-(2,2-dichlorovinyl)phosphate] resulted in reduced aflatoxigenicity and in the formation of an orange-red pigment, called versiconal acetate (**19**). Structure elucidation using ^1H and ^{13}C NMR techniques on versiconal acetate (Cox *et al.*, 1977; Steyn *et al.*, 1979a) and its 3,6-*O,O*-dimethyl derivative indicated that in polar solvents the compound exists as an equilibrium mixture of the three isomers, as shown in Fig. 3. Treatment of versiconal acetate with dilute mineral acid gave versicolorin C (**25**). The related metabolite versiconol acetate (**20**), and versiconol (**27**), were also isolated from *A. parasiticus* by Steyn *et al.* (1979a).

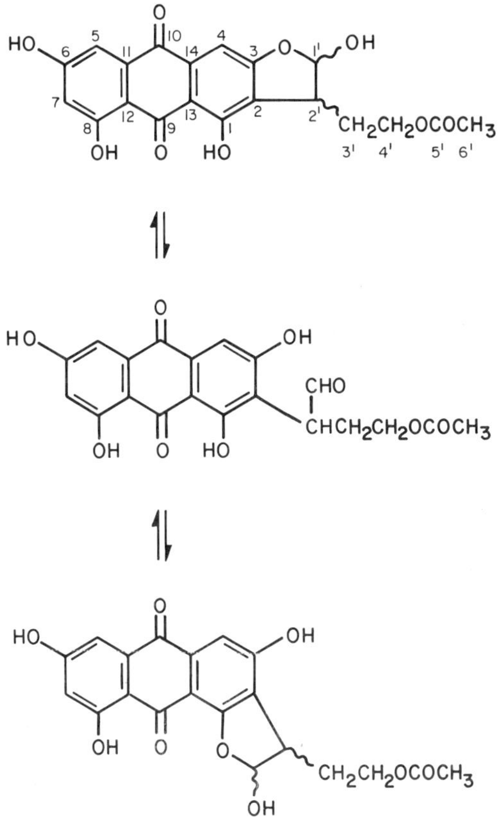

19 ISOMERS OF VERSICONAL ACETATE

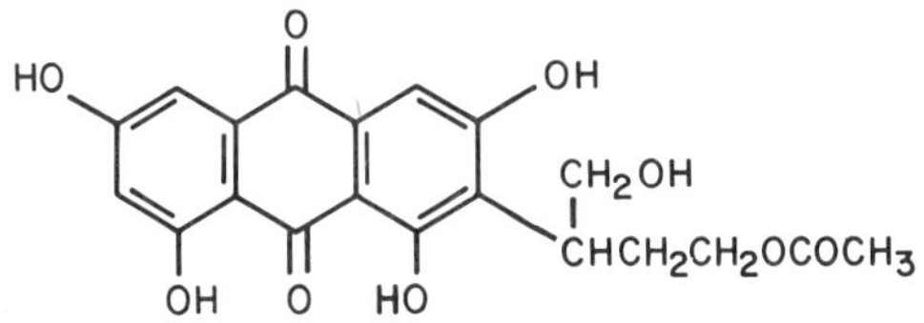

20 VERSICONOL ACETATE

Fig. 3. Structural formulas of hydroxyanthraquinones containing a branched C_6 side chain.

3. Anthraquinones Containing a C_4 Side Chain

A mixture of orange pigments from *A. versicolor* was initially called versicolorin. Extensive purification yielded an array of polyhydroxyanthraquinones, some of which are also elaborated by *A. ustus*, *A. flavus*, and *A. parasiticus*.

The presence of a five-membered vinyl ether moiety in versicolorin A (**21**) was verified by oxidative conversion into a γ-lactone group, ν_{max} 1802 cm^{-1} (Hamasaki *et al.*, 1965a). Potassium permanganate oxidation of versicolorin A trimethyl ether gave 3,5-dimethoxyphthalic acid and a 1,3,6,8-tetraoxygenated-2-carboxylanthraquinone (Hamasaki *et al.*, 1967a). 6,8-*O,O*-Dimethylversicolorin A (**22**) was isolated in the same laboratory (Hatsuda *et al.*, 1971). The levorotatory versicolorin B (**23**) and the related

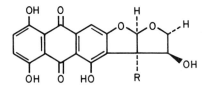

21 R = H : VERSICOLORIN A
22 R = CH₃ : 6,8-O,O-DIMETHYLVERSICOLORIN A

23 R = H : VERSICOLORIN B
24 R = CH₃ : AVERSIN

25 R = OH : VERSICOLORIN C
26 R = H : 6-DEOXYVERSICOLORIN C

27 R = CH(CH₂OH) CH₂CH₂OH : VERSICONOL
28 R = [structure] : BIPOLARIN

29 R = OH : DOTHISTROMIN
30 R = H : DEOXYDOTHISTROMIN

31 BISDEOXYDEHYDRODOTHISTROMIN

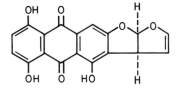

Fig. 4. Structural formulas of the C_{18}-hydroxyanthraquinones.

6,8-*O,O*-dimethylversicolorin B (aversin) (**24**) were similarly obtained from *A. versicolor*. The structure of the latter compound was proved by synthesis (Holmwood and Roberts, 1971). *A. versicolor* also produces the racemic versicolorin C (**25**) (Hamasaki *et al.*, 1965b), the structure of which was proved by X-ray crystallography (Fig. 4) (Fukuyama *et al.*, 1975a).

Versiconol (**27**) was obtained from *A. versicolor* and postulated as an intermediate in the biosynthesis of versicolorin C (Hatsuda *et al.*, 1969). Addition of (**27**) to a replacement culture of *A. versicolor* led to an increased production of versicolorin C (**25**). Bipolarin (**28**) was isolated from a *Bipolaris* sp. (Aucamp and Holzapfel, 1970) and formulated as 2(2'-tetrahydrofuranol)-1,3,6,8-tetrahydroxyanthraquinone on the basis of its ^{1}H NMR spectrum, showing a one-proton quartet at $\delta 5.33$ (J 5.5 and 6.7 Hz) arising

from Ar—C$\underline{\text{H}}$—(O—CH$_2$—) and a broad two-proton signal at $\delta 3.8$ caused by the grouping (—O—C$\underline{\text{H}}_2$—CH$_2$—). Certain compounds, such as the versicolorins, contain a branched C$_4$ moiety, owing to a rearrangement step; this rearrangement, however, has apparently not taken place in the bioformation of bipolarin.

Dothistroma pini, the fungus responsible for the necrotic disease of *Pinus radiata*, produced the phytotoxin dothistromin (**29**), deoxydothistromin (**30**), bisdeoxydehydrodothistromin (**31**), 6-deoxyversicolorin C (**26**), averufin (**8**), nidurufin (**9**), and averythrin (**18**) (Danks and Hodges, 1974). The dothistromins are red anthraquinones containing three α-hydroxy groups. Italian workers (Assante *et al.*, 1977) likewise isolated epidothistromin (3'-*epi*-**29**), averufin (**8**), and averythrin (**18**) from *Cercospora smilacis*, indicating the biogenetic interrelationships of these polyhydroxyanthraquinones.

B. Xanthones

1. Xanthones Containing an Angular Structure

Sterigmatocystin (**32**) assumes great structural importance in mycotoxin chemistry, because it was the first characterized compound which contained the unique bisdihydrofuran functionality, in this case linked to a xanthone nucleus. The structure (Fig. 5) (Bullock *et al.*, 1962) and absolute configuration were verified by X-ray crystallography (Fukuyama *et al.*, 1975c, 1976).

Sterigmatocystin (**32**) is known to be produced by isolates of *A. versicolor* (Hatsuda and Kuyama, 1954); *A. nidulans* and *Bipolaris sorokiana* (Holzapfel *et al.*, 1966a); *A. rugulosus* (Ballantine *et al.*, 1965); *A. ustus, A. aurantiobrunneus*, and *A. quadrilineatus* (Rabie *et al.*, 1977); and *A. variecolor* (Chexal *et al.*, 1975). Schroeder and Kelton (1975) reported that isolates of

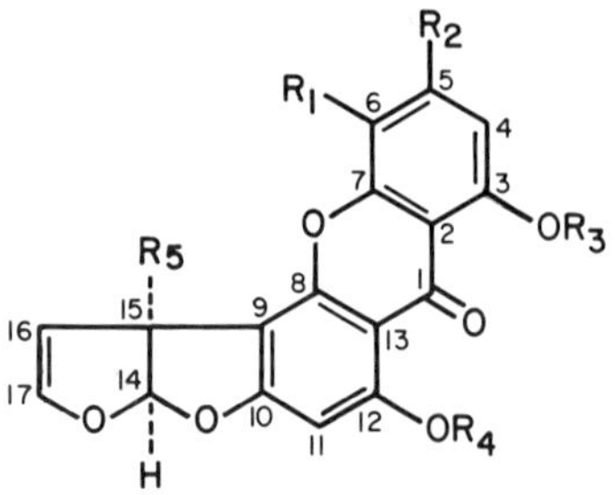

	R$_1$	R$_2$	R$_3$	R$_4$	R$_5$	
32	H	H	H	CH$_3$	H : STERIGMATOCYSTIN
33	H	H	H	H	H : DEMETHYLSTERIGMATOCYSTIN
34	H	H	CH$_3$	CH$_3$	H : O-METHYLSTERIGMATOCYSTIN
35	OCH$_3$	H	H	CH$_3$	H : 6-METHOXYSTERIGMATOCYSTIN
36	OCH$_3$	OCH$_3$	H	CH$_3$	H : 5,6 -DIMETHOXYSTERIGMATOCYSTIN
37	H	H	CH$_3$	CH$_3$	OH : ASPERTOXIN

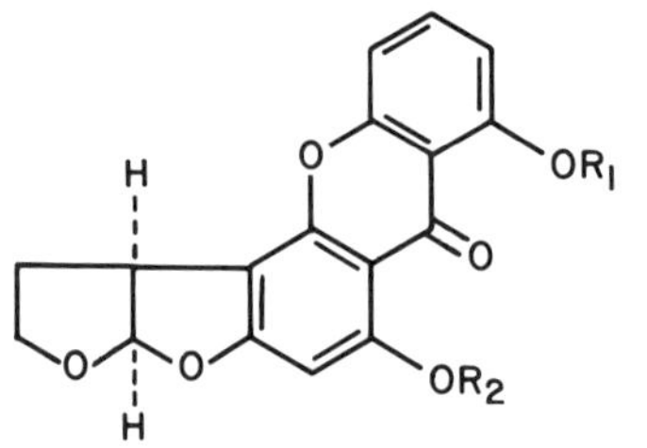

	R$_1$	R$_2$
38	H	CH$_3$: DIHYDROSTERIGMATOCYSTIN
39	H	H : DIHYDRODEMETHYLSTERIGMATOCYSTIN
40	CH$_3$	CH$_3$: DIHYDRO-O-METHYLSTERIGMATOCYSTIN

Fig. 5.   Structural formulas of the angular xanthones.

A. parasiticus and *A. flavus* produced sterigmatocystin. Steyn (1977, unpublished results) failed to obtain sterigmatocystin from these cultures.
Several derivatives of sterigmatocystin are produced by *A. versicolor*;
among these are dihydrosterigmatocystin (**38**) and dihydrodemethylsterigma-
tocystin (**39**) (Hatsuda *et al.*, 1972); demethylsterigmatocystin (**33**) (Elsworthy *et al.*, 1970); and 6-methoxysterigmatocystin (**35**) (Holker and Kagal,
1968). *Aspergillus flavus* produced dihydro-*O*-methylsterigmatocystin (**40**)
(Cole *et al.*, 1970), *O*-methylsterigmatocystin (**34**) (Burkhardt and Forgacs,
1968), and aspertoxin (**37**) (Rodricks *et al.*, 1968), whereas 5,6-dimethoxysteri-
gmatocystin (**36**) was elaborated by *A. multicolor* (Hamasaki *et al.*, 1977).

2. *Xanthones Containing a Linear Structure*

Sterigmatin (**41**), a metabolite from *A. versicolor*, was the first metabolite found with a linearly fused xanthone and bisdihydrofuran moiety (Fig. 6) (Hamasaki *et al.*, 1973; Fukuyama *et al.*, 1975b).

Steyn and Vleggaar (1974, 1975) obtained nine new linear xanthones together with averufin (**8**) and versicolorin C (**25**) from corn cultures of *A. ustus*. The linear xanthones were called austocystins (**42–50**) and frequently contain a chlorine atom, e.g., austocystin A (**42**), or an isopentyl side chain, e.g., austocystin B (**43**). The substitution pattern of the austocystins was confirmed by the results of chemical modification, as well as ^{1}H NMR techniques, particularly acetylation shifts, benzene-induced solvent shifts, and nuclear Overhauser enhancement (NOE) effects.

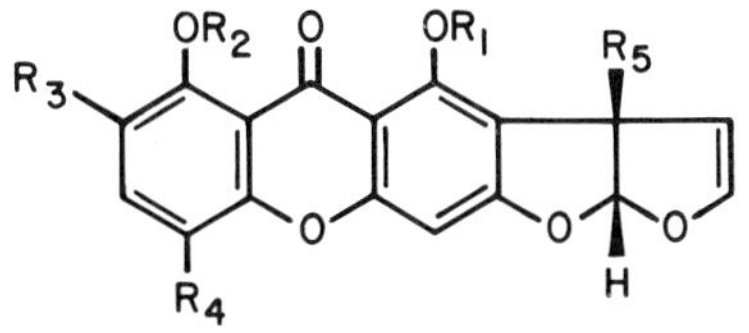

	R₁	R₂	R₃	R₄	R₅	
41	H	H	H	H	H	STERIGMATIN
42	CH₃	CH₃	Cl	H	H	AUSTOCYSTIN A
43	H	H	H	CH₂-CH₂-C(CH₃)₂OH	H	AUSTOCYSTIN B
44	CH₃	H	H	CH₂-CH₂-C(CH₃)₂OH	H	AUSTOCYSTIN C
45	H	H	H	CH₂-CH₂-C(CH₃)₂OH	OH	AUSTOCYSTIN D
46	CH₃	H	H	CH₂-CH₂-C(CH₃)₂OH	OH	AUSTOCYSTIN E
47	H	H	H	H	OH	AUSTOCYSTIN F
48	H	CH₃	Cl	H	OH	AUSTOCYSTIN G
49	H	H	H	CH₂-CH=C(CH₃)₂	OH	AUSTOCYSTIN H
50	CH₃	H	H	H	OH	AUSTOCYSTIN I

Fig. 6. Structural formulas of the linear xanthones.

C. Coumarins

Among this group of compounds, aflatoxin B₁ (**1**) is of prime importance owing to its biological properties. The structural elucidation of the aflatoxins performed by the M.I.T. group (Asao *et al.*, 1965) was largely based on interpretation of spectral data—by elegant modification, e.g., catalytic hydrogenation of aflatoxin B₁ which resulted in the uptake of three moles of hydrogen with the production of a tetrahydrodeoxoderivative; by synthesis of model compounds, e.g., 5,7-dimethoxycyclopentenonel[2,3-*c*]coumarin; and by total synthesis of aflatoxin B₁ (Büchi *et al.*, 1967). The structures of both aflatoxin B_1 (1) and aflatoxin B_2 (3) were unambiguously established by X-ray crystallography (Van Soest and Peerdeman, 1970a,b). The spatial disposition (molecular dimensions and conformation) of the bisdihydrofuran ring in aflatoxin B_1 is virtually identical to that of sterigmatocystin.

The structure of aflatoxin G_1 (5) was similarly elucidated by Asao *et al.* (1965). It contains a γ-lactone moiety as attested by the AA'XX' pattern in its NMR spectrum [$\delta 4.47$ (t), and $\delta 3.48$ (t), J 6 Hz]. The proposed structure of aflatoxin G_1 was confirmed by X-ray crystallography (Cheung and Sim, 1964).

Holzapfel *et al.*, (1966b) isolated aflatoxins M_1 (2) and M_2 (4) from moldy peanuts. The structures were deduced mainly from ^1H NMR data. Lactating cows transform aflatoxin B_1 into aflatoxin M_1. Parasiticol (7) is formed by strains of *A. parasiticus* on solid media (Stubblefield *et al.*, 1970) and by a yeast culture of *A. flavus* (Heathcote and Dutton, 1969).

Many derivatives of the aflatoxins are formed enzymatically *in vitro* and *in vivo* by reduction, oxidation, demethylation, and hydration.

III. THE BIOSYNTHETIC STUDY OF AFLATOXIN AND ITS CONGENERS

A. Conditions of Production

The origin in nature of sterigmatocystin and aflatoxin is not obvious from simple chemical analysis of their structures. The biosyntheses of only averufin (8), versiconal acetate (19), versicolorin A (21), sterigmatocystin (32), and aflatoxin B_1 (1) have been studied in detail. Each of these compounds, however, represents a specific stage in the biosynthetic sequence of aflatoxin B_1.

In biosynthetic studies, the first and most frequently employed technique for studying secondary metabolite formation involves the testing of isotopically labeled precursors (^2H, ^3H, ^{13}C, ^{14}C, ^{15}N, and ^{18}O) for specific incorporation into the metabolite(s). The earliest explorations of sterigmatocystin (Holker and Mulheirn, 1968) and aflatoxin B_1 (Biollaz *et al.*, 1970) involved the *in vivo* exposure of the enzyme systems to labeled substrates (e.g., [^{14}C]acetate and [^{14}C]methionine) followed by time-consuming carbon-by-carbon degradations of the end products as the only means available to establish the distribution of label and thus the overall biosynthetic pathways. The developments in ^{13}C techniques would reduce similar studies today to a few weeks instead of the years of concerted effort previously required. Steyn *et al.* (1975, 1979b), Pachler *et al.* (1976a), and

Gorst-Allman *et al.* (1977, 1978) prepared aflatoxin B_1 and a number of its congeners, biosynthetically labeled with singly labeled acetate or $[1,2-^{13}C]$ acetate, and established the excess of ^{13}C-label and the presence of intact acetate units by ^{13}C NMR spectroscopy. The results exemplify the utility of these techniques in biosynthetic studies (see below).

The second method employed in biosynthetic studies involves the characterization of fermentation products closely related to the secondary metabolite under investigation. This method has been extensively used and has led to the implication of averufin (**8**), the versicolorins, and sterigmatocystin (**32**) in aflatoxin biogenetic pathway. Some of the intermediates were isotopically labeled and their role in aflatoxin biosynthesis verified, e.g., sterigmatocystin by whole cell (Hsieh *et al.*, 1973) and cell-free cultures of *A. parasiticus* (Singh and Hsieh, 1976).

The use of auxotrophic mutants furnishes an elegant technique for the study of microbial biosynthesis (Queener, 1976). By this method a substance can be established as an obligatory intermediate. *In vivo*, the intermediates may never leave the enzyme surface(s) on which they are formed and are converted into the end products. It therefore becomes impossible to distinguish the order of synthesis of the individual substances. Through use of mutants, the intermediacy of averufin (**8**) (Donkersloot *et al.*, 1972), norsolorinic acid (**14**) (Detroy *et al.*, 1973), and versicolorin A (**21**) (Lee *et al.*, 1975) was verified in the aflatoxin biosynthesis; these substances were subsequently converted into aflatoxin B_1 (**1**) by resting cell cultures of a wild strain *A. parasiticus* (see below). Effects similar to those exhibited by auxotrophic mutants caused by a genetic blockage of enzyme synthesis are theoretically possible by the *in vivo* use of specific enzyme inhibitors, which lead to the accumulation of identifiable obligatory intermediate(s). Treatment of *A. parasiticus* ATCC 15517 with dichlorvos led to reduced aflatoxigenicity and the concomitant formation of versiconal acetate (**19**) (Yao and Hsieh, 1974). By application of the foregoing techniques, the biochemical events prior to the final elaboration of aflatoxin B_1 could be elucidated.

Extensive methodology is available for the production of sterigmatocystin and the aflatoxins on stationary and submerged cultures on chemically defined media (Maggon *et al.*, 1977). The amounts and relative proportions of aflatoxins B_1, B_2, G_1, and G_2 depend on the strain, balance of nutrients in the medium, and culture conditions. Lower pH and some trace metals, e.g., Mn^{2+}, Mg^{2+}, and Va^{2+} favored production of hydroxylated aflatoxins (Pai *et al.*, 1975). In biosynthetic studies, it is essential to determine the rate of metabolite production, as the precursors must not only penetrate the synthetic site but must do so at a time when the enzyme systems mediating the synthetic reactions are present and active, i.e., the late stages in the exponential phase of growth. In addition to genetic requirements, the yield of aflatoxin depends on the conditions of growth, including moisture, temperature, substrate, aeration, time of incubation, and other factors that affect the qualitative state of the fungus (Detroy *et al.*, 1971).

Maggon *et al.* (1977) reviewed the role of trace metals in aflatoxin biosynthesis. The exact step in the biosynthetic scheme at which Ba^{2+}, Cu^{2+}, and Zn^{2+} acts is not fully understood. It is probable that Cu^{2+} and Fe^{2+} are essential for the cyclization of the polyketide progenitors of the aflatoxins and biogenetically related pigments. Increased incorporation of $[^{14}C]$acetate into aflatoxins in the presence of Zn^{2+}, Mg^{2+}, Mn^{2+}, Ba^{2+}, and Ca^{2+} by resting resuspended mycelia of *A. parasiticus* was observed (Gupta *et al.*, 1975). The stimulatory effect of Zn^{2+} on aflatoxin production is well documented by Maggon *et al.* (1977). The glycolytic enzymes of *A. parasiticus* are dependent on Zn^{2+}. It was considered possible that Zn^{2+} was affecting the induction of the enzymes of secondary metabolism by the accumulation of sufficient amounts of pyruvate.

Shih and Marth (1974) studied aflatoxin, lipid synthesis, and glucose metabolism by *A. parasiticus* during incubation at 28°C for 15 days on glucose–salts medium or the yeast extract and sucrose (YES) medium with and without agitation. Generally, more growth occured in agitated cultures than in stationary cultures, but maximal yields of aflatoxin and total lipid were lower than in stationary cultures. These results suggest that the degree of aeration of the culture is important in aflatoxin biosynthesis through regulation of carbohydrate metabolism. In quiescent incubation, aflatoxin appeared in the medium (glucose–salts) after 2 days of incubation. Toxin formation increased and reached its maximum at 5 days, when the mold entered the stationary phase of growth which coincided with the end of rapid growth and the rapid uptake of oxygen. The aflatoxin concentration declined sharply between the sixth and eighth days of incubation. The pattern of formation of total lipid was similar to that of aflatoxin. These findings are in agreement with those of Detroy and Hesseltine (1970) that aflatoxin formation is associated with a shift in the metabolic capacity from the trophophase to the idiophase. These authors speculated that a sudden buildup of tricarboxylic acid intermediates, which occurs at trophophase termination, could lead to a buildup of malonyl-CoA, which could trigger secondary enzyme induction. From the similarity between aflatoxin and lipid synthesis, presumably from a common precursor (acetate), Shih and Marth (1974) postulated that the syntheses of aflatoxins and lipid were triggered by a similar mechanism and/or share a similar pathway.

During a study of aflatoxin B_1 production, Shih and Marth (1974) investigated the influence of sodium azide, an inhibitor of terminal electron transfer, which at low concentrations inhibits respiration and slightly stimulates anaerobic glycolysis in some microbial systems. They observed a selective inhibition of the respiratory system of the mold by sodium azide, as well as enhanced production of toxin and of total lipid. Shih and Marth (1974) thus concluded that the decrease in oxidative respiration during the late logarithmic growth favored an accumulation of acetate (acetyl-CoA) and NADPH which could lead to increased toxin and lipid production. The incorporation of $[1\text{-}^{14}C]$glucose into aflatoxin indicated that limiting the oxygen supply and thereby favoring glucose catabolism via the Embden–Meyerhof pathway enhanced toxin formation. It can be concluded that there is a marked correlation between glucose catabolism which occurs mainly via the Embden–Meyerhof pathway and the formation of secondary metabolites.

In a subsequent paper, Shih and Marth (1975) reported on the production of aflatoxin and its partition between the medium and the mycelium. The maximal production of total aflatoxin and of aflatoxin B_1, G_1, and G_2 occurred at 5 days, as against 7 days for aflatoxin B_2. Under these conditions, more than 60% of the total aflatoxins appeared in the mycelium after 5 days.

The basal medium used in most experiments with *A. parasiticus* was developed by Adye and Mateles (1964), and is referred to as the AM medium. The method of Hsieh and Mateles (1971) employed resting cells of *A. parasiticus* ATCC 15517 to prepare highly labeled aflatoxin from $[^{14}C]$-acetate. Resting cells were used in the labeling experiments, as these cells contain the needed enzymes required to convert the precursor into the end product with a minimum of diversion to unwanted side products. The desired precursors were added to the resting cells, and high synthetic activity was evidenced only during 40–70 hr of incubation. Glucose was required for high incorporation efficiency, whereas the concentration of labeled acetate determined the specific activity of the end product. The effect of sodium acetate on the growth and aflatoxin production of *A. parasiticus* NRRL 2999 was studied in the AMY medium (modified AM medium + 2% yeast extract). At pH 4.5 a concentration of ≥ 0.1 gm sodium acetate per 100 ml completely inhibited growth and aflatoxin production (Buchanan and Ayres, 1976). The low-salts medium (Hsieh and Yang, 1975) was employed for the static growth of mutants of *A. parasiticus* for the production of averufin (Gorst-Allman *et al.*, 1977) and versicolorin A (Gorst-Allman *et al.*, 1978). The YES medium was used for the bioproduction of versiconal acetate (Steyn *et al.*, 1979b). Hsieh and Yang (1975) also used the low-salts medium for the preparation of $[^{14}C]$sterigmatocystin, and reported a recovery of 3% of the radioactivity of the added $[1\text{-}^{14}C]$acetate in the sterigmatocystin. Rabie *et al.* (1976) evaluated five different liquid media for the production of sterigmatocystin by *A. versicolor* and *B. sorokiana*.

B. Results from ^{14}C-Labeling Experiments with Primitive Precursors

Adye and Mateles (1964) implicated phenylalanine and tyrosine as precursors in aflatoxin biosynthesis from incorporation studies. However, Donkersloot *et al.* (1968) and Heathcote *et al.* (1973) showed this finding to be erroneous; the aflatoxins therefore, are not shikimate derived.

Holker and Underwood (1964) recognized the structural similarity of aflatoxin B_1 and sterigmatocystin, and suggested that either both compounds are derived from a common biogenetic precursor, or sterigmatocystin is a precursor of aflatoxin B_1. Holker and Mulheirn (1968) supplemented cultures of *A. veriscolor* with $[1-^{14}C]$acetate. Elegant degradation of labeled sterigmatocystin (0.5% incorporation of the radioactivity) and determination of the distribution of labels gave direct values for only five carbon atoms. Their results supported the acetate–polymalonate hypothesis for the origin of the xanthone ring system and indicated an apparent difference in the level of radioactivity of the branched side chain and the xanthone nucleus. It was concluded that sterigmatocystin was formed from two separate preformed polyketide units ($C_{14} + C_4$), a hypothesis still recently supported by Heathcote *et al.* (1973). An unusual feature was that the carbon atoms involved in the joining of the dihydrofuran moiety and the xanthone system both originated in the methyl group of acetate. The same arrangement was observed in the versicolorins and aflatoxins, thus indicating a similar, albeit anomalous, polyketide origin for these compounds.

The group of Büchi (Biollaz *et al.*, 1970) made a concerted effort to solve this biosynthetic problem, and undertook the Herculean task of determining the distribution of label in aflatoxin B_1 derived from $[methyl-^{14}C]$methionine and $[1-^{14}C]$- and $[2-^{14}C]$acetates. Administration of $[methyl-^{14}C]$methionine yielded radioactive aflatoxin B_1 which on Zeisel degradation gave methyl iodide containing 97.8% of the total activity. The *O*-methylation, therefore, occurred via a transmethylation involving *S*-adenosylmethionine in which the methyl group is transferred intact.

Several ingenious experiments were designed to analyze the distribution of labels in aflatoxin B_1 derived from $[^{14}C]$acetate, e.g., in the bisdihydrofuran portion. Labeled aflatoxin B_1 was converted into the tricyclic dimethyl ether **51**. Modified Kuhn–Roth oxidation of **51** gave 2-methylbutanoic acid (**52**) (90%), propionic acid (5%), and acetic acid (5%). These acids were analyzed as the *p*-bromophenacyl esters and degraded as shown in Fig. 7. Schmidt cleavage of **52** yielded the activity of C(11); the resulting amine was oxidized to 2-butanone which on oxidation with sodium hypoiodite provided an additional source of propionic acid and iodoform C(13). Sequential degradation of propionic acid furnished the activities of C(14), C(15), and C(16). These studies established the origin of C(11), C(14), and C(16) from the methyl group of acetate and C(13) and C(15) from the carboxyl group of acetate.

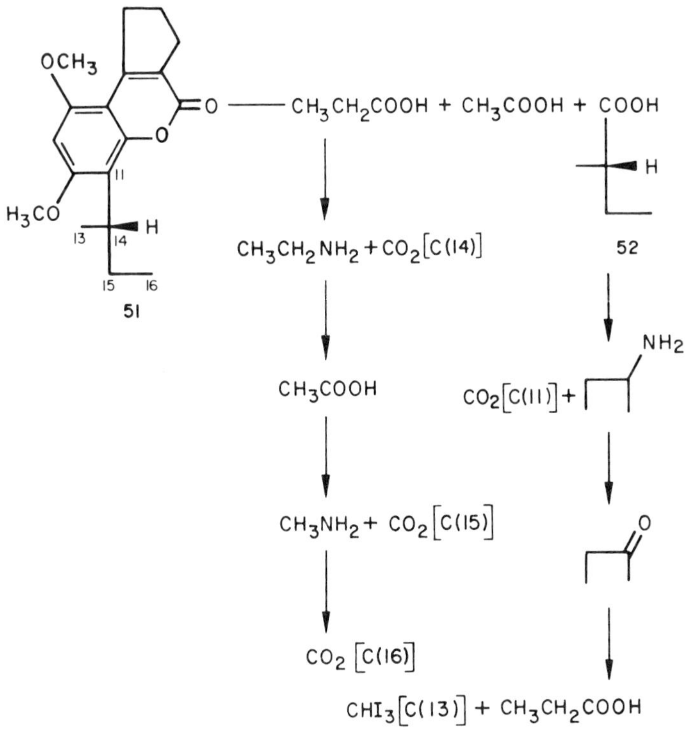

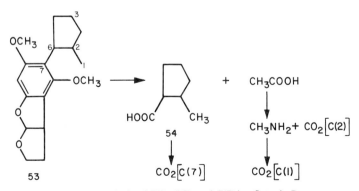

Fig. 7. Degradation of the bisdihydrofuran moiety in aflatoxin B_1.

The isotope distribution in the cyclopentenone moiety was subsequently established. Tetrahydrodeoxoaflatoxin B_1 was converted by a series of reactions into, e.g., the methycyclopentane **53** which on Kuhn–Roth oxidation gave cis-2-methylcyclopentanoic acid (**54**) and acetic acid, which established the origins of C(1), C(2), and C(7) (see Fig. 8). Oxidation of the methylcyclopentene **55** with osmic acid and potassium chlorate gave the diketone **56**

Fig. 8. Analysis of C(1), C(2), and C(7) in aflatoxin B_1.

which on selective reduction with lithium aluminum tri-*tert* butoxyhydride gave hydroxyketone **57**. Its tosylate, on hydrogenolysis with lithium aluminum hydride, was converted into the secondary alcohol **58** and degraded as shown in Fig. 9. The specific incorporations of C(1)–C(6) were thus measured directly or calculated.

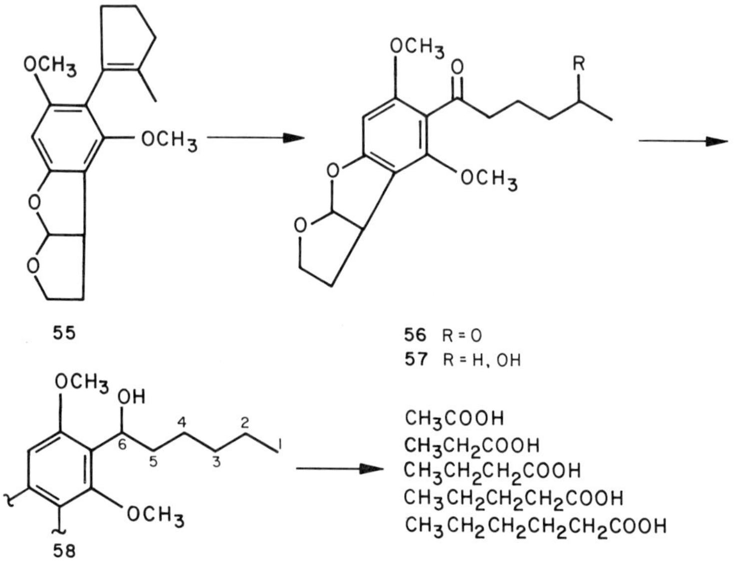

55

56 R = O
57 R = H, OH

CH₃COOH
CH₃CH₂COOH
CH₃CH₂CH₂COOH
CH₃CH₂CH₂CH₂COOH
CH₃CH₂CH₂CH₂CH₂COOH

58

Fig. 9.   Analysis of C(1)–C(6) in aflatoxin B₁.

The results obtained by Büchi established the specific incorporation of acetate and methionine. The measured and calculated radioactivities required the presence of nine labels (theoretical activity 11.1% per labeled carbon atom) in [1-¹⁴C]acetate-derived aflatoxin B₁ and seven labels (theoretical activity 14.3% per labeled carbon atom) in [2-¹⁴C]acetate-derived aflatoxin B₁. These findings are summarized in formula **59** (see Fig. 10).

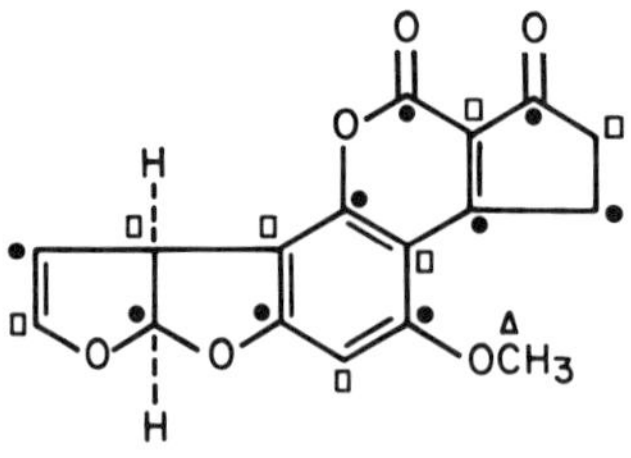

Fig. 10.   Labeling pattern of aflatoxin B₁. ●: C(1) of acetate; □: C(2) of acetate; △: CH₃SCH₂CH₂CH(NH₂)CO₂H.

59

The results indicated an unusual polyketide pathway as aflatoxin B_1 contained two atypical carbon–carbon linkages, namely, C(5)–C(6) and C(11)–C(14), in which both carbon atoms are derived from the carboxy carbon atoms and methyl carbon atoms of acetate, respectively. The degradation experiments recovered only two of the aromatic carbon atoms,

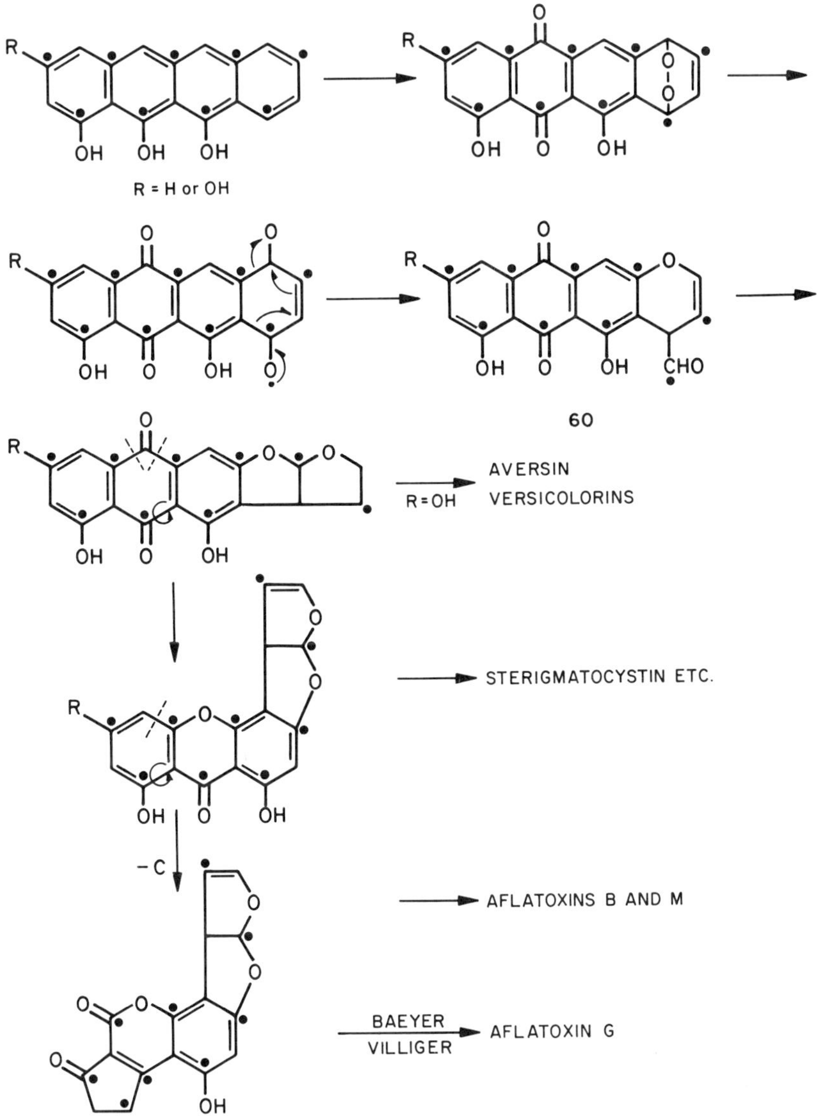

Fig. 11. Suggested biosynthesis of the bisfurans.

namely, C(7) and C(11). The ^{13}C NMR results of Steyn *et al.* (1975) and Pachler *et al.* (1976a) furnished information on the labeling of all the skeletal carbon atoms, thereby corroborating the labeling studies of the M.I.T. group and in addition proved the arrangement of intact acetate units in aflatoxin B_1. Biollaz *et al.* (1970) advanced a new hypothesis consonant with their experimental evidence. It was proposed that a C_{18}-polyhydroxynaphthacene, which is formed from a nonaketide chain by cyclization and removal of oxygen, is oxidized to an endoperoxyanthraquinone which rearranges via the diradical or zwitterion to the aldehyde (**60**). A subsequent rearrangement leads to versicolorin A (**21**). The xanthone ring as in sterigmatocystin (**32**) can be formed from the oxidative cleavage of the anthraquinone ring, rotation, cyclization, and decarboxylation. This pathway results in the elimination of one acetate methyl-derived carbon atom. The cyclization to the cyclopentenone involves another oxidative ring cleavage followed by expulsion of an acetate methyl-derived carbon atom. The postulates of Büchi are summarized in Fig. 11, and were generally accepted (Turner, 1971; Detroy *et al.*, 1971; Roberts, 1974) until the advent of definitive ^{13}C NMR studies (Steyn *et al.*, 1975).

C. Results from ^{13}C-Labeling Experiments

1. *Introduction*

The proliferation in recent years of biosynthetic studies with ^{13}C-labeled precursors is mainly due to the additional information which can be obtained, compared with studies using ^{14}C-labeled precursors. The fact that no laborious chemical degradation of the product is required to locate the ^{13}C label provided an added impetus to this development. The location of the ^{13}C isotope is determined by ^{13}C NMR spectroscopy. The principles and applications of ^{13}C NMR spectroscopy are the subject of a number of excellent monographs (Stothers, 1972; Breitmaier and Voelter, 1974; Clerc *et al.*, 1973; Wehrli and Wirthlin, 1976).

The low natural abundance of the stable, magnetically active ^{13}C isotope (1.1%) taken in conjunction with its gyromagnetic ratio $[3.98\gamma(^{13}C) = \gamma(^{1}H)]$ causes a loss in sensitivity by a factor of 5800 compared with protons at the same magnetic field strength. The lower sensitivity of ^{13}C NMR spectroscopy has been partly circumvented by proton noise decoupling (PND) as well as by pulsed Fourier transform (FT) NMR spectroscopy.

Multiplicities in a ^{13}C signal arise from coupling of the ^{13}C nucleus with neighboring ^{1}H nuclei. PND removes the (^{13}C, ^{1}H) couplings, and the resonance of the ^{13}C nucleus appears as a singlet. Every ^{13}C nucleus in a molecule gives rise to a distinct signal over a wide spectral region (ca. 200 ppm) [see Fig. 12(a) for averufin (**8**)].

In pulsed FT ^{13}C NMR spectroscopy a radiofrequency (rf) pulse instead of a varying magnetic field is employed to excite ^{13}C nuclei. A number of pulses could be applied to a sample in the same time normally used in a continuous wave recording. In this way up to a tenfold increase in sensitivity can be obtained.

The position of ^{13}C labels in a compound derived from a ^{13}C-labeled precursor is determined by comparison of the PND ^{13}C NMR spectra of the natural and the enriched compound. The incorporation of ^{13}C at certain positions in the molecule should then be evident from the intensity enhancement of the relevant ^{13}C signals.

Another valuable parameter of ^{13}C NMR spectroscopy frequently used in biosynthetic studies is (^{13}C, ^{13}C) coupling constants. In natural abundance spectra (^{13}C, ^{13}C) couplings are not observed, as the probability of two adjacent ^{13}C nuclei in the same molecule is negligible. The fate of a precursor, labeled in adjacent positions with ^{13}C, can be deduced from the (^{13}C,^{13}C) coupling constants of the final product. The intact incorporation of the precursor, e.g., [1,2-^{13}C]acetate is indicated by the appearance of peaks around the corresponding natural abundance peak. The absence of a directly bonded (^{13}C,^{13}C) coupling is an indication of a rearrangement and/or a bond cleavage in the biosynthetic sequence. The mode of folding of the polyketide progenitor of a metabolite can be deduced from experiments with doubly labeled acetate (see Fig. 14 for averufin).

Directly bonded (^{13}C,^{13}C) coupling constants are also observed in the ^{13}C NMR spectra of compounds derived from a singly labeled precursor as the result of a molecular rearrangement. Relevant examples of this phenomenon have been observed in the PND ^{13}C NMR spectra of aflatoxin B$_1$ derived from [1-^{13}C]- as well as from [2-^{13}C]acetate [see Figs. 16(a) and 16(b)].

It is obvious that ^{13}C NMR spectroscopy is of use in comprehensive biosynthetic studies only if the signals observed in the natural abundance PND ^{13}C NMR spectrum of the product are unambiguously assigned. Ideally these assignments should be independent of any preconceived biosynthetic assumptions, as the biosynthetic conclusions drawn from the ^{13}C study depend critically on the original spectral assignments.

Pertinent reviews on the use of ^{13}C NMR spectroscopy in biosynthesis are available (Grutzner, 1972; Floss, 1972; Séquin and Scott, 1974; McInnes, and Wright, 1975; Simpson, 1975; McInnes et al., 1976; White, 1976; Kunesch and Poupat, 1977).

2. Assignment Techniques in ^{13}C NMR Spectroscopy

A number of different techniques are used to assign ^{13}C NMR spectra of organic compounds. The assignment of the ^{1}H NMR spectra of aflatoxin B$_1$ and its congeners is of prime importance for a number of techniques used in our studies. The ^1H chemical shifts and $(^1H,^1H)$ coupling constants are summarized in Table I.

a. ^{13}C Chemical Shifts. Although ^{13}C chemical shifts are used to distinguish between aliphatic, olefinic, aromatic, and carbonyl carbon atoms, overlaps can occur in the chemical shift values of these ^{13}C atoms which could lead to ambiguous assignments. The use of chemical shift values derived from model compounds for assigning similar carbons in a compound is fraught with danger. The effect of methoxy-group substitution on the chemical shift of aromatic carbon atoms has been used to assign carbon atoms C(2)–C(7) in sterigmatocystin (Seto *et al.*, 1974). The shift increments (in ppm) as determined from our values for sterigmatocystin (**32**) (Pachler *et al.*, 1976a) and those reported for 6-methoxysterigmatocystin (Seto *et al.*, 1974; Tanabe, 1976), with the expected values in parentheses, are as follows: C(3), -9.0 (-6.8); C(4), -2.0 ($+2.4$); C(5), -14.8 (-15.0); C(6), $+34.3$ ($+31.3$); and C(7), -10.9 (-8.8). Although these values, with the possible exception of those for C(4), are in close agreement, a wrong assignment was still made by Seto *et al.* (1974).

b. $(^{13}C,^1H)$ Coupling Constants. Carbon-13 proton coupling constants play a pivotal role in many of the assignment techniques which will be discussed later. The values for directly bonded coupling constants $[^1J(CH)]$ reflect the specific type of carbon atom involved in the spin–spin coupling. The most important parameters in the assignment of quaternary carbon atoms are $(^{13}C,^1H)$ coupling constants over more than one bond, $^{>1}J(CH)$. In aromatic systems (e.g., anisole and phenol) the values of the $(^{13}C,^1H)$ coupling constants increase in the order $^4J < {}^2J < {}^3J \ll {}^1J$ (Ernst *et al.*, 1977).

When the hydrogen of a hydroxy group exchanges slowly on the NMR time scale (i.e., when it is strongly hydrogen bonded), a coupling is observed between the proton and the carbon atoms two and three bonds removed (Pachler *et al.*, 1975, 1976a; Chang, 1976; and Wehrli, 1975). The two-bond (^{13}COH) coupling is in the order of 5 Hz, whereas the value for $^3J(COH)$ depends on the stereochemistry of the proton of the hydroxy group: for a *trans* orientation, a value of ca. 8 Hz and for the *cis* arrangement a value of 4–5 Hz is observed. All these couplings can be readily detected by recording coupled ^{13}C spectra before and after substitution of exchangeable protons with deuterium.

This technique was used to distinguish between the two aromatic methine carbon atoms, C(4) and C(6), in sterigmatocystin (**32**) (Pachler *et al.*, 1976a). Off-resonance proton decoupling was of no avail, owing to the small difference in the C(4) and C(6) proton chemical shifts (see Table I). The C(4) resonance appeared as a doublet of triplets $[^1J(CH)$ 165 Hz, $^3J(CH)$ 7 Hz].

TABLE I

^{1}H Chemical Shifts and (^{1}H,^{1}H) Coupling Constants of Averufin (8), 3,6-O,O-Dimethylversiconal Acetate (62), Sterigmatocystin (32), and Aflatoxin B$_1$ (1)

	Averufin		3,6-O,O-Dimethylversiconal acetate[a]			Sterigmatocystin[b]			Aflatoxin B$_1$[b]		
Proton	δ[c]	J(Hz)	Proton	δ[d]	J(Hz)	Proton	δ[d]	J(Hz)	Proton	δ[d]	J(Hz)
4	6.99S		4	7.26S		4	6.74DD	J(4,5)8.2	4	2.62	} AA'BB'
5	7.10D	J(5,7)2.5	5	7.27D	J(5,7)2.4	5	7.84T	J(4,6)1.0	5	3.39	}
7	6.50D		7	6.63D		6	6.80DD	J(5,6)8.2	9	6.42S	
1'	5.24M		1'	9.68S		11	6.42S		13	6.80D	
2'	~1.8		2'	~3.9M		14	6.81D		14	4.75DT	J(13,14)7.3
3'	~1.8		3'	2.63M		15	4.78DT	J(14,15)7.0	15	5.46T	= 2.5
4'	~1.8		4'	4.06T	J(3',4')7	16	5.44T	J(15,16) = J(15,17) = 2.5	16	6.46T	J(14,15) = J(14,16)
6'	1.55S		6'	1.99S		17	6.50T	J(16,17)2.5	OCH$_3$	3.95S	J(15,16)2.5
			3-OCH$_3$	3.97S		OCH$_3$	3.98S				
			6-OCH$_3$	3.91S		OH	13.20S				
OH	12.51S		OH	12.60S							
OH	12.32S		OH	12.12S							

[a] Steyn et al. (1979a).
[b] Pachler et al. (1976).
[c] Relative to internal (CH$_3$)$_4$Si in 1:1 CDCl$_3$:(CD$_3$)$_2$SO. S, Singlet; D, doublet; T, triplet; M, multiplet.
[d] Relative to internal (CH$_3$)$_4$Si in CDCl$_3$.

One of the three-bond couplings was removed by exchange of the hydroxy-group proton with deuterium. In contrast, the C(6) carbon atom, which is five bonds removed, appeared as a doublet of doublets [^1J(CH) 167 Hz, ^3J(CH) 8 Hz] both before and after deuterium exchange.

c. Relaxation Times. The spin-lattice relaxation time (T_1) of ^{13}C atoms generally increases in the sequence methylene, methine, methyl, and quaternary carbon atoms. This parameter is very important in most pulsed FT NMR experiments, as the final signal-to-noise ratio for a specific resonance is critically dependent on the ratio of T_1 to the pulse repetition rate (Shaw, 1976). The T_1 values measured for averufin (**8**) and 3,6-*O,O*-dimethyl-versiconal acetate were ca. 1 sec for proton-bearing and ca. 20 sec for quaternary carbon atoms.

d. Proton Decoupling Techniques.

I. OFF-RESONANCE PROTON DECOUPLING. The relationship between the residual (^{13}C,^{1}H) coupling constant (J_R), measured in an off-resonance proton-decoupled ^{13}C NMR spectrum, and the power γH_2 of the rf field applied at a distance Δv from a specific proton signal, is given by

$$\Delta v = \gamma H_2 J_R / (J_0{}^2 - J_R{}^2)^{1/2}$$

if $\gamma H_2 \gg J_0$, where J_0 is the splitting observed in the single frequency (coupled) ^{13}C NMR spectrum (Pachler, 1972). A plot of the residual coupling constants J_R against different Δv values allows the correlation of specific carbon resonances with the known proton chemical shifts (Pachler *et al.*, 1976b).

II. SELECTIVE PROTON DECOUPLING. A coherent rf field applied at the exact resonance position of a specific proton will remove all the (^{13}C,^{1}H) interactions smaller than the power of the applied field from the carbon atom(s) to which this proton couples. Quaternary carbon atoms frequently exhibit (^{13}C,^{1}H) coupling to protons more than one bond removed. A selective rf field with a power larger than these couplings can therefore be used to assign quaternary carbon resonances from known proton chemical shifts. The technique, apart from its very low sensitivity, has the added disadvantage of an off-resonance proton decoupling effect on the resonances of the other carbon atoms.

III. SELECTIVE POPULATION INVERSION. Selective population inversion (SPI) is a technique which furnishes the same information as but lacks the disadvantages of selective proton decoupling. In a heteronuclear ^{13}C-{^{1}H} SPI experiment a selective rf π-pulse applied at a proton transition inverts the populations of the upper and lower energy levels. A strong nonselective rf $\pi/2$-pulse is then immediately applied in the usual way to the ^{13}C nuclei. The result of this process can be summarized as follows: The intensities of the ^{13}C transitions progressively connected to these energy levels will increase to five times their value in the normal ^{13}C spectrum, while the regressively connected transitions will appear as negative signals with maximum intensities of three times their normal value. The technique is especially advantageous in the assignment of quaternary carbon atoms with relatively long spin–lattice relaxation times (Pachler and Wessels, 1977a,b). In a repetitively pulsed SPI ^{13}C experiment, the repetition rate is determined by the spin–lattice relaxation time of the proton thereby resulting in either a large increase in the signal-to-noise or substantial time-saving in obtaining the same signal-to-noise ratio.

This technique was used in the assignment of a number of quaternary carbon resonances in the spectrum of 3,6-O,O-dimethylversiconal acetate (Steyn et al., 1979a). The C(4) proton in this compound couples with the C(2), C(3), C(10), C(13), and C(14) carbon atoms. The selective inversion of a low-field C(4) proton transition allowed these carbon atoms to be identified.

The selectivity which can be obtained with the SPI technique was demonstrated by the unambiguous assignment of the two methoxy-group proton and carbon resonances in 3,6-O,O-dimethylversiconal acetate (**61**), which differ by only 0.6 ppm and 0.2 ppm, respectively.

e. Deuterium Isotope Shifts. The replacement of a proton with a deuterium atom results in an upfield shift of ca. 0.25 ppm for directly bonded carbon atoms and 0.1 ppm for carbon atoms two bonds removed (Wehrli and Wirthlin, 1976). Wehrli (1975) reported an alpha isotope shift of 0.39 ppm for C(5) in 5-hydroxyflavanones on replacement of the hydroxy-group proton with a deuterium. Addition of a mixture of H_2O–D_2O (1:1) to a compound with exchangeable protons resulted in a doubling of specific ^{13}C resonances owing to deuterium isotope shifts (Feeney et al., 1974). The doubling can be resolved, provided that the hydrogen–deuterium exchange rate is sufficiently slow.

This technique was used to distinguish between C(1) and C(3) as well as between C(6) and C(8) of averufin (**8**) (Gorst-Allman et al., 1977) and with 3,6-O,O-dimethylversiconal acetate (Steyn et al., 1979a). The C(1) and C(8) resonances appeared as doublets because of deuterium isotope shifts of 0.25 ppm and 0.21 ppm, respectively.

f. Lanthanide-Induced Shifts. The addition of lanthanide chelates to substances containing groups susceptible to coordination gives rise to isotopic shifts in their NMR spectra (Williams, 1974). If only the pseudo-contact contribution is operative, the magnitude of the induced shifts will depend on the distance of the nuclei from the lanthanide. However, in ^{13}C spectra, the contact term makes a significant contribution, especially when europium shift reagents are used. The use of ytterbium shift reagents is recommended for ^{13}C NMR studies, as the contact contribution is small, the induced shifts are large, and line broadening is relatively small.

3. *Enrichment and Specific Incorporation*

The percentage enrichment and the specific incorporation values can, theoretically, be determined from the intensities of the different carbon resonances in a PND ^{13}C NMR spectrum. Scott *et al.* (1974) defined the percentage enrichment, i.e., % excess ^{13}C isotope at a specific location, as follows:

$$\% \text{ Enrichment} = \frac{1.1 \text{ (Integrated intensity at labeled center)}}{\text{(Integrated intensity at natural abundance)}} - 1.1$$

and

$$\text{Specific incorporation} = \frac{\% \text{ Enrichment}}{\text{Atom } \% \ ^{13}\text{C in precursor}}$$

The intensities and also the integrated intensities of a ^{13}C NMR signal depend on a number of factors. The spin–lattice relaxation time (T_1) and the NOE differ greatly for the various carbon atoms in a molecule. The addition of a relaxation agent such as chromium trisacetoacetonate which shortens spin–lattice relaxation times and which partially quenches the NOE, has been proposed (Tanabe *et al.*, 1973) to obtain more uniform peak intensities. Levy and Edlund (1975) showed that the NOE is not completely suppressed in medium and large organic molecules. The number of memory locations available for data accumulation in dedicated minicomputers used in pulsed FT NMR spectroscopy is another factor which affects the accuracy of line intensities. For an organic molecule, a spectral width of 5000 Hz at 25.2 MHz is needed to record the ^{13}C NMR spectrum. Using 8 K data points, the digital resolution after Fourier transformation is 1.25 Hz per point. As pointed out by Allerhand (1975), this results in a poorly defined absorption peak, in both height and area.

Simpson (1975) proposed the recording of the natural abundance ^{13}C spectrum and the spectrum of the ^{13}C-enriched compound under identical experimental conditions in order to obtain reliable percentage enrichment data. Gorst-Allman *et al.* (1977) found different enrichment factors when the spectra of natural abundance and enriched averufin (**8**) were recorded at the same concentration under identical experimental conditions using either a short pulse spacing or a long pulse spacing equal to three times the longest T_1. A much wider scatter of enrichment factors was obtained using short pulsing conditions. Similar results were obtained by Cattel *et al.* (1973).

The percentage enrichment can, according to Wright *et al.* (1977), be accurately determined from the intensities of the satellites and center lines in a $[1,2\text{-}^{13}\text{C}]$acetate-enriched precursor. The possibility of geminal and vicinal $(^{13}\text{C},^{13}\text{C})$ coupling is proportional to the percentage enrichment, and complicates the calculation (London *et al.*, 1975). Jones and Phillips (1974) also criticized this method, especially when applied to strongly coupled $(^{13}\text{C},^{13}\text{C})$ systems and to quaternary carbon atoms. Enrichment values should be used with great caution except when employed to determine the location of ^{13}C incorporation.

4. ^{13}C Data and Assignments

a. Averufin (8). A number of ^{13}C NMR studies of averufin (**8**) have been published. Fitzell *et al.* (1975) reported a partial assignment for averufin as well as the ^{13}C NMR spectrum of $[1\text{-}^{13}\text{C}]$acetate-derived averufin. Berger and Jadot (1975, 1976) also studied this compound and the $[1\text{-}^{13}\text{C}]$-acetate-derived analogue. The ^{13}C assignments obtained by the authors are based on the chemical shifts of model compounds, and differ on a number of crucial points from those obtained by Gorst-Allman *et al.* (1977).

The assigned natural abundance PND 25.2 MHz ^{13}C NMR spectrum of averufin is shown in Fig. 12(a), and the chemical shifts from the study by Gorst-Allman *et al.* (1977) are collected in Table II. The assignment of the ^{13}C resonances was accomplished as reported below.

The signals of the methyl carbon $[\text{C}(6'), \delta27.5]$, the three methylene carbon atoms $(\delta15.6, \delta27.1, \text{and } \delta35.5)$, and the single aliphatic methine carbon atom $[\text{C}(1'), \delta66.3]$ were distinguished by their multiplicities in the off-resonance proton-decoupled ^{13}C NMR spectrum. The resonances of the three methylene carbon atoms were assigned on the basis of chemical shift considerations. Shift increments, determined for methyl, phenyl, and methoxy groups in monosubstituted cyclohexanes (Clerc *et al.*, 1973), were added to the appropriate chemical shifts for the carbon atoms in tetrahydropyran to give the following values (experimental values in parentheses): $\text{C}(2'), \delta33.5 (\delta27.1)$; $\text{C}(3'), \delta20.9 (\delta15.6)$; and $\text{C}(4'), \delta39.9 (\delta35.5)$. These values, though consistently higher than the experimental results, suggested the assignments made in Table II. The $(^{13}\text{C},^{13}\text{C})$ coupling constants observed in the PND ^{13}C NMR spectrum of $[1,2\text{-}^{13}\text{C}]$acetate-derived averufin confirmed these assignments. The resonance assigned to $\text{C}(1')$ showed a $^{1}J(\text{CC})$ coupling of 34.8 Hz which was also observed at $\delta27.1 [\text{C}(2')]$. The only aliphatic quaternary carbon atom, $\text{C}(5')$, resonated at $\delta100.9$, a value in agreement with the chemical shift of carbon atoms in similar environments (Pachler *et al.*, 1976a). Selective irradiation at the frequency of the methyl protons changed the pattern of the resonance at $\delta100.9$, thereby confirming the assignment.

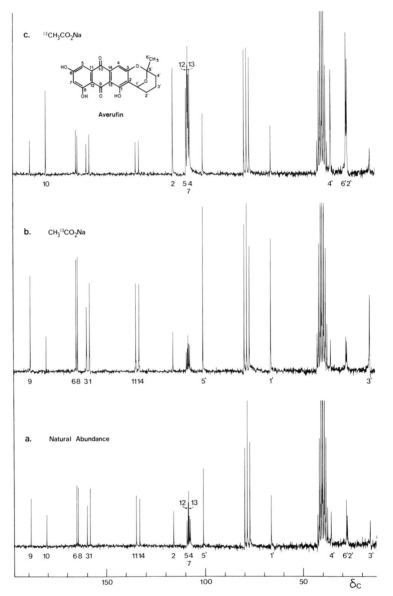

Fig. 12. Proton noise decoupled 25.2 MHz ^{13}C NMR spectra of averufin (**8**). Spectral width 5000 Hz; pulse delay 40 sec; 90 rf pulse (18 μsec); transients 1024 (a) natural abundance, (b) derived from [1-^{13}C]acetate, (c) derived from [2-^{13}C]acetate. [From Gorst-Allman *et al.* (1977), *J. Chem. Soc. Perkin Trans. 1*, 2181–2188. Copyright permission from The Chemical Society, London.]

^{13}C NMR Data for Averufin (8), Versicolorin A (21), 3,6-O,O-Dimethylversiconal Acetate (62), Sterigmatocystin (32), and Aflatoxin B$_1$ (1)

Carbon atom	Averufin[a] δ[e]	Averufin J(CC)(Hz)	Versicolorin A[b] δ[f]	Versicolorin A J(CC)(Hz)	3,6-O,O-Dimethylversiconal acetate[c] δ[e]	acetate J(CC)(Hz)	Sterigmatocystin[d] δ[f,g]	Sterigmatocystin J(CC)[h](Hz)	Aflatoxin B$_1$[d] δ[e]	Aflatoxin B$_1$ J(CC)(Hz)
1	158.1*	64.1	158.2*	62.7	161.7*	62.6	180.9*	58	155.2*	S
2	115.8	65.3	120.4	62.6	119.5	71.1	108.8		117.4	60
3	159.9*	65.2	163.4*	~61.5	163.4*	70.6	162.1*		201.3*	40
4	107.9	65.1	101.6	63.9	103.0	64.3	110.0	70	35.1	40
5	109.1	62.1	108.8	62.4	108.6	66.0	135.4*	59	29.0*	S
6	164.9*	63.3	165.0*	62.7	166.2*	65.3	105.7	58	177.1*	60
7	108.0	70.0	107.8	69.8	106.0	70.6	154.7*	S[i]	104.0	64
8	164.1*	70.1	164.0*	69.6	165.0*	70.0	153.7*		161.6*	71
9	188.7*	57.7	188.7*	58.5	189.6*	58.0	106.4		90.6	71
10	180.7	53.6	180.4	54.6	181.0	54.8	164.3*		165.8*	61
11	134.6*	53.8	134.6*	53.8	134.5*	54.4	90.4	72	107.9	61
12	108.6	58.3	108.4	58.8	109.7	57.4	163.0*		153.0	64
13	108.2	64.2	111.3	~61.0	110.7	62.6	105.7		113.6*	33
14	132.9*	65.0	135.1*	63.1	134.3*	63.9	113.1*	34	47.9	33
15 or 1'	66.3*	34.8	112.8*	33.2	199.6*	38.5	47.9	34	102.7*	75
16 or 2'	27.1	34.6	47.2	33.0	44.8	38.7	102.4*	76	145.4	75
17 or 3'	15.6*	31.6	101.2*	75.0	26.5*	39.1	145.1	76		
4'	35.5	31.8	145.3	74.9	62.3	38.8				
5'	100.9*	48.8			170.6*	60.0				
6'	27.5	49.0			20.8	59.5				
OCH$_3$ or 3-OCH$_3$					56.4		56.6		56.6	
6-OCH$_3$					56.1					
Solvent	CDCl$_3$:(CD$_3$)$_2$SO(1:1)		(CD$_3$)$_2$SO at 95°C		CDCl$_3$		CDCl$_3$		CDCl$_3$	

[a] Gorst-Allman et al. (1977). Asterisk indicates carbon atom derived from [1-^{13}C]acetate. [b] Gorst-Allman et al. (1976a). [c] Steyn et al. (1979b). [d] Pachler et al. (1976a). [e] Relative to internal (CH$_3$)$_4$Si. [f] Relative to internal (CH$_3$)$_4$Si. Measured from internal (CD$_3$)$_2$SO and corrected by using the expression δ[(CH$_3$)$_4$Si] = δ[(CD$_3$)$_2$SO] + 39.7. [g] [1-^{13}C]acetate enrichment data from Tanabe et al. (1970). [h] Seto et al. (1974). [i] S, enhanced singlet.

By correlating the residual splittings (J_R) observed in a series of off-resonance proton-decoupled ^{13}C NMR spectra with the known chemical shifts of the aromatic protons (see Table I), the signal at $\delta108.0$ was assigned to C(7). An observed ($^{13}C,OH$) coupling to C(7) confirmed the assignment of this carbon atom. The resonances at $\delta107.6$ and $\delta109.1$ were attributed to C(4) and C(5), respectively. The splitting patterns in the NOE single-frequency spectrum were used to assign the last two resonances to individual carbon atoms. The C(5) signal was a doublet of doublets centered at $\delta109.1$ [$^1J(CH)$ 166.4 Hz, $^3J(CH)$ 4.9 Hz], and that of C(4) was a doublet at $\delta107.6$ [$^1J(CH)$ 168.4 Hz]. The two carbonyl carbon atoms [C(9) and C(10)] resonated at $\delta180.7$ and $\delta188.7$. The resonance at $\delta180.7$ exhibited triplet fine structure, which simplified on irradiation at the frequency of either H(4) or H(5), assigning it to C(10) and the resonance at $\delta188.7$ to C(9).

The aromatic quaternary carbon atoms can be divided into three different groups: (a) oxygen-bearing carbon atoms [C(1), C(3), C(6), C(8); $\delta158–165$]; (b) carbon atoms *ortho* to aryloxy substituents [C(2), C(12), C(13); $\delta108.2$, $\delta108.6$, $\delta115.8$]; and (c) carbon atoms C(11) and C(14), which resonate at $\delta132.9$ and $\delta134.6$. To assign these carbon atoms, extensive use was made of (C,H) couplings over more than one bond (Ernst *et al.*, 1977) and of selective proton decoupling experiments.

The resonances of the carbon atoms of group (a) showed extensive fine structure. Two of the resonances appeared as triplets at $\delta159.9$ [$^{>1}J(CH)$ 2.7 Hz] and $\delta164.9$ [$^{>1}J(CH)$ 2.3 Hz], and the other two as doublets [$\delta158.1$, $^{>1}J(CH)$ 1.8 Hz; $\delta164.1$, $^{>1}J(CH)$ 3.4 Hz]. Selective decoupling of H(1') caused a collapse of the resonance at $\delta158.1$ to a singlet and changed the triplet at $\delta159.9$ to a doublet. The latter resonance also changed to a doublet on decoupling of H(4). The peaks at $\delta158.1$ and 159.9 were therefore assigned to C(1) and C(3), respectively. The triplet at $\delta164.9$ with two-bond couplings to H(5) and H(7) was assigned to C(6), and the doublet at $\delta164.1$ to C(8). Decoupling of H(7) changed the signal at $\delta164.9$ to a doublet and resulted in the collapse of the signal at $\delta164.9$ to a singlet, thus confirming the assignments.

Irradiation of H(1') changed the quartet at $\delta115.8$ to a triplet. This signal was assigned to C(2), the only carbon atom in group (b) less than four bonds away from H(1'). Selective decoupling of H(7) changed the triplet at $\delta108.6$ to a doublet, whereas the doublet at $\delta108.2$ collapsed when H(4) was irradiated; these resonances were therefore assigned to C(12) and C(13), respectively.

The two resonances at $\delta134.6$ and $\delta132.9$ caused by C(11) and C(14) could not be assigned individually from the natural abundance spectrum of averufin. The two signals were assigned to C(11) and C(14), respectively, on the basis of the observed ($^{13}C,^{13}C$) coupling in [$1,2-^{13}C$]acetate-derived averufin.

The PND spectrum of [1-^{13}C]acetate-labeled averufin [Fig. 12(b)] showed ten enhanced carbon signals: C(1′), C(3′), C(5′), C(1), C(3), C(6), C(8), C(9), C(11), and C(14). The remaining ten carbon atoms are derived from [2-^{13}C]acetate [see Fig. 12(c)]. All the carbon resonances in the PND spectrum of [1,2-^{13}C]acetate-derived averufin (Fig. 13) exhibited satellite peaks arising from (^{13}C,^{13}C) couplings. The measurement of the couplings to C(12) and C(13) was prevented by overlap with the C(4), C(5), and C(7) resonances. These values could, however, be obtained from a low-power PND partially relaxed FT ^{13}C NMR spectrum (Oldfield et al., 1975) (see insert, Fig. 13). The ^1J(CC) values in Table II proved that averufin is derived

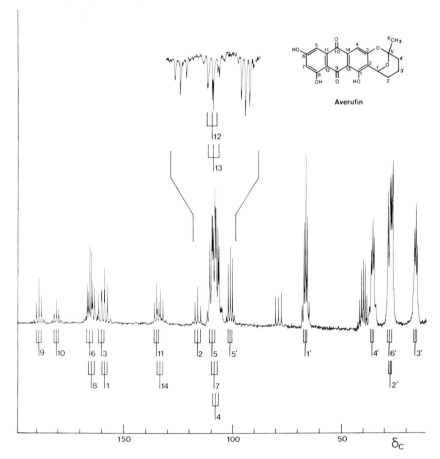

Fig. 13. Proton noise decoupled 25.2 MHz ^{13}C NMR spectrum of averufin (**8**) derived from [1,2-^{13}C]acetate. Spectral width 5000 Hz, pulse delay 1 sec; 90° rf pulse (50 μsec); transients 20 K. Insert: low power off-resonance proton-decoupled partially relaxed spectrum. [From Gorst-Allman et al. (1977), J. Chem. Soc. Perkin Trans. 1, 2181–2188. Copyright permission from The Chemical Society, London.]

from ten intact acetate units: C(6′)–C(5′), C(4′)–C(3′), C(2′)–C(1′), C(2)–C(3), C(4)–C(14), C(10)–C(11), C(5)–C(6), C(7)–C(8), C(12)–C(9), and C(13)–C(1). The results are summarized in Figs. 14 and 21.

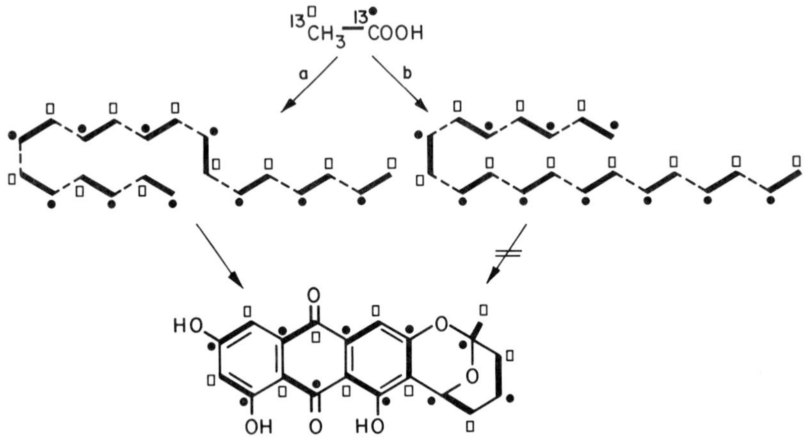

Fig. 14. Alternative arrangements of the acetate units in the biosynthesis of averufin. ● : C(1) of acetate; □ : C(2) of acetate.

b. Versicolorin A (21). The only ^{13}C NMR biosynthetic study of versicolorin A was described by Gorst-Allman *et al.* (1978). Cox *et al.* (1977) and Berger and Jadot (1976) reported ^{13}C data for versicolorin C (**25**). The chemical shifts and ^1J(CC) values for [1,2-^{13}C]acetate-derived versicolorin A are given in Table II, and the labeling results are shown in Fig. 21.

c. Versiconal Acetate (19). Cox *et al.* (1977) concluded from a ^{13}C NMR study of versiconal acetate (**19**) that the compound exists in (CD$_3$)$_2$SO solution as an equilibrium mixture of the two hemiacetal forms as shown in **19**. The authors based the structure of versiconal acetate mainly on the resonance at δ113.0 ppm, which they assigned to a five-membered ring hemiacetal carbon atom. Fitzell *et al.* (1977) studied this compound in (CD$_3$)$_2$CO solution and claimed that it exists predominantly as the linear hemiacetal. A signal at δ116.2 was assigned to C(1′). A detailed study by Steyn *et al.* (1979a) showed that versiconal acetate is a solvent-dependent equilibrium mixture. The hemiacetal carbon atom, C(1′), should resonate at ∼ 108 ppm. The other values observed for this carbon atom must be due to the average value of this carbon atom for the hemiacetal and aldehyde structures. Selective methylation of versiconal acetate gave the 3,6-*O,O*-dimethyl derivative which in CDCl$_3$ exists as the aldehyde **61** (see Fig. 15). The ^{13}C resonances of this compound were assigned by Steyn *et al.* (1979a) (Table II).

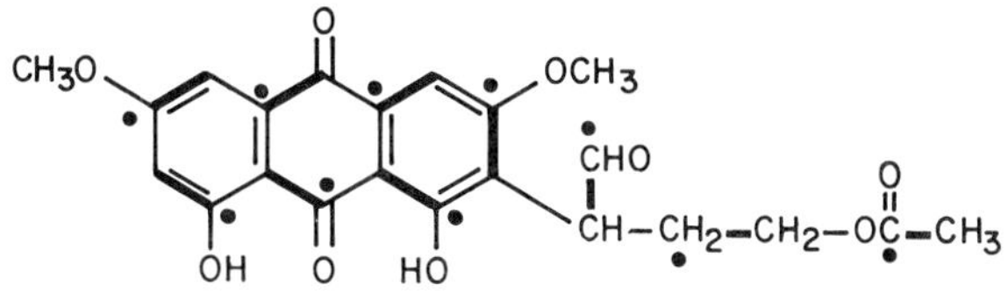

61

Fig. 15.   Structural formula of 3,6-O,O-dimethylversiconal acetate.

The results from ^{13}C-labeling studies using [1-^{13}C]- and [1,2-^{13}C]acetates are collected in Table II and shown in **61** (Steyn *et al.*, 1979b) and in Fig. 21.

The biosyntheses of the related metabolite versiconol acetate (**20**) and of versiconol (**27**) were also reported by Steyn *et al.* (1979b).

d. Sterigmatocystin (32).   The biosynthesis of sterigmatocystin was initially studied by Tanabe *et al.* (1970) employing [1-^{13}C]- and [2-^{13}C]-acetates as precursors. Although only a partial assignment of the resonances in the natural abundance ^{13}C NMR spectrum of sterigmatocystin was reported, the study confirmed the acetate origin of the metabolite. The (^{13}C,[13]C) coupling observed between C(15) and C(9) in the PND spectrum of [2-^{13}C]acetate-derived sterigmatocystin indicates the unusual head-to-head linkage of two acetate units.

On the basis of their ^{13}C assignments for sterigmatocystin and the observed coupling constants, [1]J(CC), in the PND ^{13}C NMR spectrum of [1,2-^{13}C]-acetate-enriched sterigmatocystin, Seto *et al.* (1974) proposed an erroneous arrangement of intact acetate units. A reinvestigation of the assignment of the ^{13}C NMR spectrum of sterigmatocystin by Pachler *et al.* (1975, 1976a) showed the previous assignment of Seto *et al.* (1974) to be incorrect. The revised distribution of intact acetate units is shown in Fig. 21.

e. Aflatoxin B₁ (1).   The natural abundance ^{13}C NMR spectrum of aflatoxin B$_1$ was completely assigned by Steyn *et al.* (1975) and Pachler *et al.* (1976a). This assignment, which differed from that of Hsieh *et al.* (1975), was subsequently confirmed by Cox and Cole (1977). The ^{13}C chemical shifts as well as the (^{13}C,[13]C) coupling constants obtained from the ^{13}C NMR spectrum of [1,2-^{13}C]acetate-derived aflatoxin B$_1$ are given in Table II.

The signals from proton-bearing carbon atoms were assigned by correlating the residual splittings (J_R) in off-resonance proton-decoupled ^{13}C spectra with the known proton chemical shifts (see Table I). The magnitude of the observed directly bonded (^{13}C,[1]H) coupling constants supported these assignments.

When a selective π-pulse in an SPI experiment was applied at 3 Hz to higher field of the H(9) resonance, the signals at δ104.0 [doublet, $>$[1]J(CH) 6 Hz] and $\delta 107.9$ [doublet of doublets, $^{>1}J(CH)$ 9 and 3 Hz] were affected, thereby assigning them to C(7) and C(11). Selective decoupling of the C(14) proton removed the 3 Hz coupling from the $\delta 107.9$ resonance, thereby assigning it to C(11).

If chemical shift values are taken into consideration, C(2) ($\delta 117.4$) is the only other carbon atom which could resonate in the 90–120 ppm region. The corresponding carbon atom in coumarin, C(3), resonates at $\delta 116.3$ (Lapper, 1974), whereas the β-carbon atom in styrene resonates at $\delta 112.3$ (Stothers, 1972).

Selective decoupling of the C(4) protons resulted in the collapse of the multiplets at $\delta 201.3$ and $\delta 177.1$ to triplets with couplings of 3 Hz and 7 Hz, respectively. Conversely, decoupling of the C(5) protons simplified the same multiplets to triplets with couplings of 6 Hz and 3 Hz, respectively. The resonance at $\delta 201.3$ is characteristic of a carbon atom at an oxo group and was assigned to C(3), and the resonance at $\delta 177.1$ was allocated to C(6). Selective irradiation of H(13) changed the resonance at $\delta 165.8$, attributed to C(10), from a doublet of doublets [$^{>1}J(CH)$ 7 and 3 Hz] to a doublet with a splitting ca. 3 Hz and in addition affected the resonances of C(14), C(15), and C(16).

In the single-frequency NOE ^{13}C NMR spectrum, the remaining singlet resonances at $\delta 153.0$ and $\delta 155.2$ and the multiplet with at least a quartetlike fine structure at $\delta 161.6$ were ascribed to C(1), C(8), and C(12). As C(1) is four bonds removed from the nearest proton and as C(12) has only one proton three bonds removed, it follows that the resonance at $\delta 161.6$ is due to C(8). The assignments of C(1) ($\delta 155.2$) and C(12) ($\delta 153.0$) are based on the results of a Eu(fod)$_3$-induced shift experiment [tris(2,2-dimethyl-6,6,7,7,8,8,8-heptafluoro-3,5-octanedione)europium(III)]. Complexation occurred at the C(3) oxo group, causing a downfield shift of the C(1) resonance ($\delta 155.2$), whereas the C(12) resonance ($\delta 153.0$) remained unaffected.

The [1-^{13}C]acetate-derived aflatoxin B$_1$ spectrum [Fig. 16(a)] shows nine enhanced carbon signals. Seven enhanced carbon signals were observed in the spectrum of [2-^{13}C]acetate-derived aflatoxin B$_1$ [Fig. 16(b)]. The labeling pattern of aflatoxin B$_1$ derived from the two singly labeled ^{13}C acetates is consonant with the reported results from [^{14}C]acetate (Biollaz *et al.*, 1970). The observed directly bonded ($^{13}C, ^{13}C$) coupling constants of 34 Hz between C(5) and C(6) (Hsieh *et al.*, 1975) and of 44 Hz between C(11) and C(14) in the spectra of [1-^{13}C]- and [2-^{13}C]acetate-derived aflatoxin B$_1$ [see Figs. 16(a) and (b)] are indicative of rearrangements involving bond fission during the biosynthetic process.

The PND ^{13}C NMR spectrum of [1,2-^{13}C]acetate-enriched aflatoxin B$_1$ [Fig. 16(c)] and the values of $^1J(CC)$ proved that it contains seven intact acetate units: C(2)–C(6), C(3)–C(4), C(7)–C(12), C(8)–C(9), C(10)–C(11)

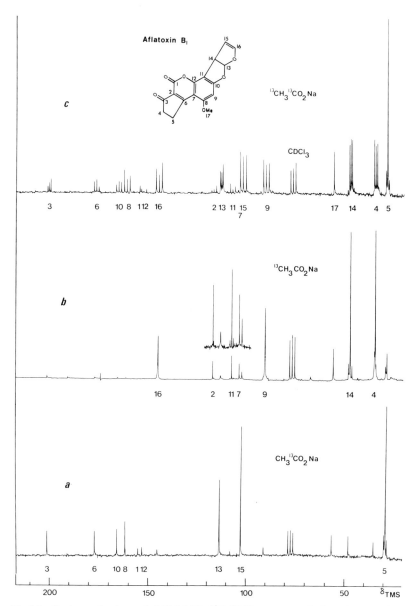

Fig. 16.   Proton noise decoupled 25.2 MHz ^{13}C NMR spectrum of aflatoxin B$_1$ (**1**) derived from (a) [1-^{13}C]acetate, spectral width 5500 Hz, pulse delay 5 sec, 80° rf pulse, transients 40 K; (b) [2-^{13}C]acetate, spectral width 5500 Hz, pulse delay 1 sec, 80° rf pulse, transients 32 K; (c) [1,2-^{13}C]acetate, spectral width 5500 Hz, pulse delay 5 sec, 80° rf pulse, transients 32 K. [From Pachler *et al.* (1976a), *J. Chem. Soc. Perkin Trans. 1*, 1182–1189. Copyright permission from The Chemical Society, London.]

C(13)–C(14), and C(15)–C(16). The C(1) and C(5) resonances were enhanced but showed no (^{13}C,^{13}C) coupling, thus confirming that two bond fissions with the concomitant loss of two methyl acetate-derived carbon atoms occur in the biosynthesis of aflatoxin B_1. The data from the ^{13}C labeling studies are summarized in Fig. 21.

IV. THE SEQUENCE OF THE AFLATOXIN BIOSYNTHETIC PATHWAY: ELUCIDATION BY USING BLOCKED MUTANTS, ENZYME INHIBITORS, AND CONVERSION OF POTENTIAL PRECURSORS

The biochemical events prior to the elaboration of the aflatoxins were clarified by the use of mutants, and enzyme inhibitors and by incorporation studies of potential precursors. Norsolorinic acid (14), averufin (8), versiconal acetate (19) (from biosynthetic inhibitors), and versicolorin A (21) comply with two of the postulated requirements for an intermediate; i.e., they are overproduced by a mutant blocked in aflatoxin synthesis and furthermore are converted into aflatoxin by the wild-type culture of *A. parasiticus*. In view of the low incorporation of acetate into aflatoxin B_1 [relative specific activity (RSA) = 0.24 vs. a maximum of 9.0], the high RSA values and the higher quantities of aflatoxins derived from the above-mentioned four precursors (14, 8, 19, and 21), as compared to acetate, provide strong evidence for their conversion into the aflatoxins without the intermediary formation of acetate (Singh and Hsieh, 1977).

Mutations of aflatoxin-producing strains of *A. parasiticus* were accomplished by ultraviolet irradiation (Lee *et al.*, 1971) and by treatment with the mutagen *N*-methyl-*N*-nitro-*N*-nitrosoguanidine (Detroy *et al.*, 1973). These mutants had altered biosynthetic capacities, as indicated by the impairment of aflatoxin production and the accumulation of norsolorinic acid (14) in the mycelium. In mutant J-B-8, the synthesis of norsolorinic acid paralleled growth, whereas aflatoxin formation typically occurred as growth began to decline (Detroy *et al.*, 1973). Incubation of [^{14}C]norsolorinic acid (14) with resting cells of the parent strain of *A. parasiticus* led to its conversion into aflatoxin B_1 (1) (Hsieh *et al.*, 1976a). Labels from norsolorinic acid were incorporated into aflatoxin B_1 in significantly lower yield than those from averufin, presumably because norsolorinic acid required conversion into averufin before its conversion into aflatoxin B_1.

Donkersloot *et al.* (1972) induced mutations of the conidia of *A. parasiticus* ATCC 15517 by treatment with *N*-methyl-*N*-nitro-*N*-nitrosoguanidine. One mutant (W49 ≡ ATCC 24551) in which aflatoxin production was drastically reduced, however, accumulated averufin (**8**) in the mycelium. Only traces of averufin were found in the wild-type mycelium. $[^{14}C]$Averufin was efficiently converted into aflatoxin B_1 by incubation with resting cells of the wild-type strain (Lin *et al.*, 1973; Lin and Hsieh, 1973), indicating its intermediacy in the pathway leading from acetate to aflatoxin B_1. Hsieh *et al.* (1976b) converted $[1\text{-}^{13}C]$acetate-derived averufin into aflatoxin B_1 by the mycelium of *A. parasiticus*. The excess ^{13}C indicated that the formed aflatoxin B_1 had the same enrichment pattern as that derived from $[1\text{-}^{13}C]$acetate. Recently, de Jesus *et al.* (1979; unpublished results) converted $[1,2\text{-}^{13}C]$acetate-derived averufin into aflatoxin B_1 by incubation with the wild-type strain of *A. parasiticus*. This aflatoxin B_1 contained the same distribution of ^{13}C labels and directly bonded ($^{13}C,^{13}C$) coupling constants as that derived from $[1,2\text{-}^{13}C]$-acetate (see Fig. 21). This experiment explicitly verified the crucial role of averufin in the aflatoxin biosynthesis, as the carbon atoms derived from the aliphatic side chain and the anthraquinonoid nucleus contributed equally to the aflatoxin B_1 molecule, except the methoxymethyl carbon atom. Singh and Hsieh (1977) showed that the reduced aflatoxigenicity of the averufin-accumulating mutant was due to a defect in the enzyme responsible for the conversion of averufin into versiconal acetate. In the presence of versiconal acetate, the mutant produced about twice as much aflatoxin B_1 as it did in the presence of acetate. Furthermore, addition of versicolorin A and sterigmatocystin substantially increased the yield of aflatoxin by the mutant (Singh and Hsieh, 1977).

Dichlorvos possesses a strong inhibitory effect on aflatoxin biosynthesis in *A. flavus* and *A. parasiticus*, presumably by specific enzyme inhibition. Dichlorvos inhibited 90% of the aflatoxin production by *A. parasiticus* ATCC 15517 (Hsieh, 1973). An early step in the secondary metabolic pathway was inhibited, as only additions of dichlorvos prior to the initiation of toxin production, which occurs 40 hr after incubation effectively stopped the toxin synthesis. The reduction in aflatoxin synthesis was accompanied by the excretion of versiconal acetate (**19**). Yao and Hsieh (1974) reported the efficient conversion of $[^{14}C]$versiconal acetate (13.7%) into aflatoxin B_1 by a nitrogen-free resting cell medium of *A. parasiticus*. Averufin is converted into versiconal acetate, and not into aflatoxin B_1, in the presence of dichlorvos (Yao and Hsieh, 1974).

Singh and Hsieh (1977) likewise observed the inhibition of versiconal acetate conversion into aflatoxin by dichlorvos. However, the conversion of versicolorin A (**21**), and therefore also that of sterigmatocystin (**32**), into the aflatoxins, was not affected. These findings indicated that **21** and **32** lay beyond the step in the biosynthetic sequence inhibited by dichlorvos and that versicolorin A is most probably derived from versiconal acetate.

Mutants of *A. parasiticus* (NRRL A-16,462) were obtained by ultraviolet irradiation (Bennett and Goldblatt, 1973). One white-spored mutant (1-11-105wh-1) displayed impaired aflatoxin production and aberrant pigmentation. The major pigment, versicolorin A, was formed in very low yield by the nonmutant strain (Lee *et al.*, 1975). [^{14}C]Versicolorin A (**21**) was converted very efficiently (46%) by wild-type cultures of *A. parasiticus* into aflatoxin B$_1$ (Lee *et al.*, 1975). Singh and Hsieh (1977) concluded that this mutant (1-11-105wh-1) was deficient in aflatoxin production because of blocking of the enzyme catalyzing the conversion of versicolorin A into sterigmatocystin. In fact, this mutant incorporated 54% of the radioactivity of sterigmatocystin into aflatoxin B$_1$, and the conversion was not inhibited by dichlorvos.

Dutton and Anderson (1978) removed the cell walls of *A. flavus* by enzymatic digestion with *Trichoderma viride*. The formed protoplasts are capable of *de novo* aflatoxin biosynthesis. [^{14}C]Versicolorin A added to the protoplasts was incorporated into aflatoxin B$_1$. The racemic versicolorin C is formed by aflatoxin-producing strains of *A. flavus* (Heathcote and Dutton, 1969). Although Heathcote *et al.* (1976) reported that versicolorin C was not converted into the aflatoxins by *A. flavus* CMI 91019B, Dutton and Anderson (1978) reported its apparent conversion into aflatoxin by protoplast preparations.

Holker and Underwood (1964) postulated sterigmatocystin (**32**) as a precursor of aflatoxin B$_1$. This proposal was supported by the similarity between the label distributions (^{13}C and ^{14}C) of the two compounds and by the isolation of *O*-methylsterigmatocystin (**34**) (Burkhardt and Forgacs, 1973) and of aspertoxin (**37**) (Rodricks *et al.*, 1968) from aflatoxin-producing strains of *A. flavus*. Although Schroeder and Kelton (1975) reported that a large number of isolates of *A. flavus* produced both aflatoxin B$_1$ and sterigmatocystin, Steyn (1977, unpublished results) could not confirm these findings. Elsworthy *et al.* (1970) converted 6-hydroxydihydrosterigmatocystin (^{14}C label in the *O*-methyl group) with cultures of *A. parasiticus* (7 days at 25°C) into aflatoxins. The total incorporations were as follows: B$_1$, 0.06%; B$_2$, 1.94%; G$_1$, 0.06%; and G$_2$, 0.41%. On the basis of these results, it was postulated that 6-hydroxydihydrosterigmatocystin could be a direct precursor of aflatoxins B$_2$ and G$_2$. Hsieh *et al.* (1973) reported the conversion of [^{14}C]sterigmatocystin by the resting mycelium of *A. parasiticus* ATCC 15517 into aflatoxin B$_1$, whereas Singh and Hsieh (1976) achieved this conversion in a cell-free system in the presence of NADPH. The synthetic activity was shown by the time course of the conversion and the linear dependence of the aflatoxin B$_1$ yield on enzyme concentrations. Optimum activity was obtained at pH 7.5–7.8 at 27°C. The NADPH dependence of the sterigmatocystin-to-aflatoxin reaction indicates that the enzyme catalyzing the reaction is, most probably, an oxygenase. The enzymatic conversion of sterigmatocystin into aflatoxin B_1 confirmed their biosynthetic relationship. Heathcote et al. (1976) studied the conversion of ^{14}C-labeled aflatoxins by A. flavus CMI 91019B into related metabolites. They concluded that aflatoxin B_1 may be converted into most of the other aflatoxins e.g., B_2, B_{2a}, G_1, G_2, and G_{2a}. Furthermore, aflatoxin B_1 and G_1 were not converted into the aflatoxin M series, but in contrast, aflatoxin M_1 acted as a precursor of both aflatoxin B_1 and G_1. These authors concluded that the later stages of the aflatoxin biosynthesis probably follow the order $M_1 \rightarrow B_1 \rightarrow G_1$. Biollaz et al. (1970) suggested that aflatoxin B_1 is a precursor of aflatoxin M_1, as the benzylic carbon [C(14)] was derived from the acetate methyl group. The conclusion of Biollaz et al. (1970) was corroborated by the findings of Maggon and Venkitasubramanian (1973) that aflatoxins M_1, B_{2a}, and G_{2a} are not precursors of aflatoxins B_1 and G_1. Maggon and Venkitasubramanian (1973) also presented unambiguous evidence that aflatoxin B_1 is the biogenetic precursor of aflatoxin G_1, and they postulated that the conversion may involve a keto-lactonase system.

Hsieh et al. (1976a) attempted to incorporate radioactivity into aflatoxin B_1 from four tritiated anthraquinone and anthrone derivatives to simulate the proposed C_{18} compounds (Biollaz et al., 1970). None of the four compounds was readily convertible into aflatoxin B_1. These findings clearly indicated that a C_{18} naphthacene precursor is no longer tenable.

V. BIOSYNTHETIC SCHEME

Biogenetic studies on aflatoxin B_1 have shown that the basic skeleton of the molecule is derived from the acetate–polymalonate pathway and that methionine contributes the methoxymethyl group (Biollaz et al., 1970; Pachler et al., 1976a). Fundamental aspects of the biosynthesis of polyketides were adequately reviewed by Birch (1967), Packter (1973), and Money (1973). It is probable that the enzymes of aflatoxin biosynthesis and of other polyketides are similarly arranged in discrete particles in the postmitochondrial fraction (Maggon et al., 1977). The enzyme activities involved in aflatoxin biosynthesis may be divided into two main phases: (a) construction of the anthraquinone precursor (e.g., averufin) by the polyketide synthetase, and (b) the cleavage and rearrangement phase, which involves enzymes having different substrate specificities. Gatenbeck (1960) established the acetate–polymalonate origin of anthraquinones, which involves condensation of an enzyme-bound carboxylic acid derivative (acetyl) with a variable number of malonate units (nine units for averufin). Direct evidence for a specific carrier protein in polyketide biosynthesis is not available; Weinberg (1970) proposed that metal chelation, e.g., Zn^{2+}, may be involved in the stabilization of the intermediates on the carrier protein. The polyketide synthetase leads to enzyme-bound β-polyketothiol esters, which undergo intramolecular condensation–aromatization and secondary transformations. Polyketides are evidently limited to polycarbonyl compounds of no more than ten carbonyl groups, hence the sharp cutout at the C_{20} level. Although most work on aromatic polyketides was done on whole cells, considerable progress has been made on the enzymology of systems which produce phenolic compounds by this pathway, e.g., 6-methylsalicylic acid synthetase (Dimroth *et al.*, 1970; Scott *et al.*, 1971), and on the synthesis of polyketide-type aromatic systems by biogenetically modeled routes (Harris and Harris, 1977).

The biosynthesis of the anthraquinonoid C_{20} compounds is defined by the detailed analysis of averufin (Gorst-Allman *et al.*, 1977), as shown in Fig. 14. These data established both an acetate–polymalonate pathway with the labels occupying alternating positions in the molecule and the directional mode of folding, (a) (see Fig. 14), of the polyketide progenitor. This polyketide is probably common to all the metabolites depicted in Figs. 1–6. This supposition was corroborated by recent findings on the arrangement of intact acetate units in compounds derived from averufin, namely, versiconal acetate (Steyn *et al.*, 1979b), versicolorin A (Gorst-Allman *et al.*, 1978), and sterigmatocystin and aflatoxin B_1 (Pachler *et al.*, 1976a). From these results and those obtained from the use of mutants and feeding of putative intermediates, it is possible to present a scheme for the aflatoxin biosynthesis (see Fig. 21).

Several mechanisms have been proposed for the conversion of the C_6 side chain of averufin into the C_4 side chain in, e.g., versicolorin A, with the concomitant rearrangement leading to the unique head-to-head coupling of the dihydrofuran ring and the aromatic system. Thomas (1972) proposed a Baeyer–Villiger oxidation on an acetylfuran intermediate; Kingston *et al.* (1976), however, suggested that the key rearrangement step occurred through a pinacol-type rearrangement of the open-chain form of nidurufin (9). Tanabe *et al.* (1976) favored a Favorsky rearrangement which involved a cyclopropanone intermediate. Gorst-Allman *et al.* (1977) advocated an epoxide intermediate for this rearrangement (see Fig. 17). This mechanism involves ring opening and hydration of averufin, followed sequentially by dehydration and epoxidation. Rearrangement of the epoxide affords the branched benzylic aldehyde. The terminal acetyl can be removed by an enzymatic Baeyer–Villiger oxidation. Versiconal acetate (19) is a compound of this nature; both its structure (Steyn *et al.*, 1979a) and biosynthesis (Steyn *et al.*, 1979b) support an intermediary epoxide. The biosynthesis

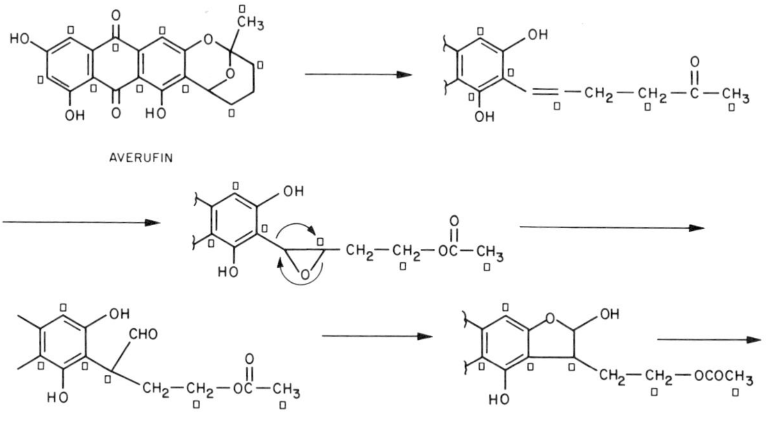

AVERUFIN

VERSICONAL ACETATE (19)

Fig. 17. Proposed structural rearrangement of averufin into versiconal acetate. □ : C(2) of acetate.

of versiconol acetate (**20**) is naturally very closely related to that of versiconal acetate, as the former is obtained by reduction of the aldehyde group.

Mild acid treatment of versiconal acetate causes a rearrangement to versicolorin C (both these compounds are racemic mixtures). Versiconal acetate is released only during genetic blockage (dichlorvos) of aflatoxin-producing fungi. Under normal aflatoxin-producing conditions, a versiconal acetate-type compound should apparently retain its chirality on the enzyme surface before transformation into versicolorin A. The biosynthesis of versicolorin A (Gorst-Allman *et al.*, 1978a) (see Fig. 21) constitutes direct proof of its role in aflatoxin biosynthesis and additionally for the biosynthesis of all the compounds in Fig. 4. Fungi dissimilar to, e.g., *A. versicolor*, namely, *D. pini* (Danks and Hodges, 1974) and *Cercospora smilacis* (Assante *et al.*, 1977) produced not only the dothistromins and 6-deoxyversicolorin C (*D. pini*) but some C_{20}-anthraquinones, e.g., averufin, averythrin, and nidurufin. The co-occurrence of these metabolites attests to similar biochemical reactions (Shaw *et al.*, 1978) in the secondary metabolism of these diverse fungi.

Anthraquinones are metabolically active and are frequently transformed by fungal enzymes into xanthones, e.g., ravenelin (Birch *et al.*, 1976) and tajixanthone (Holker *et al.*, 1974), and into secalonic acids (Franck, 1969), (Kurobane *et al.*, 1978). The biosynthetic relationship between versicolorin A and sterigmatocystin is indicated by their structural similarity, their co-occurrence in several fungi, and also the fact that their absolute configurations are identical (Gorst-Allman *et al.*, 1978). In aflatoxin biosynthesis, a versicolorin, probably versicolorin A, is converted into sterigmatocystin by oxidative decarboxylation and elimination of an acetate-derived methyl carbon atom. In the biosynthetic sequence the *O*-methylation step lies beyond versicolorin A but before sterigmatocystin. The ^{13}C assignments of sterigmatocystin by Seto *et al.* (1974) involved the crucial interchange of the C(4) and C(6) resonances; this led to an erroneous arrangement of acetate units in the central ring of sterigmatocystin and an incorrect folding, (b) of the original polyketide precursor of averufin (see Fig. 14). The ^{13}C NMR study of sterigmatocystin by Pachler *et al.* (1976a) allowed only one arrangement of acetate units consonant with its role in aflatoxin biosynthesis (see Fig. 21). The biosynthesis of sterigmatocystin illustrates the origin of the compounds in Fig. 5. The linear xanthones in Fig. 6, namely, sterigmatin and the austocystins, are presumably formed in a similar fashion. A key intermediate in this pathway is the postulated benzophenone carboxylic acid **62** (Fig. 18). Rotation about (a) in **62** would lead to the sterigmatocystins, whereas no rotation or rotation about (b) would lead to the metabolites in Fig. 6. The production of the versicolorins, sterigmatocystin, and sterigmatin by *A. versicolor*, and the production of averufin, versicolorin C, austocystins, and sterigmatocystin by *A. ustus* supply evidence for these postulates. The structural diversity of the austocystins is due to extensive secondary modifications (e.g., hydroxylation, chlorination, and isoprenylation) which can occur at several stages during the biosynthetic route.

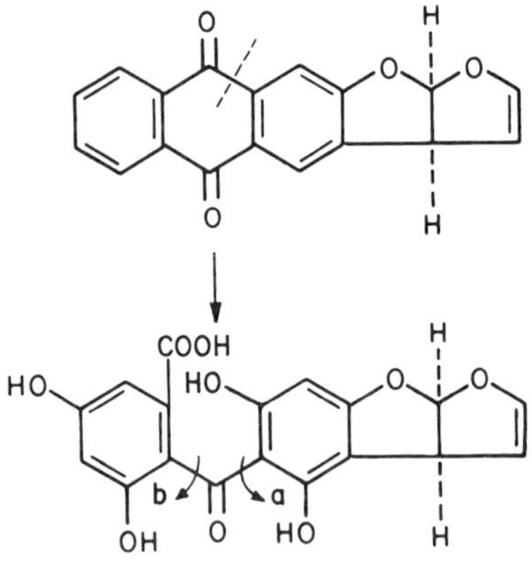

Fig. 18. Formation of angular and linear xanthones from a common intermediate.

(62)

Labeling experiments with [1,2-^{13}C]acetate established enrichment arising from rotation about the twofold axis of symmetry in the trisubstituted ring of an intermediate, e.g., **63** in the case of secalonic acid A (Kurobane *et al.*, 1978). This rotation, which interchanges carbon atoms on opposite sides of the axis, can occur only if, at some stage, **63** is not bound rigidly to an enzyme surface (Kurobane *et al.*, 1978). A similar rotation step was proposed for the biosynthesis of the xanthone ravenelin (Birch *et al.*, 1976). The ^{13}C NMR spectral data of sterigmatocystin (Seto *et al.*, 1974) and of aflatoxin B_1 (Pachler *et al.*, 1976a) indicate rotation only about axis (a) of

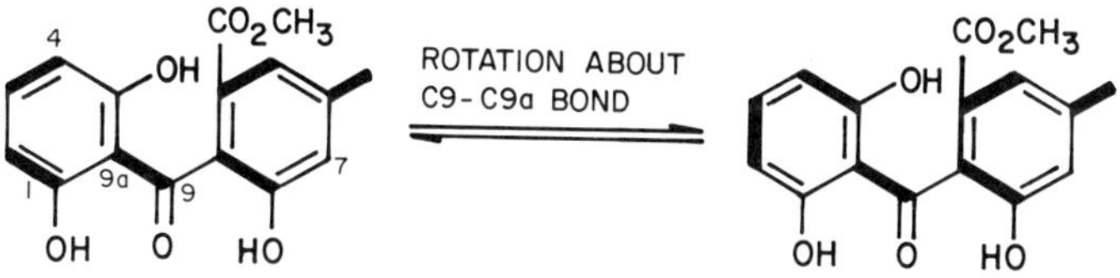

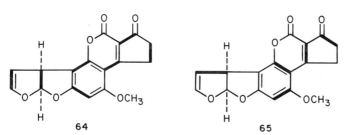

ROTATION ABOUT
C9 - C9a BOND

63

Fig. 19. Proposed intermediate in the formation of the secalonic acids.

the intermediate **62**; however, a minimal rotation about axis (b) cannot be completely excluded by these data.

The conversion of sterigmatocystin into aflatoxin B_1 involves the loss of another acetate-derived methyl group. Aflatoxin B_1 biosynthesized according to Biollaz *et al.* (1970) required the arrangement **64** or **65** of intact acetate units (see Fig. 20). The ^{13}C studies of aflatoxin biosynthesis, using singly and doubly labeled acetate (see Fig. 21) (Pachler *et al.*, 1976a), established the presence of three intact acetate units in the central ring of aflatoxin B_1; this ring is therefore derived from the outer ring of an aromatic precursor (averufin). A C_{13}-naphthacene precursor is no longer tenable; Hsieh *et al.* (1976a) observed only a very low incorporation of naphthacenequinones and benzanthrenes into aflatoxin B_1. The ^{13}C NMR data and the facile incorporation of several C_{20}-anthraquinones into sterigmatocystin (Hsieh *et al.*, 1978) and into aflatoxin B_1 eliminated the involvement of a formal C_4 unit linked to a C_{14} unit (Holker and Mulheirn, 1968) or the mevalonate (Moody, 1964) and kojic acid-based postulates (Heathcote *et al.*, 1965).

64   **65**

Fig. 20. Arrangement of acetate units in aflatoxin B_1 according to the Biollaz proposal.

Ranganathan and Ranganathan (1976) and Maggon *et al.* (1977) proposed schemes for the biosynthesis of the aflatoxins. Each scheme suffered from severe discrepancies from the well-documented data. Ranganathan and Ranganathan (1977) postulated that the C_6 side chain of C_{20}-anthraquinones is converted into an aromatic ring, with the subsequent loss of a two-carbon unit. This scheme does not accommodate the requisite bond cleavage leading to the head-to-head linkage of the two acetate units in, e.g., the versicolorins, sterigmatocystins, and aflatoxins, for coupling of the dihydrofuran ring and the aromatic system. The scheme of Maggon *et al.* (1977) implicated the loss of C(7), an acetate-derived carboxyl-carbon atom, in the conversion of sterigmatocystin into aflatoxin B_1. This proposal leads to eight intact acetate units in aflatoxin B_1. This postulate is not compatible with the unambiguous ^{13}C-derived findings of Steyn *et al.* (1975) and Pachler *et al.* (1976a).

The biosynthetic scheme of aflatoxin B_1 (Fig. 21) is currently accepted (Simpson, 1977) and illustrates the formation of all the coumarins in Fig. 1. Biollaz *et al.* (1970) proposed that aflatoxin M_1 was derived from aflatoxin B_1 by an oxidative process, as C(14) is derived from an acetate methyl carbon atom. However, Heathcote *et al.* (1976) by studying the interconvertibility of the aflatoxins, put forward aflatoxin M_1 as a precursor of aflatoxin B_1, whereas Maggon and Venkitasubramanian (1973) reported results in agreement with the proposal of the M.I.T. group. Some strains of *A. flavus* have been reported to produce only aflatoxin B_2 (Papa, 1977). In contrast, strains producing only aflatoxins G_1 or G_2 have not been reported. These findings provide evidence that aflatoxin G_1 is derived from aflatoxin B_1, probably by an enzymatic Baeyer–Villiger-type oxygen insertion between C(3) and C(4). Parasiticol is probably derived from aflatoxin G_1 by hydrolytic reaction followed by decarboxylation. This process may be related to the microbial degradation and disappearance of aflatoxins from mold cultures.

Several enrichment experiments established the primitive biogenetic precursors of the aflatoxins. The directional mode of folding of the original polyketide and the anomalous nature of the aflatoxin biosynthesis were deduced from ^{13}C NMR spectroscopy, hence illustrating the utility of this technique. The sequence of the aflatoxin biosynthesis was elucidated by the identification of advanced intermediates, the use of blocked mutants and enzyme inhibitors, and conversion of potential precursors by whole cell and cell-free systems into the aflatoxins. Certain facets of aflatoxin biosynthesis require further attention; among these are the nature of the polyketide synthetase; the exact mechanism by which primary metabolites induce the enzymes of aflatoxin production; the loss of the C(6) phenolic hydroxy group during the conversion of the polyhydroxyanthraquinones (e.g., averufin,

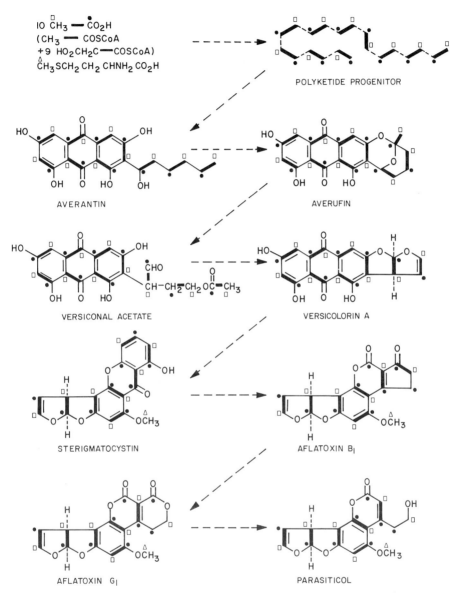

Fig. 21. Proposed biosynthetic scheme of aflatoxins and related compounds.

versiconal acetate, and versicolorin A) into xanthones (e.g., sterigmatocystin and austocystin A)—in polyketide biogenesis deoxygenation usually occurs prior to aromatization of the polyketide precursor; and the processes involved in the catabolism of aflatoxin B_1 during fermentation.

It is evident that the aflatoxins, which are secondary metabolites *par excellence*, not only significantly contributed to the present comprehension of chemical carcinogenesis, but led to a better understanding of secondary metabolism, particularly polyketide biosynthesis.

REFERENCES

Adye, J., and Mateles, R. I. (1964). *Biochim. Biophys. Acta.* **86**, 418–420.
Allerhand, A. (1975). *Pure Appl. Chem.* **41**, 247–273.
Anderson, H. A., Thomson, R. H., and Wells, J. W. (1966). *J. Chem. Soc. C*, pp. 1727–1729.
Asao, T., Büchi, G., Abdel-kader, M. M., Chang, S. B., Wick, E. L., and Wogan, G. N. (1965). *J. Am. Chem. Soc.* **87**, 882–886.
Assante, G., Camarda, L., Merlini, L., and Nasini, G. (1977). *Phytochemistry* **16**, 125–126.
Aucamp, P. J., and Holzapfel, C. W. (1970). *J. S. Afr. Chem. Inst.* **23**, 40–56.
Ballantine, J. A., Hassal, C. H., and Jones, G. (1965). *J. Chem. Soc.* 4672–4678.
Bennett, J. W., and Goldblatt, L. A. (1973). *Sabouraudia* **11**, 235.
Berger, Y., and Jadot, J. (1975). *Bull Soc. R. Sci. Liege* **44**, 310–313.
Berger, Y., and Jadot, J. (1976). *Bull. Soc. Chim. Belg.* **85**, 271–276.
Berger, Y., Jadot, J., and Ramaut, J. (1976). *Bull. Soc. Chim. Belg.* **85**, 161–166.
Biollaz, M., Büchi, G., and Milne, G. (1970). *J. Am. Chem. Soc.* **92**, 1035–1043.
Birch, A. J. (1967). *Science* **156**, 202–206.
Birch, A. J., Baldas, J., Hlubucek, J. R., Simpson, T. J., and Westerman, P. W. (1976). *J. Chem. Soc. Perkin Trans. 1*, 898–904.
Birkinshaw, J. H., Roberts, J. C., and Roffey, P. (1966). *J. Chem. Soc. C*, pp. 855–857.
Breitmaier, E., and Voelter, W. (1974). "^{13}C NMR Spectroscopy." Verlag Chemie, Weinheim.
Buchanan, R. L., and Ayres, J. C. (1976). *J. Food Sci.* **41**, 128–132.
Büchi, G., Foulkes, D. M., Kurono, M., Mitchell, G. F., and Schneider, R. S. (1967). *J. Am. Chem. Soc.* **89**, 6745–6753.
Bullock, E., Roberts, J. C., and Underwood, J. G. (1962). *J. Chem. Soc.* 4179–4183.
Burkhardt, H. J., and Forgacs, J. (1968). *Tetrahedron* **24**, 717–720.
Butler, W. H. (1974). *In* "Mycotoxins" (I. F. H. Purchase, ed.), pp. 1–28. Elsevier, Amsterdam.
Campbell, T. C., and Hayes, J. R. (1976). *Toxicol. Appl. Pharmacol.* **35**, 199–222.
Cattel, L., Grove, J. F., and Shaw, D. (1973). *J. Chem. Soc. Perkin Trans. 1*, 2626–2629.
Chang, C. (1976). *J. Org. Chem.* **41**, 1881–1883.
Cheung, K. K., and Sim. G. A. (1964). *Nature (London)* **201**, 1185–1188.
Chexal, K. K., Holker, J. S. E., Simpson, T. J., and Young, K. (1975). *J. Chem. Soc. Perkin Trans. 1*, 543–548.
Ciegler, A. C. (1975). *Lloydia* **38**, 21–34.
Clerc, J. T., Pretsch, E., and Sternhell, S. (1973). "[13]C-Kernresonanzspektroskopie." Akad. Verlagsges., Frankfurt.
Cole, R. J., Kirksey, J. W., and Schroeder, H. W. (1970). *Tetrahedron Lett.*, pp. 3109–3112.
Cox, R. H., and Cole, R. J. (1977). *J. Org. Chem.* **42**, 112–114.
Cox, R. H., Churchill, F., Cole, R. J., and Dorner, J. W. (1977). *J. Am. Chem. Soc.* **99**, 3159–3161.
Danks, A. V., and Hodges, R. (1974). *Aust. J. Chem.* **27**, 1603–1606.
Detroy, R. W., and Hesseltine, C. W. (1970). *Can. J. Microbiol.* **16**, 959–963.
Detroy, R. W., Lillehoj, E. B., and Ciegler, A. (1971). *In* "Microbial Toxins" (A. Ciegler, S. Kadis, and S. J. Ajl, eds.), Vol. VI, pp. 4–178. Academic Press, New York.

Detroy, R. W., Freer, S., and Ciegler, A. (1973). *Can. J. Microbiol.* **19**, 1373–1378.
Dimroth, P., Walter, H., and Lynen, F. (1970). *Eur. J. Biochem.* **13**, 98–110.
Donkersloot, J. A., Hsieh, D. P. H., and Mateles, R. I. (1968). *J. Am. Chem. Soc.* **90**, 5020–5021.
Donkersloot, J. A., Mateles, R. I., and Yang, S. S. (1972). *Biochem. Biophys. Res. Commun.* **47**, 1051–1055.
Dutton, M. F., and Anderson, M. S. (1978). *Experientia* **34**, 22–23.
Elsworthy, G. C., Holker, J. S. E., McKeown, J. M., Robinson, J. B., and Mulheirn, L. J. (1970). *J. Chem. Soc. Chem. Commun.*, 1069–1070.
Ernst, L., Wray, V., Chertkov, V. A., and Sergeyev, N. M. (1977). *J. Magn. Resonance* **25**, 123–139.
Essigmann, J. M., Croy, R. G., Nadzan, A. M., Busby, Jr. W. F., Reinhold, V. N., Büchi, G., and Wogan, G. N. (1977). *Proc. Natl. Acad. Sci. U.S.A.* **74**, 1870–1874.
Feeney, J., Partington, P., and Roberts, G. C. K. (1974). *J. Magn. Resonance* **13**, 268–274.
Fitzell, D. L., Hsieh, D. P. H., Yao, R. C., and La Mar, G. N. (1975). *J. Agric. Food Chem.* **23**, 442–444.
Fitzell, D. L., Singh, R., Hsieh, D. P. H., and Motell, E. L. (1977). *J. Agric. Food Chem.* **25**, 1193–1197.
Floss, H. G. (1972). *Lloydia* **35**, 399–417.
Franck, B. (1969). *Angew. Chem. Int. Ed. Engl.* **8**, 251–260.
Fukuyama, K., Tsukihara, T., Katsube, Y., Hamasaki, T., and Hatsuda, Y. (1975a). *Bull. Chem. Soc. Jpn.* **48**, 2648–2652.
Fukuyama, K., Tsukihara, T., Katsube, Y., Hamasaki, T., Hatsuda, Y., Tanaka, N., Ashida, T., and Kakudo, M. (1975b). *Bull. Chem. Soc. Jpn.* **48**, 1639–1640.
Fukuyama, K., Tsukihara, T., Katsube, Y., Tanaka, N., Hamasaki, T., and Hatsuda, Y. (1975c). *Bull. Chem. Soc. Jpn.* **48**, 1980–1983.
Fukuyama, K., Hamada, K., Tsukihara, T., Katsube, Y., Hamasaki, T., and Hatsuda, Y., (1976). *Bull. Chem. Soc. Jpn.* **49**, 1153–1154.
Gatenbeck, S. (1960). *Sven. Kem. Tidskr.* **72**, 188–203.
Goldblatt, L. A. (1969). "Aflatoxin: Scientific Background, Control and Implications." Academic Press, New York.
Gorst-Allman, C. P., Pachler, K. G. R., Steyn, P. S., Wessels, P. L., Scott, De B. (1977). *J. Chem. Soc. Perkin Trans. 1*, 2181–2188.
Gorst-Allman, C. P. Steyn, P. S., Wessels, P. L., and Scott, De B. (1978). *J. Chem. Soc. Perkin Trans. 1*, 961–964.
Grutzner, J. B. (1972). *Lloydia* **35**, 375–398.
Gupta, S. R., Prasanna, H. R., Viswanathan, L., and Venkitasubramanian, T. A. (1975). *Z. Lebensm. Unters. Forsch.* **157**, 19–22.
Hamasaki, T., and Hatsuda, Y. (1977). *In* "Mycotoxins in Human and Animal Health" (J. V. Rodricks, C. W. Hesseltine, and M. A. Mehlman, eds.), pp. 597–607. Pathotox Publishers, Park Forest South, Illinois.
Hamasaki, T., Hatsuda, Y., Terashima, N., and Renbutsu, M. (1965a). *Agric. Biol. Chem.* **29**, 166–167.
Hamasaki, T., Hatsuda, Y., Terashima, N., and Renbutsu, M. (1965b). *Agric. Biol. Chem.* **29**, 696–697.
Hamasaki, T., Hatsuda, Y., Terashima, N., and Renbutsu, M. (1967a). *Agric. Biol. Chem.* **31**, 11–17.
Hamasaki, T., Renbutsu, M., and Hatsuda, Y. (1967b). *Agric. Biol. Chem.* **31**, 1513–1514.
Hamasaki, T., Matsui, K., Isono, K., and Hatsuda, Y. (1973). *Agric. Biol. Chem.* **37**, 1769–1770.
Hamasaki, T., Nakagomi, T., Hatsuda, Y., Fukuyama, K., and Katsube, Y. (1977). *Tetrahedron Lett.*, pp. 2765–2766.
Harris, T. M., and Harris, C. M. (1977). *Tetrahedron* **33**, 2159–2185.

Hatsuda, Y., and Kuyama, S. (1954). *J. Agric. Chem. Soc. Jpn.* **28**, 989.
Hatsuda, Y., Hamasaki, T., Ishida, M., and Yoshikawa, S. (1969). *Agric. Biol. Chem.* **33**, 131–133.
Hatsuda, Y., Hamasaki, T., Ishida, M., and Kiyama, Y. (1971). *Agric. Biol. Chem.* **35**, 444.
Hatsuda, Y., Hamasaki, T., Ishida, M., Matsui, K., and Hara, S. (1972). *Agric. Biol. Chem.* **36**, 521–522.
Heathcote, J. G., and Dutton, M. F. (1969). *Tetrahedron* **25**, 1497–1500.
Heathcote, J. G., Child, J. J., and Dutton, M. F. (1965). *Biochem. J.* **95**, 23.
Heathcote, J. G., Dutton, M. F., and Hibbert, J. R. (1973). *Chem. Ind. (London)*, 1027–1030.
Heathcote, J. G., Dutton, M. F., and Hibbert, J. R. (1976). *Chem. Ind. (London)*, 270–272.
Holker, J. S. E., and Kagal, S. A. (1968). *J. Chem. Soc. Chem. Commun.*, 1574–1575.
Holker, J. S. E., and Mulheirn, L. J. (1968). *J. Chem. Soc. Chem. Commun.*, 1576–1577.
Holker, J. S. E., and Underwood, J. G. (1964). *Chem. Ind. (London)*, 1865–1866.
Holker, J. S. E., Kagal, S. A., Mulheirn, L. J., and White, P. M. (1966). *J. Chem. Soc. Chem. Commun.* **24**, 911–913.
Holker, J. S. E., Lapper, R. D., and Simpson, T. J. (1974). *J. Chem. Soc. Perkin Trans. 1*, 2135–2140.
Holmwood, G. M., and Roberts, J. C. (1971). *J. Chem. Soc. C*, pp. 3899–3902.
Holzapfel, C. W., Purchase, I. F. H., Steyn, P. S., and Gouws, L. (1966a). *S. Afr. Med. J.* **40**, 1100–1107.
Holzapfel, C. W., Steyn, P. S., and Purchase, I. F. H. (1966b). *Tetrahedron Lett.*, pp. 2799–2803.
Hsieh, D. P. H. (1973). *J. Agric. Food Chem.* **21**, 468–470.
Hsieh, D. P. H., and Mateles, R. I. (1971). *Appl. Microbiol.* **22**, 79–83.
Hsieh, D. P. H., and Yang, S. L. (1975). *Appl. Microbiol.* **29**, 17–20.
Hsieh, D. P. H., Lin, M. T., and Yao, R. C. (1973). *Biochem. Biophys. Res. Commun.* **52**, 992–997.
Hsieh, D. P. H., Seiber, J. N., Reece, C. A., Fitzell, D. L., Yang, S. L., Dalezios, J. I., La Mar, G. N., Budd, D. L., and Motell, E. (1975). *Tetrahedron* **31**, 661–663.
Hsieh, D. P. H., Lin, M. T., Yao, R. C., and Singh, R. (1976a). *J. Agric. Food Chem.* **24**, 1170–1174.
Hsieh, D. P. H., Yao, R. C., Fitzell, D. L., and Reece, C. A. (1976b). *J. Am. Chem. Soc.* **98**, 1020–1021.
Hsieh, D. P. H., Singh, R., Yao, R., and Bennett, J. W. (1978). *Appl. Environ. Microbiol.* **35**, 980–982.
Jemmali, M. (1976). *Bull. Inst. Pasteur (Paris)* **74**, 435–460.
Jones, R. B., and Phillips, L. (1974). *Annu. Rep. Prog. Chem., Sect. B.* **71**, 17–34.
Katsube, Y., Tsukihara, T., Tanaka, N., Ando, K., Hamasaki, T., and Hatsuda, Y. (1972). *Bull. Chem. Soc. Jpn.* **45**, 2091–2096.
Kingston, D. G. I., Chen, P. N., and Vercellotti, J. R. (1976). *Phytochemistry* **15**, 1037–1039.
Koller, G., and Russ., H. (1937). *Monatsh. Chem.* **70**, 54–72.
Kunesch, G., and Poupat, C. (1977). *In* "Isotopes in Organic Chemistry" (E. Buncel and C. C. Lee, eds.), Vol. 3, pp. 105–170. Elsevier, Amsterdam.
Kurobane, I., Vining, L. C., McInnes, A. G., Walter, J. A., and Wright, J. L. C. (1978). *Tetrahedron Lett.*, pp. 1379–1382.
Lapper, R. D. (1974). *Tetrahedron Lett.*, pp. 4293–4296.
Lee, L. S., Bennet, J. W., Goldblatt, L. A., and Lundin, R. E. (1971). *J. Am. Oil Chem. Soc.* **41**, 93–94.
Lee, L. S., Bennett, J. W., Cucullu, A. F., and Stanley, J. B. (1975). *J. Agric. Food Chem.* **23**, 1132–1133.
Levy, G. C., and Edlund, U. (1975). *J. Am. Chem. Soc.* **97**, 4482–4485.
Lin, M. T., and Hsieh, D. P. H. (1973). *J. Am. Chem. Soc.* **95**, 1668–1669.

Lin, M. T., Hsieh, D. P. H., Yao, R. C., and Donkersloot, J. A. (1973). *Biochemistry* **12**, 5167–5171.

Lin, J–K., Miller, J. A., and Miller, E. C. (1977). *Cancer Res.* **37**, 4430–4438.

London, R. E., Kollman, V. H., and Matwijoff, N. A. (1975). *J. Am. Chem. Soc.* **97**, 3565–3573.

Maggon, K. K., and Venkitasubramanian, T. A. (1973). *Experientia* **29**, 1210–1211.

Maggon, K. K., Gupta, S. K., and Venkitasubramanian, T. A. (1977). *Bacteriol. Revs.* **41**, 822–855.

Martin, C. N., and Garner, R. C. (1977). *Nature (London), New Biol.* **267**, 863–865.

McInnes, A. G., and Wright, J. L. C. (1975). *Acc. Chem. Res.* **8**, 313–320.

McInnes, A. G., Walter, J. A., Wright, J. L. C., and Vining, L. C. (1976). *Topics in C-13 NMR Spectry.* **2**, 123–178.

Money, T. (1973). *In* "Biosynthesis-Specialist Periodical Reports" (T. A. Geissman, senior reporter), Vol. 2, pp. 183–214. Chemical Society, London.

Moody, D. P. (1964). *Nature (London)* **202**, 188.

Oldfield. E., Norton, R. S., and Allerhand, A. (1975). *J. Biol. Chem.* **250**, 6368–6380.

Pachler, K. G. R. (1972). *J. Magn. Resonance* **7**, 442–443.

Pachler, K. G. R., and Wessels, P. L. (1977a). *Org. Magn. Resonance* **9**, 557–558.

Pachler, K. G. R., and Wessels, P. L. (1977b). *J. Magn. Resonance* **28**, 53–61.

Pachler, K. G. R., Steyn, P. S., Vleggaar, R., and Wessels, P. L. (1975). *J. Chem. Soc. Chem. Commun.*, pp. 355–356.

Pachler, K. G. R., Steyn, P. S., Vleggaar, R., Wessels, P. L., and Scott, De B. (1976a). *J. Chem. Soc. Perkin Trans. 1*, 1182–1189.

Pachler, K. G. R., Wessels, P. L., Dekker, J., Dekker, J. J., and Dekker, T. G. (1976b). *Tetrahedron Lett.*, pp. 3059–3062.

Packter, N. M. (1973). "Biosynthesis of Acetate-Derived Compounds." Wiley (Interscience), New York.

Pai, M. R., Bai, N. J., and Venkitasubramanian, T. A. (1975). *Appl. Microbiol.* **29**, 850–851.

Papa, K. E. (1977). *Appl. Environ. Microbiol.* **33**, 206.

Purchase, I. F. H., and Steyn, M. (1973). *Toxicol. Appl. Pharmacol.* **24**, 162–164.

Queener, S. W. (1976). *Microbiology*, pp. 512–516.

Rabie, C. J., Lübben, A., and Steyn, M. (1976). *Appl. Environ. Microbiol.* **32**, 206–208.

Rabie, C. J., Steyn, M., and van Schalkwyk, G. C. (1977). *Appl. Environ. Microbiol.* **33**, 1023–1025.

Ranganathan, D., and Ranganathan, S. (1976). "Art in Biosynthesis." pp. 155–160. Academic Press, New York.

Roberts, J. C. (1974). *Fortschr. Chem. Org. Naturst.* **31**, 119–151.

Roberts, J. C., and Roffey, P. (1965). *J. Chem. Soc. C*, pp. 3666–3672.

Rodricks, J. V., Lustig, E., Campbell, A. D., Stoloff, L., and Henery-Logan, K. R. (1968). *Tetrahedron Lett.*, 2975–2978.

Roebuck, B. D., and Wogan, G. N. (1977). *Cancer Res.* **37**, 1649–1656.

Roffey, P., Sargeant, M. V., and Knight, J. A., (1967). *J. Chem. Soc. C.*, pp. 2328–2331.

Schroeder, H. W., and Kelton, W. H. (1975). *Appl. Environ. Microbiol.* **30**, 589–591.

Scott, A. I., Phillips, G. T., and Kircheis, U. (1971). *Bioorg. Chem.* **1**, 380–399.

Scott, A. I., Townsend, C. A., Okada, K., Kajiwara, M., Cushley, R. J., and Whitman, P. J. (1974). *J. Am. Chem. Soc.* **96**, 8069–8080.

Séquin, U., and Scott, A. I. (1974). *Science* **186**, 101–107.

Seto, H., Cary, L. W., and Tanabe, M. (1974). *Tetrahedron Lett.*, pp. 4491–4494.

Shank, R. C. (1976). *In* "Mycotoxins and other Fungal Related Food Problems" (J. V. Rodricks, ed.), Vol. 149, pp. 51–57. *Adv. Chem. Ser.*, American Chemical Society.

Shaw, D. (1976). "Fourier Transform N. M. R. Spectroscopy." Elsevier, Amsterdam.

Shaw, G. J., Chick, M., and Hodges, R. (1978). *Phytochemistry* **17**, 1743–1745.

Shih, C–N., and Marth, E. H. (1974). *Biochim. Biophys. Acta.* **338**, 286–296.

Shih, C–N, and Marth, E. H. (1975). *Z. Lebensm. Unters. Forsch.* **158**, 215–224.

Simpson, T. J. (1975). *Chem. Soc. Rev.* **4**, 497–522.

Simpson, T. J. (1977). *In* "Biosynthesis–Specialist Periodical Reports" (J. D. Bu'Lock, senior reporter), Vol. 5, pp. 21–24. Chemical Society, London.

Singh, R., and Hsieh, D. P. H. (1976). *Appl. Environ. Microbiol.* **31**, 743–745.

Singh, R., and Hsieh, D. P. H. (1977). *Arch. Biochem. Biophys.* **178**, 285–292.

Steyn, P. S., and Vleggaar, R. (1974). *J. Chem. Soc. Perkin Trans 1* 2250–2254.

Steyn, P. S., and Vleggaar, R. (1975). *J. S. Afr. Chem. Inst.* **28**, 375–377.

Steyn, P. S., Vleggaar, R., Wessels, P. L., and Scott, De B. (1975). *J. Chem. Soc. Chem. Commun.* 193–195.

Steyn, P. S., Vleggaar, R., and Seegers, J. C. (1977). *Zesz. Probl. Postepow Nauk Roln.* **189**, 163–168.

Steyn, P. S., Vleggaar, R., Wessels, P. L., Cole, R. J., and Scott, De B. (1979a). *J. Chem. Soc. Perkin Trans. 1*, 451–459.

Steyn, P. S., Vleggaar, R., Wessels, P. L., and Scott, De B. (1979b). *J. Chem. Soc. Perkin Trans. 1*, 460–463.

Stoloff, L. (1977). *In* "Mycotoxins in Human and Animal Health" (J. V Rodricks, C. W. Hesseltine, and M. A. Mehlman, eds.), pp. 8–28. Pathotox Publishers, Park Forest South, Illinois.

Stothers, J. B. (1972). "Carbon-13 NMR Spectroscopy." Academic Press, New York.

Stubblefield, R. D., Shotwell, O. L., Shannon, G. M., Weisleder, D., and Rohwedder, W. K. (1970). *J. Agric. Food Chem.* **18**, 391–393.

Swenson, D. H., Lin, J–K., Miller, E. C., and Miller, J. A. (1977), *Cancer Res.* **37**, 172–181.

Tanabe, M. (1976). *In* "Biosynthesis–Specialist Periodical Reports" (J. D. Bu'Lock, senior reporter), Vol. 4, pp. 204–247. Chemical Society, London.

Tanabe, M., Hamasaki, T., Seto, H., and Johnson, L. (1970). *J. Chem. Soc. Chem. Commun.*, pp. 1539–1540.

Tanabe, M., Suzuki, K. T., and Jankowski, W. C. (1973). *Tetrahedron Lett.*, pp. 4723–4726.

Tanabe, M., Uramoto, M., Hamasaki, T., and Cary L. (1976). *Heterocycles* **5**, 355–365.

Thaxton, J. P., Tung, H. T., and Hamilton, P. B. (1974). *Poult. Sci.* **53**, 721–725.

Thomas, R. (1972). Personal communication to M. O. Moss, *in* "Phytochemical Ecology" (J. B. Harborne, ed.), p. 140. Academic Press, New York.

Turner, W. B. (1971). "Fungal Metabolites." p. 182. Academic Press, New York.

Van der Watt, J. J. (1974). *In* "Mycotoxins" (I. F. H. Purchase, ed.), pp. 369–382. Elsevier, Amsterdam.

Van Rensburg, S. J., Van der Watt, J. J., Purchase, I. F. H., Pereira Coutinho, L., and Markham, R. (1974). *S. Afr. Med. J.* **48**, 2508a–2508d.

Van Soest, T. C., and Peerdeman, A. F. (1970a). *Acta Cryst.* **26**, 1940–1947.

Van Soest, T. C., and Peerdeman, A. F. (1970b). *Acta Cryst.* **26**, 1956–1963.

Venkitasubramanian, T. A. (1977). *In* "Mycotoxins in Human and Animal Health" (J. V. Rodricks, C. W. Hesseltine, and M. A. Mehlman, eds.), pp. 83–98. Pathotox Publishers, Park Forest South, Illinois.

Wehrli, F. W. (1975). *J. Chem. Soc. Chem. Commun.*, pp. 663–664.

Wehrli, F. W., and Wirthlin, T. (1976). "Interpretation of Carbon-13 NMR Spectra." Heyden, London.

Weinberg, E. D. (1970). *Adv. Microb. Physiol.* **4**, 1–44.

White, R. J. (1976). *Process Biochem.* **11**, 9–12.

Williams, D. H. (1974). *Pure Appl. Chem.* **40**, 25–40.

Wilson, B. J., Campbell, T. C., Hayes, A. W., and Hanlin, R. T. (1968). *Appl. Microbiol.* **16**, 819–821.

Wogan, G. N. (1966). *Bacteriol. Rev.* **30**, 460–470.

Wogan, G. N., Paglialunga, S., and Newberne, P. M. (1974). *Fd. Cosmet. Toxicol.* **12**, 681–685.

Wong, J. J., Singh, R., and Hsieh, D. P. H. (1977). *Mutat, Res.* **44**, 447–450.

Wright, J. L. C., Vining, L. C., McInnes, A. G., Smith, D. G., and Walter, J. A. (1977). *Can. J. Chem.* **55**, 678–685.

Yao, R. C., and Hsieh, D. P. H. (1974). *Appl. Microbiol.* **28**, 52–57.

5

The Biosynthesis of the Ergochromes

I. INTRODUCTION

The ergochromes are a group of light yellow mycotoxins which were first isolated from ergot, the sclerotia of the filamentous fungus *Claviceps purpurea*, and later also were isolated from mold fungi and lichens. Isolation

The Biosynthesis of Mycotoxins
Copyright © 1980 by Academic Press, Inc.
All rights of reproduction in any form reserved.
ISBN 0-12-670650-6.

and structure determination of the ergochromes are described in several reviews (Eglinton *et al.*, 1958; Franck, 1965, 1969, 1972; Turner, 1971; Gröger, 1972; Franck and Flasch, 1973; van Rensburg and Altenkirk, 1974). For the main component of the ergochromes from ergot, namely, secalonic acid A, chemical degradation in combination with spectroscopic investigations established the structure as a dimeric xanthone derivative (**1**) (Franck *et al.*, 1964; Hooper *et al.*, 1971). The ergochromes are an interesting group of natural products, owing to their unusual chiral and biological properties, production by dissimilar microorganisms, and biosynthesis.

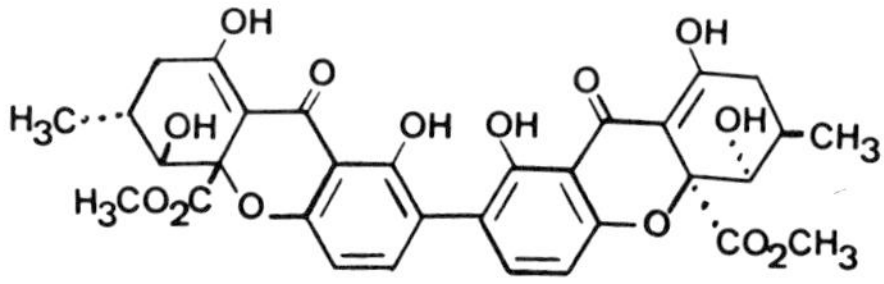

The ergochromes contain from six to ten chiral centers. As this gives rise to the occurrence of mixtures of diastereoisomers that are not easily separated, the investigation of the ergochromes, which had already begun 100 years ago (Dragendorff *et al.*, 1877), was initially fraught with severe difficulties. With the aid of modern chromatographic separation methods, 13 stereochemically pure ergochromes could be isolated by several research groups, and their structures including absolute configurations were completely determined (Table I). It is remarkable with respect to enzyme evolution and very unusual among natural products with several chiral centers that the occurrence of both enantiomers of ergochromes have been observed. Thus, for instance, Steyn (1970) was able to show that the ergochrome secalonic acid D (**2**), which he had isolated from *Penicillium oxalicum*, differs from secalonic acid A (**1**) by having opposite configurations at all its chiral carbon atoms, and is, therefore, the enantiomer. The same relationship was observed by Howard *et al.* (1973) for secalonic acid B and secalonic acid E, isolated from *Phoma terrestris*.

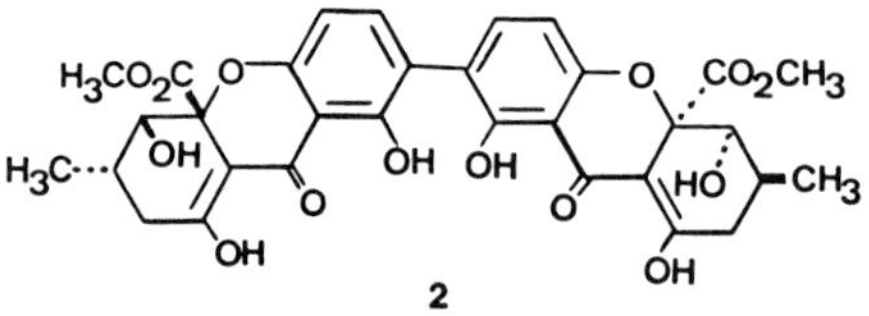

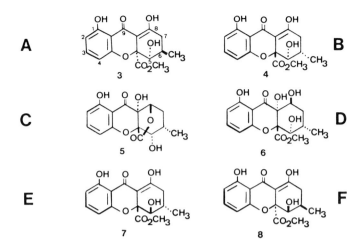

A

3

B

4

C

5

D

6

E

7

F

8

TABLE I

Names, Structures, and Occurrence of Pure Ergochromes

Systematic name	Original name	Structure	Occurrence[m]
Ergochrome AA	Secalonic acid A	$3-3 = 1^{a-c}$	a, b, c
Ergochrome BB	Secalonic acid B	$4-4^{a,b}$	a
Ergochrome AB	Secalonic acid C	$3-4^{a,c}$	a
Ergochrome CC	Ergoflavin	$5-5^{d-f}$	d
Ergochrome AC	Ergochrysin A	$3-5^{g,h}$	a
Ergochrome BC	Ergochrysin B	$4-5^{g,h}$	a
Ergochrome AD	—	$3-6^{i}$	a
Ergochrome BD	—	$4-6^{i}$	a
Ergochrome CD	—	$5-6^{i}$	a
Ergochrome DD	—	$6-6^{i}$	a
Ergochrome EE	Secalonic acid D	$7-7 = (2)^{j}$	e
Ergochrome FF	Secalonic acid E	$8-8^{k}$	f
Ergochrome BE	Secalonic acid F	$4-7^{l}$	g

[a] Franck et al. (1966)
[b] ApSimon et al. (1965b)
[c] Hooper et al. (1971)
[d] Eglinton et al. (1958)
[e] ApSimon et al. (1965a)
[f] McPhail et al. (1966)
[g] Franck and Baumann (1966a)
[h] Aberhart et al. (1965)
[i] Franck and Baumann (1966a)
[j] Steyn (1970)
[k] Howard et al. (1973)
[l] Andersen et al. (1977)
[m] Occurrences: a, Claviceps purpurea of various origin (Franck et al., 1964, 1966); b, Aspergillus ochraceus (57 strains) (Yamazaki et al., 1971); c, Lichen Parmelia entotheiochroa and three further species (Yosioka et al., 1968); d, Claviceps purpurea (Freeburn, 1912; Eglinton et al., 1958); e, Penicillium oxalicum (five strains) (Steyn, 1970); f, Phoma terrestris (Howard et al., 1973); g, Aspergillus aculeatus (Andersen et al., 1977).

The structure determination revealed that all the known ergochromes are dimers of the monoxanthones A–F, linked at C(2). This made possible a simple, systematic nomenclature, which characterizes the ergochromes by an additional specification "AA," "AB," or "BB," according to the types of their monomeric units A, B, etc. (Franck et al., 1964, 1966). These systematic names are shown in Table I with their frequently used original names, the corresponding structures, and the occurrence of the ergochromes.

The ergochromes were reported as the toxic principle of numerous rice and corn (maize) fungi (Yamazaki et al., 1971; Steyn, 1970). Maize meal infected with P. oxalicum caused extensive liver necrosis (Steyn, 1970). The LD_{50} is about 40 mg/kg (i.p. on mice) and thus a little less than the value of the highly toxic aflatoxins (6 mg/kg; i.p. in rats; Butler, 1964). At this dose level and with smaller doses, secalonic acid A (1) revealed phlogistic activity in rats and mice (Harada et al., 1974). It is of special interest that carcinostatic activity comparable with that of 5-fluorouracil and mitomycin has been claimed for secalonic acid D (2) and two of its derivatives in an application for a patent (Ishida et al., 1974).

The investigation of ergochrome biosynthesis with labeled precursors revealed that these mycotoxins are formed from anthraquinones by oxidative ring cleavage, a hitherto unknown biosynthetic procedure (Franck et al., 1966, 1968; Gröger et al., 1968). This review summarizes previous and recent investigations on the biosynthesis of ergochromes and related secoanthraquinones, and in addition the application of the knowledge thus gained to biomimetic reactions.

II. HYPOTHESES ON ERGOCHROME BIOSYNTHESIS

A. Some General Aspects of Acetogenin Biosynthesis

In ergot, the ergochromes are accompanied by small amounts of the two anthraquinone carboxylic acids, endocrocin (9) and clavorubin (10) (Franck and Reschke, 1960; Franck and Zimmer, 1965). This finding gave rise to the assumption that ergochromes might be derived during biosynthesis from anthraquinones by an oxidative ring opening according to the reaction sequence described by structures 11–13 (Franck, 1964; ApSimon et al., 1965). The anthraquinone biosynthesis by microorganisms is closely related to the in vivo formation of fatty acids, e.g., palmitic acid (14). One molecule of acetyl-coenzyme A (acetyl-CoA) as a starting unit condenses with seven molecules of malonyl-coenzyme A (malonyl-CoA), whereby the formed carbonyl group is reduced after each reaction step. If these reductions fail

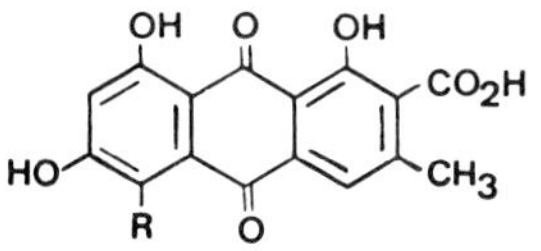

9 R = H
10 R = OH

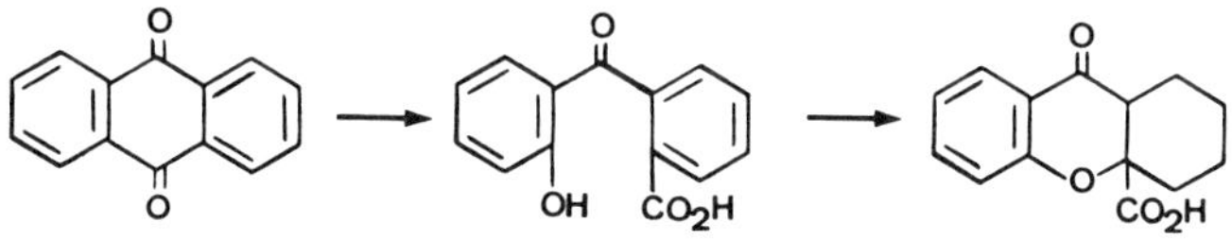

11   12   13

to occur, aromatic condensation products can be formed by intramolecular aldol condensations and by dehydrations of the polyketide via various conformations, e.g., **15** and **16**. These relationships have been excellently reviewed (Turner, 1971; Bentley, 1975).

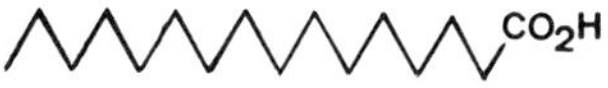

14

Acetyl-CoA + 7 Malonyl-CoA

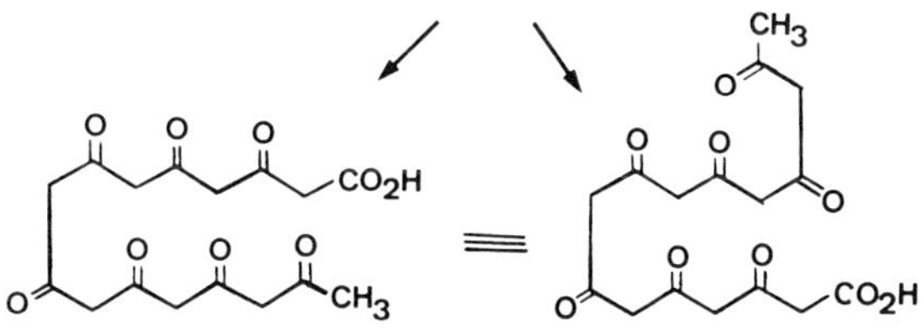

15   16

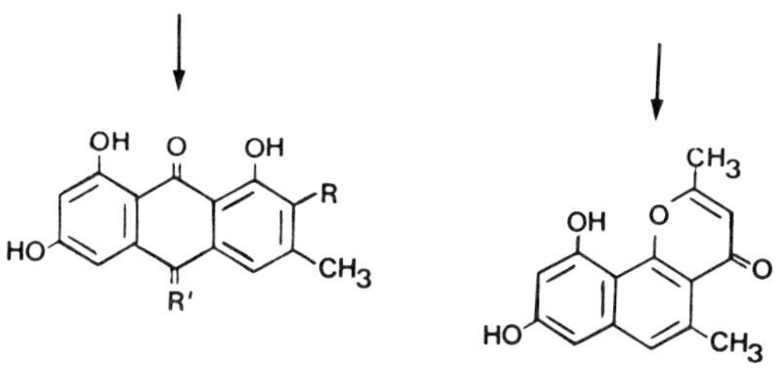

17 R = CO$_2$H; R' = O
18 R = H; R'=H$_2$
19 R = H; R'=O

20

It is not known if the formation of the polyketide chain and its cyclization proceed successively or as one process. The incorporation of smaller ketide units or of partly cyclized, possible intermediates of anthraquinone biosynthesis, e.g., **21** or **22**, has not yet been investigated successfully. Furthermore, no information is available on the mechanism of the conformationally controlled enzymatic cyclization of the polyketide chain to give either endocrocin (**17**) or emodin (**19**) via **15**, or to give the benzochromone eleutherin (**20**) via **16**.

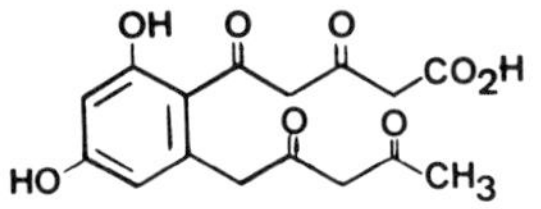

In this connection, the behavior of polyketides, synthesized by Harris *et al.* (1976) is of particular interest. For 2,4,6,8,10,12,14-heptaoxodecapentane a central protecting ketal group (**23**) favors the formation of a hairpin-type conformation similar to **15**, which gives the anthraquinone derivative. On the other hand, ketal groupings at both ends of this highly reactive synthetic polyketide give rise to a reaction sequence leading to eleutherin (**20**). From this result it might be concluded that during anthraquinone biosynthesis the polyketide precursor is brought into a hairpin-type conformation by fixing its central keto group to a certain area of the enzyme.

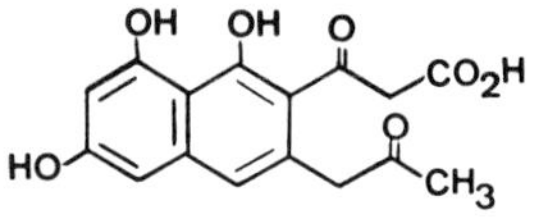

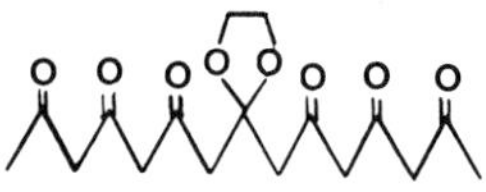

B. Anthraquinones and Benzophenones as Possible Precursors of Ergochromes

The benzophenone **26** was considered a key compound in the biosynthesis of the ergochromes, e.g., secalonic acid A (**1**). It could be transformed to secalonic acid A (**1**) via the dienone **27** by oxidative ring closure, stereospecific enone reduction, and oxidative dimerization. The necessary structural requirements for two oxidations proceeding by the phenol oxidation mechanism are present.

The benzophenone **26** may arise from the structurally related anthraquinones endocrocin (**17**) or emodin (**19**), by an oxidative cleavage of the C(10)–C(10a) bond. However, this assumption appeared tenuous, as metabolism of anthraquinones had not previously been observed. Therefore, other authors (ApSimon *et al.*, 1965; Davis *et al.*, 1969) considered the possibility that the ergochromes and other benzophenone derivatives could be formed by condensation of two monobenzene units, **24** and **25**. Thus, in the case of ergochrome biosynthesis, the two building units would first have to condense to the anthraquinone. However, this would contradict the well-confirmed evidence that anthraquinones of this type are generated from only one polyketide chain.

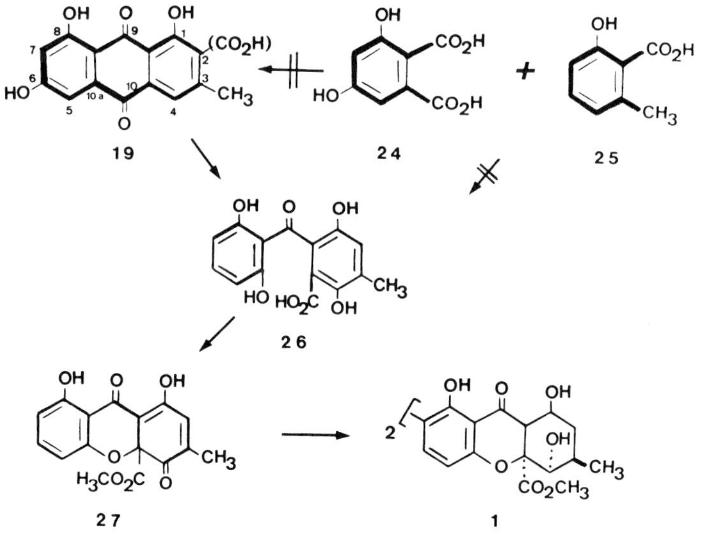

The experimental examination of these hypotheses involved initially the investigation of the role of acetate and selected anthraquinones as precursors in the ergochrome biosynthesis. After gaining positive evidence for a precursor function of anthraquinones, the mechanism of subsequent transformations, that is, the sequence of the following reaction steps, had to be determined: (a) ring opening; (b) reductive elimination of the hydroxygroup at C(6); (c) hydroxylation at C(4); (d) Xanthone ring closure; (e) reduction of the dienone system; and (f) dimerization.

III. METHODOLOGY

A. Selection and Cultivation of Ergochrome-Producing Fungi

For the investigation of ergochrome biosynthesis, microorganisms were required which produce ergochromes steadily and which accept labeled precursors efficiently. Lichens as *Parmelia entotheiochroa*, which grow extremely slowly, and *C. purpurea*, with its almost inaccessible sclerotia, could not be considered. Therefore, numerous *Claviceps* strains of various origin were examined for their ability to produce ergochromes in surface cultures on synthetic nutrient solutions. A strain of *Claviceps* which was collected in Japan from *Elymus mollis* proved especially efficient, with a production of 83 mg of an ergochrome mixture in one 250 ml surface culture (Gröger, 1959; Franck *et al.*, 1968). This production was suitable for initial biogenetic investigations, but the strain lost its ability for ergochrome production, and in spite of concerted efforts, including the examination of further *Claviceps* strains, it was not possible to prepare cultures of this fungus with reproducible ergochrome production.

The fungi *Aspergillus ochraceus* (Yamazaki *et al.*, 1971) and *P. oxalicum* (Steyn, 1970) from the American Type Culture Collection (ATCC) were then examined systematically for their capability to produce ergochrome D (Franck *et al.*, 1978). One strain of *P. oxalicum* (ATCC 10476), grown on sterilized, unpeeled rice as nutrient, reliably produced sufficient secalonic acid D (**2**), differing in this respect from two related strains (ATCC 1126 and 16501). As was shown by trial experiments, labeled precursors were incorporated by fungi on this solid nutrient, which becomes completely intermingled with mycelium, at the same rate as on liquid cultures. The examined strain of *A. ochraceus* (ATCC 18641) yielded no secalonic acid D (**2**) on a variety of solid and liquid nutrients.

B. Isolation and Separation of Ergochromes

Because of their low solubility in water, the ergochromes are almost exclusively found in the mycelium of the fungus, from which they can be easily extracted with organic solvents. The freeze-dried mycelium is first thoroughly milled and then extracted with petroleum ether. These steps are followed by exhaustive extraction with chloroform and chloroform–methanol, evaporation of the extracts, extraction of the residue with boiling chloroform, and intensive washing of the final extract with water. The resulting chloroform solution of the ergochrome mixture can be used directly for chromatographic separation. Silica gel impregnated with tartaric acid is most effective for separation of the ergochromes, which are partly diastereomeric and therefore very similar in their chromatographic behavior (Franck and Gottschalk, 1964). Even multicomponent ergochrome mixtures can be separated efficiently on this system, with chloroform containing 1–5% methanol. The natural color of the ergochromes suffices for their detection. Figure 1 displays schematically a thin layer chromatogram of the ergochromes found in ergot.

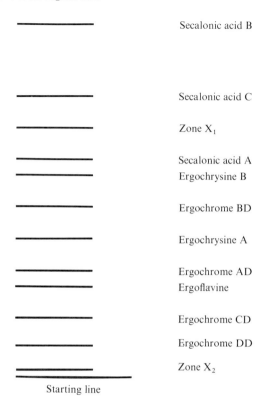

Secalonic acid B

Secalonic acid C

Zone X_1

Secalonic acid A
Ergochrysine B

Ergochrome BD

Ergochrysine A

Ergochrome AD
Ergoflavine

Ergochrome CD

Ergochrome DD

Zone X_2

Starting line

Fig. 1.   Thin layer chromatogram of an ergochrome mixture (chloroform: methanol, 100:1) on silica gel, impregnated with tartaric acid. From Franck, 1969.

C. Preparation of Labeled Precursors by Biological, Chemical, and Radiochemical Synthesis

As the labeled precursors needed for the investigation of ergochrome biosynthesis are natural products of the acetogenin type, they can be obtained most easily by feeding labeled acetate to suitable microorganisms. However, this procedure suffers from two disadvantages: the labeling is largely unspecific, and the percentage of incorporation is low, because of the diverse utilization of acetate in metabolism. Thus, in the case of the biosynthetic preparation of the differently ^{14}C-labeled emodins **28** and **29** by feeding sodium [2-^{14}C]- and [1-^{14}C]acetate, respectively, to liquid cultures of *Penicillium islandicum* (Gröger, 1968), the specific incorporation amounted to 0.003–0.014%. In this labeling procedure, the metabolite skyrine (**32**) obtained from *P. islandicum* is transformed into emodin, e.g., **28**, by reductive cleavage. The specific incorporation of sodium [2-^{3}H$_3$]acetate into emodin (**30**) was similar.

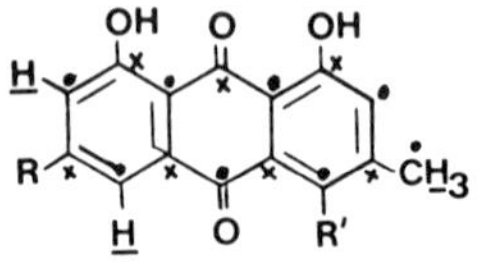

28 , • = ^{14}C, R=OH,R'=H
29 , x = ^{14}C, R=OH,R'= H
30 , H = ^{3}H, R=OH, R'=H
31 , H = ^{2}H, R= H,R'=OH

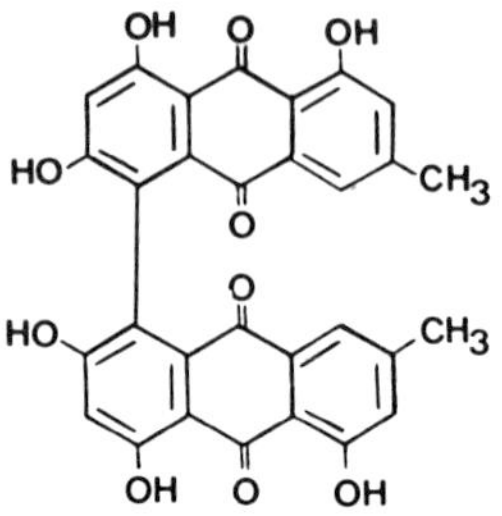

32

The concentration of labeled acetate in the nutrient during these feeding experiments was about $10^{-4}\%$, the usual level in applications of radioactive precursors. As the detection of stable isotopes requires higher enrichments, these conditions were unsuitable for them. Therefore, the effect of using much higher, almost unphysiological, concentrations on the specific incorporation of acetate into anthraquinones was investigated (Franck and Schrameyer, 1978). It was found that growth and pigment production of the fungus were not noticeably affected by concentrations of up to 0.5% sodium acetate in the nutrient. After feeding sodium [2-^{2}H$_3$]acetate in concentrations of 0.23 and 0.57% to the fungal culture, the isotope content of the deuteriated anthraquinone islandicin (**31**), determined by mass spectrometry, corresponded to specific incorporations of as high as 11.8 and 15.9%. Similar incorporations could be achieved with sodium [1-^{13}C]acetate. This finding suggests promising possibilities for taking better advantage of the very convenient use of stable isotopes in biosynthetic research. Besides the antraquinones, labeled secalonic acid A (**1**), secalonic acid B, and other ergochromes were prepared by feeding sodium [1-^{14}]-, [2-^{14}C]-, [2-^{3}H$_3$]-, and [1,2-^{13}C]acetates (Franck, *et al.*, 1968; Kurobane and Vining, 1978).

As an additional approach in preparing a ^{3}H-labeled anthraquinone, the radiochemical labeling of emodin (33) was undertaken (Gröger *et al.*, 1968). Reaction with 10 Ci tritium gas for 3 wk (Wilzbach conditions) (Wenzel and Schulze, 1962) yielded, after exchange of the labile tritium and intensive purification, crystalline emodin (**33**) with specific tritium radioactivity of 11.6 mCi/mmole. As usual with Wilzbach tritiations (Evans, 1974), the radioactivity was predominantly located on the aromatic nucleus, and the C-methyl radioactivity as determined by Kuhn–Roth oxidation amounted to only 8.5% of the overall radioactivity.

33

34, ∇ = ^{14}C, R = CO_2H
35, × = ^{14}C, R = H
36, • = ^{14}C, R = H

37, R,R' $\sqcup_2$ = H
38, R,R' = H
39, R = H, R' = OH
40, R,R' = OH

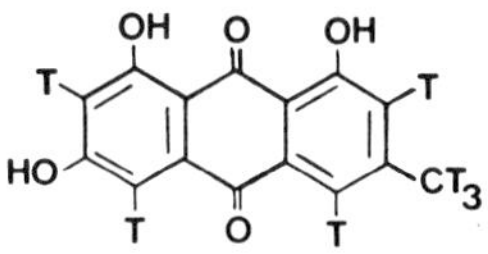

The relatively easy methods of biosynthetic and radiochemical labeling cannot be considered for precursors which have not been isolated as natural products, or for which a definite, specific labeling is desired. This was the case with the precursors [10-^{14}C]endocrocin (**34**), [3-^{14}C]emodin (**35**), [methyl-^{14}C]emodin (**36**), [*U*-^{14}C]chrysophanol (**37**), and with the bisanthraquinonyls [*U*-^{14}C]dianhydrorugulosin (**38**), [*U*-^{14}C]iridoskyrin (**39**), and [*U*-^{14}C]dicatenarin (**40**), needed for the study of biosynthetic mechanisms. Their preparation required labeling by chemical syntheses or partial syntheses from other uniformly labeled natural products. Synthesis of the anthraquinones **34**–**36** with ^{14}C in specific positions was achieved by the Friedel–Crafts condensations (a)–(c), (Fig. 2, structures **41**–**51**) (Franck and Flasch, 1970; Franck *et al.*, 1970). The resulting benzophenone carboxylic acids (yields referred to are for the radioactive educt) yielded the corresponding anthraquinones on cyclization in fuming sulfuric acid–boric acid and subsequent demethylation.

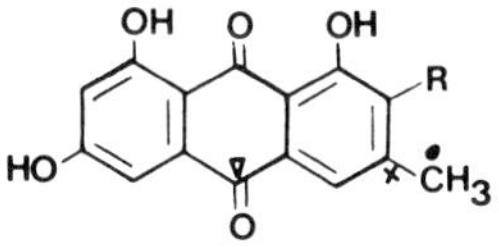

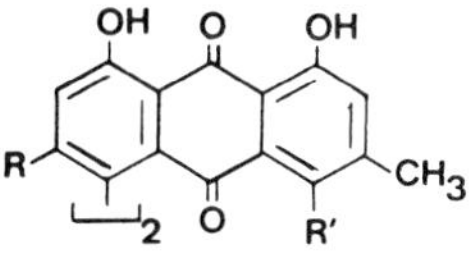

A different condensation principle (d) (Fig. 2) was applied by Steglich and Reiniger (1970) for the synthesis of specifically labeled [^{14}C]endocrocin (**17**) and endocrocinanthrone. The biphenylmethane **51** is formed from an aryl-*β*-diketone (**50**) and [1,5-^{14}C]dimethylacetonedicarboxylate, and then cyclized with polyphosphoric acid. The labeled educts **41** and **45** used in the condensation reactions (a) and (b) (Fig. 2) were prepared from 3,5-dimethoxy-[*carboxyl*-^{14}C]benzoic acid and [1-^{14}C]benzoic acid, using common synthetic methods. A different method was employed for reaction (c) (Fig. 2).

In reaction (b) (Fig. 2) the radioactive yield was only 8% because, contrary to normal Friedel–Crafts reactions, the radioactive *m*-[3-^{14}C]cresol could

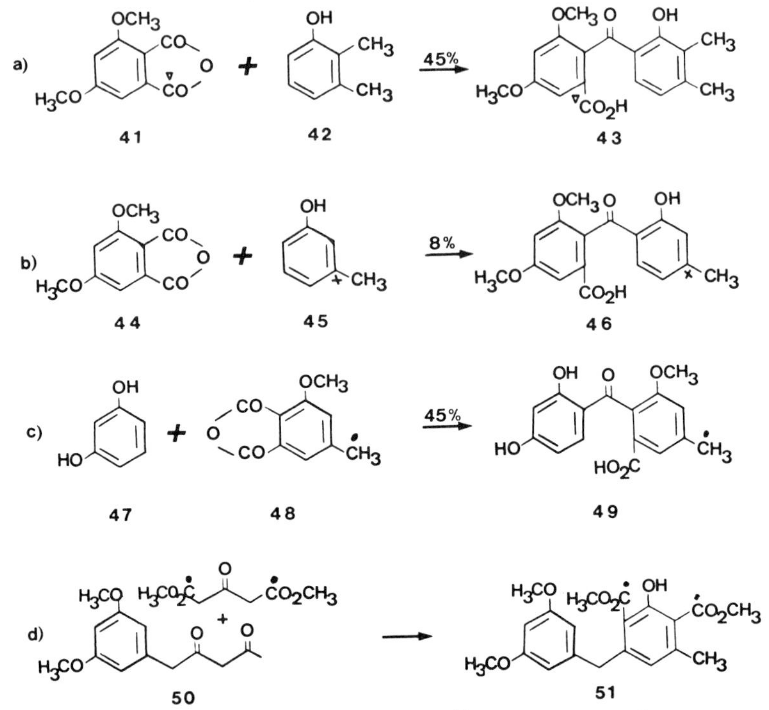

Fig. 2. Condensation reactions for the synthesis of ^{14}C-labeled anthraquinone precursors.

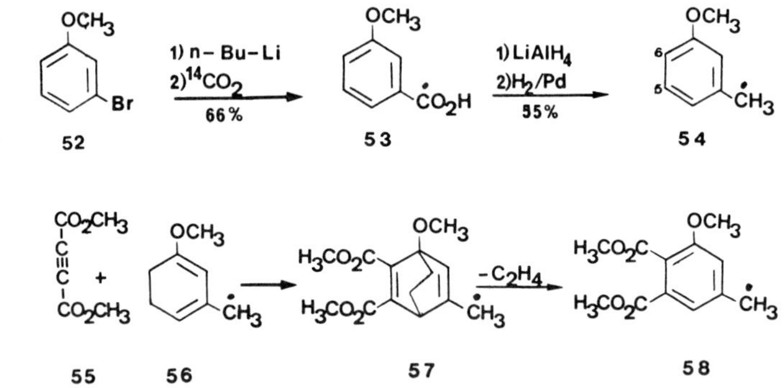

not be added in excess. An inverse Friedel–Crafts reaction, employing a ^{14}C-labeled phthalic anhydride component **48** and the resorcinol **47** in excess, was investigated for the synthesis of the benzophenone (**49**). This was made possible via a Diels–Alder reaction and a subsequent retrocleavage. Starting from *m*-methoxybromobenzene (**52**), 3-[*methyl*-^{14}C]methylanisole (**54**) was prepared via 3-methoxy-[*carboxyl*-^{14}C]benzoic acid (**53**) by the reactions shown. To transform **54** into the phthalic acid **58**, C(5) and C(6) had to be replaced by a C_4-dicarboxylic acid. This replacement was achieved by thermal isomerization of the Birch reduction product of **54** to give the cyclohexadiene **56**, and by Diels–Alder reaction with dimethylacetylenedicarboxylate (**55**) for 1 hr at 200°C. This reaction was accompanied by elimination of ethylene from the initial cycloaddition product (**57**) to form the labeled phthalic acid, **58**. The overall radioactive yield of **58** based on $^{14}CO_2$ for this reaction sequence was 3.2%, the average yield per step 60%.

The bisanthraquinonyls iridoskyrin (**39**), dianhydrorugulosin (**38**), and dicatenarin (**40**) were prepared by partial synthesis from other labeled biosynthetic products (Franck and Flohr, 1977). Rubroskyrin (**59**) (Shibata *et al.*, 1968) was isolated in addition to uniformly labeled skyrin (**32**), after feeding sodium [1-^{14}C]acetate to liquid cultures of *P. islandicum*, and transformed into [U-^{14}C]iridoskyrin (**39**) by acid-catalyzed dehydration. Dehydration of labeled rugulosin (**60**) (Shibata *et al.*, 1968) obtained from cultures of *Talaromyces wortmannii* after feeding of sodium [2-^{14}C]acetate produced [U-^{14}C]-dianhydrorugulosin (**38**). In this case, dehydration was accomplished with thionylchloride in pyridine.

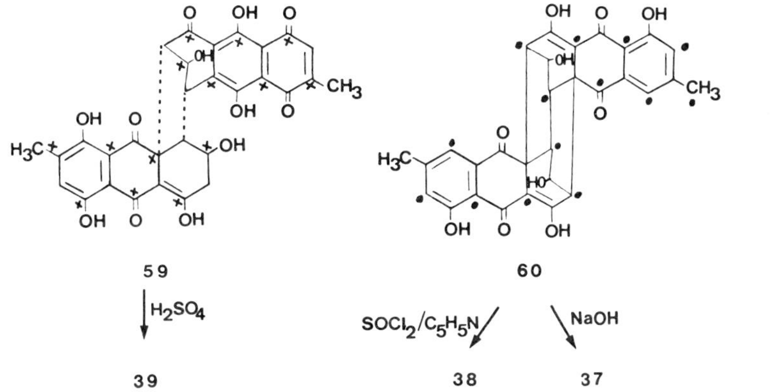

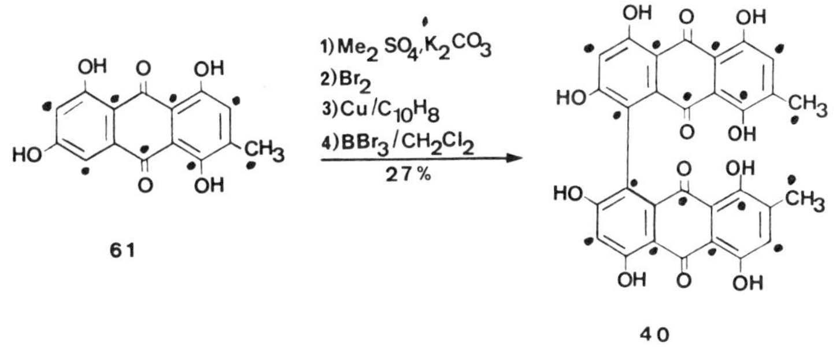

On cleavage with alkali, rugulosin (60) gave a good yield of the otherwise not easily accessible [U-^{14}C]chrysophanol (37). For [U-^{14}C]dicatenarin (40), a partial synthesis starting from the labeled monomeric anthraquinone catenarin (61) from *Helminthosporium catenarium* was considered. Selective bromination of catenarin tetramethyl ether yielded the 5-bromo compound, which after Ullmann condensation and demethylation gave the desired dicatenarin (40).

D. Feeding Procedures

In the investigation of ergochrome biosynthesis with labeled precursors, three problems which determine the success of the feeding experiments had to be considered: (a) permeability of the cell wall for the precursor, (b) solubility of the labeled precursor, and (c) variation and comparability of incorporation results obtained by different cultures of the same organism. Exploratory feeding experiments with ergochrome-producing fungi unexpectedly revealed that anthraquinones, despite their low solubility, were taken up by the intact cells and incorporated with specific rates of 0.3–1.5% (Franck and Flasch 1973). Such incorporation rates are sufficient for biosynthetic investigations. Thus it was unnecessary to forgo the very informative *in vivo* experiments with whole organisms and to work with cell-free systems or isolated enzymes.

As a result of their low solubility in water, the labeled anthraquinones, and other precursors of similar solubility, had to be applied to the fungal cultures together with solubility mediators or as suspensions. In practice, this took place by injecting labeled emodin (19) either as a sterilized solution of 50–100 mg in a mixture of 2 gm Tween 20 (polyhydroxyethylene sorbitan ester of long-chain fatty acids) and 125 ml propylene glycol, or as a suspension of 25 mg **19** obtained by sonic oscillation in 25 ml Czapek–Thom nutrient solution, under the mycelium cover of well-developed fungal cultures. Equally good results were achieved by spraying the sterilized precursor suspension on the solid rice nutrient before inoculation with the fungus. As mentioned earlier, the mycelium penetrates so thoroughly into the nutrient that complete contact with the precursor is obtained.

As the incorporation depends to a certain degree on the growth conditions, comparisons of the incorporations of labeled precursors in different cultures must be treated with reservation. In order to differentiate precursors with similar incorporation rates independently from growth variations, it was necessary to feed them in competition to the same culture. For this, the precursor mixtures were labeled either with different isotopes, e.g., ^{14}C, ^{3}H, or with the same isotope at different positions, as, for instance, with [3-^{14}C]-emodin (35) and [*methyl*-^{14}C]emodinanthrone (18). After feeding a mixture of the two precursors to the same fungal culture, the incorporations of the precursors can be derived from the ^{14}C and ^{3}H radioactivities, or from the ^{14}C radioactivity of different fragments of the biosynthetic product.

E. Determination of Isotope Positions

The isotope positions in a metabolite from an incorporation experiment can be ascertained for ^{13}C by NMR spectroscopy and for ^{3}H and ^{14}C by chemical degradation. Both approaches were applied in the elucidation of the biosynthesis of the ergochromes.

The advantage of the easy location of the isotopes in ^{13}C-labeled compounds is offset by the disadvantage that ^{13}C NMR evaluation needs a specific incorporation of at least 0.1%, and preferably 0.5–1%, because of the fairly high natural abundance of ^{13}C, i.e., 1.1% (^{14}C = 10^{-10}%). As a result of this problem, it is necessary to provide precursors with ^{13}C enrichment of about 90% at the required positions, as is possible by chemical synthesis. The application of ^{13}C is excluded, therefore, should the required precursor be derived from biosynthetic labeling, for then, depending on the incorporation, ^{13}C enrichments of less than 5% can be expected. Incorporation experiments with acetate are excellently suited for ^{13}C-labeling in biosynthetic studies.

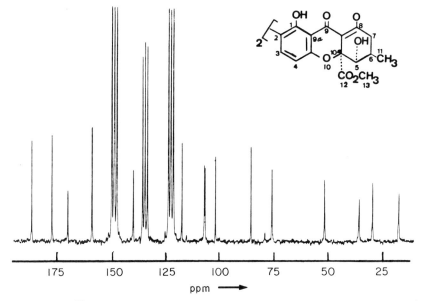

Fig. 3. The ^{13}C NMR spectrum of secalonic acid A (**1**) in pyridine (TMS = 0). From Franck and Güneysu, 1977.

Figure 3 shows the ^{13}C NMR spectrum of secalonic acid A (1) without isotope enrichment and Table II the assignment of the resonances, which were independently determined by Kurobane *et al.* (1978) and Franck and Güneysu (1976). The two research groups arrived at the same assignments of the 16 signals of the symmetrical molecule which are based upon proton off-resonance decoupling, additivity rules, and ^{13}C NMR spectra of derivatives of secalonic acid.

TABLE II

^{13}C Chemical Shifts of Secalonic Acid A (1) in Pyridine (TMS = 0)^a

Carbons	ppm	Carbons	ppm
C(1),(1′)	159.74	C(8),(8′)	178.32
C(2),(2′)	118.01	C(8a),(8a′)	102.42
C(3),(3′)	140.56	C(9),(9′)	187.68
C(4),(4′)	107.61	C(9a),(9a′)	107.29
C(4a),(4a′)	159.87	C(10a),(10a′)	86.04
C(5),(5′)	76.42	C(11),(11′)	18.19
C(6),(6′)	30.43	C(12),(12′)	170.91
C(7),(7′)	36.52	C(13),(13′)	52.50

^{a} TMS-tetramethylsilane.

In order to determine the isotope distribution after feeding experiments with radioactive precursors, the chemical degradation reactions, summarized in Fig. 4 (structures 62–65), were used. The carbon atoms C(6) and C(11) could be analyzed easily for measurement of radioactivity by Kuhn–Roth oxidation. They were, therefore, preferentially selected as labeled sites.

Schmidt degradation of the acetic acid derived from the Kuhn–Roth reaction yielded CO_2 and methylamine. The latter was condensed with *O*-benzylisovanilin for purification and weight increase purposes and reduced with sodium borohydride to give methyl-(4-methoxy-3-benzyloxy)amine (63), according to a useful procedure described by Barton *et al.* (1966). A degradation with acetic anhydride–pyridine and thereafter with concentrated HBr, described by Whalley *et al.* (1955), degrades secalonic acid A (1) and similar ergochromes into 2,2′,4,4′-tetrahydroxybiphenyl (64), two molecules of CO_2, and 5-hydroxy-3-methylbenzoic acid (65). The carboxy group of 65 is afterward split off as CO_2 by Schmidt degradation. With these reactions, the radioactivities of the carbon atoms of the Kuhn–Roth-derived acetic acid [C(6) and C(11)], of the carboxy group C(12), and of the carbonyl group [C(9)] of an ergochrome can be determined separately, whereas those of the remaining carbon atoms can be determined in groups.

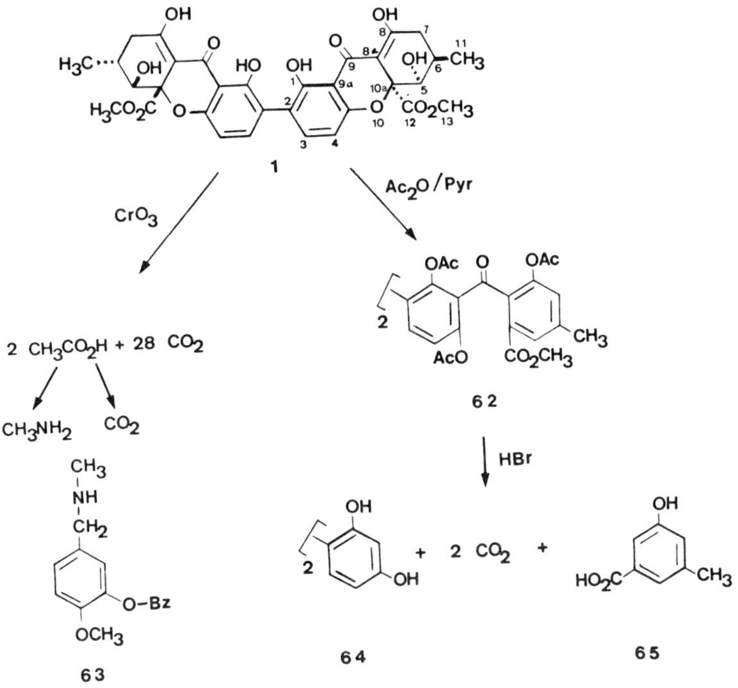

Fig. 4.   Chemical degradation of secalonic acid A (1) for location of radioactive isotopes.

IV. INVESTIGATION OF ERGOCHROME BIOSYNTHESIS WITH LABELED PRECURSORS

A. Acetates

The first indications of the validity of the hypothesis that ergochromes are biosynthesized by ring cleavage of anthraquinones were obtained by feeding sodium $[1\text{-}^{14}C]\text{-}$, $[2\text{-}^{14}C]\text{-}$, and $[2\text{-}^{3}H]$acetates to surface cultures of *C. purpurea* (Franck, *et al.*, 1968). In accord with a biosynthesis via a polyketide intermediate **15**, the ^{14}C atoms of labeled acetate should be arranged after incorporation in alternating positions in the anthraquinone (**66**). The ergochromes (**67**) arising from it should show an analogous isotope distribution, with the carboxy carbon atom C(12) derived from the methyl group of an acetate unit. After feeding of sodium $[2\text{-}^{3}H]$acetate, the tritium is to be expected in the methyl group of the ergochromes and in only one position on the xanthone skeleton, for it is eliminated from all remaining positions of the original polyketide by condensation and elimination re-actions. Therefore, the isotope concentrations at carbon atoms C(6), C(11),

C(9), and C(12), which could be determined separately with the degradation reactions mentioned above (see Fig. 4), were particularly instructive for the investigation of ergochrome biosynthesis.

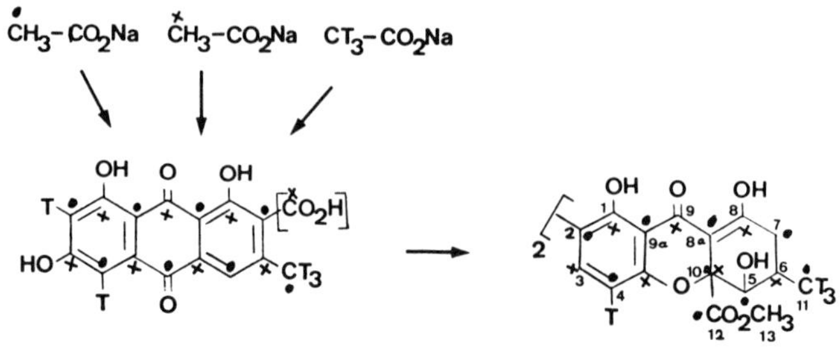

66   67

TABLE III

Radioactive Carbon Atoms of the Ergochromes AB 3–4 and AC 3–5 and Their Degradation Products, Obtained after Feeding of Sodium [2-^{14}C]- and [1-^{14}C]Acetate^a

		Radioactive carbon atoms after feeding of:			
		[2-^{14}C]Acetate		[1-^{14}C]Acetate	
Substance	C atom position	Calculated	Found^b	Calculated	Found^b
Ergochrome AB	C(1)–(13)	16	16.6	14	15.4
	Kuhn–Roth degradation				
CH_3CO_2H	C(6),(11)	1	1	1	1
CO_2	C(6)	0	0.01	1	1
CH_3NH_2	C(11)	1	1	0	—
	HBr degradation				
CO_2	C(9)	0	0.09	1	0.58
5-Hydroxy-2-methyl benzoic acid (65)	C(5),(6),(7),(8),(8a), (10a),(11),(12)	5	4.6	3	2.3
CO_2	C(12)	1	0.64	0	0.07

^{a} See Fig. 4. From Franck et al., 1968.
^{b} Relative to the radioactivity of the acetic acid as 1.

The results from incorporation experiments with sodium [2-^{14}C]- and [1-^{14}C]acetate are summarized in Table III. The isotope distributions of all carbon atoms which relate the biosynthetic mechanism corresponded within experimental errors to the values expected, when the ergochromes are formed by oxidative ring opening of an anthraquinone, e.g., 66. Analogous incorporation results were obtained for ergochrome AC (3–5) (Franck et al., 1968).

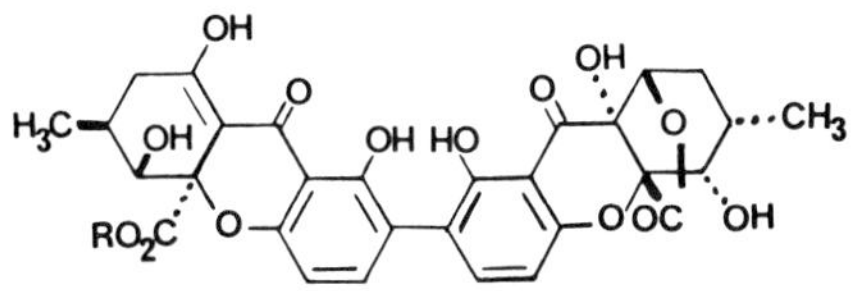

68a R= CH₃
68b R= H

TABLE IV

Distribution of ^{3}H in Ergochrome BC (68a) from *C. purpurea* after Feeding Sodium [2-^{3}H]Acetate

Substance	Atoms ^{3}H per molecule	
	Calculated	Found[a]
Ergochrome BC (68a)	8	9.7
Demethylergochrome BC (68b)	8	8.4
CH₃CO₂H from Kuhn–Roth		
degradation	3	3
H atoms at the ring system (difference)	2	2.4

[a] Relative to the radioactivity of the acetic acid as 3.

The ergochrome BC (68a) isolated from *C. purpurea* after feeding sodium [2-^{3}H]acetate showed the expected ^{3}H distribution (Table IV) (Hüper, 1967). In order to separate the ^{3}H radioactivity of the methoxy group, ergochrome BC (68a) was transformed into the demethyl compound (68b) with HBr–acetic acid. Relative to the radioactivity of the acetic acid as equal to 3, the demethylergochrome BC (68b) contains, within experimental error, eight tritium atoms, of which six belong to the two *C*-methyl groups and one belongs to each of the two phenyl groups of the molecular halves.

B. Anthraquinones

Feeding experiments were performed with *C. purpurea* and *P. oxalicum* (Table V) (Franck and Flasch, 1973; Gröger et al., 1968) to obtain direct proof for the role of anthraquinones in ergochrome biosynthesis. The evaluation shows that ergochromes arise from emodin (71) by ring opening. The specific incorporations of emodin into the four ergochromes (0.38–1.5%) are comparatively high, indicating that the cell walls of the fungi are apparently permeable to emodin. However, the incorporation of endocrocin (72), which had earlier been regarded as a biogenetic precursor for emodin and further anthraquinones, is small ($\leq 0.005\%$). This finding is of general importance. It indicates that in anthraquinone biosynthesis from acetate

TABLE V

Feeding of Radioactive Precursors to *C. purpurea* and *P. oxalicum*

Precursor	Organism	Radioactive products	Specific incorporation (%)
[*U*-^{14}C]Emodin (**71**)	*C. purpurea*	Ergochrome BB (**70**)	0.38
		Ergochrome BC (**68**)	0.60
[*U*-^{3}H]Emodin (**71**)	*C. purpurea*	Ergochrome AC (**3**)–(**5**)	1.3
		Ergochrome BC (**68**)	1.5
[10-^{14}C]Endocrocin (**72**)	*C. purpurea*	Ergochrome BB (**70**)	0.0005
		Ergochrome BC (**68**)	0.005
[*U*-^{14}C]Emodin (**71**)	*P. oxalicum*	Ergochrome EE (**2**)	0.53
[10-^{14}C]Endocrocin (**72**)	*P. oxalicum*	Ergochrome EE (**2**)	0.005
[*U*-^{14}C]Shikimic acid (**69**)	*C. purpurea*	—	—

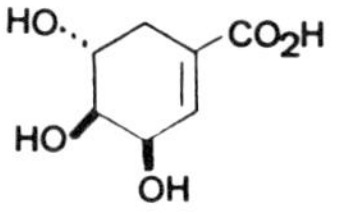

69

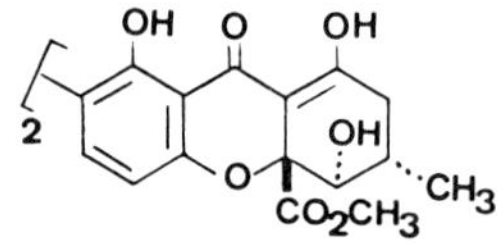

70

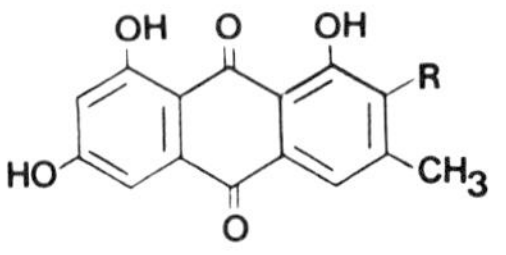

71   R = H
72   R = CO$_2$H

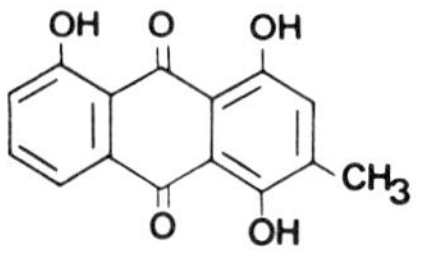

73

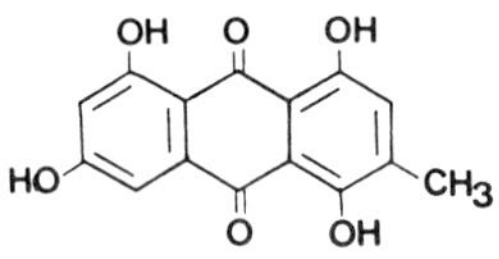

74

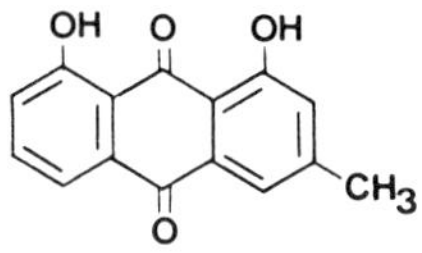

75

units, the elimination of the terminal carboxy group occurs during the poly-ketide condensation. Thus, endocrocin (**72**) seems to occur on a branch of anthraquinone biosynthesis. Steglich *et al.* (1972) also provided evidence that endocrocin (**72**) is not transformed into emodin (**71**) or related anthraquinones, by their investigation of the biosynthesis of anthraquinone pigments from *Dermocybe* species. The nonincorporation of shikimic acid (69) precludes the less probable participation of this building unit in ergochrome biosynthesis.

The objection that the radioactivity of the labeled emodins is not directly incorporated into the ergochromes, but goes via degradation into radioactive acetic acid, could be invalidated by examination of the lipids formed during the incorporation (Gröger *et al.*, 1968). In this case, the radioactivity should be located predominantly in the lipid fraction, as after feeding labeled acetate. However, the total lipid radioactivity amounted to only 0.14% of that of the ergochromes.

During the ergochrome biosynthesis from emodin (71), its hydroxy group at C(6) has to be eliminated and an additional hydroxy group introduced at C(4). Therefore, not only emodin (71) but the natural products islandicin (73), catenarin (74), and chrysophanol (75), whose arrangement of hydroxy groups corresponds partly or completely to that of an ergochrome half, had to be taken into consideration. As the incorporation of the three additional anthraquinones might differ little from that of emodin (71), competitive feeding experiments were performed. For this investigation, two component mixtures of $[U\text{-}^3H]$emodin (71) and of one of the other $[U\text{-}^{14}C]$anthraquinones were added to a culture of *P. oxalicum*, and the ^3H and ^{14}C activities of the isolated ergochrome EE (2) were determined (Franck *et al.*, 1978). Table VI gives the results of these experiments.

Experiment 1 (Table VI) reveals that during incorporation of $[U\text{-}^3H]$-emodin (71) into ergochrome EE (2), the loss of ^3H activity, located predominantly in the methyl group, is negligible (about 3%). The single

TABLE VI

Competitive Incorporation of Four Anthraquinones in Ergochrome EE (2) by *P. oxalicum*[a]

Experiment	Anthraquinone	Specific incorporation (%)	Ratio b/a
1	(a) $[U\text{-}^3H]$Emodin (71)	0.418	1.03
	(b) $[U\text{-}^{14}C]$Emodin (71)	0.432	
2	(a) $[U\text{-}^3H]$Emodin (71)	0.541	0.301
	(b) $[U\text{-}^{14}C]$Islandicin (73)	0.163	
3	(a) $[U\text{-}^3H]$Emodin (71)	0.37	0.022
	(b) $[U\text{-}^{14}C]$Catenarin (74)	0.008	
4	(a) $[U\text{-}^3H]$Emodin (71)	0.96	3.56
	(b) $[U\text{-}^{14}C]$Chrysophanol (75)	3.42	

[a] Franck *et al.*, 1980b.

incorporation of [U-^{3}H]emodin (71) shows a variation between 0.37 and 0.96%, caused by growth differences. The specific incorporations relative to emodin [ratio (b/a) in Table VI] prove that chrysophanol (75) is incorporated 3.56 times more effectively than emodin (71), whereas islandicin (73) is evidently a poorer precursor, in spite of its ergochrome-type hydroxylation pattern. Catenarin (74) is excluded as a precursor because of its insignificant incorporation. These results indicate that ergochrome biosynthesis proceeds via chrysophanol (75), with the introduction of the additional hydroxy group at C(4) at a later stage, e.g., after ring cleavage.

C. Anthrones

Once it was established that chrysophanol (75) and emodin (71) are biogenetic precursors of the ergochromes, it was considered important to investigate the incorporation of the corresponding anthrones. Anthrones are precursors of the anthraquinones during their biosynthesis from acetate units. Moreover, they have been successfully subjected to an oxidative *in vitro* ring opening to benzophenone derivatives (Franck *et al.*, 1967; Franck and Berger-Lohr, 1975). To be able to detect small differences in specific

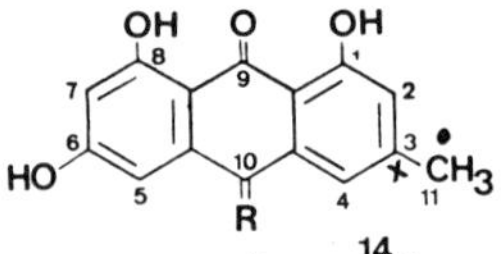

76 R = O, x = ^{14}C
77 R = H$_2$, • = ^{14}C

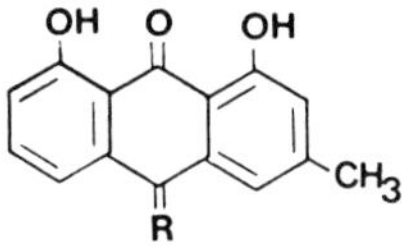

78 R = O
79 R = H$_2$

TABLE VII

Competitive Incorporation of Anthraquinones and Anthrones into Ergochrome EE (2) by *P. oxalicum*[a]

Experiment	Anthraquinones and anthrones	Specific incorporation (%)	Ratio (b/a)
1	(a) [3-^{14}C]Emodin (76)	0.37	4.5
	(b) [11-^{14}C]Emodinanthrone (77)	1.68	
2	(a) [U-^{3}H]Chrysophanol (78)	3.75	1.3
	(b) [U-^{14}C]Chrysophanol (78)	4.81	
3	(a) [U-^{3}H]Chrysophanol (78)	4.14	} 0.9
	(b) [U-^{14}C]Chrysophanolanthrone (79)	3.71	} 0.7[b]

[a] Franck *et al.*, 1980a; Fels, 1978.
[b] Corrected for ^{3}H loss during chrysophanol incorporation.

incorporations, differently labeled anthraquinones and anthrones were fed in competition (Table VII) (Franck *et al.*, 1974; G. Fels, unpublished data). In experiment 1 (Table VII), the precursors emodin (**76**) and emodin-anthrone (**77**) were labeled with the same isotope (^{14}C) in two different positions [at C(3) and C(11)] by the synthetic procedures described above. After incorporation, the corresponding carbon atoms of the ergochrome EE (**2**) could be analyzed as acetic acid by Kuhn-Roth oxidation. The specific incorporations were derived from the activities of the two carbon atoms, determined separately by Schmidt degradation of the acetic acid. The results show that emodinanthrone (**77**) is incorporated into ergochrome EE (**2**) 4.5 times more effectively than emodin (**76**).

The competitive incorporation of chrysophanol (**78**) and chrysophanol-anthrone (**79**) was carried out by using different isotopes (^3H and ^{14}C) for the two precursors. It was shown that chrysophanol and chrysophanolanthrone differ slightly in their specific incorporations (4.14 and 3.71%, respectively).

D. Bisanthraquinonyls

The most interesting reaction of ergochrome biosynthesis is the oxidative ring cleavage of the anthraquinone precursor. To establish whether it occurs before or after dimerization of the anthraquinone units, the incorporation of appropriately labeled benzophenone derivatives or bisanthraquinonyls might be investigated. As the labeled bisanthraquinonyls (**32, 38**–**40**) were available from the methods, mentioned before, they were used for biosynthetic experiments (Franck and Flohr, 1977).

32 R = OH, R' = H
38 R, R = H
39 R = H, R' = OH
40 R, R' = OH

Addition of a mixture of [*U*-^3H]emodin (**71**) and [*U*-^{14}C]skyrin (**32**) to *P. oxalicum* gave an ergochrome EE (**2**) with a specific incorporation of 0.47 and 0.13%, respectively, for [*U*-^3H]-**71** and [*U*-^{14}C]-**32**. Thus the incorporation of skyrin (**32**) is at least 3.61 times less than that of emodin (**71**) and 12.9 times less than that of chrysophanol (**75**). In the case of the three other bisanthraquinonyls (**38**–**40**), the incorporations were below 0.005% and thus insignificant. On the basis of these results, an ergochrome biosynthesis via the bisanthraquinonyls is improbable, although possible. Their nonincorporation might be caused by the fact that the 5,5-connection, although preferred with anthraquinone natural products, is unsuitable for ergochrome biosynthesis.

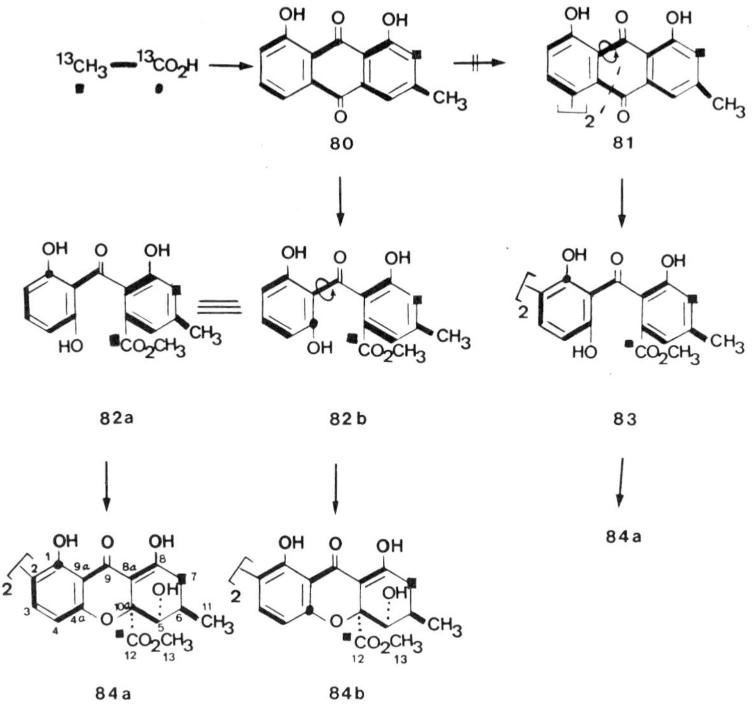

Recently, Kurobane and Vining (1978) were able to show, by feeding [1,2-^{13}C]acetate to the secalonic acid A-producing mold fungus *Pyrenochaeta terrestris*, that in agreement with the results obtained by feeding labeled bisanthraquinonyls, the oxidative ring cleavage proceeds at the monomeric anthraquinone before its dimerization. This investigation was based on the consideration that during the oxidative ring cleavage of an anthraquinone precursor, e.g., chrysophanol (**80**), a benzophenone (**82**) is formed in which each of the two hydroxy groups of the symmetrically substituted benzene nucleus can participate in the xanthone ring closure. It is, therefore, possible to detect whether both of these ring closures occur, if the anthraquinone precursor **80** is labeled by incorporation of [1,2-^{13}C]-acetate. Three kinds of secalonic acid A, which differ in the arrangement of intact ^{13}C,^{13}C units, can then be expected. These are **84a**, **84b**, and the hybrid which contains one molecular half of each of the two label isomers. In case of dimerization of the anthraquinone before ring cleavage (**81**), only the secalonic acid A with the label pattern **84a** can be formed. The proton noise decoupling (PND) ^{13}C NMR spectrum of the secalonic acid A isolated after feeding [1,2-^{13}C]acetate to *P. terrestris* revealed characteristic (^{13}C,^{13}C) spin couplings, which enabled the identification of eight

($^{13}C,^{13}C$) pairs. The ^{13}C enrichments of the intact acetate units in ring A [C(1)–C(2), C(2)–C(3), C(3)–C(4), C(4)–C(4a)] were only half as high as those of the four units in rings B and C. Therefore, a rotation about the twofold axis of symmetry of the trisubstituted ring in the monomeric benzophenone (82) occurs during biosynthesis, thus giving secalonic acids A with differently labeled xanthone units corresponding to 84a and 84b.

E. Ergochromes

To obtain information on the interconversion of the ergochromes and their biogenetic sequence, it was necessary to feed to fungi different labeled ergochromes, obtained by biosynthesis. For such experiments, a fungus producing many different ergochromes was needed. Only *C. purpurea* could be considered, although its ergochrome production varies substantially in amount and number of the components. Furthermore, it seemed doubtful that labeled ergochromes could give significant incorporation, owing to their molecular weight (> 600). This property placed them among the largest precursor molecules which had been fed to microorganisms. As Table VIII shows, incorporations of up to 0.9% were achieved after feeding ergochromes to *C. purpurea* (Franck and Flasch, 1973). This is remarkably high for biosynthetic experiments with intact cells.

The results of experiment 1 (Table VIII) allow the assumption that the biosynthesis of the isolated ergochromes proceeds via the following sequence: BB → BD → BC → CC. This presumes, however, that the dilution of the radioactive ergochromes, formed during the feeding experiment by

TABLE VIII

Specific Incorporation for the Isolated Ergochromes after Feeding Radioactive Ergochromes to *C. purpurea*

	Isolated ergochromes		
Fed ergochromes	Experiment 1 ergochrome BB	Experiment 2 ergochrome BC	Experiment 3 ergochrome CC
Ergochrome BB 4–4	1.3%	0.002%	No radioactive ergochromes isolated
Ergochrome BD 4–6	0.90%	—	
Ergochrome BC 4–5	0.34%	0.19%	
Ergochrome CC 5–5	0.12%	0.025%	

inactive ergochromes already present in the culture, is nearly similar. Experiments 2 and 3 (Table VIII) are also in agreement with the biogenetic sequence. The results reveal that there is practically no retrotransformation of ergochrome BC into BB, and that ergochrome CC is at the end of the sequence.

F. Discussion and Results

The described incorporation experiments with labeled precursors result in a fairly complete picture of ergochrome biosynthesis, which is displayed in Fig. 5. In Fig. 5 the structures within brackets are probable intermediates, but have not yet been proven by direct incorporation. The key compound of the ergochrome biosynthesis is chrysophanol (75). By regioselective ring cleavage, it is transformed into the benzophenone carboxylic acid 85 (see Fig. 5), which has to be hydroxylated at C(3) to give 86 (see Fig. 5) for the subsequent oxidative cyclization. Stereoselective intramolecular cyclization of the biradical 87 (see Fig. 5) by attack of the aryloxy group at the dienone part from above or below, followed by reduction and further reactions, gives the ergochrome halves 3–6. They can be subsequently dimerized to the various ergochromes.

It is remarkable that besides the main precursor chrysophanol (75), emodin (71) and islandicin (73) are also incorporated into ergochromes. The incorporations are, respectively, 3.6 and 11.8 times less than for chrysophanol (75), but still significant. As emodin (71) and islandicin (73) arise from the same polyketide precursor (15), their incorporation represents an offshoot of ergochrome biosynthesis, the participation of which was precisely established (see Table VI). Only few comparative incorporations with differently labeled precursors have been carried out in other natural product areas. Therefore, it is still uncertain to what extent such branching of biosynthetic pathways occurs.

According to investigations on the biogenetic sequence of the ergochromes using biosynthesized labeled ergochromes, ergochrome BB (secalonic acid B) (4)–(4) is the precursor of the ergochromes DD (6)–(6) and CC (5)–(5), which are produced by hydration of the olefinic double bond and lactone ring closure. The fact that no analogous transformation products of ergochrome AA (secalonic acid A) (1) = (3) − (3) have so far been isolated may be explained by stronger steric hindrance of its enzymatic hydration compared to the diastereomeric ergochrome BB. Similarly, no biogenetic transformation products corresponding to the ergochromes CC and DD are known for the ergochrome EE (2), isolated as the only metabolite of this type from *P. oxalicum* (Steyn, 1970). Ergochrome EE is the enantiomer of ergochrome AA (1).

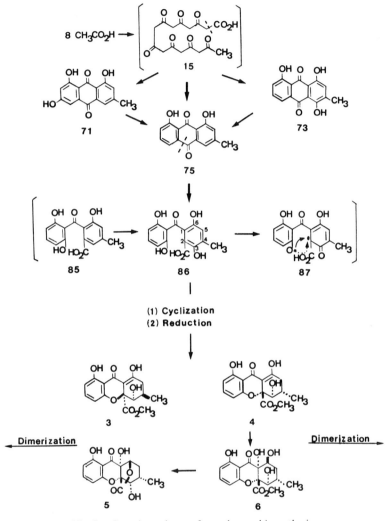

Fig. 5.   Complete scheme of ergochrome biosynthesis.

V. BIOSYNTHESIS OF RELATED SECOANTHRAQUINONES

After the proof that ergochrome biosynthesis occurs by oxidative ring cleavage of anthraquinones (Franck *et al.*, 1966, 1968, Gröger *et al.*, 1968), this previously unknown biogenetic reaction was established for further natural products, which are also secoanthraquinones (Table IX).

TABLE IX

Biosynthesis of Secoanthraquinones from Labeled Anthraquinones

Anthraquinone precursor	Fungus	Isolated secoanthraquinone	Specific incorporation (%)
[Methoxy-^{14}C]questin (91)	P. frequentans	Sulochrin (95)[a]	3.97
[U-^{14}C]Emodin (71)	A. terreus	Dihydrogeodin (96)[b]	0.29
		Geodin (94)[b]	0.27

[a] Gatenbeck and Malmström (1969).
[b] Fujimoto et al. (1975).

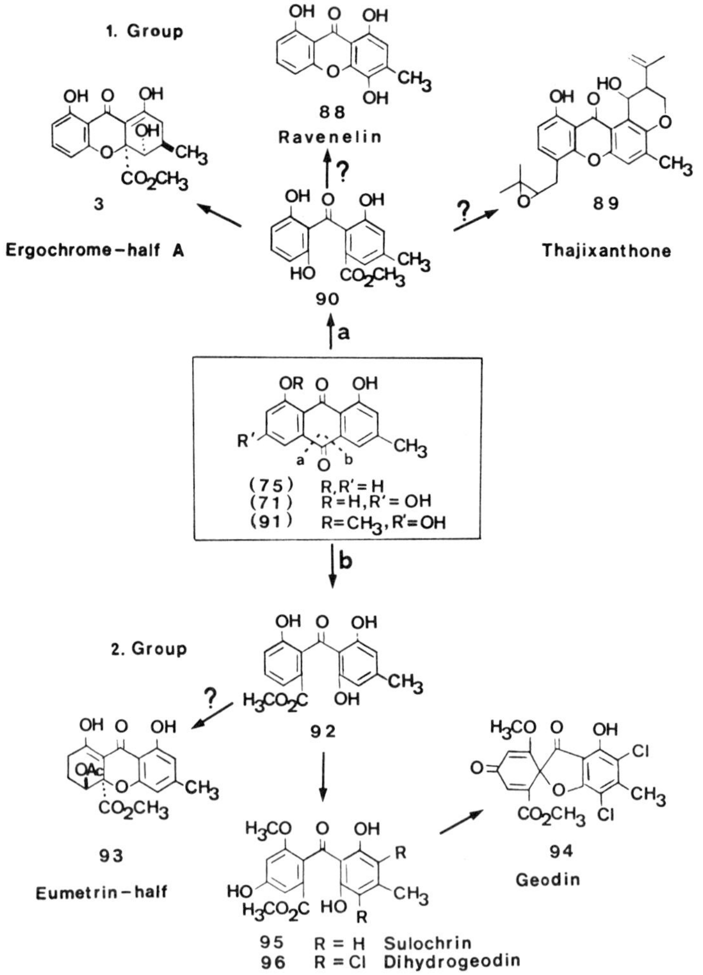

Fig. 6. Proved and hypothetical biosynthetic pathways for two groups of secoanthraquinones from anthraquinones.

According to Gatenbeck and Malmström (1969), the benzophenone sulochrin (95) of *Penicillium frequentans* is formed from questin (8-*O*-methylemodin) (91) (3.97% incorporation). [*U*-^{14}C]Emodin (71) was converted into the antibiotic geodin (94) and its reduction product dihydrogeodin (96) by *Aspergillus terreus* (Fujimoto *et al.*, 1975). Here the incorporations, although clearly significant, are less than for sulochrin, because of more reaction steps and the introduction of two chlorine atoms.

For the formation of the secoanthraquinones sulochrin (95), dihydrogeodin (96), and geodin, the cleavage of the anthraquinone precursor 75 to give the benzophenone 92, in contrast to ergochrome biosynthesis, must be assumed to be between the quinone carbonyl atom C(10) and the methyl-substituted phenyl nucleus (cleavage b). Figure 6 describes the biosynthetic pathways for some secoanthraquinones. Cleavage of the anthraquinones chrysophanol (75) and emodin (71) at (a) and (b) (square in Fig. 6) leads to the isomeric benzophenones 90 and 92 which are themselves precursors for two groups of secoanthraquinones. The ergochromes and possibly the xanthone natural products ravenelin (88) (Raistrick *et al.*, 1936) and taji-xanthone (89) (Chexal *et al.*, 1974) belong to the first group. Sulochrin (95), geodin (94), dihydrogeodin (96), and perhaps the eumetrins, isolated by Shibata *et al.* (1973) from the lichen *Usnea bayleyi*, constitute the second group. (See Fig. 6 for structures 88–96.)

The eumetrin A$_1$ (98) is constructed of one molecular half (3) of ergochrome AA (1) and another similar tetrahydroxanthone unit with interchanged substituents. In this secoanthraquinone, which is also very interesting from a biogenetic point of view, possibly the two benzophenones 90 and 92, formed by oxygenolysis of chrysophanol (75), are combined. The tajixanthone 99 found in *Aspergillus variecolor* could be developed from 90 by

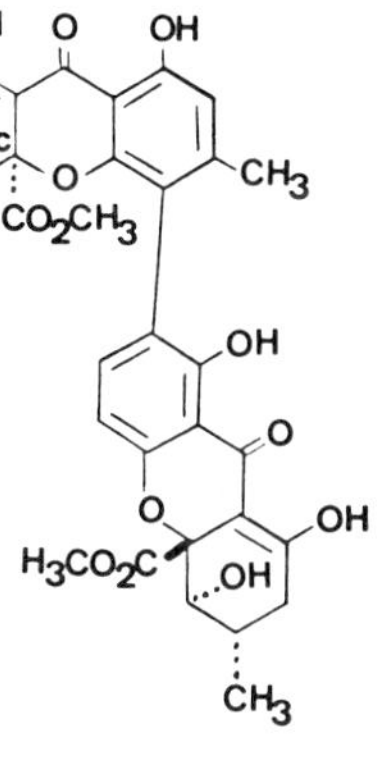

98

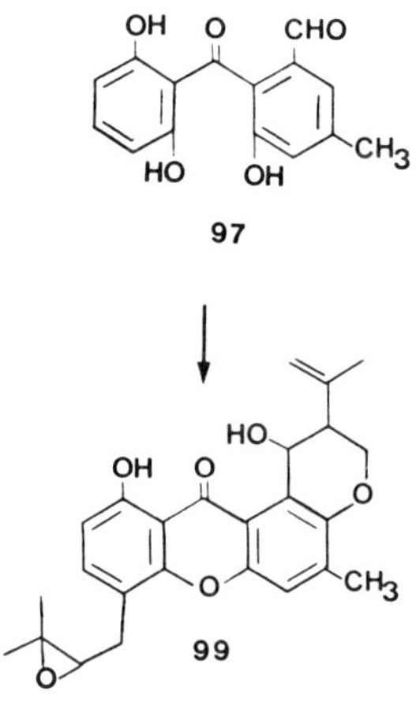

97

99

transforming the methoxycarbonyl to an aldehyde group to give **97**, by two prenylations and further oxidative steps.

VI. BIOMIMETIC REACTIONS

A. Oxygenolysis of Anthraquinones

The simulation of biosynthetic steps by model reactions *in vitro* is useful for mechanistic understanding and development of biomimetic procedures. This is especially so when an unusual reaction with hitherto unknown synthetic possibilities is involved. This was the case with the oxidative ring cleavage of anthraquinones during the biosynthesis of the ergochromes and other secoanthraquinones. Formally, this conversion resembles the Baeyer–Villiger oxidation of ketones. However, numerous hydroxyanthraquinones, including emodin (**71**), did not react on treatment with pertrifluoroacetic acid and other organic peracids, while benzophenone was cleaved under these conditions in high yield (Franck *et al.*, 1967).

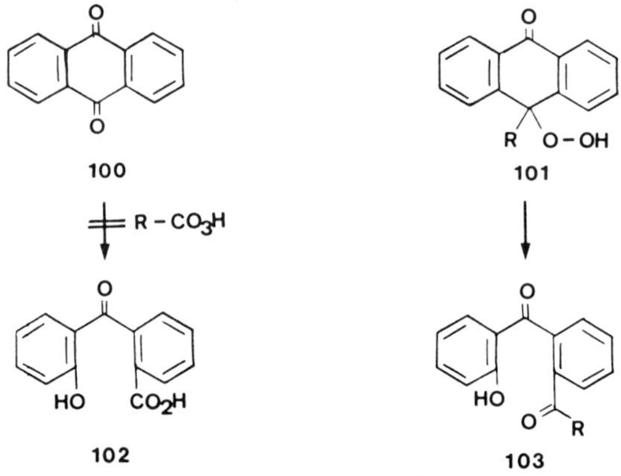

Money (1963) discussed another chemical approach for oxidative cleavage, in connection with biogenetic hypotheses, which involved starting from anthrones, the intermediates in anthraquinone biosynthesis from acetate units. The anthrone might be autoxidized to the hydroperoxide (**101**, R = H) and then rearranged by acid catalysis to the benzophenone (**103**, R = H). On the basis of this speculation, it was possible to perform the oxidative cleavage for the first time by converting 10-methylanthrone hydroperoxide (**101**, R = CH$_3$) in 4.5% yield into (**103**, R = CH$_3$) (Franck *et al.*, 1967).

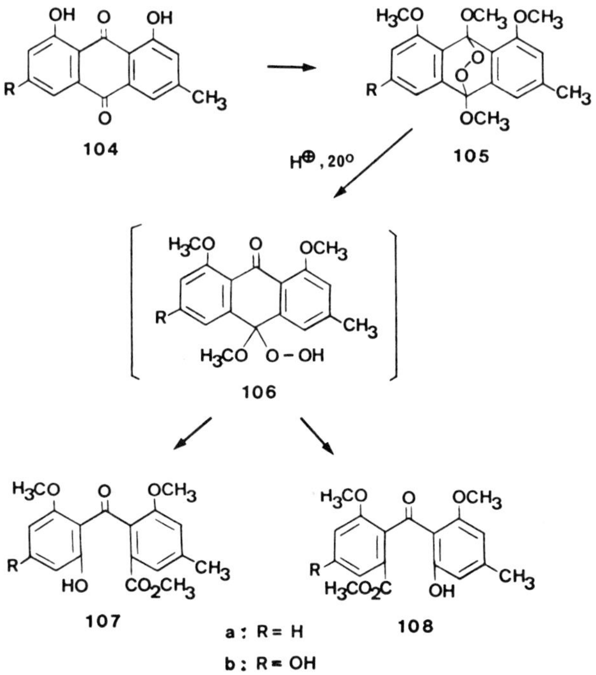

To achieve ring cleavage to a benzophenonecarboxymethyl ester as in ergochrome biosynthesis, a 10-methoxyanthrone hydroperoxide (**101**, R = OCH$_3$) had to be used as starting material. From chrysophanol (**104a**) and emodin (**104b**), the biogenetic precursors of the ergochromes, the endoperoxides **105a** and **105b** could be prepared via the [4 + 2]cycloaddition of singlet oxygen to leucopermethyl ethers. From these endoperoxides, two sets of isomeric benzophenone carboxymethyl esters (**107a, 107b** and **108a, 108b**) were obtained in 70–72% yield, by acid-catalyzed rearrangement with sulfuric acid in acetone via the intermediary hydroperoxides **106a** and **106b** (Franck and Berger-Lohr, 1975). These ring-cleavage reactions probably simulate closely the corresponding step of ergochrome biosynthesis. They also provide the most promising synthetic access to the benzophenone precursors of ergochrome biosynthesis.

B. Oxidative Cyclization of Benzophenones

The benzophenone **109** appears to be most suitable as a starting compound for the biomimetic synthesis of a molecular half of the ergochromes. It could give the xanthone by an intramolecular Michael addition after oxidation of its hydroquinone unit to the corresponding *p*-quinone. However, oxidations with the more easily accessible model compound **110** revealed that, under the applied conditions (aqueous $FeCl_3$), the spirodienone **114** is formed in 86% yield, instead of the desired xanthone derivative **112** (Franck and Zeidler

109 110 111

112 113 114

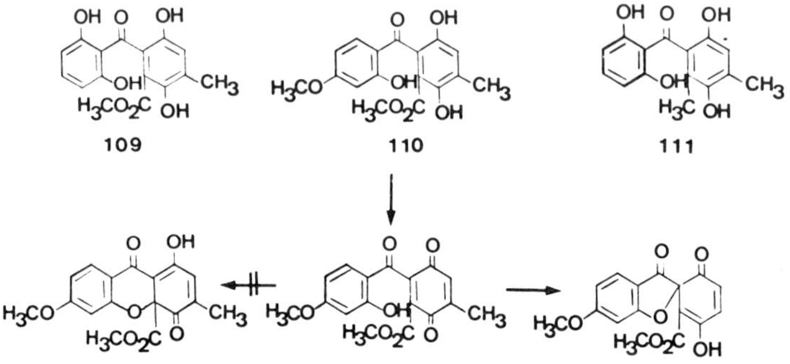

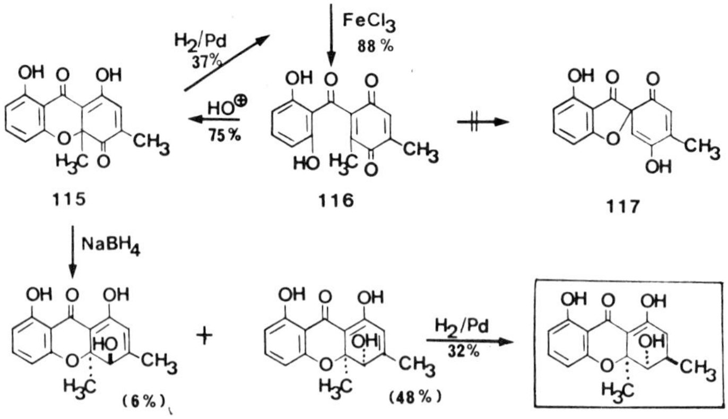

1973). While assuming that this reaction is caused by the spacial demand of the voluminous methoxycarbonyl group, the oxidation of the dimethylhydroquinone (**111**) was investigated (Franck *et al.*, 1973). Oxidation with $FeCl_3$ produced the crystalline *p*-quinone **116** which condensed under weakly alkaline conditions to give exclusively xanthone **115**. Catalytic hydrogenation of **115** did not lead to the conformationally favored tetrahydroxanthone, **120**, or to another diastereomeric racemate, but by allyl ether hydrogenolysis it gave the educt (**111**). The stereoselective reduction of the dienone (**115**) could, however, be achieved in two steps. Thus, of the two diastereomeric dienol racemates (**118** and **119**) obtained on treatment with

115 116 117

118 119 120

sodium borohydride, the predominantly formed species (119) was hydro-genated to give the desired tetrahydroxanthone (120). In this fashion, the synthesis of the racemic tetrahydroxanthone 120 with the same relative configurations at all three chiral carbon atoms, as in one molecular half (3) of secalonic acid A (1), was achieved. Species 120 differs from 3 only in that it has a methoxycarbonyl for a methyl group and is, therefore, a 10-methylhemisecalonic acid A. As in the case of the biomimetic ring cleavage of anthraquinones, the oxidative cyclization of benzophenones shows that the course of ergochrome biosynthesis, as derived from incorporation experiments, is in its important steps, understandable from the mechanistic point of view and can be simulated *in vitro*.

ACKNOWLEDGMENT

The research from the author's laboratory was supported by the *Landesamt für Forschung in Nordrhein-Westfalen*, and the *Fonds der Chemischen Industrie*.

REFERENCES

Aberhart, D. J., Chen, Y. S., DeMayo, P., and Stothers, J. B. (1965). *Tetrahedron* 21, 1417.
Andersen, R., Büchi, G., Kobbe, B., and Demain, A. L. (1977). *J. Org. Chem.* 42, 352.
ApSimon, J. W., Corran, J. A., Creasey, N. G., Marlow, W., Whalley, W. B., and Sim, K. Y. (1965a). *J. Chem. Soc.*, p. 4144.
ApSimon, J. W., Corran, J. A., Creasey, N. G., Sim, K. Y., and Whalley, W. B. (1965b). *J. Chem. Soc.*, p. 4130.
Barton, D. H. R., Hesse, R. H., and Kirby, G. W. (1966). *J. Chem. Soc.*, p. 6379.
Bentley, R. (1975). *In* "Biosynthesis, A Specialist Periodical Report" (T. A. Geissman, ed.), Vol. 3, p. 181. The Chemical Society, London.
Butler, W. H. (1964). *Brit. J. Cancer* 18, 756.
Chexal, K. K., Fouweather, Ch., Holker, J. S., Simpson, T. J., and Young, K. (1974). *J. Chem. Soc. Perkin Trans. 1*, p. 1584.
Davies, J. S., Davies, V. H., and Hassal, C. H. (1969). *J. Chem. Soc. C*, p. 1873.
Dragendorff, G., and Podwyssotski, V. (1877). *Naunyn–Schmiedebergs Arch. Exp. Pathol. Pharmakol.* 6, 153.
Eglinton, G., King, F. E., Lloyd, G., Loder, J. W., Marshall, J. R., Robertson, A., and Whalley, W. B. (1958). *J. Chem. Soc.*, p. 1833.
Evans, E. A. (1974). "Tritium and its Compounds." Butterworth, London.
Fels, G. (1978). Personal communication.
Flohr, G. (1977). Ph. D. thesis, Münster, West Germany.
Franck, B. (1964). (*Angew. Chem.* 76, 864; *Angew. Chem. Int. ed.* 3, 763.
Franck, B. (1965). *In* "Beiträge zur Biochemie und Physiologie von Naturstoffen. Festschrift K. Mothes". (D. Gröger, H.-B. Schröter, and H. R. Schütte, eds.), p. 153. Fischer, Jena.
Franck, B. (1969). *Angew. Chem.* 81, 269; *Angew. Chem. Int. Edit.* 8, 251.

Franck, B. (1972). "Abhandlungen Rhein-Westf-Akademie," p. 43. Westdeutscher Verlag, Opladen.
Franck, B., and Baumann, G. (1966a). *Chem. Ber.* **99**, 3863.
Franck, B., and Baumann, G. (1966b). *Chem. Ber.* **99**, 3875.
Franck, B., and Berger-Lohr, B. (1975). *Angew. Chem.* **87**, 845; *Angew. Int. Edit.* **14**, 818.
Franck, B., and Flasch, H. (1973). *Fortschr. Chem. Org. Naturstoff.* **30**, 151.
Franck, B., and Gottschalk, E. M. (1964). *Angew. Chem.* **76**, 438; *Angew. Chem. Int. Edit.* **3**, 441.
Franck, B., and Reschke, T. (1960). *Chem. Ber*, **93**, 347.
Franck, B., and Zeidler, U. (1973). *Chem. Ber.* **106**, 1182.
Franck, B., and Zimmer, I. (1965). *Chem. Ber.* **98**, 1514.
Franck, B., Gottschalk, E. M., Ohnsorge, U., and Hüper, F. (1966a). *Chem. Ber.* **99**, 3842.
Franck, B., Hüper, F., Gröger, D., and Erge, D. (1966b). *Angew. Chem.* **78**, 752; *Angew. Chem. Int. Edit.* **5**, 728.
Franck, B., Radtke, V., and Zeidler, U. (1967). *Angew. Chem.* **79**, 935; *Angew. Chem. Int. Edit.* **6**, 952.
Franck, B., Hüper, F., Gröger, D., and Erge, D. (1968). *Chem. Ber.* **101**, 1954.
Franck, B., Ohnsorge, U., and Flasch, H. (1970). *Tetrahedron Lett.*, p. 3773.
Franck, B., Stöckigt, J., Zeidler, U., and Franckowiak, G. (1973). *Chem. Ber.* **106**, 1198.
Franck, B., Backhaus, H., and Rolf, M. (1980a). *Tetrahedron Lett.* (in press).
Franck, B., Bringmann, G., and Flohr, G. (1980b). *Angew. Chem.* (in press).
Freeburn, A. (1912). *Pharmacol. J.* **34**, 568; *Chem. Zentralbl.* **83**, II, 39.
Fujimoto, H., Flasch, H., and Franck, B. (1975). *Chem. Ber.* **108**, 1224.
Gatenbeck, S., and Malmström, L. (1969). *Acta Chem. Scand.* **23**, 3493.
Gröger, D. (1972a). In "Mycotoxins" (I. F. H. Purchase, ed.), p. 82. Elsevier, Amsterdam.
Gröger, D. (1972b). In "Microbial Toxins" (S. Kadis, A. Ciegler, and S. J. Ajl, eds.), Vol. VIII, p. 348. Academic Press, New York.
Gröger, D., Erge, D., Franck, B., Ohnsorge, U., Flasch, H., and Hüper, F. (1968). *Chem. Ber.* **101**, 1970.
Güneysu, A. (1976). Masters thesis, Münster, West Germany.
Harada, M., Yano, S., Watanabe, H., Yamazaki, M., and Miyaki, K. (1974) *Chem. Pharm. Bull. (Jpn)* **22**, 1600.
Harris, T. M., Harris, C. M., and Hindley, K. B. (1974). *Fortschr. Chem. Org. Naturstoff.* **31**, 217.
Harris, T. M., Webb, A. D., Harris, C. M., Wittek, P. I., and Murray, T. P. (1976). *J. Am. Chem. Soc.* **98**, 6065.
Hooper, J. W., Marlow, W., Whalley, W. B., Borthwick, A. D., and Bowden, R. (1971). *J. Chem. Soc.*, p. 3580.
Howard, C. C., and Johnstone, R. A. W. (1973). *J. Chem. Soc. Perkin Trans. 1*, p. 2440.
Hüper, F. (1967). Ph.D. thesis, Münster, West Germany.
Ishida, T., Ohoishi, J., Yoshida, K. Akashi, K., and Takeda, I. (1973) Japan. Patent Appl. 73 50.658.09; *Chem. Abs.* **82**, 423 (1975).
Kurobane, I., and Vining, L. C. (1978). *Tetrahedron Lett.*, p. 1379.
McPhail, A. T., Sim, G. A., Asher, J. D. M., Robertson, J. M., and Silverton, J. V. (1966). *J. Chem. Soc. B*, p. 18.
Money, T. (1963). *Nature (London)* **199**, 592.
Raistrick, H., Robinson, R., and White, D. E. (1936). *Biochem. J.*, p. 1303.
Schrameyer, M. (1976). Ph.D. thesis, Münster, West Germany.
Shibata, S., Ogihara, Y., Seo, S., and Kitagawa, I. (1968). *Tetrahedron Lett.*, p. 3179.
Steglich, W., and Reininger, W. (1970). *Chem. Commun.*, p. 178.
Steglich, W., Arnold, R., Lösel, W., and Reininger, W. (1972). *Chem. Commun.* p. 102.
Steyn, P. S. (1970). *Tetrahedron* **26**, 51.

Turner, W. B. (1971). "Fungal Metabolites." Academic Press, New York.
Wenzel, M., and Schulze, P. E. (1962). "Tritium-Markierung." de Gruyter, Berlin.
Yamazaki, M., Maebayashi, Y., and Miyaki, K., (1971). *Chem. Pharm. Bull. (Jpn.)* **19**, 199.
Yang, D. -M., Takeda, N., Iitaka, Y., Sankawa, U., and Shibata, S. (1973). *Tetrahedron* **29**, 519.
Yosioka, I., Nakanishi, T., Izumi, S., and Kitagawa, I. (1968). *Chem. Pharm. Bull. (Jpn.)* **16**, 2090.

6

The Biosynthesis
of Neurotropic Mycotoxins

MIKIO YAMAZAKI

I. INTRODUCTION

Outbreaks of poisoning from the ingestion of mycotoxins occur frequently in domestic animals, because they occasionally consume moldy
feeds in bulk. In contrast, acute exogenic toxicosis from mycotoxins in
humans is relatively uncommon, for humans usually refuse moldy food.
Therefore, the deleterious effects, including cancer, caused by the chronic
consumption of mycotoxins are of more importance to man than acute
poisoning. Carcinogenic mycotoxins have thus attracted the primary
interest of many investigators. However, the importance of neurotropic
mycotoxins should also be emphasized because of their violent and sometimes lethal effects in cases of acute mycotoxicoses.

Ergotism caused by the eating of ergot-contaminated rye bread may be
the earliest-reported and most formidable instance of mycotoxicosis in man.
The ergot toxins are fully described in Chapter 2 of this book.

In addition to the ergot toxins, some other mycotoxins also exhibit
neurotoxic activity. Aspects of the chemistry and biosynthesis of these toxins

193

The Biosynthesis of Mycotoxins
Copyright © 1980 by Academic Press, Inc.
All rights of reproduction in any form reserved.
ISBN 0-12-670650-6.

are described in this chapter. Aflatoxins (Chapter 4), cyclopiazonic acid (Chapter 11), and patulin (Chapter 7), which are also reported to have tremorgenic activity, are excluded from this review.

II. CITREOVIRIDIN

Mycotoxicological investigations were undertaken by Japanese scientists prior to the discovery of aflatoxins. In 1891, a Japanese doctor found that an extract of certain moldy rice, available in Tokyo, caused neurological symptoms in experimental animals. From these findings he suggested that the principal cause of cardiac beriberi in man, which was recognized as a heart disease of the most violent type, might be the chronic consumption of moldy rice. In the 1940's, *Penicillium toxicarium* (subsequently identified as *Penicillium citreo-viride*) was found to be toxinogenic when grown on rice grains. An alcoholic extract of the fungal material was lethal in mammals and other vertebrates. After a single parenteral injection of the extract, animals exhibited a progressive paralysis of the ascending type, transient convulsive signs, fluctuation of tendon reflex, cardiovascular damage, and respiratory failure; death frequently occurred within a day. The signs and symptoms and their development in the experimental animals closely resembled the clinical manifestations of cardiac beriberi (Uraguchi, 1969, 1971). A principal metabolite, citreoviridin, of the toxinogenic fungus was subsequently isolated and its chemical structure was determined as 1 by Sakabe *et al.* (1964).

Citreoviridin 1, $C_{23}H_{30}O_6CH_3OH$, was shown to contain one methoxy group and six double bonds. Permanganate oxidation of this compound in pyridine afforded a carboxylic acid (2), which contained one methyl, one methoxy, and one carboxy group. Infrared (ir) and ultraviolet (uv) absorption spectra of 2 indicated that this acid contained an α-pyrone moiety. The substitution on the pyrone ring was evident from the nuclear magnetic resonance (NMR) spectral data.

Partial catalytic hydrogenation of citreoviridin followed by oxidation afforded methyl pyruvate and an oily methyl ester (3). The uv spectrum of citreoviridin (388 nm, ε 48,000) suggested that the pyrone chromophore was conjugated with a polyene moiety. The partial structure of citreoviridin was therefore proposed as 4.

Ozonolysis of the di-*p*-nitrobenzoate derivative of citreoviridin gave an aldehyde (5). Oxidation of this aldehyde with permanganate in pyridine gave the corresponding acid (6). Hydrolysis of the acid with alkali followed by acidification afforded a γ-lactone (7).

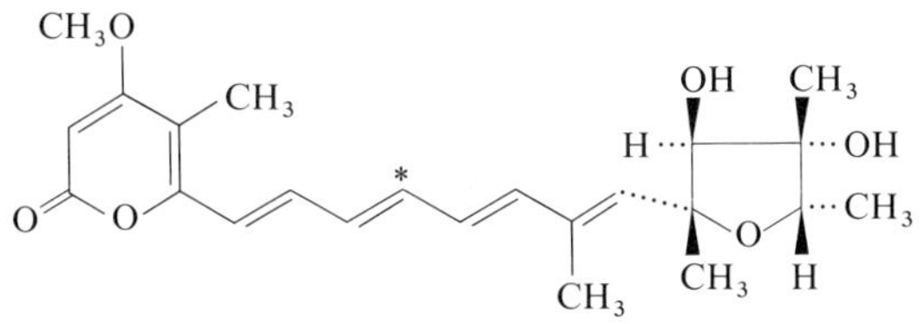

The structure and stereochemistry of the aldehyde was determined mainly from the slow consumption of periodate and the NMR data of this compound. The structure of citreoviridin was conclusively established as **1** (Sakabe *et al.*, 1964).

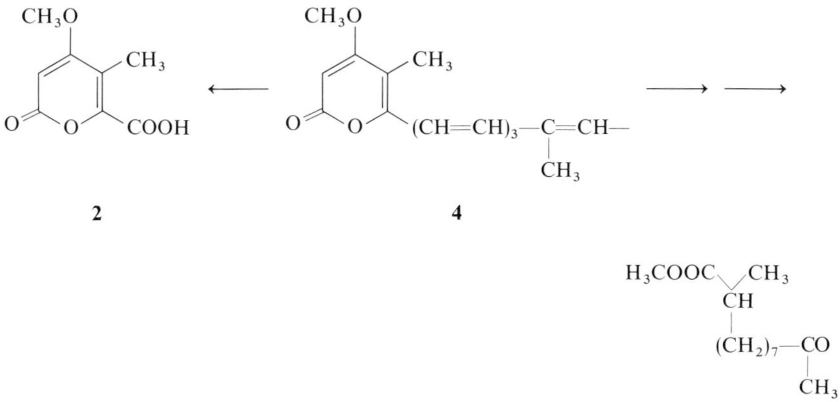

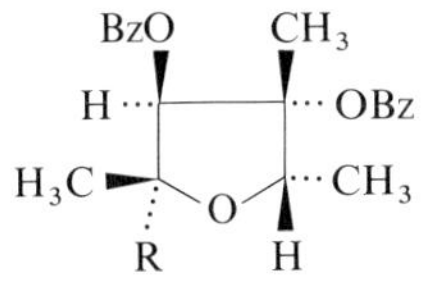

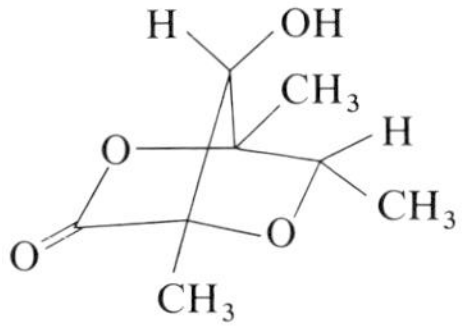

Citreoviridin was completely stable toward heating in chloroform–methanol for 24 hr. However, treatment of a dilute solution of citreoviridin in diffused light with a catalytic amount of iodine at room temperature gave a mixture of citreoviridin and isocitreoviridin in a ratio of 7:3. It was presumed that a change in geometry from *trans* to *cis* had occurred at the double bond marked with an asterisk in the structure of citreoviridin (**1**). Injection of a single dose of isocitreoviridin (100 mg/kg) had no effect on rats, whereas at this dosage level, citreoviridin caused the death within 2 hr of all the experimental animals (Nagel *et al.*, 1972a).

Penicillium ochrosalmoneum (*Eupenicillium ochrosalmoneum*), when cultured on rice, produced citreoviridin. *Penicillium pulvillorum* also produced citreoviridin in high yield, when cultured on cornmeal (Nagel *et al.*, 1972a).

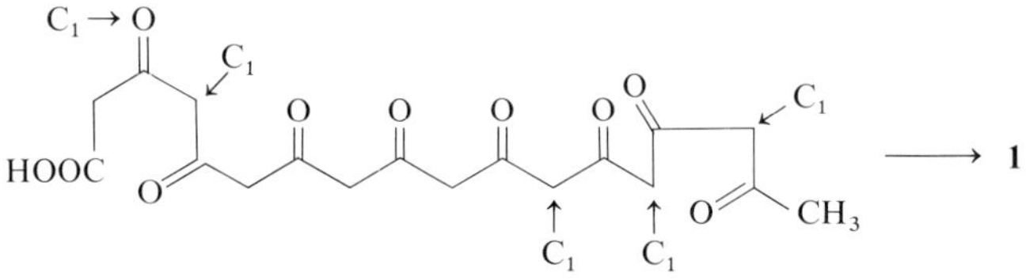

$$\text{8} \longrightarrow \textbf{1} \tag{2}$$

The polyene structure of citreoviridin suggested that this compound is derived from a polyketide e.g. (**8**) through the "acetate polymalonate condensation pathway" with the introduction of five C_1-units from methionine. In the biosynthetic studies, a strain of *Penicillium pulvillorum* was grown in Ushinsky medium at 25°C in stationary culture. Radioactive precursors were added to the culture 9–10 days after inoculation when the production of citreoviridin started to increase rapidly. Citreoviridin was then isolated and purified. The incorporation ratios obtained from [*methyl*-^{14}C]methionine and [2-^{14}C]acetate were 70% and 5%, respectively. The radioactive citreoviridin was degraded as shown in Scheme 1.

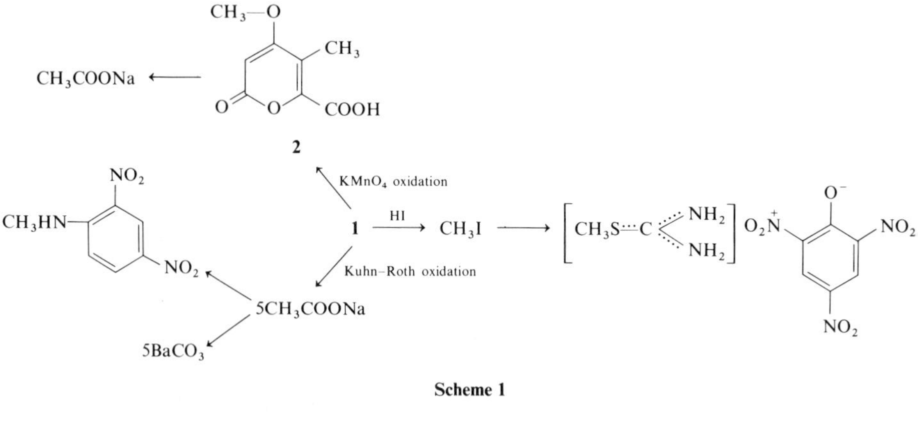

Scheme 1

The methoxy group represented 20.4% of the total activity of citreoviridin labeled by [*methy*-^{14}C]methionine, indicating that four of the five methyl groups other than the methoxy group were derived from methionine. Acetic acid which was obtained by Kuhn–Roth oxidation of citreoviridin was shown to contain 80.8% of the total activity, and all the activity was located in the methyl group of the acetic acid. The α-pyronecarboxylic acid (2), obtained by oxidation of citreoviridin, showed specific activity equal to 39.7% of that of the starting material, indicating that the methyl group attached to the pyrone ring should be derived from the methyl group of methionine. However, acetic acid obtained by Kuhn–Roth oxidation from [2-^{14}C]acetate-derived citreoviridin had a specific activity of 51.8% (theoretical value: 5/9 = 55.5% of that of citreoviridin). The finding that the acid (2) obtained by oxidation of [2-^{14}C]acetate-derived citreoviridin had 31% of the activity of 1 gave support to the above findings. Thus, it was concluded by Nagel *et al.* (1972b) that citreoviridin was formed from an unbranched polyketide chain probably derived from one acetate and eight malonate units which contained one *O*-methyl and four *C*-methyl groups derived from the methyl group of methionine.

III. MALTORYZINE

In the period from September to November in 1954, many dairy cattle became ill and died after being fed malt sprout. The animals that ingested toxic malt sprout exhibited tremors, loss of appetite, weakness in the legs, lumbar paralysis, and decreased lactation. Histopathological examination showed a marked disturbance of circulation as evidenced by congestion of various organs, petechiae in serous membranes, and hemorrhage in small vessels of the brain (Ohkubo *et al.*, 1955).

After investigation of the microflora in the malt sprout, Iizuka and Iida (1962) identified *Aspergillus oryzae* var. *microsporus* as the causal fungus. The fungus was grown on a Czapek–Dox medium containing malt sprout extract in tank culture. After incubation for 2.5 days at 30°C, crystals of maltoryzine were obtained from the culture broth. When injected intraperitoneally (i.p.), maltoryzine showed an LD_{50} of 3 mg/kg in mice; the mice also exhibited muscular paralysis (Iizuka, 1974).

Maltoryzine (9), $C_{11}H_{14}O_4$, reacted negatively with ninhydrin. Schiff's, and Gibbs reagents, whereas positive reactions were obtained with ferric chloride, methyl red, and 2,4-dinitrophenylhydrazine. Its uv spectrum, $\lambda_{(max)}$ (ε), 220 (12,900), 280 (1290), and 320 nm (129), indicated that the compound contained the oxygenated benzoyl group. The ir spectrum of 9 indicated the presence of the hydroxy (3300 cm^{-1}) and carbonyl (1700 cm^{-1})

groups, as well as conjugated double bonds (1600 and 1500 cm^{-1}). Ozonolysis of the methylated maltoryzine in chloroform afforded one mole of
acetic acid and an acidic substance (10), $C_{12}H_{14}O_6$. Hydrolysis of 10 with
1 N KOH in ethanol gave one mole of acetic acid and 2,3,6-trimethoxy-
benzoic acid (11). Hydrolysis of 10 with 1 N H_2SO_4 gave one mole of
carbon dioxide and a carbonyl compound, indicating that the acid (10)
obtained by ozonolysis was 2,3,6-trimethoxybenzoyl acetic acid. Based on
the above results, the chemical structure of maltoryzine (9) was proposed
(Scheme 2).

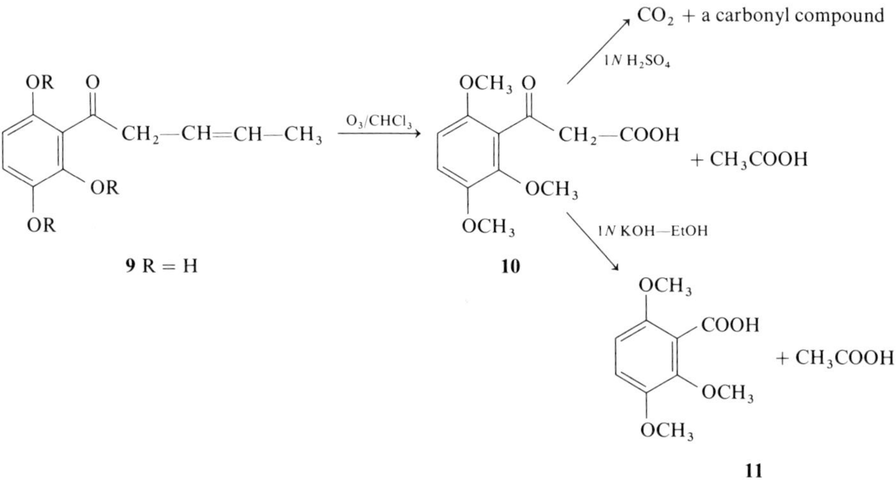

Scheme 2

The carbon skeleton of maltoryzine appears to be derived from polyketide 12. The oxygenation pattern in the phenol ring and side chain of this
compound, however, differed from the general biogenetic principles of
polyketide formation (Turner, 1971). No evidence to support the biosynthesis of maltoryzine has yet been obtained.

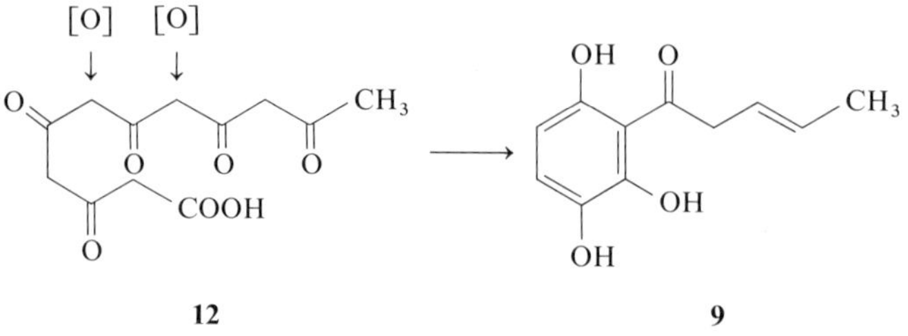

IV. ASPERGILLIC ACID AND RELATED PYRAZINE OXIDES

During a survey of aflatoxin-producing fungi in Japanese industrial seed molds, about 70 strains were isolated which possessed the ability to produce aspergillic acid, β-nitropropionic acid, and oxalic acid in liquid culture (Yokozuka *et al.*, 1969). No aflatoxin-producing fungi were identified. Aspergillic acid, was first isolated in 1942 as an antibiotic. White and Hill (1943) reported that aspergillic acid caused convulsions in animals. The largest dose of aspergillic acid reported to be tolerated was about 4 mg/20 gm mouse (per os), although this dose was lethal to a few of the mice. With doses of >5 mg/20 gm mouse, the animals went into convulsions within 5–10 min and died. Intraperitoneal injection of the sodium salt of this compound (dosage 3 mg/20 gm mouse) caused rapid onset of convulsions and death within 10 min (White and Hill, 1943).

Aspergillic acid (**13**), $C_{12}H_{20}N_2O_2$, was first suggested to contain its two oxygen atoms as a carboxy group. The postulate was subsequently negated, for deoxyaspergillic acid was obtained through dry distillation of aspergillic acid with copper chromate catalyst (Dutcher, 1947a). Coloration of aspergillic acid with ferric chloride and formation of a green cupric salt suggested that this compound is a hydroxamic acid. The formation of deoxyaspergillic acid from aspergillic acid on reduction was explained as the hydroxy group on the nitrogen atom being replaced by a hydrogen atom. Dutcher (1947b) found that bromination of aspergillic acid gave bromoaspergillic acid. On reduction of bromoaspergillic acid with zinc and acetic acid, a dioxopiperazine was obtained. It was demonstrated by Dunn *et al.* (1949a,b) that a mixture of DL-leucine and DL-isoleucine was obtained on vigorous hydrolysis of the dioxopiperazine with hydrogen bromide. It was thus concluded that the structure of aspergillic acid should be presented as **13**.

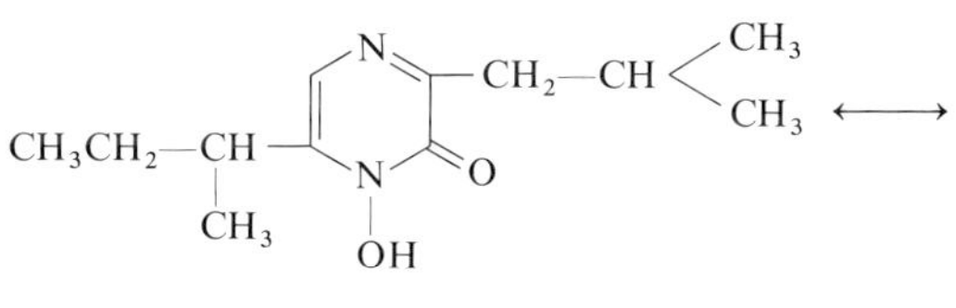

13

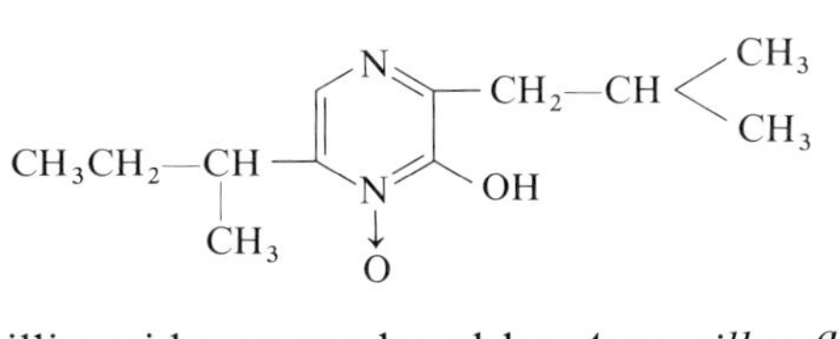

(4)

Labeled aspergillic acid was produced by *Aspergillus flavus* grown on a medium supplemented separately with radioactive leucine and isoleucine.

TABLE I

Incorporation of Labeled Leucine and Isoleucine into Mycelium and Aspergillic Acid
by *Aspergillus flavus*

	Specific activity (μCi/mmole)				
	Mycelium		Aspergillic acid		
Labeled precursors	Leucine	Isoleucine	Aspergillic acid	Leucine	Isoleucine
DL-[1-^{14}C]Leucine (4.36 μCi)	1.04	0.01	1.19	1.21	0.02
D-[1-^{14}C]Leucine (1.57 μCi)	0.53	0.01	0.62	—	—
L-[U-^{14}C]Leucine (4.84 μCi)	0.84	0.02	1.26	—	—
L-[U-^{14}C]Isoleucine (4.58 μCi)	0.19	1.68	2.29	0.22	2.32

The radioactive aspergillic acid was degraded by the methods used in its structural elucidation to yield leucine and isoleucine. The results of the measurement of radioactivity of aspergillic acid and the degradation products are summarized in Table I (MacDonald, 1961).

DL-[1-^{14}C]Leucine was efficiently incorporated into aspergillic acid. Subsequent hydrolysis of aspergillic acid indicated that all the activity was present in leucine, as shown in Table I. Eighty-seven percent of the activity of the labeled leucine as determined by decarboxylation with ninhydrin was found to be present in the carboxy group of the amino acid, whereas less than 2% was located in the rest of the molecule. As well as DL-[1-^{14}C]leucine, L-[U-^{14}C]isoleucine was also efficiently incorporated into aspergillic acid. Most of the radioactivity was found to be located in the isoleucine moiety in the aspergillic acid molecule. These results indicate that aspergillic acid was formed by the fungus from one molecule of leucine and one molecule of isoleucine.

L-leucine + L-isoleucine ⟶

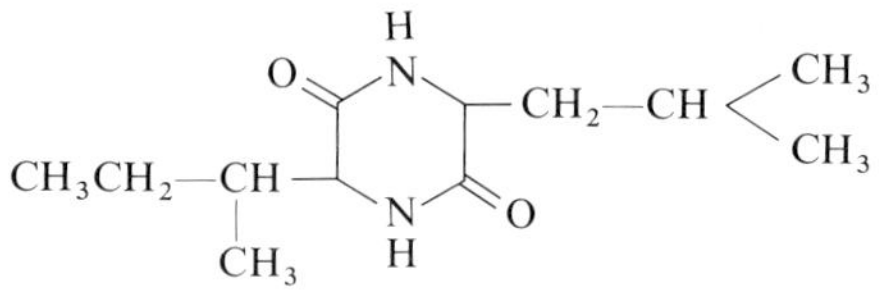

⟶ **13**

(5)

Hydroxyaspergillic acid, an antibiotic isolated from *A. flavus*, (Dutcher, 1958), was also shown to be derived from leucine and isoleucine, based on feeding experiments with ^{14}C-labeled L-leucine and L-isoleucine. When the fungus was grown on a medium containing [^{14}C]aspergillic acid, a significant amount of radioactivity was found in hydroxyaspergillic acid. However, feeding experiments with labeled hydroxyaspergillic acid did not produce labeled aspergillic acid. In the early stages of fungal growth, a greater amount of aspergillic acid was found than hydroxyaspergillic acid. However, the amount of aspergillic acid decreased in the later stage of

growth, whereas more hydroxyaspergillic acid was formed. The above result indicates that aspergillic acid is possibly a precursor of hydroxyaspergillic acid (MacDonald, 1965b).

Neoaspergillic acid and neohydroxyaspergillic acid are antibiotics, first
isolated from cultures of *Aspergillus sclerotiorum* (Weiss *et al.*, 1958). When
the fungus was cultivated on a yeast extract medium containing L-[1-^{14}C]-
leucine, the radioactive precursor was incorporated without significant
randomization into both neoaspergillic and neohydroxyaspergillic acid. On
cultivation of fungus on a medium containing radioactive neoaspergillic
acid, radioactivity was found in the isolated neohydroxyaspergillic acid.
Neohydroxyaspergillic acid was, however, not converted into neoaspergillic
acid. The fungus was found to have the ability to oxidize deoxyneoaspergillic
acid (flavacol) to neoaspergillic acid in replacement culture. These results
suggest that flavacol is oxidized to neoaspergillic acid and that neoaspergillic acid is a precursor of neohydroxyaspergillic acid (Mietlich and Mac-
Donald, 1965).

Cook and Slater (1954) obtained pulcherriminic acid (**14**) at first as an
acid component of a red pigment, pulcherrimin, from *Candida pulcherrima*.
MacDonald (1963) subsequently obtained this acid directly from the same
fungus. The structure proposed by MacDonald was essentially the same as
that proposed by Cook and Slater (1956), although the properties of pulcherriminic acid obtained by both research groups were not entirely identical.

It was demonstrated by a trapping experiment that cyclo-L-leucyl-L-leucine
was an effective intermediate in the pulcherriminic acid biosynthesis [Eq.
(6)]. L-[1-^{14}C]Leucine was efficiently incorporated into pulcherriminic acid.
These results indicated that cycloleucylleucine, perhaps derived directly from
L-leucine, is a precursor of pulcherriminic acid in *C. pulcherrima* (Mac-
Donald, 1965a).

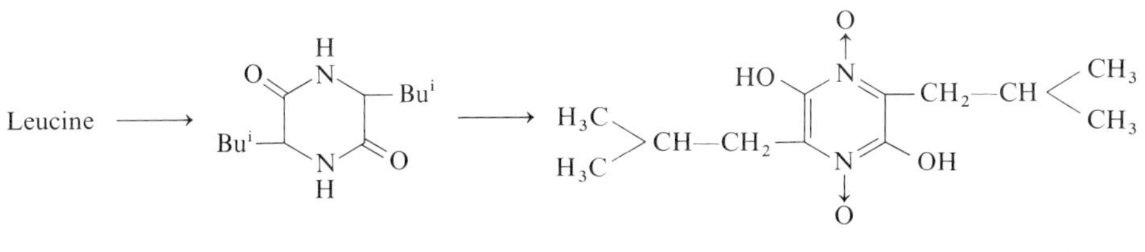

14   (6)

It has been generally demonstrated that pyrazine 1-oxides are biologically
active but that the deoxy derivatives are not. The hydroxamic acid moiety
of these compounds is probably a major structural requirement for the
exhibition of their biological activity, because the compounds containing
the hydroxamic acid moiety show an antibiotic effect on microorganisms
and a convulsive effect on animals. The naturally occurring fungal pyrazine
1-oxides are shown in Table II.

TABLE II

Naturally Occurring Pyrazine 1-Oxides

Valine–Leucine	
Mutaaspergillic acid 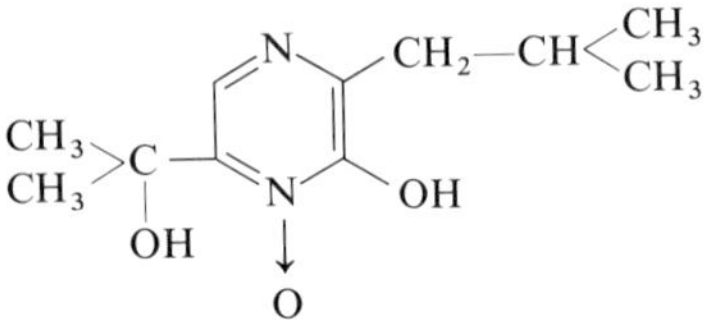	2-Hydroxy-3-isobutyl-6-isopropylpyrazine-1-oxide 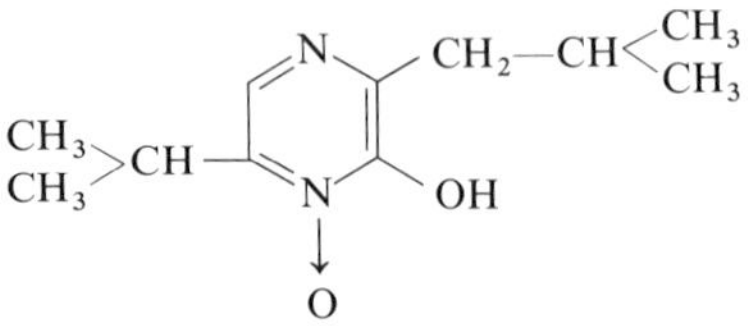

m.p. 173°–174°

$C_{11}H_{18}N_2O_3$

LD_{50} 100 mg/kg

A. oryzae[a]

m.p. 94°–95°

$C_{11}H_{18}N_2O_2$

3/3 125 mg/kg mice
0/3 62.5 mg/kg

A. sojae[b]

Isoleucine–Leucine	
Aspergillic acid 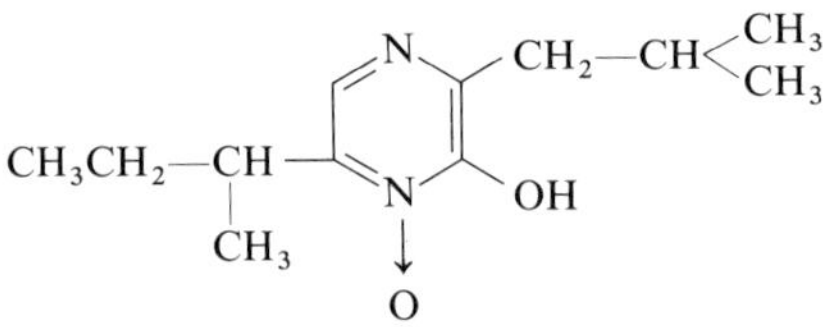	Hydroxyaspergillic acid 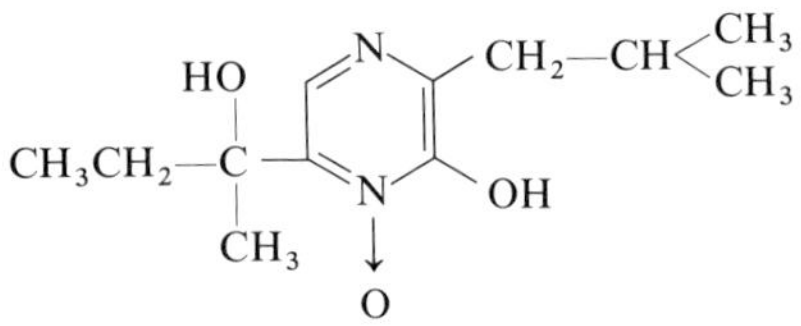

m.p. 97°–99°

$C_{12}H_{20}N_2O_2$

LD_{50} 100 mg/kg mice

A. flavus[c]
A. sojae[d]

m.p. 148–150°

$C_{12}H_{20}N_2O_3$

LD_{50} 100 mg/kg

A. flavus[e]
A. oryzae[f]   *A. sojae*[b]

Leucine–Leucine	
Neoaspergillic acid 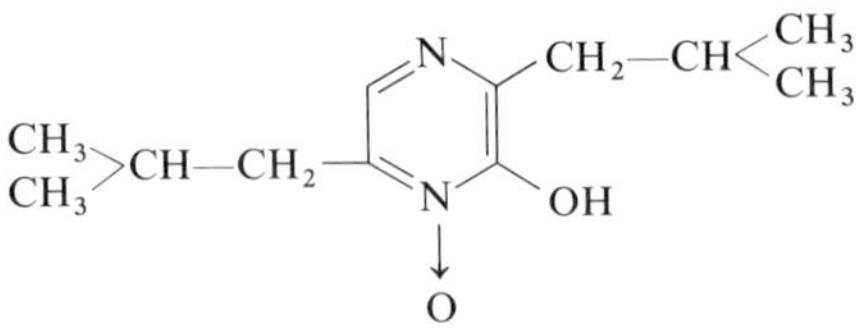	Neohydroxyaspergillic acid 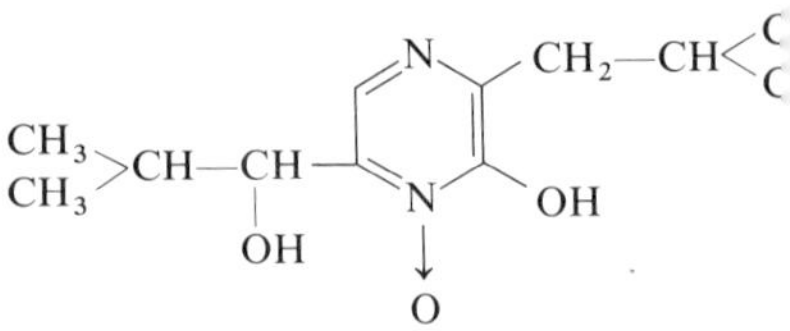

m.p. 125°–126°

$C_{12}H_{20}N_2O_2$

A. flavus[g]
A. ochraceus[h,l]   *A. scleotiorum*[i,j]

m.p. 164°–166°

$C_{12}H_{20}N_2O_3$

A. scleotiorum[k]

202

TABLE II (*continued*)

Naturally Occurring Pyrazine 1-Oxides

Leucine–Leucine	
β-Hydroxyneoaspergillic acid 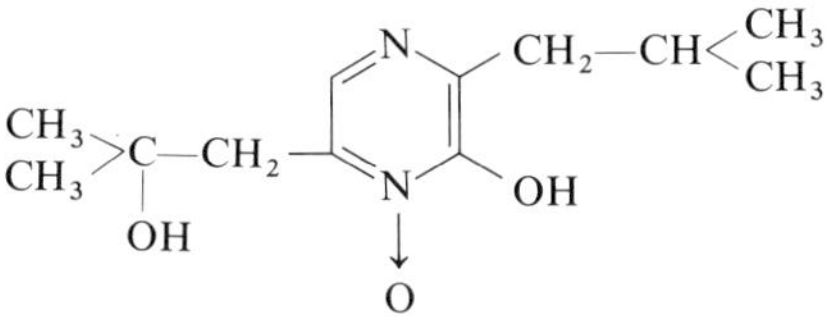	Pulcherriminic acid 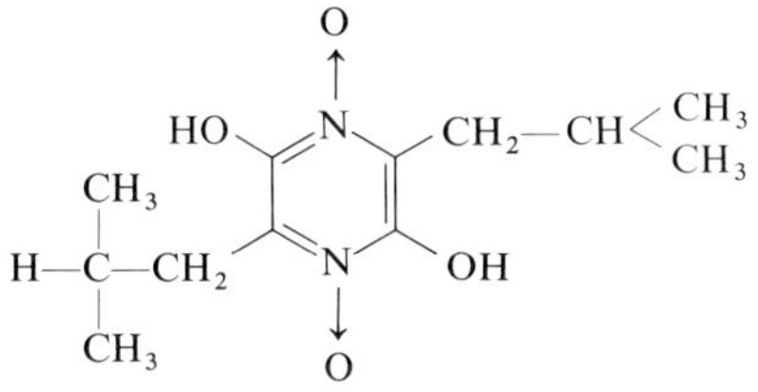

m.p. 143.5°–144°

$C_{12}H_{20}N_2O_3$

A. ochraceus[l]

m.p. 162°–164°

$C_{12}H_{20}N_2O_4$

Candida pulcherrima[m]

Isoleucine–Isoleucine	
2-Hydroxy-3,6-di-*sec*-butylpyrazine-1-oxide 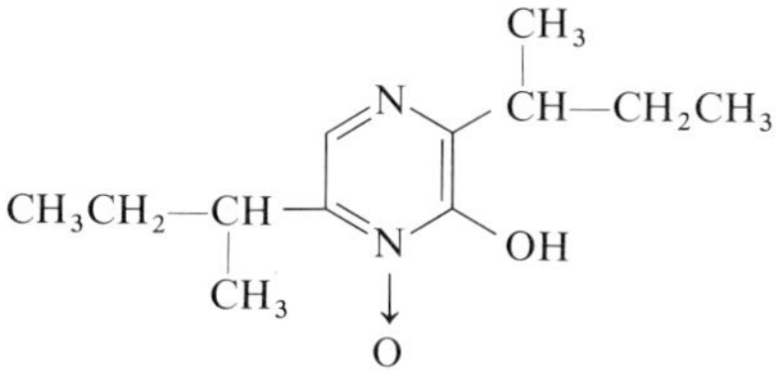	2-Hydroxy-3-*sec*-butyl-6-(1-hydroxy-1-methyl-propyl)-pyrazine-1-oxide 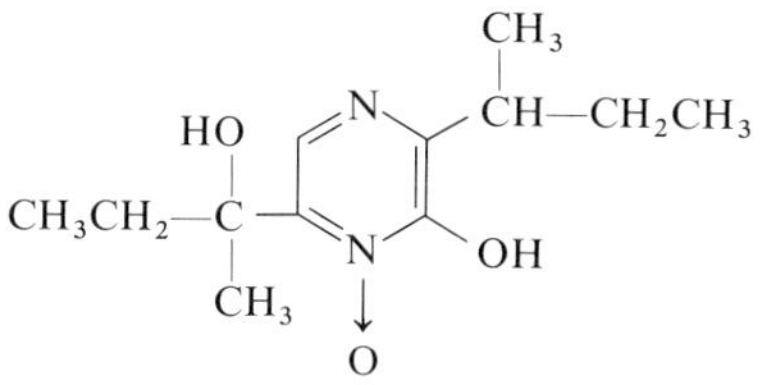

m.p. oil

$C_{12}H_{20}N_2O_2$

3/3 250 mg/kg mice
0/3 125 mg/kg

A.

m.p. 120°–121°

$C_{12}H_{20}N_2O_3$

3/3 125 mg/kg mice
0/3 62.5 mg/kg

A. sojae[b]

[a] From Nakamura (1960).
[b] From Sasaki *et al.* (1963).
[c] From White and Hill (1943).
[d] From Yokotsuka *et al.* (1968).
[e] From Menzel *et al.* (1943) and Dutcher (1958).
[f] From Nakamura and Shiro (1959).
[g] From Dunn *et al.* (1949b).
[h] From Yamazaki *et al.* (1972).
[i] From Micetich and MacDonald (1964).
[j] From MacDonald *et al.* (1964).
[k] From Weiss *et al.* (1958).
[l] From Maebayashi *et al.* (1977).
[m] From MacDonald (1965).

V. FUMITREMORGIN, VERRUCULOGEN, AND ROQUEFORTINE

Yamazaki *et al.* (1971) found, during a survey of toxigenic food-borne fungi in Japan, the presence of certain strains of *Aspergillus fumigatus*, which caused vigorous tremor and convulsions in experimental animals. Two new indole-containing metabolites, designated fumitremorgin A and B, were isolated from extracts of this fungus. Fumitremorgin A (**15**), $C_{32}H_{41}N_3O_7$, and fumitremorgin B (**16**), $C_{27}H_{33}N_3O_5$, caused severe tremor and convulsions. The ED_{50} values for causing tremor in mice by i.p. administration were 0.177 mg/kg for fumitremorgin A and 3.5 mg/kg for fumitremorgin B. The LD_{50} of fumitremorgin A in mice by intravenous administration was 0.185 mg/kg (Yamazaki *et al.*, 1979a).

The uv absorption spectra of fumitremorgin A and B resembled those of certain synthetic model compounds, which indicated the presence of a 6-methoxyindole moiety in these toxins. The 2,3,6-substituted indole system was established by the NMR spectral data of **15** and **16**. The presence of the dioxopiperazine ring in the molecule was indicated by the strong i.r absorption bands at 1685 and 1665 cm^{-1} and the absence of the amide-II bands. Proline and 6-methoxyindole moieties were shown to be present in the dioxopiperazine structure by NMR spectroscopy; proline was actually detected after hydrolysis of fumitremorgin A and B.

The presence of two isoprenyl units in fumitremorgin B was clearly demonstrated by its NMR and mass spectra. A two-proton doublet at 4.52 ppm, assigned to the methylene protons adjacent to the nitrogen atom, was coupled with an olefinic hydrogen at 5.04 ppm. This result indicated that one of the two isoprenyl groups of fumitremorgin B is located on position 1 of the indole ring. The location of the other isoprenyl group was established by the signal at 5.97 ppm, which was assigned to a methine proton adjacent to the nitrogen atom. The results of the NMR spectral analysis of the di- and tetrahydro derivatives of fumitremorgin B were completely consistent with those obtained on the parent compound (Yamazaki, 1973; Yamazaki *et al.*, 1974).

Spectroscopic analysis of fumitremorgin A and its derivatives by Yamazaki *et al.* (1975b, 1980) elucidated its structure. The structure of fumitremorgin A was also determined by X-ray diffraction analysis, (Eickman *et al.*, 1975); this result verified the structure obtained from chemical and spectroscopic evidence.

In 1972, a new tremorgenic mycotoxin was obtained in the United States from a strain of *Penicillium verruculosum* isolated from peanuts. The toxin was named verruculogen, and a close resemblance to fumitremorgin was evident. Oral administration of this toxin to mice caused tremor and convulsions; and the toxin's LD_{50} was 126.7 mg/kg in mice. Intraperitoneal injection was 40 times more effective than oral administration in producing tremors in mice, and LD_{50} (i.p.) was 2.4 mg/kg (Cole *et al.*, 1972).

Verruculogen (**17**), $C_{27}H_{33}N_3O_7$, afforded a reduction product, TR-2 (**21**) $C_{22}H_{27}N_3O_7$, and a volatile isovaleraldehyde on catalytic hydrogenation with palladium on carbon in ethanol. The uv and NMR spectra (in the region of δ 6–9 ppm) of verruculogen and the reduction product were almost identical, indicating that the indole nucleus of verruculogen was not altered by reduction (Cole and Kirksey, 1973). The relative stereochemistry of verruculogen was subsequently deduced by Foyes *et al.* (1974) from a single-crystal X-ray diffraction study. The close structural and spectral properties, combined with the similar biological activity of verruculogen and fumitremorgin B, argued strongly for the similar stereochemistry of these metabolites. Immediately after determination of the stereochemistry of verruculogen, the crystal structure, including the absolute configuration of fumitremorgin B, was determined by X-ray diffraction analysis. The levorotatory optical activity of proline, which was obtained by hydrolysis of fumitremorgin B, established its absolute configuration (Yamazaki *et al.*, 1975a).

Recently, a new verruculogen-related compound was isolated from the culture broth of *P. verruculosum*. This compound, acetoxyverruculogen (**18**), $C_{29}H_{35}N_3O_9$, gave spectral data similar to those of verruculogen, except for the observation which indicated the presence of an acetoxy group in this compound [v_{max}^{Nujol} 1735, 1235 cm^{-1}; m/e 527 ($M^+ - COCH_2$); $\delta_H^{CDCl_3}$ 2.10 ppm. (3H, singlet); $\delta_C^{CDCl_3}$ 20.9, 170.0 ppm]. Hydrolysis of **16** afforded hydroxyproline, suggesting the position of the acetoxyl group in the proline moiety of this compound. Structure **18**, including the stereochemistry, was finally determined by X-ray diffraction analysis (Tanabe, 1976).

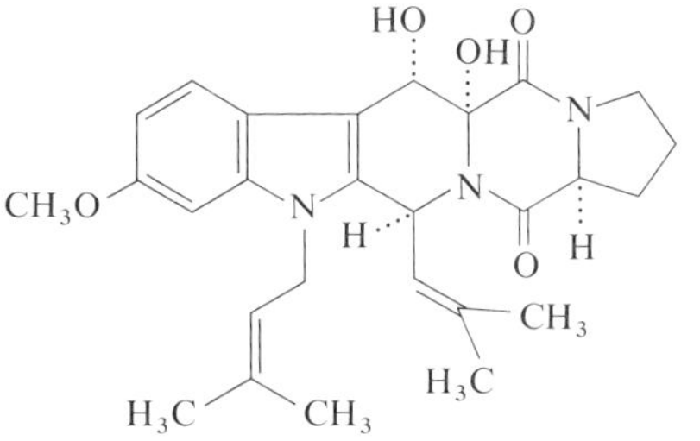

16

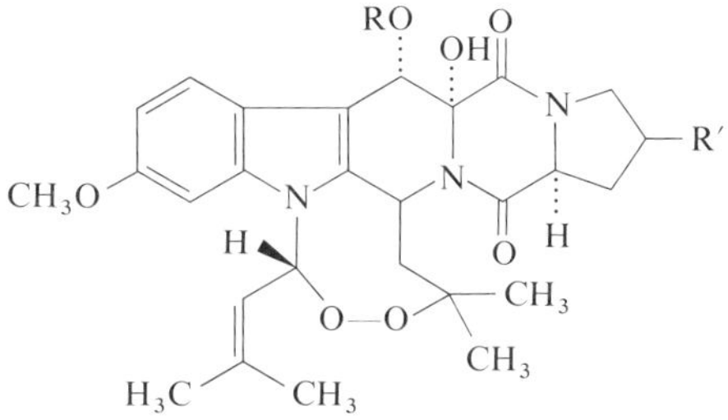

15 R = CH₂—CH=C(CH₃)₂ R′ = H

17 R = H, R′ = H
18 R = H, R′ = OCOCH₃

Fumitremorgin C (**19**), the simplest member of this group of toxins, was isolated from the culture extract of *A. fumigatus*, obtained from silage. The structure of fumitremorgin C was determined by X-ray analysis (Cole, 1976). TR-2 (**21**) was originally isolated as a hydrogenation product of verruculogen and was later found in the culture extract of *P. verruculosum* and *A. fumigtus* (Cole *et al.*, 1977a). Epoxyfumitremorgin C (**20**) together with fumitremorgin C were also isolated from the same fungus by Cole (1976).

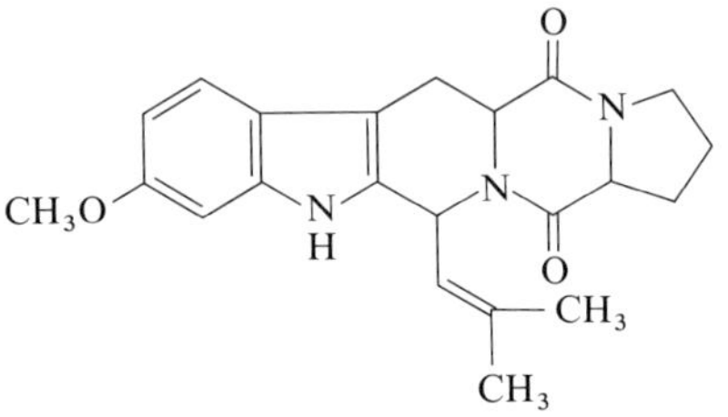

19

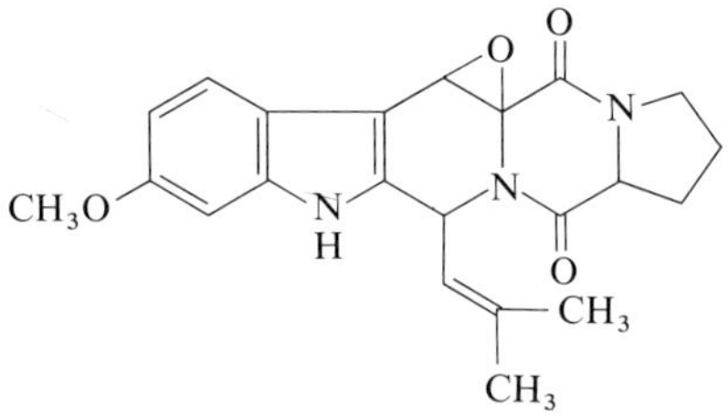

20

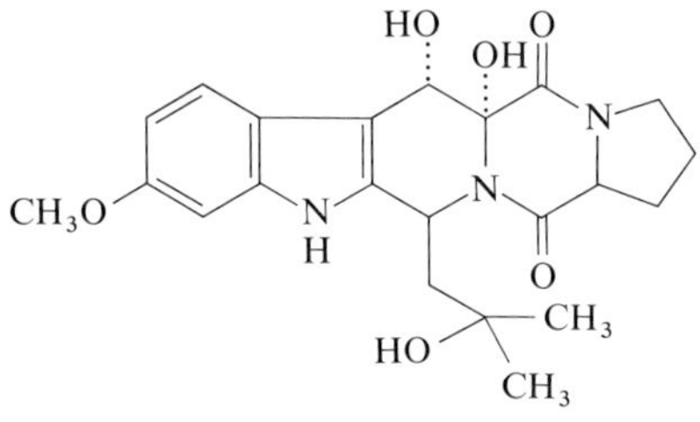

21

In 1976, two new nitrogen-containing metabolites were isolated from the mycelium of *Penicillium roqueforti*. The major metabolite was designated roquefortine and assigned structure **22** based on chemical and spectroscopic evidence. The minor metabolite was shown to be a stereoisomer of a known alkaloid, fumigaclavin A. Roquefortine possessed neurotoxic properties and caused convulsions in experimental animals. The LD_{50} to male mice was 15–10 mg/kg on i.p. injection (Scott *et al.*, 1976).

The fungus *P. roqueforti* is of interest to agricultural and food scientists owing to its use in the production of roquefort cheese and other blue cheeses. Roquefortine is a natural contaminant, as it was detected in all 16 samples of blue cheese that were produced in seven countries (Scott and Kennedy, 1976). Scott *et al.* (1977) reported that an optimum yield of roquefortine was obtained on cultivation of the fungus in a medium containing sucrose (15%) and yeast extract (2%) for 16 days at 25°C.

Roquefortine (**22**), $C_{22}H_{23}N_5O_2$, afforded a dihydroroquefortine on catalytic reduction in acetic acid. The presence of the indole ring system in roquefortine was suggested from their ^1H and ^{13}C NMR spectral data and by comparison with data for the corresponding carbon atoms of hodgkinsine and 16-epivindoline (Scott *et al.*, 1976a).

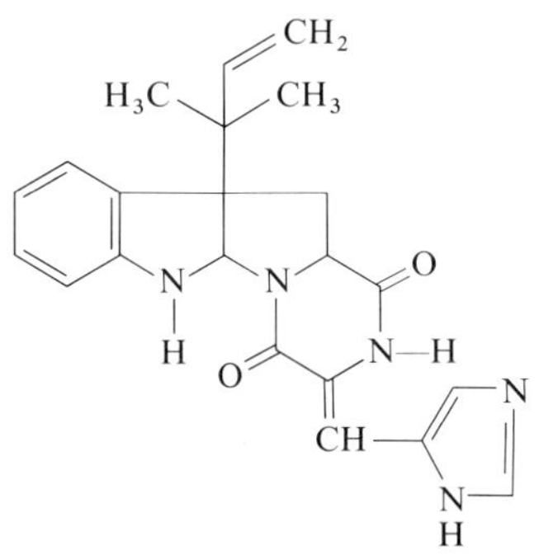

22 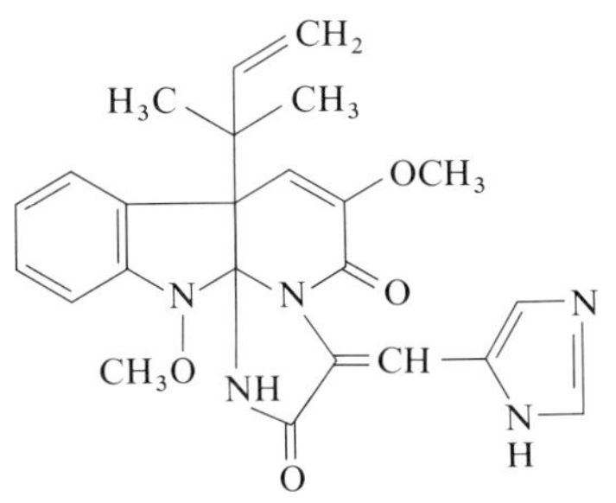   23

The isoprenyl group in roquefortine was shown to be an inverted 1,1-dimethylallyl group by comparison of the relevant portions of the ^1H and ^{13}C NMR spectra of roquefortine and dihydroroquefortine. Reduction of roquefortine with zinc in acetic acid afforded two amorphous dihydro derivatives. On hydrolysis with hydrochloric acid, histidine was obtained from both these reduced derivatives but not from roquefortine itself. Roquefortine should accordingly contain the didehydrohistidine unit. It is of interest to note that oxaline (**23**), $C_{24}H_{25}N_5O_4$, a metabolite biogenetically related to roquefortine, has been isolated from the toxigenic strains of *Penicillium oxalicum* (Nagel *et al.*, 1976).

As described above, fumitremorgin and verruculogen consist of a dioxopiperazine ring perhaps derived from tryptophan and proline with isoprene units, whereas roquefortine arises by the coupling of tryptophan and dehydrohistidine. The presence of a tryptophan-containing dioxopiperazine ring system is the distinctive structural feature of these tremorgenic mycotoxins, which elicit severe tremor and convulsions in animals. It is of interest to note that roquefortine contains the same ring system as that found in the dethio derivatives of sporidesmins, known mycotoxins which cause facial eczema in cattle and sheep in New Zealand (Leigh and Taylor, 1976 and references cited therein).

When *A. fumigatus* was grown in a synthetic basal medium in stationary culture, the production of fumitremorgins was extremely poor. However, the addition of L-tryptophan to the culture medium caused an abundant production of the toxin, as shown in Table III (Yamazaki *et al.*, 1971).

TABLE III

Influence of L-Tryptophan on the Production of Fumitremorgin

Medium	Final pH	Dry mycelia (g/liter)	Crude toxin (mg/liter)
Basic	4.8	8.3	Trace
Basic + L-Trp (125 mg)	4.8	9.1	19.2
Basic + L-Trp (250 mg)	4.2	8.6	49.3

This result strongly suggested that tryptophan is an efficient precursor of fumitremorgin, and forms the dioxopiperazine ring with proline. In fact, $[3-^{14}C]$tryptophan and L-$[U-^{14}C]$proline added to the culture were significantly incorporated into fumitremorgin A and B, as was also the case with $[2-^{14}C]$mevalonic acid (Table IV) (Yamazaki *et al.*, 1975c).

TABLE IV

Incorporation of Labeled Precursors into Fumitremorgins A and B

Precursor	Total radioactivity Fumitremorgin A	Fumitremorgin B
DL-$[3-^{14}C]$Tryptophan (0.09 mCi)	3.28×10^5	2.30×10^4
L-$[U-^{14}C]$Proline (0.1 mCi)	5.22×10^5	2.73×10^4
$[2-^{14}C]$Mevalonic acid (0.025 mCi)	2.76×10^5	2.48×10^4

Analogous to fumitremorgin biosynthesis, tryptophan and proline with two isoprene units certainly participate in the biosynthesis of verruculogen. In addition, tryptophan and histidine with one isoprene unit probably participate in the biosynthesis of roquefortine, although the experimental result has not yet been obtained.

Sodium $[1,2-^{13}C]$acetate added to the culture medium of *P. verruculosum* was incorporated into verruculogen. Intact acetate units were located at

C(5)–C(6), C(8)–C(9), C(21)–C(22), C(23)–C(24), C(28)–C(29), and C(3)–
C(31). The above data from ^{13}C NMR spectroscopy, indicated that two
acetate units were incorporated into the proline moiety through the pathway of *de novo* synthesis of proline: acetate → TCA cycle → glutamic acid →
proline, and that the other four units were incorporated into two isoprenyl
groups in the verruculogen molecule. In addition to the six directly bonded
(^{13}C, ^{13}C) couplings observed in the ^{13}C NMR spectrum of verruculogen,
a new (^{13}C, ^{13}C) coupling in the acetyl group was observed in the spectrum
of acetoxyverruculogen (**18**) (Uramoto *et al.*, 1977).

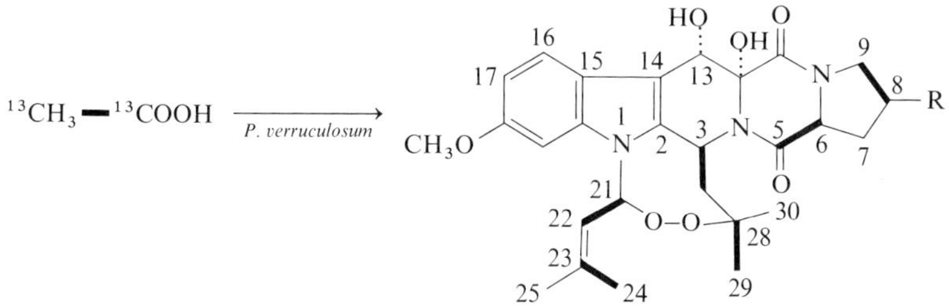

$$^{13}CH_3 \text{—} ^{13}COOH \xrightarrow{P.\ verruculosum} \tag{7}$$

17 R = H
18 R = OCOCH$_3$

It is important to note that the orientation of the isoprene unit on position
2 of the indole ring of fumitremorgins A and B is "normal," whereas in
roquefortine, the isoprene unit is present in a novel arrangement on position
3 of the indole nucleus. In echinulin and related naturally occurring tryptophan-containing dioxopiperazine metabolites, the linkage of the isoprene unit on position 2 of the indole ring is generally "inverted." It should
be noticed that the linkage of the isoprene unit is normal only in the fumitre-
morgin-related metabolites; the reason remains obscure (Sammes, 1975).
   In a model reaction, an acid-catalyzed rearrangement of the isoprene
chain was observed from position 1 to 2 of the indole nucleus together with
a partial rearrangement of the allyl chain. Treatment of 3-methyl-*N*-(1,1-
dimethylallyl)indole with trifluoroacetic acid gave two 2-alkylated indole
compounds, an "inverted" and a "normal" type. The finding indicated the
possible participation of an initial isoprenylation at the nitrogen atom of the
indole ring followed by a rearrangement to position 2 with an inversion of
the migrating isoprene group in the biosynthesis of echinulin-type metabolites. However, the rearrangement from 1-isoprenylindole to a 2-γ,γ-
dimethylallyl-type compound in the reaction indicated a possible mechanism
for the biosynthesis of fumitremorgin-type metabolites (Casnati, 1970;
Casnati *et al.*, 1974).

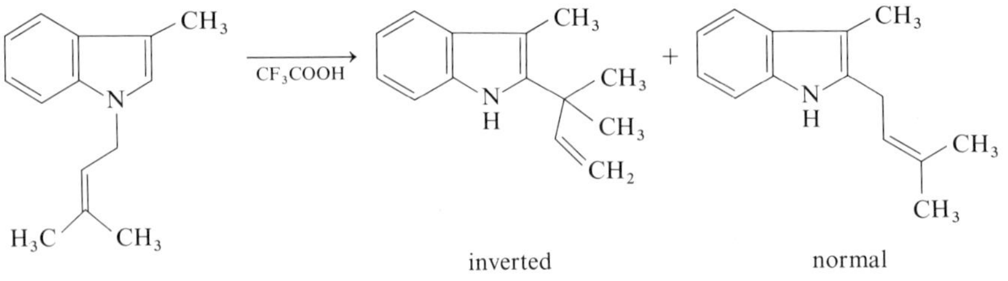

(8)

VI. PAXILLINE, PASPALINE, AND RELATED METABOLITES

A neurological disorder has been known to occur in cattle and horses on consumption of Dallis grass (*Paspalum dilatatum*) infected with an ergot-related fungus, *Claviceps paspali*. Dallis grass poisoning is also called "paspalum staggers." Clinical signs of this poisoning are tremors which are exaggerated by enforced movement, hyperexcitability, and ataxia. Three tremorgenic metabolites were isolated by Cole *et al.* (1977b) from sclerotia of *C. paspali* obtained from *Paspalum dilatatum*. One of the metabolites was identical with paspalinine (**24**), which had been previously isolated from *C. paspali*. The remaining two metabolites contain either an additional isoprene or hydroxyisoprene unit attached to position 5 on the indole nucleus, ie., 3-methyl-2-butenylpaspalinine (**25**) and 3-hydroxy-3-methyl-1-butenylpas-palinine (**26**), respectively.

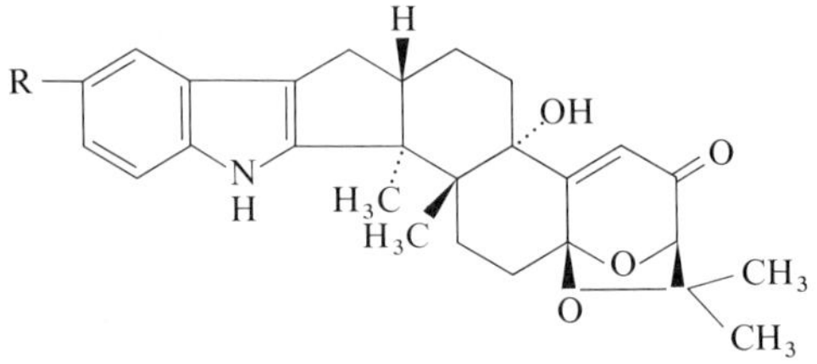

From the dried mycelium of *C. paspali*, paspaline (**27**) and paspalicine (**28**) were previously isolated, both of which contain a 2,3-disubstituted indole nucleus (Fehr and Acklin, 1966).

A new tremorgenic metabolite, paxilline (**29**), was isolated from *Penicillium paxilli* obtained from insect-damaged pecans in the State of Georgia (Cole *et al.*, 1974). Paxilline caused tremor to cockerels about 0.5 to 2 hr after dosing. Some cockerels died at 100 mg/kg; all died at 250 mg/kg and 500 mg/kg. Clinical signs in mice appeared about 30 min after i.p. administration. The outstanding signs included tremor and hypersensitivity to sound stimuli.

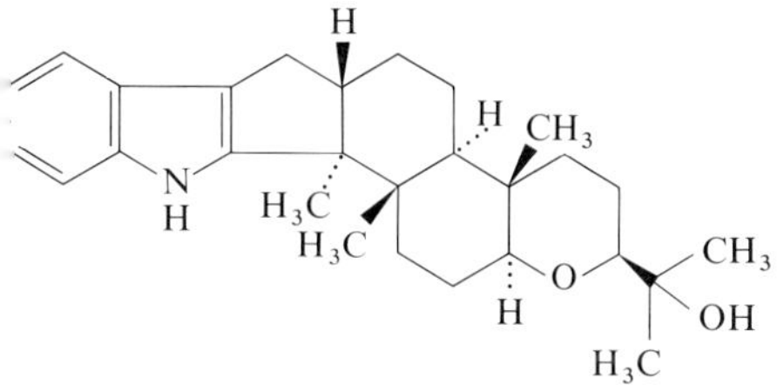

27

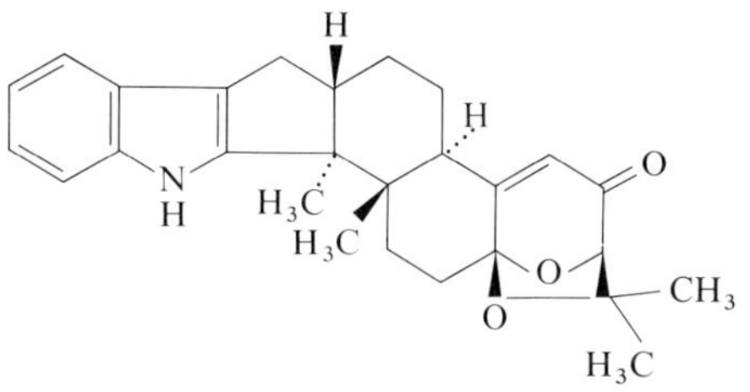

28

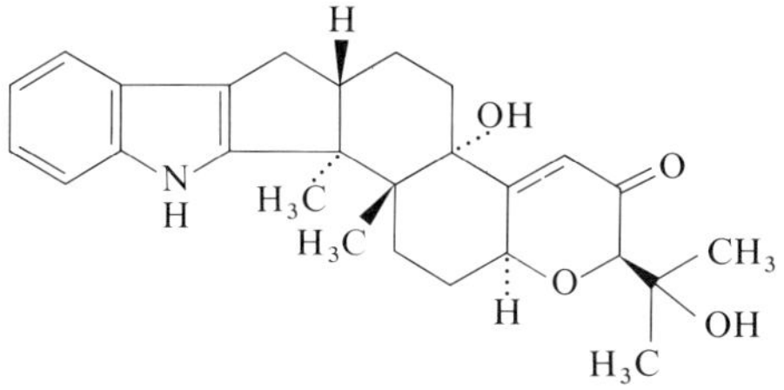

29

Paxilline (**29**), $C_{27}H_{33}NO_4$, showed a uv spectrum characteristic of 2,3-substituted indole compounds with no double bonds in conjugation with the indole ring. The structure of paxilline was finally determined by X-ray diffraction analysis as **29** (Springer *et al.*, 1975).

Tanabe (1976) and Acklin *et al.* (1976) studied the biosynthesis of paxilline by employing ^{13}C-labeled precursors and ^{13}C NMR spectroscopy. Tanabe proposed a biosynthetic scheme (scheme 3) for paxilline based on the results obtained from labeling experiments with $[1,2-^{13}C]$acetate and analysis of the product.

Acklin *et al.* (1976) also carried out the biosynthetic study using $[1-^{13}C]$-, $[2-^{13}C]$-, and $[1,2-^{13}C]$acetates as precursors. The distribution pattern of the ^{13}C atoms from acetate (singly and doubly labeled) for paspaline (**27**), paspalicine (**28**), and paspalinine (**24**) is shown in Eq. (9).

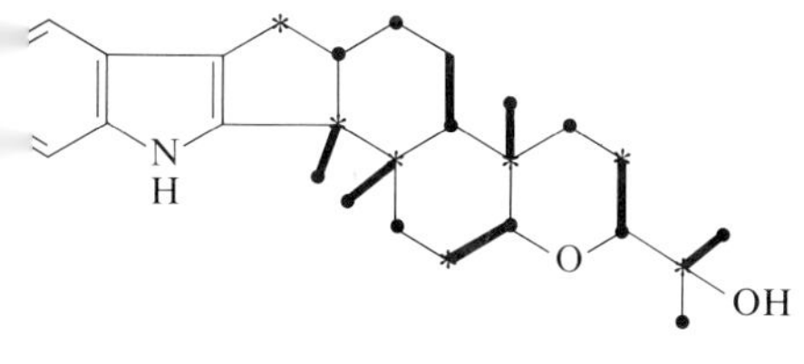

27

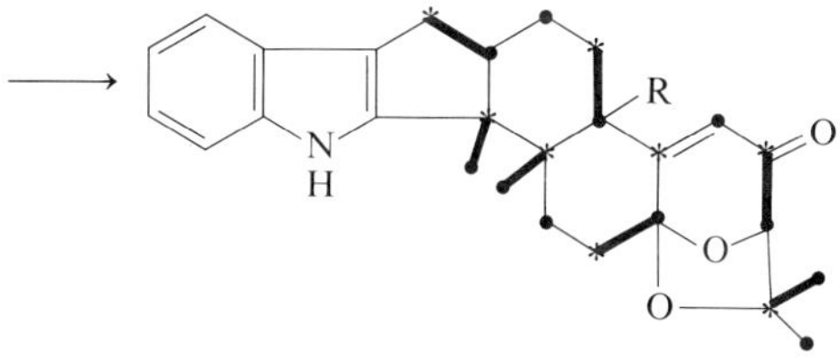

28 R = H
24 R = OH

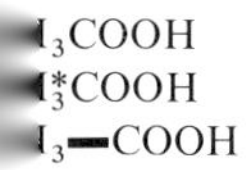

$_3$COOH
$^*_3$COOH
$_3$—COOH

(9)

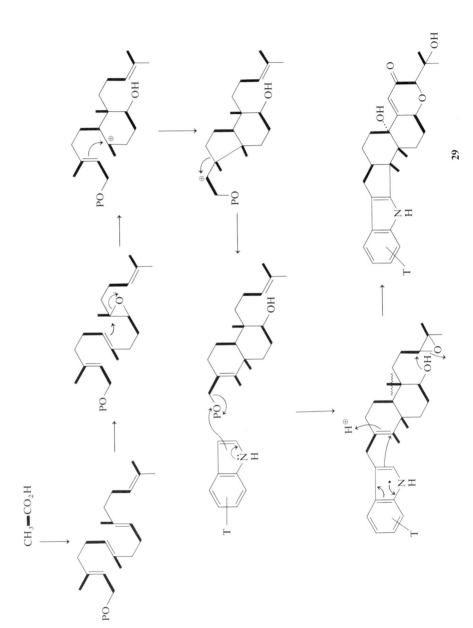

VII. TRYPTOQUIVALINES

Two tremor-producing metabolites, tryptoquivaline and tryptoquivalone, were isolated by Clardy *et al.* (1975) from a toxinogenic strain of *Aspergillus clavatus* obtained from rice. Büchi *et al.* (1973) obtained small amounts of the highly toxic cytochalasin E and two nontoxic metabolites, kotanin and demethylkotanin from the same fungus.

Tryptoquivaline (**30**), $C_{29}H_{30}N_4O_7$, afforded a deacetyl methanolysis product (**31**) [Eq. (10)]. Compound **31** was characterized as the *p*-bromobenzoate and *p*-bromophenylurethane. Crystals suitable for X-ray crystallography were obtained from the *p*-bromophenylurethane derivative. The structure of tryptoquivaline as determined by X-ray analysis was shown to be **30**.

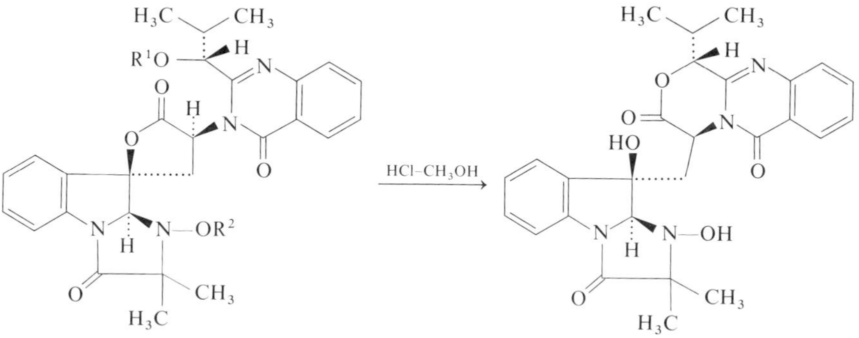

30 $R^1 = OCCH_3$, $R^2 = H$
33 $R^1 = H$, $R^2 = OCCH_3$

31

(10)

Tryptoquivalone (**32**), $C_{26}H_{24}N_4O_6$, gave a positive triphenyltetrazolium chloride test and was converted into a 2,4-dinitrophenylhydrazone, indicating that it contained hydroxylamine and carbonyl groups. The structure of tryptoquivalone was suggested as **32** from the above information and its spectral data (Clardy *et al.*, 1975).

Yamazaki *et al.* (1976) isolated six metabolites closely related to tryptoquivaline from *A. fumigatus*, which is also a producer of fumitremorgin A and B. The substances were tentatively named FTC–FTH. FTC, $C_{29}H_{30}N_4O_7$, was shown by Yamazaki to be **33** but recently shown to be identical to tryptoquivaline (**30**). FTD (**40**), $C_{28}H_{28}N_4O_7$, exhibited uv and ir spectra virtually identical to those of FTC. Signals very similar to those of FTC were observed in its NMR spectrum, except for the absence of the two methyl singlets, which appeared in the spectrum of FTC. Instead, a three-proton doublet appeared at 1.56 ppm in the spectrum of FTD. The structure of FTD, at first suggested to be **46**, was recently revised to **40** (Yamazaki *et al.*, 1979b). Yamazaki *et al.* (1977) reported the *S* configuration for position 15 in FTD, for hydrolysis of FTD after reduction with zinc in acetic acid gave L-(+)-alanine.

The structures **34**–**37** were assigned for FTE–FTH from analysis of their spectral data. A single aromatic proton was characteristically observed in their NMR spectra instead of signals of the hydroxyisobutyl group which appeared in the spectrum of FTC and FTD. Furthermore, they isolated and characterized two new tryptoquivaline-related metabolites, FTI (**38**) and FTJ (**39**), from *A. fumigatus* (Yamazaki *et al.*, 1978). Büchi *et al.* (1977) also isolated four new tryptoquivaline-related metabolites from *A. clavatus*, which were called nortryptoquivaline (**40**), deoxytryptoquivaline (**41**), deoxynortryptoquivaline (**42**), and deoxynortryptoquivalone (**43**). More recently, Yamazaki *et al.* (1979a) isolated tryptoquivalines L (**44**), M (**45**), and N,

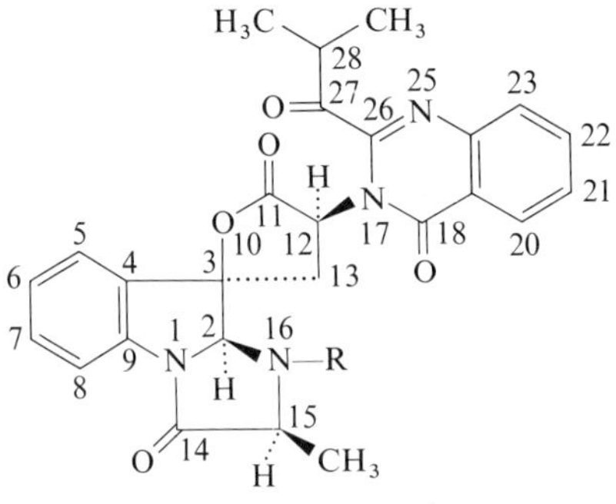

32 R = OH
43 R = H

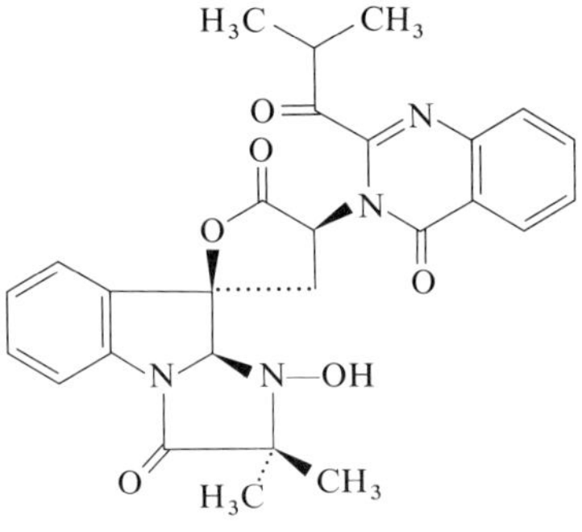

38

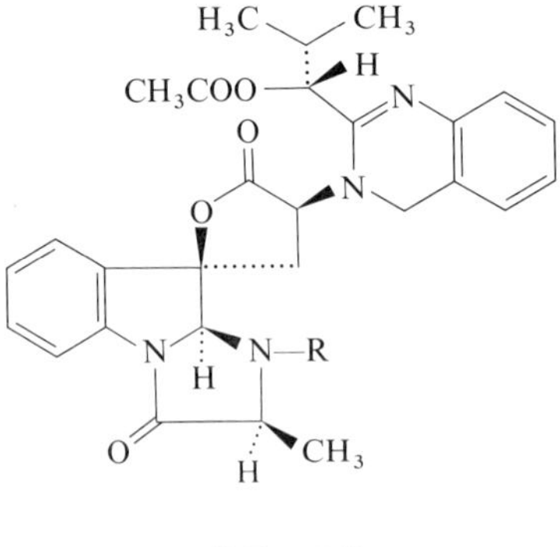

40 R = OH
42 R = H

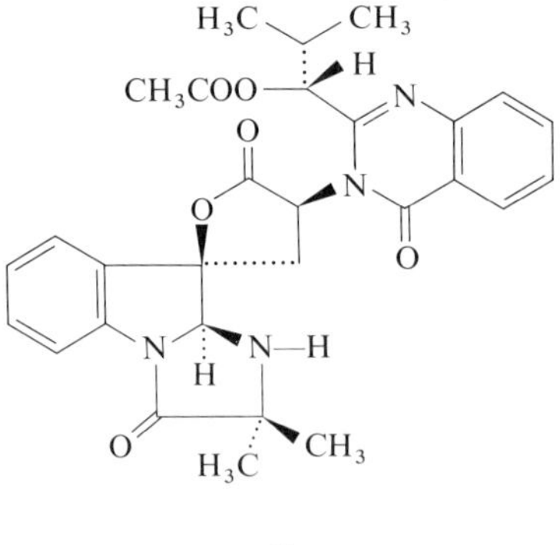

41

from *A. fumigatus*. Tryptoquivaline N was shown to be identical to deoxy-nortryptoquivalone (**43**).

Thus, six and eleven tryptoquivaline-related metabolites were isolated from *A. clavatus* and *A. fumigatus*, respectively, and their structures have been established. Yamazaki *et al.* (1977) proposed to rename their metabolites from *A. fumigatus*, i.e., FTE–FTM, to tryptoquivalines E–M.

Büchi *et al.* (1973) reported that tryptoquivaline and tryptoquivalone were tremor-producing toxins, and that the four newly isolated metabolites were also toxic (Büchi *et al.*, 1977). However, details of their toxicity have not been described. Yamazaki *et al.*, (1976) examined the tremorgenicity of the tryptoquivalines isolated in their laboratory and recognized no detectable tremorgenic activity from these metabolites. No antimicrobial activity was exhibited by tryptoquivaline and tryptoquivalone against 29 strains of yeast, two molds, and 46 bacteria (Demain *et al.*, 1976).

It is of interest that the optical rotations of tryptoquivalines F, H, and L were opposite (negative) to those of J, E, and G (positive), respectively, although their chemical structures were identical except the stereochemistry with each other. Yamazaki *et al.* (1978) found that tryptoquivalines F, H, and L were obtained by treatment with 0.1% KOH in methanol from J, E, and G, respectively [Eqs. (11)–(13)]. This fact indicated that tryptoquivalines F, H, and L could be derived from J, E, and G, respectively, in the fungus, although the possibility remains that the metabolites having negative rotations are artifacts. When the reaction was carried out in deuteriated solvents, reaction products deuteriated at position 12 were obtained, indicating that epimerization at position 12 occurred with alkali, converting tryptoquivalines J, E, and G into F, H, and L, respectively (Yamazaki *et al.*, 1979b).

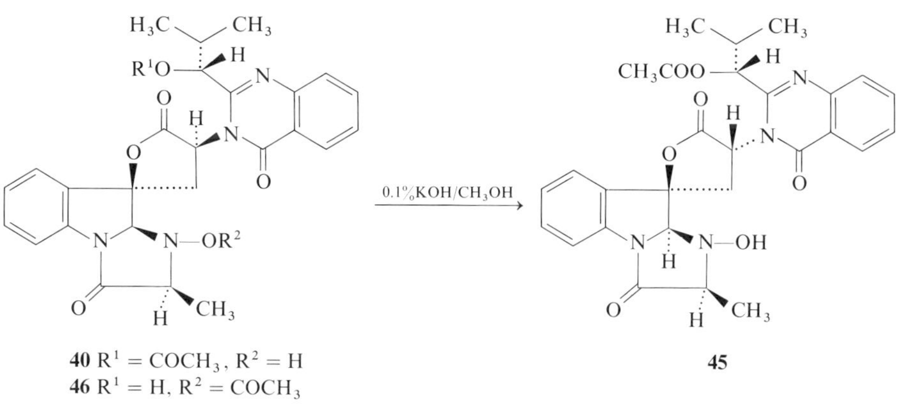

40 $R^1 = COCH_3$, $R^2 = H$
46 $R^1 = H$, $R^2 = COCH_3$

45

(11)

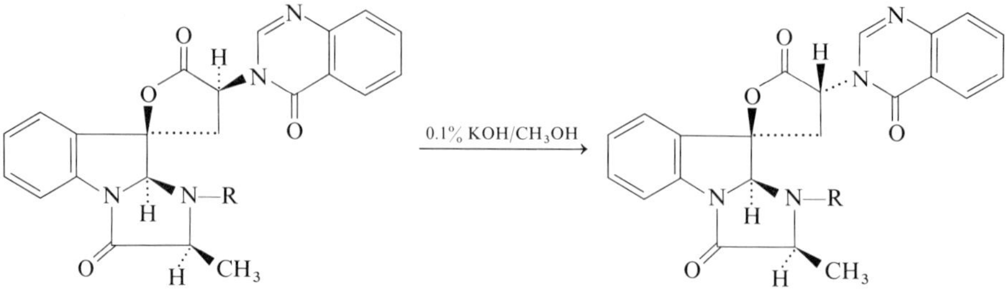

34 R = OH
39 R = H

37 R = OH
35 R = H

(12)

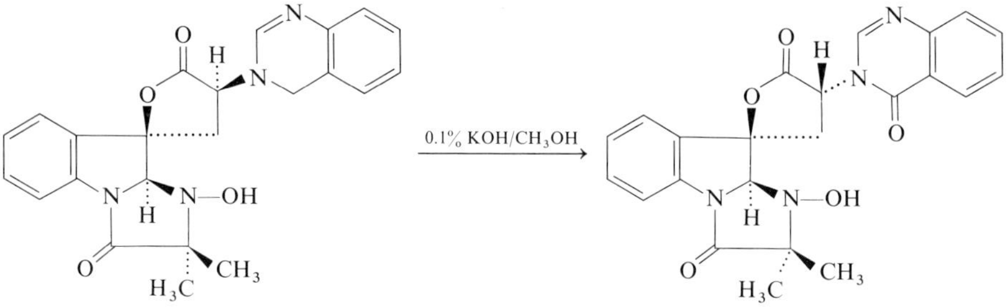

36

44

(13)

These novel metabolites may be derived from four amino acids: tryptophan, anthranilic acid, valine, and alanine (or methylalanine). Deoxynortryptoquivalone (**43**) may be the first metabolite formed in the pathway of the tryptoquivaline biosynthesis. By oxidation of the secondary amine to the hydroxylamine, nortryptoquivalone (= tryptoquivalone) (**32**) would be formed from **43**. If the isobutyl side chain is lost by further oxidation, tryptoquivaline J (**39**) and E (**34**) would be derived from these tryptoquivalones, respectively. On the other hand, if reduction occurred on the carbonyl in the side chain, deoxynortryptoquivaline (**42**) and nortryptoquivaline (FTD) (**40**) would be derived, respectively, from these tryptoquivalones. The geminal dimethyl group at position 15 appeared to be formed by the participation of methylalanine in the biosynthesis, and the actual incorporation of ^{14}C-labeled methylalanine into tryptoquivaline (FTC) and tryptoquivaline I has been demonstrated (M. Yamazaki, unpublished work).

A hypothetical scheme for the biosynthesis of these tryptoquivaline-related metabolites is proposed in Scheme 4.

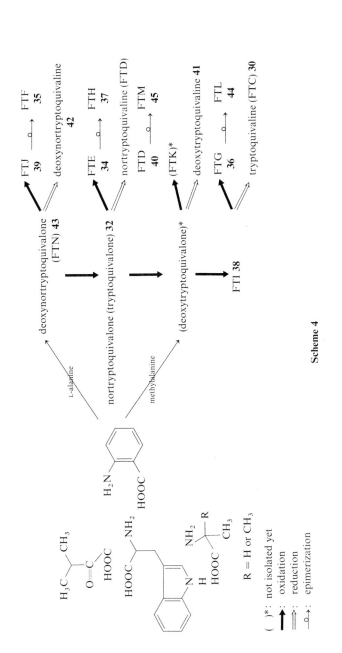

Scheme 4

VIII. SLAFRAMINE

A toxicity problem associated with second-cutting red clover hay was reported in 1959 in Missouri. Cattle and sheep which were fed such hay slobbered excessively, went off feed, developed diarrhea and stiff joints, and sometimes died. A similar disorder in ruminants was investigated in Illinois in 1961; however, the causal agent was not identified. Similar cases were reported in Wisconsin in 1962 and 1963; this finally led to the isolation of a toxinogenic strain of *Rhizoctonia leguminicola*, the cause of the black patch disease of red clover. It was concluded that the salivation factor was contained in the mycelium of the *R. leguminicola* and that it was not a product of red clover per se (Rainey *et al.*, 1965; Aust and Broquist, 1965).

After incubation of the fungus for 30 days in stationary culture, the mycelial mats were collected and extracted with water or ethanol. Slaframine was isolated from the extract as a picrate. The physiological action of slaframine was very much like those of physostigmine or pilocarpine and was reversed by atropine. The parasympathomimetic action of this compound suggested that it might be an anticholine esterase or acetylcholinelike substance (Aust, 1969). Although slaframine was very potent in stimulating salivation *in vivo*, it showed very little or no cholinergic action *in vitro*. Slaframine was subsequently found to be activated by the liver microsomes in the presence of NADPH to a form capable of stimulation *in vitro* of the guinea ileum. The active metabolite seemed to have a high affinity for the receptor and to exert its activity by binding to and stimulating cholinergic fibers. Addition of atropine blocked the salivation activity if administered to the organ bath prior to the active metabolite but did not reverse the activity, indicating that the cholinergic system was involved in the occurrence of excess salivation (Spike and Aust, 1971).

Slaframine (**47**), $C_{10}H_{18}N_2O_2$, contained a secondary acetoxy group. Treatment of **47** with boiling 1 N NaOH for 2 min gave crystalline deacetylslaframine, $C_8H_{16}N_2O$, which was devoid of the physiological activity. The presence of a primary amino group was indicated by a purple ninhydrin test and by Van Slyke analysis on slaframine hydrochloride. Slaframine gave an N-acetyl derivative, $C_{12}H_{20}N_2O_3$, by acetylation with acetic anhydride. Treatment of the acetyl derivative with cyanogen bromide gave the ring-opened product (**48**), $C_{13}H_{20}BrN_3O_3$. Compound **48** gave a reduced compound (**49**) on sequential treatment with NaI and LiAlH$_4$ [Eq. (14)]. The presence of a tertiary amine was indicated by the positive test with Dragendorff's reagent. NMR spindecoupling experiments performed on N-acetylslaframine hydrochloride established the structure of slaframine as 1-acetoxy-6-aminooctahydroindolizine (**47**) (Gardiner *et al.*, 1968).

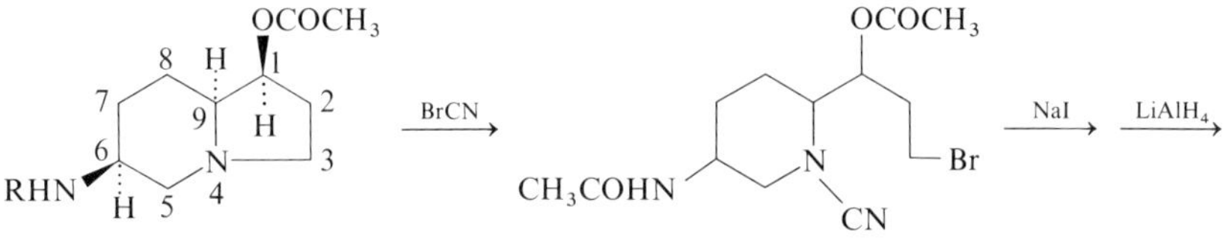

47   48

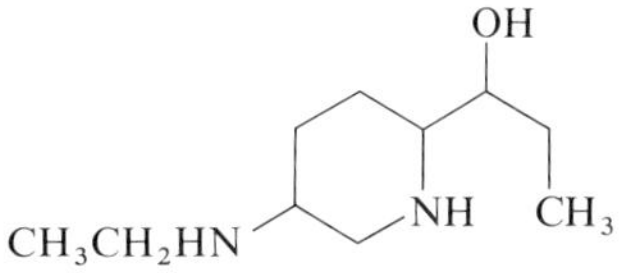

(14)

49

The proton at position 6 (multiplet) was coupled to H(5) (axial). The equatorial orientation of H(6) was indicated by its half-bandwidth of 7 Hz. The amino group was thus located at the position 6 in an axial orientation. The relative configuration of the hydrogens at C(1) and C(9) was assigned *cis* by comparison of the NMR spectrum of *N*-acetylslaframine to those of the synthetic isomeric 1-acetoxyoctahydroindolizines with known relative stereochemistries. Treatment of *N*-acetyl-O-deacetylslaframine with α-phenylbutyric anhydride gave residual α-phenylbutyric acid with a negative rotation (Gardiner *et al.*, 1968). Aust *et al.* (1966) thus concluded that slaframine contains the (1*S*, 9*S*) configuration.

$[1\text{-}^{14}C]$Lysine, $[6\text{-}^{14}C]$lysine, $[1\text{-}^{14}C]$aminoadipate, and $[carboxyl\text{-}^{14}C]$ pipecolate were incorporated into slaframine during growth of *R. leguminicola* on a hay infusion medium. Addition of unlabeled pipecolate markedly reduced incorporation of the other precursors into slaframine, indicating that pipecolate was most effectively involved in the slaframine biosynthesis. A cell-free extract of the fungus was found to contain saccharopine dehydrogenase. This finding indicated that saccharopine (**50**) [Eq. (15)] could be involved in the early stage of the metabolism of lysine (Snyder and Broquist, 1968).

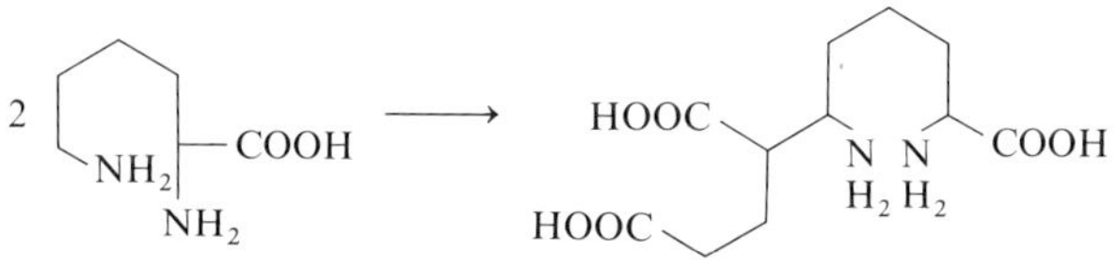

(15)

50

From the mycelium of *R. leguminicola* cultured on $[^{3}H]$pipecolate, two previously unrecognized tritiated basic substances, named compounds I and

II, were isolated. When the fungus was grown on a medium containing ^{3}H-labeled compounds I and II, compound II was incorporated into slaframine 10 times more efficiently than compound I. Thus, the pathway of the slaframine biosynthesis was postulated as follows by Guengerich (1971).

Lysine → saccharopine → aminoadipic semialdehyde → Δ^1-piperideine →

pipecolate → compound I → compound II → slaframine

REFERENCES

Acklin, W., Weibel, F., and Arigoni, D. (1976). In "Mycotoxins in Human and Animal Health" (J. V. Rodricks, ed.), pp. 583–595. Pathotox Pub., Illinois.
Aust, S. D. (1969). Biochem. Pharmacol. 18, 929–932.
Aust, S. D., and Broquist, H. P. (1965). Nature (London) 205, 204–205.
Aust, S. D., Broquist, H. P., and Rinehart, Jr., K. L. (1966). J. Am. Chem. Soc. 88, 2879–2880.
Büchi, G., Kitamura, Y., Yuan, S-S., Wright, H. E., Clardy, J., Demain, Al L., Glinsukon, T., Hunt, N., and Wogan, G. N. (1973). J. Am. Chem. Soc. 95, 5423–5425.
Büchi, G., Luk, K-C., Kobbe, B., and Townsend, J. M. (1977). J. Org. Chem. 42, 244–246.
Casnati, G., and Pochini, A. (1970): J. Chem. Soc., Chem. Commun., pp. 1328–1329.
Casnati, G., Marchelli, R., and Pochini, A. (1974). J. Chem. Soc., pp. 754–757.
Clardy, J., Springer, J. P., Büchi, G., Matsuo, K., and Wightman, R. (1975). J. Am. Chem. Soc. 97, 663–665.
Cole, R. J. (1976). Proc. US–Jpn. Conf. on Mycotoxins in Human and Animal Health, University of Maryland, College Park.
Cole, R. J., and Kirksey, J. W. (1973). J. Agr. Food Chem. 21, 927–929.
Cole, R. J., Kirksey, J. W., Moore, J. H., Blankenship, B. R., Diener, U. L., and Davis, N. D. (1972). Appl. Microbiol. 24, 248–256.
Cole, R. J., Kirksey, J. W., and Wells, J. M. (1974). Can J. Microbiol. 20, 1159–1162.
Cole, R. J., Kirksey, J. W., Dorner, J. W., Wilson, D. M., Johnson, Jr., J. C., Johnson, A. N., Bedell, D. M., Springer, J. P., Chexal, K. K., Clardy, J., and Cox, R. H. (1977a). Agr. Food Chem. 25, 826–830.
Cole, R. J., Dorner, J. W., Lansden, J. A., Cox, R. H., Pape, C., Cunfer, B., Nicholson, S. S., and Bedell, D. M. (1977b). J. Agr. Food Chem. 25, 1197–1201.
Cook, A. H., and Slater, C. A. (1954). J. Inst. Brew. 51, 213
Cook, A. H., and Slater, C. A. (1956). J. Chem. Soc., pp. 4133
Demain, A. L., Hunt, N. A., Malik, V., Kobbe, B., Howkins, H., Matsuo, K., and Wogan, G. N. (1976). Appl. Environ. Microbiol. 31, 138–140.
Dunn, G., Gallagher, J. J., Newbold, G. T., and Spring, F. S. (1949a). J. Chem. Soc., pp. 126–131.
Dunn, G., Newbold, G. T., and Spring, F. S. (1949b). J. Chem. Soc., pp. 131–133.
Dutcher, J. D. (1947a). J. Biol. Chem. 171, 321–339.
Dutcher, J. D. (1947b). J. Biol. Chem. 171, 341–353.
Dutcher, J. D. (1958). J. Biol. Chem. 232, 785–795.
Eickman, N., Clardy, J., Cole, R. J., and Kirksey, J. W. (1975). Tetrahedron Lett., pp. 1051–1054.
Fehr, Th., and Acklin, W. (1966). Helv. Chim. Acta 49, 1907–1910.
Foyes, J., Lokensgard, D., Clardy, J., Cole, R. J., and Kirksey, J. W. (1974). J. Am. Chem. Soc., 96, 6785–6787.

Gardiner, R. A., Rinehart Jr, K. L., Snyder, J. J., and Broquist, H. P. (1968). *J. Am. Chem. Soc.* **90**, 5639–5640.
Guengerich, F. P. (1971). *Federation Proc.* **30**, 1067.
Iizuka, H. (1974). *In* "Mycotoxins" (I. F. H. Purchase, ed.), p. 411. Elsevier, Amsterdam.
Iizuka, H., and Iida, M. (1962). *Nature (London)* **196**, 681–682.
Leigh, C., and Taylor, A. (1976). *In* "Mycotoxins and Other Fungal Related Food Problems" (J. V. Rodricks, ed.), pp. 228–275 and references cited therein: *Adv. in Chemistry Series 149*, Am. Chem. Soc., Washington D.C.
MacDonald, J. C. (1961). *J. Biol. Chem.* **236**, 512–514.
MacDonald, J. C. (1963). *Canad. J. Chem.* **41**, 165.
MacDonald, J. C. (1965a). *Biochem. J.* **96**, 533–538.
MacDonald, J. C. (1965b). *J. Biol. Chem.* **237**, 1977–1981.
MacDonald, J. C., Mictich, R. G., and Haskins, R. H. (1964). *Can J. Microbiol.* **10**, 90.
Maebayashi, Y., Sumita, M., Fukushima, K., and Yamazaki, M. (1977). *Chem. Pharm. Bull. (Tokyo)* **26**, 1320.
Menzel, A. E. O., Wintersteiner, O., and Rake, G. (1943). *J. Bacteriol.* **46**, 109.
Micetich, R. G., and MacDonald, J. C. (1964). *J. Chem. Soc.*, p. 1507.
Micetich, R. G. and MacDonald, J. C. (1965). *J. Biol. Chem.* **240**, 1692–1695.
Nagel, D. W., Steyn, P. S., and Scott, D. B. (1972a). *Phytochemistry* **11**, 627–630.
Nagel, D. W., Steyn, P. S., and Ferreira, N. P. (1972b). *Phytochemistry* **11**, 3215–3218.
Nagel, D. W., Pachler, K. G. R., Steyn P. S., Vleggaar, R., and Wessels, P. L. (1976). *Tetrahedron* **32**, 2625–2631.
Nakamura, S. (1960). *Bull. Agric. Chem. Soc. Jpn.* **24**, 629.
Nakamura, S., Shiro, T. (1959). *Bull. Agric. Chem. Soc. Jpn.* **23**, 418.
Ohkubo, Y., Urakawa, N., Hayama, T., Seto, Y., Miura, T., Kano, Y., Motoyoshi, S., Yamamoto, S., Ishida, K., Iizuka, H., and Iida, M. (1955). *Japan. J. Vet. Sci.* **17**, 145–151.
Rainey, D. P., Smalley, E. B., Crump, M. H., and Strong, F. M. (1965). *Nature (London)* **205**, 203–204.
Sakabe, N., Goto, T., and Hirata, Y. (1964). *Tetrahedron Lett.*, pp. 1825–1830.
Sammes, P. G. (1975). *Fortschritte Chem. Org. Naturstoffe.* **32**, 51–118.
Sasaki, M., Asao, Y., and Yokotsuka, T. (1963). *Nogei. Kagaku. Kaishi. (Tokyo)* **42**, 346.
Scott, P. M., and Kennedy, B. P. C. (1976). *J. Agr. Food Chem.* **24**, 865–868.
Scott, P. M., Merrien, M-A., and Polonsky, J. (1976). *Experientia* **32**, 140–142.
Scott, P. M., Kennedy, B. P. C., Harwig, J., and Blanchfield, B. J. (1977). *Appl. Envir. Microbiol.* **33**, 249–253.
Snyder, J. J. and Broquist, H. P. (1968). *Federation Proc.* **27**, 764.
Spike, T. E. and Aust, S. D. (1971). *Biochem. Pharmacol.* **20**, 721–728.
Springer, J. P., Clardy, J., Wells, J. M., Cole, R. J., and Kirksey, J. W. (1975). *Tetrahedron Lett.*, pp. 2531–2534.
Tanabe, M. (1976). *Proc. U.S. Jpn. Joint Seminar on Biosynthesis of Natural Products*, Honolulu, Hawaii.
Turner, W. B. (1971). *"Fungal Metabolites,"* p. 138. Academic Press, New York.
Uraguchi, K. (1969). *J. Stored Prod. Res.* **5**, 227–236.
Uraguchi, K. (1971). *In* "International Encyclopedia of Pharmacology and Therapeutics" (H. Raskova ed.), Section 71, pp. 143–298. Pergamon Press, Oxford.
Uramoto, M., Cary, L., Tanabe, M., Hirotsu, K., and Clardy, J. (1977). *Proc. Ann. Meeting, Kanto Branch, Agr. Chem. Soc. of Japan*, Tokyo, Japan.
Weiss, U., Strelitz, F., Flon, H., and Asheshov, I. N. (1958). *Arch. Biochem. Biophys.* **74**, 150–.
White, E. C., and Hill, J. H. (1943). *J. Bacteriol.* **45**, 433–443.

222   Mikio Yamazaki

Yamazaki, M., Suzuki, S., and Miyaki, K. (1971). *Chem. Pharm. Bull., (Tokyo)* **19**, 1739–1740.
Yamazaki, M., Maebayashi, Y. and Miyaki, K. (1972). *Chem. Pharm. Bull. (Tokyo)* **20**, 2274.
Yamazaki, M. (1973). *Proc. 24th IUPAC Congress,* Hamburg, Germany.
Yamazaki, M., Sasago, K., and Miyaki, K. (1974). *J. Chem. Soc. Chem. Commun.,* pp. 408–409.
Yamazaki, M., Fujimoto, H., Akiyama, T., Sankawa, U., and Iitaka, Y. (1975a). *Tetrahderon Lett.,* pp. 27–28.
Yamazaki, M., Fujimoto, H., and Kawasaki, T. (1975b). *Tetrahedron Lett.,* pp. 1241–1244.
Yamazaki, M., Fujimoto, H., Kawasaki, T., Okuyama, E., and Kuga, T. (1975c). *Proc. 19th Symp. on Chemistry of Natural Products, Hiroshima, Japan.*
Yamazaki, M., Fujimoto, H., and Okuyama, E. (1976). *Tetrahedron Lett.,* pp. 2861–2864.
Yamazaki, M., Fujimoto, H., and Okuyama, E. (1977). *Chem. Pharm. Bull. (Tokyo)* **25**, 2554–2560.
Yamazaki, M., Fujimoto, H., and Okuyama, E. (1978). *Chem. Pharm. Bull. (Tokyo)* **26**, 111–117.
Yamazaki, M., Suzuki, S., and Kukita, K. (1971a). *J. Pharm. Dyn. (Tokyo)* **2**, 119–125.
Yamazaki, M., Okuyama, E., and Maebayashi, Y. (1979b). *Chem. Pharm. Bull. (Tokyo)* **27**, 1611–1617.
Yamazaki, M., Fujimoto, H., and Kawasaki, T. (1980). *Chem. Pharm. Bull. (Tokyo)* **28**, 245–254.
Yokotsuka, T., Asao, Y., and Sasaki, M. (1968). *Nogei. Kagaku. Kaishi. (Tokyo)* **42**, 346.
Yokotsuka, T., Oshita, K., Kikuchi, T., Sasaki, M., and Asao, Y. (1969). *Nogei Kagaku Kaishi (Tokyo)* **43**, 189–196.

7

The Biosynthesis of Patulin
and Penicillic Acid

LOLITA O. ZAMIR

The Biosynthesis of Mycotoxins
Copyright © 1980 by Academic Press, Inc.

I. INTRODUCTION

Patulin (**1**) and penicillic acid (**2**) are secondary metabolites which are synthesized primarily by *Penicillium* and *Aspergillus* species. The patulin isolated has been given various names: patulin, claviformin, clavacin, clavatin, expansin, leucopin, mycoin C, penicidin, and tercinin (Florey *et al.*, 1949; Scott, 1974; Singh, 1967; Wilson and Hayes, 1973; Wilson, 1976). Patulin and penicillic acid are produced by different fungal species, but the biological reactions leading to these two natural products are very similar. In this chapter, only the physical properties of patulin and penicillic acid relevant to biosynthetic studies will be discussed.

A. Patulin

Patulin (Fig. 1) was discovered by Birkinshaw *et al.* (1943), and its chemical structure elegantly proved and synthesized by Woodward and Singh (1949, 1950). The oxime was independently prepared by another route (Serratosa, 1961). A recent crystallographic study by Hubbard *et al.* (1977) confirmed the structure of patulin and gave the bond distances and angles of the patulin molecule. Patulin isolated from natural sources has one asymmetric center on carbon 1. Patulin is, however, racemic. One explanation could be that the center at C(1) may racemize easily during work-up. Another possibility could be that the hemiacetal formation is not enzyme controlled.

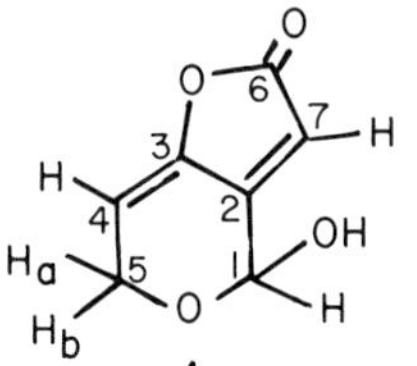

Fig. 1.   Structure of patulin.

The 100 MHz ^{1}H NMR spectra of patulin will be described in some detail (Zamir, 1973). After exchange of the hydroxy proton with deuterium, the spectrum of patulin shows five kinds of protons. The methylene protons are centered at $\delta 4.38$ and $\delta 4.82$ as a typical AB pattern with J 17 Hz. The methine region shows the presence of three hydrogens, one which appears as a singlet 1-H whereas the other two show a fine splitting pattern (Fig. 2). When the methylene region is expanded, a further weak splitting of each of the doublets (J 0.6–1.0 Hz) is observed. This spectrum fits quite well with the patulin structure, where $J \sim 4$ Hz is probably the coupling constant between H(4) and $H_a(5)$ or $H_b(5)$, and $J \sim 3$ Hz is the coupling between H(4) and $H_b(5)$ or $H_a(5)$. The coupling between $H_a(5)$ or $H_b(5)$ and H(7) is 1.0 and

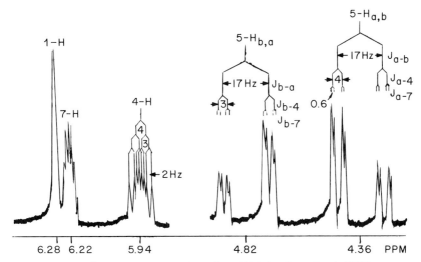

Fig. 2. ^{1}H NMR spectrum of patulin at 100 MHz. From Zamir (1973).

0.6 Hz. By expanding the methine region, we find a broad singlet which corresponds to proton H(1) because it has no vicinal protons. The vinylic methine protons H(4) and H(7) are resolved into two groups of fine splitting structures which are centered at δ5.94 and δ6.22, respectively. H(4) shows eight lines which are interpreted as splitting by $H_a(5)$ ($J \sim 4$ Hz), then by $H_b(5)$ ($J \sim 3$ Hz); the splitting with proton H(7) is reflected by a further splitting ($J_{4-7} \sim 2$ Hz). Analogously, the proton H(7) shows a fine splitting arising from both coupling with proton H(4) and long-range coupling with the methylene protons.

The mass spectrum of patulin at different ionizing energies has been analyzed in detail by Zamir (1973). Patulin is a very intricate molecule possessing a functional group on every carbon; therefore, a large number of fragmentation peaks are observed (Fig. 3). The analysis is derived from the numerous metastable peaks and the high-resolution mass spectrum. The major fragments involve elimination of water (m/e 136) or of the fragment C_2H_4O (m/e 110), or decarbonylation (m/e 126).

B. Penicillic Acid

Penicillic acid (Fig. 4) was first isolated from *Penicillium puberulum* grown on corn by Alsberg and Black (1913). The discovery of a different strain, *Penicillium cyclopium* Westling, producing large amounts of penicillic acid, has enabled the elucidation of the molecular structure (Birkinshaw *et al.*, 1936; Birkinshaw and Raistrick, 1942). The synthesis of penicillic

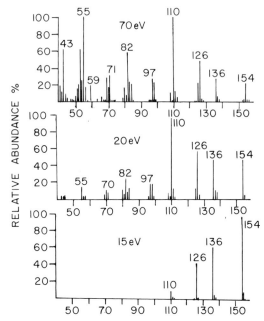

Fig. 3. Mass spectrum of patulin at different ionizing energies. From Zamir (1973).

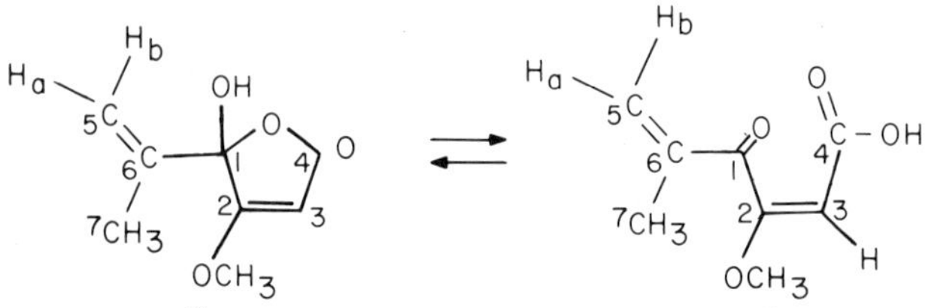

Fig. 4. Structure of the two tautomeric forms of penicillic acid.

acid as well as of dihydropenicillic acid has been accomplished by Raphael (1947, 1948, 1950). Penicillic acid exists in two tautomeric forms (Birkinshaw *et al.*, 1936): the cyclic lactol and the open-chain form; these are shown in Fig. 4. The pH of the solution determines the equilibrium position. In base, the open acid form predominates; in neutral solution, the cyclic lactol is the main tautomer.

The Fourier transform (FT) 90.02 MHz ^{1}H NMR spectra of penicillic acid has been described in detail (Al-Rawi *et al.*, 1974; Elvidge *et al.*, 1977) (Fig. 5). The methyl group at C(7) and the methoxyl at C(2) appear as singlets centered at $\delta 1.77$ and $\delta 3.9$, respectively. The methine proton at C(3) shows at

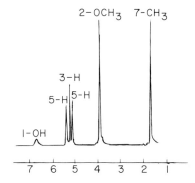

Fig. 5. Fourier transform 90.02 MHz ^{1}H NMR spectrum of penicillic acid. Spectrum provided by J. Elvidge. [From Elvidge *et al.* (1977) with permission from the author and *J. Chem. Soc.*]

$\delta 5.27$. The 5-methylene signals appeared at $\delta 5.19$ and $\delta 5.49$. The chemical shifts, as well as the allylic coupling constants, could not distinguish with certainty between the 5-methylene peaks. The assignments of H_a and H_b at C(5) derived from the use of the shift reagent Eu(thd)$_3$ [shorthand for tris(2,2,6,6-tetramethylheptane-3,5-dionato)europium(III)] (Elvidge *et al.*, 1977). The higher-field 5-methylene signal was assigned to H_b *trans* to the C-methyl group.

The FT ^{13}C NMR spectrum of penicillic acid has been analyzed in some detail by Seto *et al.* (1974). An unusual feature is the assignment of C(2) at a very low-field position ($\delta 178.17$). The interpretation invokes the deshielding of C(2) by two β-oxygens, as well as that caused by the attachment of the methoxy group (Seto *et al.*, 1974). The C(1) and C(5) signals were not resolved.

C. Biological Activities of Patulin and Penicillic Acid

The patulin- and penicillic acid-producing strains are widely spread in food as contaminants. Patulin has been found in many batches of commercial apple juice in Canada and in the United States (Stoloff, 1975). The amounts range from 9 to 150 mg/liter. It has been shown that the patulin originates from cider mills where decayed apples are not sorted out or where apples are stored in large bins for long periods. The storage rot of various fruits is caused by the patulin-producing species *Penicillium expansum* (Scott *et al.*, 1977). Patulin is also detected in molded bread, fermented sausage, and animal food (Ukai *et al.*, 1954; Reiss, 1972, 1973; Alperden *et al.*, 1973). Penicillic acid is found in moldy tobacco (23 μg/100 gm), rice, many commercial corn samples (5–230 μg/kg), dried beans, and barley grains (Snow *et al.*, 1972; Thorpe *et al.*, 1974). The toxicity of penicillic acid was established very early during its first isolation by Alsberg and Black (1913). Nevertheless, patulin was at one time considered a possible cure for the common cold (Boyd, 1944). Patulin has since been recognized to be useless against the common cold and to be very toxic (Stansfield *et al.*, 1944; Capitaine and

Balouet, 1974). Patulin, like penicillic acid, inhibits the growth of gram-negative and gram-positive bacteria; however, neither patulin nor penicillic acid can be used as antibiotics, for they have been shown to be very toxic and carcinogenic (Dickens, 1967; Ciegler et al., 1977). Patulin has also been found to be teratogenic (Ciegler et al., 1976) and to inhibit the aerobic respiration of bacteria and higher plants (Dickens, 1967). The lethal dose LD_{50} of patulin for mice is 5.7 mg/kg (Dailey et al., 1977). The LD_{50} of penicillic acid for mice is 110 mg/kg by subcutaneous injection (Wilson and Hayes, 1973; Sansing et al., 1976). The modes of action of patulin and of penicillic acid are still unknown, and the molecular basis for their toxicity remains to be established.

II. BIOGENETIC THEORIES

A. Patulin

The aromatic metabolite 6-methylsalicylic acid (6-MSA) (4) was first discovered in the culture of *Penicillium patulum* by Ehrensvard (1955). Among all the systems investigated in the past 20 years, 6-MSA biosynthesis has been most extensively studied, and has been considered as a model for many other polyketides. This is probably due in part to the availability of 6-MSA from several sources (fungi, bacteria, plants) and to the involvement of 6-MSA in the very first biosynthetic experiment. Birch and co-workers (1955) have fed [1-^{14}C]acetate to *P. patulum*, isolated 6-MSA, degraded it, and found the appropriate labeling (Fig. 6). This investigation represents the first experimental proof of the polyacetate rule. The aromatic origin of patulin has been demonstrated by Bu'lock and Ryan (1958), and Tanenbaum and Bassett (1958), by feeding 6-MSA labeled with ^{14}C in known positions to *P. patulum*. The 6-MSA sample was isolated from [1-^{14}C]acetate feeding and was found to be labeled at the carbon atoms numbered 2, 4, 6, and 8 (Fig. 6). The numbering in 6-MSA follows the sequence of acetic acid residues. The patulin resulting from this feeding was degraded and the radioactivity (Fig. 6) was found at carbons 2, 4, and 6.

Many biogenetic pathways have been proposed for the conversion of 6-MSA to patulin. In addition to 6-MSA (4) and patulin (1), *P. patulum* produces a variety of phenolic metabolites, some of which are represented in Fig. 7: 6-formylsalicylic acid (5), m-cresol (6), m-hydroxybenzyl alcohol (7), gentisyl alcohol (8), gentisaldehyde (9), gentisic acid (10), and toluquinol (11).

Early biogenetic theories have involved the intermediacy of 6-formylsalicylic acid (5) (Fig. 7) in patulin formation. Hydroxylation of 5 to yield a hypothetical metabolite, 5-hydroxy-6-formylsalicylic acid, and subsequent

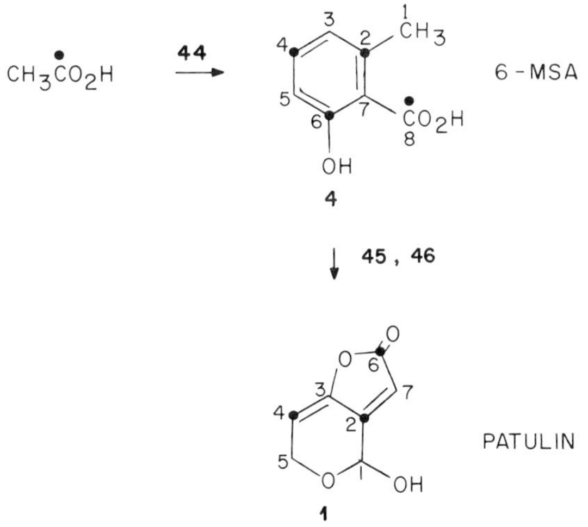

$$CH_3CO_2H \xrightarrow{\ 44\ }$$

6 - MSA

4

45 , 46

PATULIN

1

Fig. 6.   Aromatic origin of patulin, modified after Birch *et al.* (1955), Bu'lock and Ryan (1958), and Tanenbaum and Bassett (1958).

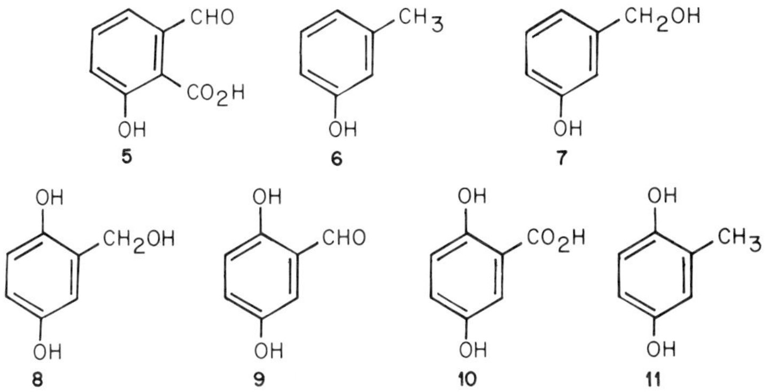

5   6   7

8   9   10   11

Fig. 7.   Some aromatic metabolites of *P. patulum.*

decarboxylation would give gentisaldehyde (9). Gentisaldehyde was then assumed to be oxidatively cleaved to patulin. This putative pathway was not supported by experimental studies. Another early scheme postulated that 6-MSA and patulin originate from a common open-chain C_8 precursor

Patulin $\leftarrow$ open-chain $C_8 \rightleftharpoons \cdots \rightleftharpoons$ 6-MSA

However, it would have been unlikely that after the aromatic 6-MSA is produced it would recleave to a C_8 open-chain form. An early feeding experiment (Tanenbaum and Bassett, 1959) showed that labeled gentisic acid

(10) was not incorporated into patulin. The discovery of *m*-cresol (6) (Fig. 7) in *P. patulum* suggested that 6-formylsalicylic acid was not necessarily on the pathway to patulin. Bu'lock and co-workers (1965) indicated by a general metabolic grid the various possible interrelationships among the aromatic compounds in *P. patulum*. Gentisaldehyde (9) has also been assumed to be the last aromatic compound to be cleaved to patulin. The biosynthetic experiment that demonstrated the conversion of trideuterio-*m*-cresol to patulin ruled out 6-formylsalicylic acid intermediacy (Zamir, 1973; Scott *et al.*, 1967; Scott *et al.*, 1973). A kinetic pulse-labeling study (Forrester and Gaucher, 1972a,b) suggests that the major pathway for patulin biosynthesis involves *m*-hydroxybenzyl alcohol (7), *m*-hydroxybenzaldehyde, gentisyl alcohol (8), and gentisaldehyde (9) (Fig. 7). Feeding experiments with deuterated intermediates (Scott *et al.*, 1973) and mass spectral analysis of the products have enabled us to propose a biogenetic scheme.

B. The Last Step in the Biogenesis of Patulin

Prior to 1978 no intermediates were isolated between the aromatic metabolites and patulin. It was therefore suggested that the cleavage intermediate was tightly bound to the enzyme. For almost three decades gentisaldehyde (9) (Fig. 7) was assumed to be the last aromatic precursor in

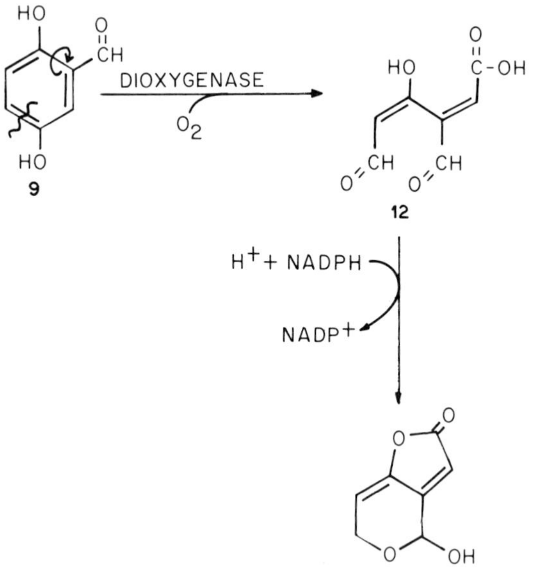

Fig. 8.   Mechanism of the conversion of gentisaldehyde to patulin. [From Zamir (1973) and Scott *et al.* (1973) with permission from the senior author and *Bioorg. Chem.*]

patulin biosynthesis, but no experimental proof was offered. Indeed, this assumption was validated by the positive incorporation of ^{14}C-labeled and deuterated gentisaldehyde into patulin in 1972–1973 (Forrester and Gaucher, 1972a,b; Scott *et al.*, 1973). The mechanism of the conversion of gentisaldehyde is shown in Fig. 8 (Zamir, 1973 and Scott *et al.*, 1973). According to Fig. 8, gentisaldehyde (**9**) is first cleaved by an oxygenase to give **12**. The next step involves a stereospecific reduction catalyzed by a dehydrogenase and NADPH to give patulin (**1**).

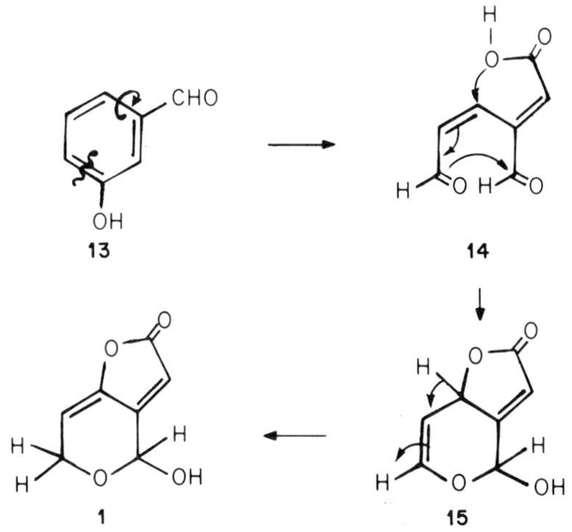

Fig. 9.   Mechanism of the conversion of *m*-hydroxybenzaldehyde to patulin. [From Zamir (1973) and Scott *et al.* (1973) with permission from the authors and *Bioorg. Chem.*]

m-Hydroxybenzaldehyde (**13**) was suggested by Zamir (1973) and Scott *et al.* (1973) as a plausible last aromatic precursor (Fig. 9). This biogenetic scheme first involves an oxygenase to cleave *m*-hydroxybenzaldehyde to **14** (Fig. 9). Lactonization will give **15** (Fig. 9). Enzymatic prototropy will then generate patulin (**1**). According to this mechanism, no reduction is needed to convert *m*-hydroxybenzaldehyde (**13**) to patulin (**1**). However, because there is probably only one major pathway leading to patulin, and because the enzyme catalyzing the conversion of gentisaldehyde to patulin has been isolated, *m*-hydroxybenzaldehyde is probably not the last aromatic intermediate in patulin biosynthesis. A hydroxylated quinone intermediate,**16** (Fig. 10), was postulated (Wikholm and Moore, 1972) in the conversion of gentisaldehyde (**9**) to patulin (**1**). However, the experimental result obtained by Zamir (1973) and Scott *et al.* (1973) that three deuteriums in the aromatic ring of gentisaldehyde were incorporated into patulin disproves this hypothesis.

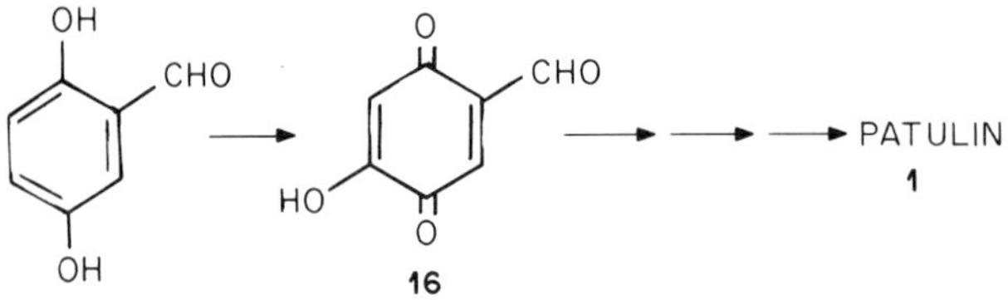

Fig. 10. Postulated mechanism of the conversion of gentisaldehyde to patulin, modified after Wikholm and Moore (1972).

C. Penicillic Acid

The isopropylidene side chain in penicillic acid suggests a terpenoid origin. The insignificant incorporation (0.03%) of [2-^{14}C]mevalonic acid lactone into penicillic acid (Birch *et al.*, 1958) rules out this possibility. Birch and co-workers (1958) have demonstrated the acetate bioorigin of penicillic acid and were the first to suggest the cleavage of an aromatic compound, orsellinic acid (**17**). The labeling distribution in penicillic acid after the feeding of [1-^{14}C]acetic acid to *P. cyclopium* Westling is shown in Fig. 11. The radioactivity is located at C(2), C(4), and C(6).

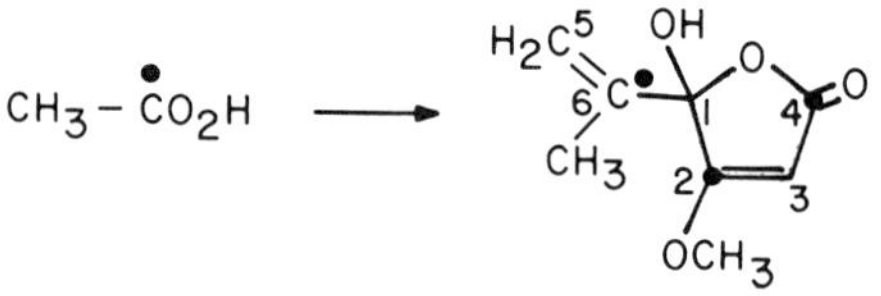

Fig. 11. Labeling distribution in penicillic acid, modified after Birch *et al.* (1958).

D. The Last Step in the Biogenesis of Penicillic Acid

Birch and co-workers (1958) have suggested that orsellinic acid (**17**) is probably the aromatic precursor of penicillic acid. Their prediction involves cleavage at site a (see Fig. 12). Mosbach (1960) has demonstrated that orsellinic acid is converted to penicillic acid but through cleavage at site b (see Fig. 12). Indeed, the doubly labeled orsellinic acid (**17**) which was fed showed retention of the radioactivity at carbon 2 and not at carbon 4 in penicillic acid (Fig. 12).

There are two main mechanisms that can explain the cleavage of orsellinic acid at site b to give penicillic acid (Al-Rawi *et al.*, 1974; Elvidge, *et al.*, 1977; Axberg and Gatenbeck, 1975a,b; Better and Gatenbeck, 1976). Both mechanisms invoke specific methylation of one of the hydroxy groups and

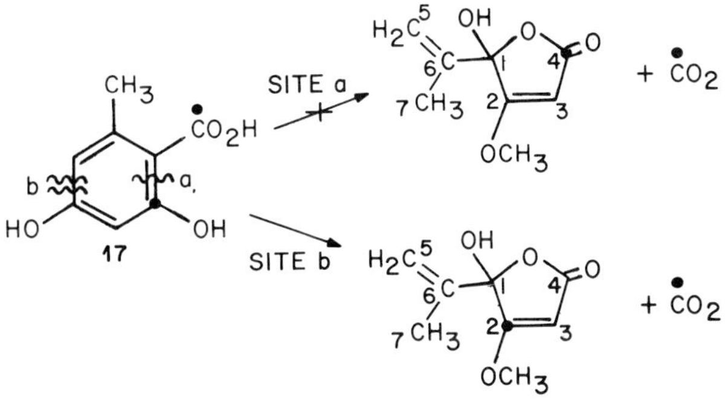

Fig. 12. Cleavage site of orsellinic acid, modified after Mosbach (1960).

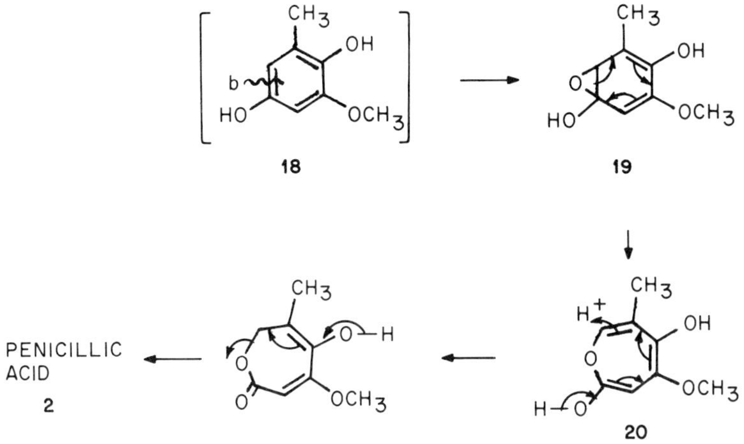

Fig. 13. Mechanism of the conversion of orsellinic acid to penicillic acid, modified after Al-Rawi *et al.* (1974) and Elvidge *et al.* (1977).

oxidative decarboxylation at an early stage to give the aromatic compound **18** (Fig. 13). Cleavage of **18** at site b is then assumed to be catalyzed by a monooxygenase to give the corresponding arene oxide, **19**, which is then converted to the oxepin (**20**). Tautomerism, opening of the seven-membered ring, and lactolization then lead to penicillic acid (**2**) (Al-Rawi *et al.*, 1974; Elvidge *et al.*, 1977). It is interesting to note that this biogenetic sequence does not involve oxidation of compound **18** and therefore needs no reduction at a later stage.

A different mechanism has been proposed by Axberg and Gatenbeck (1975a,b). The aromatic intermediate (**18**) (Figs. 13 and 14) is oxidized to the

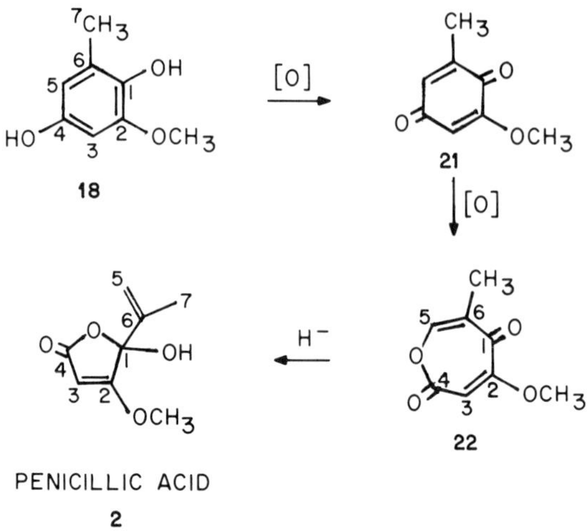

234 Lolita O. Zamir

Fig. 14. Mechanism of the conversion of orsellinic acid to penicillic acid, modified after Axberg and Gatenbeck (1975).

corresponding quinone (21) (Fig. 14). Oxidation of compound 21 by a monooxygenase would yield the seven-membered ring quinoid intermediate, 22. Subsequent reactions must include a reduction of the potential aldehyde at C(5). Dehydration and lactolization would generate penicillic acid (2). Experimental evidence supports the mechanism outlined in Fig. 14: involvement of the quinone and necessity of a reduction step. It is interesting to notice that in both patulin and penicillic acid nature favors the higher oxidation state intermediate requiring a reduction at a later stage.

III. METHODOLOGY FOLLOWED DURING THE STUDY

The combination of the studies on patulin and on penicillic acid represents almost all the methods known in biosynthetic investigations: ^{14}C-precursors and analysis of the labels, kinetic pulse labeling, ^{2}H precursors and mass spectrometry, ^{13}C NMR, ^{3}H NMR, and the use of enzymes. I will summarize very briefly the results of these different methods, as well as their advantages and drawbacks.

A. [14]C Precursors and Analysis of the Labels

This is the oldest method used; however, it will always remain a very important tool in biosynthetic investigations. It involves synthesizing a precursor with one or two radioisotopes (^{14}C or ^{3}H). This putative precursor is then fed to the fungi. The resulting product is then purified and an aliquot is analyzed with a scintillation counter, in order to check if it is radioactive and therefore if the precursor was incorporated. The next step is to locate the radioactive carbons. This is usually done by chemical degradations. The great advantage of this method is its sensitivity. ^{14}C or ^{3}H can be easily traced even if very small quantities of the end products are obtained or if the incorporation is very low. A significant positive incorporation in fungal studies is above 0.1% (in plant work a positive incorporation could be 0.05%!). This method is, therefore, of utmost importance as a preliminary tool to check if the precursor is incorporated and to determine the best feeding conditions. Its drawback is that, in order to locate the radioactive carbons, the only method known is to resort to tedious, and sometimes very difficult, chemical degradations. This method has enabled the proof of the aromatic origin of patulin (Bu'lock and Ryan, 1958; Tanenbaum and Bassett, 1958) and penicillic acid (Mosbach, 1960), as well as the distinction between two possible cleavage sites in the penicillic acid study (Mosbach, 1960).

B. Kinetic Pulse Labeling

Forrester and Gaucher (1972a,b) have introduced the interesting technique of kinetic pulse labeling in fungal studies for the metabolites of *P. patulum*. It gives the sequence of appearance of metabolites and therefore can be regarded as a rapid qualitative probe. The method consists in feeding radio-active acetate and other radioactive putative precursors, and following their metabolism with time. The advantage of this method is that the sequential appearance of the metabolites can suggest an overall biosynthetic pathway. In addition, this is the only technique in which transient intermediates can be distinguished from side or end products. If successful, it is probably an excellent preliminary study.

C. ^{2}H Precursors and Mass Spectrometry

Scott and co-workers (1967, 1973) have used deuterated precursors to delineate patulin biosynthesis. The method involves preparing deuterated putative intermediates, feeding them to the fungi, and isolating the enriched products. The compounds are then purified by the usual organic methods and analyzed by mass spectrometry. The advantages of this technique are (a) it is much easier to synthesize precursors with ^{2}H rather than ^{14}C; (b) mass spectrometry analyses require only a minute amount of product; (c) ^{2}H is a nontoxic stable isotope; and (d) deuterated precursors can give valuable information on prochiral centers. In the case of racemic patulin, some of the enriched deuterated patulin showed optical activity (Zamir, 1973; Scott and Yalpani, 1967; Scott, et al., 1973). This interesting result will be discussed in Section V.

D. ^{13}C NMR

As a result of the technological advances of the last decade, FT ^{13}C NMR has come to be used (and reviewed) extensively to confirm biosynthetic pathways previously investigated with radioisotopic methods. The method consists in feeding to the fungi substrates labeled with ^{13}C at specific locations in the molecule. After isolation of the ^{13}C-enriched product and its purification, the ^{13}C positions are traced by comparing the ^{13}C NMR of the ^{13}C-enriched product with the ^{13}C NMR of the "cold" ("natural", non-enriched) analogue.

Recently, Seto, et al. (1973) introduced a very useful technique employing double-labeled ^{13}C precursors. Sodium [1,2-^{13}C]acetate, as well as "cold" sodium acetate, is added to a polyketide-producing organism. The idea is based on observing the (^{13}C,^{13}C)coupling of intact acetate units in the product. The cold sodium acetate prevents additional (^{13}C,^{13}C)couplings which can complicate the ^{13}C NMR interpretation. An alternative method (Seto et al., 1973) for confirming this result is to feed a 1:1 mixture of ^{13}CH$_3$COONa:CH$_3$^{13}COONa. No cold sodium acetate is added, as a high incorporation of ^{13}C is needed to detect (^{13}C,^{13}C)couplings of "in-between" intact acetate units. The two methods complement each other and give the folding pattern of the polyketide chain. This technique has been used extensively, to distinguish between alternative foldings of polyketide chains. This method has been used for penicillic acid (Seto et al., 1974) and griseo-fulvin (Simpson and Holker, 1977), which is a cometabolite of patulin. The advantages of the use of FT ^{13}C NMR in biosynthesis are nontoxicity of the stable isotope, easy location of the ^{13}C atoms with no need for tedious chemical degradations, and the use of the doubly labeled acetate technique, the only method that can indicate a polyketide chain-folding pattern. The disadvantage is the need for a good yield of substrate formation, as well as an incorporation of the order of 1% or higher.

E. ^{3}H NMR

The technique of tritium NMR was reported by Bloxsidge et al., (1971). The first application of this method in biosynthesis involved penicillic acid (Al-Rawi et al., 1974; Elvidge et al., 1977). The triton has a spin of $\frac{1}{2}$, and its sensitivity to detection is even higher than the proton's. Bloxsidge et al.

(1971) describe the microcell assembly used to conform with radiochemical safety. In order to measure the ^{3}H NMR detection sensitivity, a standard [7α,7β-^{3}H]dehydroepiandrosterone with varying radioactivities has been used (0.12mCi; 1.2mCi; 12mCi per 100 μl NMR cell). This experiment has shown that the detection of ^{3}H is possible with as little as 1 mCi of tritium per labeled site in a molecule. The advantages of this method are (a) the sensitivity of ^{3}H is higher than that of ^{2}H; (b) the proton–chemical shift information can be used to interpret the ^{3}H NMR spectra; (c) as with the case of ^{2}H, information on prochiral hydrogens can be obtained; and (d) FT ^{13}C NMR and ^{3}H NMR data can complement each other. Possible disadvantages include: (a) a special microcell assembly is required; (b) the radioactivity hazard of tritium must be considered; and (c) in the unlikely event of the microbulb and NMR tube breaking, the rf–coil assembly must be removable to decontaminate the spectrometer.

F. The Use of Enzymes

Whole-cell feeding experiments imply adding labeled putative precursors (radioactive or stable isotope label) to the whole organism, which is grown on a synthetic media. The products and intermediates are then isolated, purified, and analyzed by the various methods. This type of experiment enables one to propose a plausible biosynthetic pathway. Isolation and purification of the enzymes responsible for each step of the pathway enable verification at the enzymatic level. The *in vitro* conversion of a putative precursor by the pure enzyme to the product constitutes unambiguous proof of the biosynthetic reaction. The ultimate proof of a biosynthetic pathway depends, therefore, on the characterization of the enzymes involved in each step of the pathway. The only major drawback is that the procedure is extremely difficult, and the detailed enzymology for polyketide-derived compounds deserves further study. The problems are (a) instability of the enzymes, (b) lack of reproducibility, and (c) variability of activity in different enzymatic preparations (some of these enzymes are membrane bound and easily deactivated by isolation). Despite the difficulties involved, some of the enzymes involved in the biosynthesis of patulin and penicillic acid have been partially purified and characterized.

IV. ORIGIN OF THE AROMATIC PRECURSORS

The biosynthesis of patulin, as well as that of penicillic acid, can be summarized as acetate → aromatic compound → product. In this section we will concentrate on the first step: the origin of the aromatic precursor.

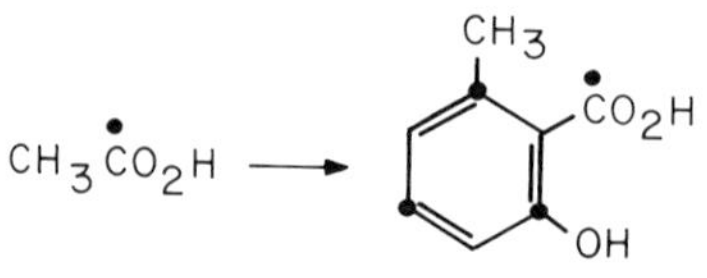

Fig. 15. Polyacetate origin of 6-MSA. [From Birch *et al.* (1955) with permission from the authors and *Aust. J. Chem.*]

A. Acetate → 6-Methylsalicylic Acid

The polyacetate origin of 6-MSA (4) has been demonstrated by Birch and co-workers (1955). [1-^{14}C]Acetate has been fed to *P. patulum* cultures. The degradation of the resulting 6-MSA has shown the labeling distribution depicted in Fig. 15.

The involvement of the chain-elongating malonyl group has been proved by the feeding of [2-^{14}C]diethylmalonate to *P. patulum* (Bu'lock *et al.*, 1962). Indeed, degradation of the resulting 6-MSA has shown it to be formed from one acetyl starter and three malonyl units. The discovery of coenzyme A in cultures of *P. patulum* and the conversion of radioactive acetyl-CoA by a crude enzymatic extract into 6-MSA has confirmed the obligatory intermediacy of acetyl-CoA (Tanenbaum and Bassett, 1959; Bassett and Tanenbaum, 1960). Lynen and Tada (1961) and Lynen (1967a,b), proposed a mechanism for the biosynthesis of 6-MSA by analogy with Lynen's hypothesis for the biosynthesis of fatty acids involving acetyl-CoA, malonyl-CoA, and NADPH in a multienzyme complex. This hypothesis can be considered a model for the biogenesis of all the polyketide-derived aromatics. The isolation of a partially pure cell-free extract (Lynen and Tada, 1961; Lynen, 1967a,b) has enabled one to confirm that malonyl-CoA and NADPH are required, in addition to acetyl-CoA, for the synthesis of 6-MSA. Since then, three major groups have purified 6-MSA synthetase to various degrees: (1) Lynen and Tada (1961), Lynen (1967a,b), Dimroth *et al.* (1970, 1972, 1976); (2) Light (1967), Light and Hager (1968); (3) Scott *et al.* (1971, 1974), Scott (1974), Scott and Beadling (1974). I will first review Lynen's hypothesis (shown in Fig. 16) and will then discuss the known experimental evidence which verifies it.

The multienzyme, by analogy with fatty acids, has two sulfhydryl groups: one at the periphery of the enzyme (S_p) and one at the center (S_c). Acetylation of the sulfhydryl group (S_p) with acetyl-CoA releases coenzyme A. A similar reaction between malonyl-CoA and S_cH gives the first step: the acetyl group and the malonyl unit are attached on the enzyme. Decarboxylation of the malonyl group, combined with condensation with the acetyl unit, produces the acetoacetyl group on S_c. Because S_c is where the malonyl unit can be attached, the acetoacetyl group has to be transacetylated to S_p. The second malonyl group is loaded onto S_c. Further condensation and decarboxylation

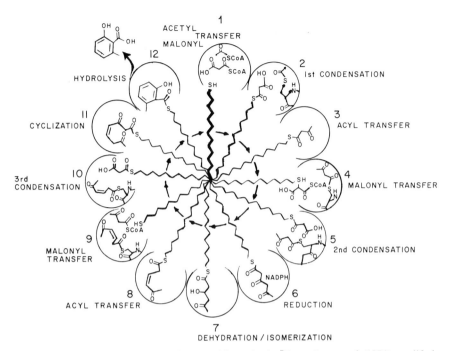

1 ACETYL TRANSFER MALONYL

12 HYDROLYSIS

2 1st CONDENSATION

11 CYCLIZATION

3 ACYL TRANSFER

10 3rd CONDENSATION

4 MALONYL TRANSFER

9 MALONYL TRANSFER

5 2nd CONDENSATION

8 ACYL TRANSFER

6 REDUCTION

7 DEHYDRATION / ISOMERIZATION

Fig. 16. Hypothetical scheme of 6-MSA biosynthesis. [From Scott *et al.* (1974), modified from Dimroth *et al.* (1970), with permission from the authors, *Bioorg. Chem., and Eur. J. Biochem.*]

generate the C_6-polyketo species on the central sulfhydryl group. At this level, Lynen postulates a reduction of one of the keto groups (aided by NADPH), followed by a dehydration, leading directly to the *cis* double bond. To add the third malonyl, the C(6) species is transferred to the peripheral sulfhydryl group. Further reactions involve addition of malonyl-CoA, condensation, internal aldol reaction, and dehydration to give 6-MSA bound as an acyl derivative to the multienzyme. Hydrolysis will regenerate the synthetase and liberate 6-MSA. The idea is that all the reactions occur on that multienzyme with the peripheral SH as part of a flexible long arm (4′-phosphopantotheine) which brings the groups closer to the active site. It is very similar to the multienzyme proposed by Lynen for the fatty acids biosynthesis. The experimental evidence in favor of this scheme is discussed below.

1. Sulfhydryl Groups on the Multienzyme

6-MSA synthetase is inhibited by N-ethyl maleimide and by iodoacetamide (Dimroth *et al.*, 1970; Scott *et al.*, 1971); this suggests that the synthetase contains sulfhydryl groups in the active sites. The presence of two SH groups is inferred (Dimroth *et al.*, 1972) by inhibition kinetics of the 6-MSA synthetase with iodoacetamide and *N*-ethylmaleimide at different pH values. Yeast fatty acid synthetase had also been shown to contain 2 SH sites (Lynen, 1967a,b).

2. Flexible Arm on the Multienzyme

The 4′-phosphopantotheine residue has been identified as part of the enzyme (Dimroth *et al.*, 1972). This identifies the same "acyl carrier" flexible arm which has been isolated in fatty acid synthetase from yeast and *Escherichia coli*.

3. Analogy between 6-Methylsalicylic Acid Synthetase and Yeast Fatty Acid Synthetase

(a) The 6-MSA synthetase isolated from *P. patulum* has many similarities to the fatty acid synthetase from yeast or from *P. patulum*. All these three enzymes are stable multienzymes of high molecular weight.

(b) All the three enzymes are inhibited by iodoacetamide and *N*-ethylmaleimide (Dimroth *et al.*, 1970; Holtermüller *et al.*, 1970; Lynen, 1967a,b; Scott *et al.*, 1971, 1974). Electron microscopy showed a great similarity between the 6-MSA synthetase and the fatty acid multienzyme isolated from yeast (Lynen *et al.*, 1968).

(c) The specificity of acetyl-CoA as a starter group has been checked by substituting it with propionyl-CoA, butyryl-CoA, or hexanoyl-CoA (Dimroth *et al.*, 1976). The higher homologue 6-ethylsalicylic acid is produced by 6-MSA synthetase with propionyl-CoA at 13% of the rate of 6-MSA synthesis with acetyl-CoA. This marked reduction in rate shows the specificity of acetyl-CoA as a primer and also shows that 6-MSA is the *in vivo* product. 6-Ethylsalicylic acid is probably a forced metabolite induced by propionyl-CoA.

(d) The 6-MSA synthetase contains an acyl transferase activity (Dimroth *et al.*, 1976). Similarly to fatty acid, 6-MSA synthesis is postulated to start with the transfer of an acetyl unit from acetyl-CoA to the peripheral SH group of the enzyme. This transferase activity has been proved by measuring the translocation of acetyl from acetyl-CoA to pantetheine. This same method has been developed for fatty acid synthetase.

(e) Incubation of 6-MSA synthetase with iodoacetamide, malonyl-CoA, and NADPH without any acetyl-CoA results in 6-MSA synthesis (Dimroth *et al.*, 1976). The rate of synthesis, as expected, is slower than with acetyl-CoA, malonyl-CoA, and NADPH, and slower than without the —SH inhibitor iodoacetamide. This experimental result shows that the addition of iodoacetamide induces a malonyl-CoA decarboxylase activity. The same conclusion has been obtained with fatty acid synthetase.

(f) The main difference between 6-MSA biosynthesis and fatty acids is that the former needs only one reduction for three condensation reactions. In addition, in order to generate 6-MSA, the intermediate after the dehydration must have a *cis* double bond and not the *trans* double bond found in fatty acid biosynthesis. The timing of the reduction and dehydration reactions is, therefore, crucial. Does it occur at a 6-carbon intermediate or at an 8-carbon moiety?

4. Reduction Step in 6-Methylsalicylic Acid Biosynthesis

No intermediate has been found from acetyl-CoA to 6-MSA, and this leads to the assumption that the intermediates stay bound to the SH group of the enzyme. Different research groups (Dimroth *et al.*, 1970; Lynen, 1967a, b; Scott *et al.*, 1971, 1974 found that incubation of 6-MSA synthetase with acetyl-CoA and malonyl-CoA without NADPH leads to the accumulation of triacetic acid lactone (**23**) (TAL in Fig. 17). This experimental result has first been considered as evidence that the reduction occurs at the triacetic acid [C(6)] level (Lynen, 1967a,b; Dimroth *et al.*, 1970). Scott *et al.* (1971, 1974) explain why this experiment does not prove the reduction timing. In fatty acids, the reduction step occurs at the C(4) intermediate, but omission of NADPH also leads to triacetic acid lactone. In addition, the fatty acid synthetase from *E. coli* (Brock and Bloch, 1966), as well as 6-MSA synthetase from *P. patulum*, produces a small amount of TAL in the presence of NADPH. Therefore, TAL can be considered a derailment product (Fig. 17) which does not reflect the reduction timing.

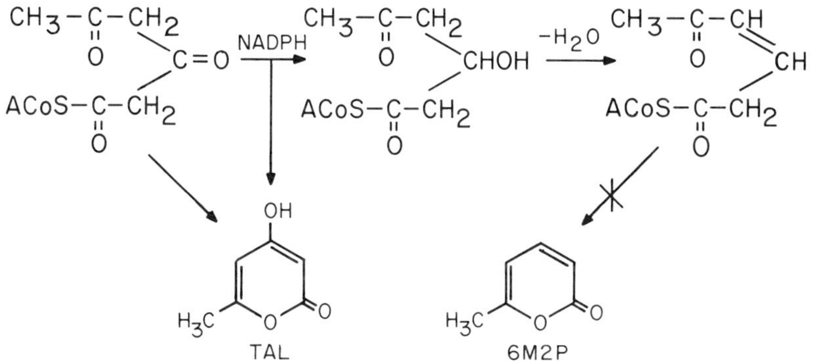

Fig. 17. Derailment products of 6-MSA synthetase. Abbreviations defined in text; modified after Scott *et al.* (1971) and Dimroth *et al.* (1976).

A model compound, ethyl 3,5-diketohexanoate, has been shown to be reduced by NADPH in the 6-MSA synthetase cell-free system (Dimroth *et al.*, 1972). This result could be considered as evidence for reduction at the 6-carbon level; however, experimental details for this conversion are not yet available. 6-Methyl-2-pyrone (**24**) (6M2P in Fig. 17) has been predicted (Dimroth *et al.*, 1976) as a derailment product arising after reduction and dehydration of the C_6 species and prior to the addition of the third malonyl-CoA. A drastic reduction in malonyl-CoA concentration has not permitted the detection of 6-methyl-2-pyrone. This compound would have indicated that in this species ketohexenoic acid might be involved.

5. Dehydration Step in 6-MSA Biosynthesis

Scott *et al.* (1971, 1974) have found that the enzymatic synthesis of 6-MSA could be inhibited by the following acetylenic inhibitors: 3-hexynoyl-*N*-acetylcysteamine, 2-hexynoyl-*N*-acetylcysteamine, and 3-pentynoyl-*N*-acetylcysteamine at very low concentrations (10^{-5} M). This result is similar to the studies obtained by Brock and Bloch (1966), who found that 3-decynoyl-*N*-acetylcysteamine at low concentrations inhibits the unsaturated fatty acid synthetase of *E. coli*. The mechanism of action has been shown to be the inhibition of the enzyme β-hydroxydecanoyl thioester dehydrase. 3-Decynoyl-*N*-acetylcysteamine has been shown by Brock and Bloch (1966)

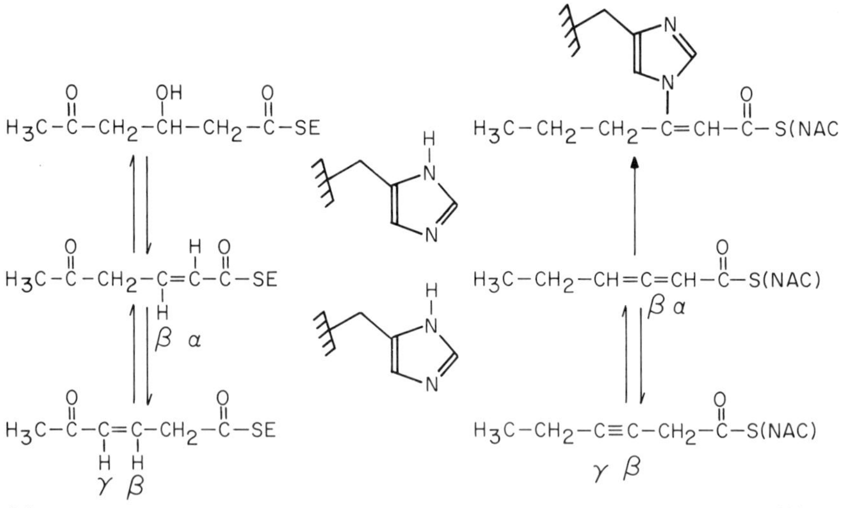

Fig. 18.   Mechanism of action of the 6-MSA dehydrase. [From Scott *et al.* (1974) with permission from the senior author and *Bioorg. Chem.*]

to bind covalently to a histidine site on the enzyme. It has also been shown that the acetylenic inhibitor is probably converted to the allene, which then binds to the histidyl site of the enzyme. By analogy, Scott *et al.* (1974) suggests the same mechanism for their inhibitors (Fig. 18). After reduction, the C(6) intermediate is dehydrated to α,β-enoyl, which then isomerizes to the β,γ substrate. The allene, as well as the acetylenic inhibitors therefore, will block this dehydration.

In order to clarify the timing of this dehydration, Scott *et al.* (1974) have studied the oxidation of NADPH to NADP$^+$ in the presence of the acetylenic inhibitor. These studies show that (a) at an acetylenic inhibitor concentration ($10^{-4}M$) which completely blocks 6-MSA synthesis, there is still a noticeable oxidation of NADPH to NADP$^+$; and (b) when N-ethylmaleimide is used at a concentration that completely blocks 6-MSA synthesis, there is no oxidation of NADPH to NADP$^+$. This experimental evidence suggests that the acetylenic inhibitor must act after the reduction step. These inhibition studies can, therefore, be considered indirect proof that the reduction step does not occur at the C(8) carbon, but probably at the C(6) stage.

In conclusion, 6-MSA is perhaps the only system that has been so extensively investigated at the enzymatic level. The various steps involved in its biosynthesis are, however, not verified and more research is needed.

B.   Acetate → Orsellinic Acid

Early studies (Birch *et al.*, 1958) of the biosynthesis of penicillic acid in *P. cyclopium* with [2-^{14}C]acetate have postulated the intermediacy of orsellinic acid (**17**). Orsellinic acid is the classic example of an aromatic compound produced by the polyketide pathway. Indeed, it is formed by aldol condensation of a tetraacetyl unit with no further modifications (Fig. 19).

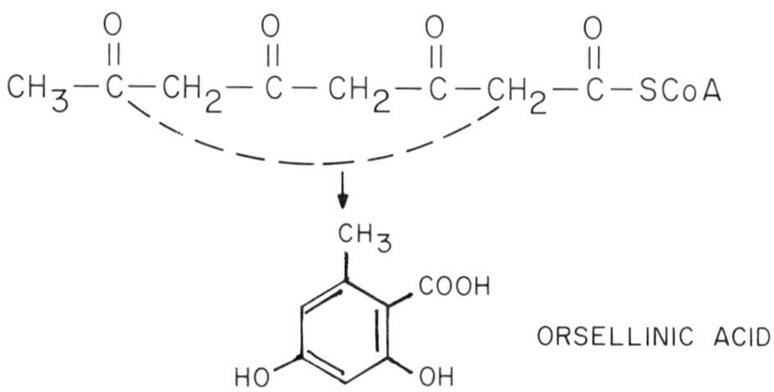

Fig. 19.   Origin of orsellinic acid.

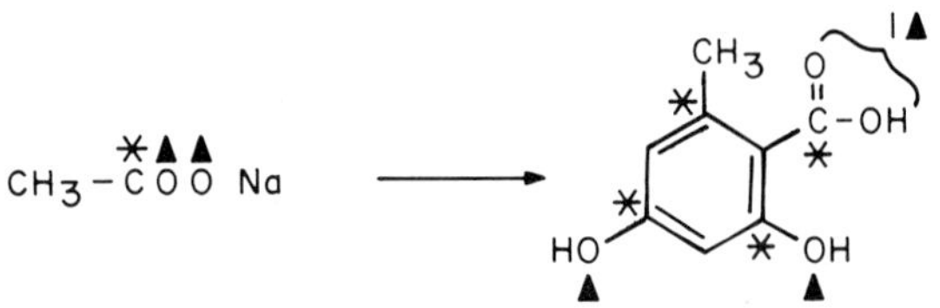

Fig. 20. Labeling distribution of CH_3-$^{14}C^{18}O^{18}O$Na-derived orsellinic acid, modified after Gatenbeck and Mosback (1959). $* = {}^{14}C$, ▲ $= {}^{18}O$.

Orsellinic acid has been known for a long time in lichens; however, it has first been found to be a fungal product in the culture filtrate of *Chaetomium cochliodes* Pall (Mosbach, 1959). Orsellinic acid is the center of a crucial basic experiment performed by Gatenbeck and Mosbach (1959). These investigators have demonstrated that a polyketo acid can be the intermediate between acetate and aromatic compounds. The feeding of $CH_3{}^{14}C^{18}O^{18}O$Na to the fungi has shown that ^{18}O is retained in orsellinic acid. The two hydroxyls incorporated one ^{18}O, whereas the carboxylic acid which arises from hydrolysis of bonds —CO—SCoA shows one ^{18}O distributed between the two oxygens (Fig. 20). This experiment also shows that there is no exchange of the oxygens at the polyketo stage. Orsellinic acid has been shown to be a cometabolite of penicillic acid in *Penicillium barnense* (Mosbach, 1960) and *P. cyclopium* (Bentley and Kiel, 1961). The condensation of one acetyl and three malonyl units is proved by degradation of [1-^{14}C]acetate and [2-^{14}C]malonic acid-derived orsellinic acid (Mosbach, 1960, 1961; Birkinshaw and Gowland, 1962). Orsellinic acid is biogenetically the simplest acetate-originated aromatic compound; however, isolation and purification of the synthesizing enzyme has proved to be extremely difficult. Indeed, the only partial purification reported at present is of the order of fivefold (fivefold purer than the first crude extract) (Gaucher and Shepherd, 1968). Acetyl-CoA is required in the cell-free synthesis of orsellinic acid from malonyl-CoA. The instability of the enzyme has hindered further study.

V. SECONDARY TRANSFORMATIONS OF THE AROMATIC PRECURSORS

A. 6-Methylsalicylic Acid → Gentisaldehyde

The development phases which are associated with secondary metabolism are reviewed in Chapter 1 of this volume and will not be dealt with here.

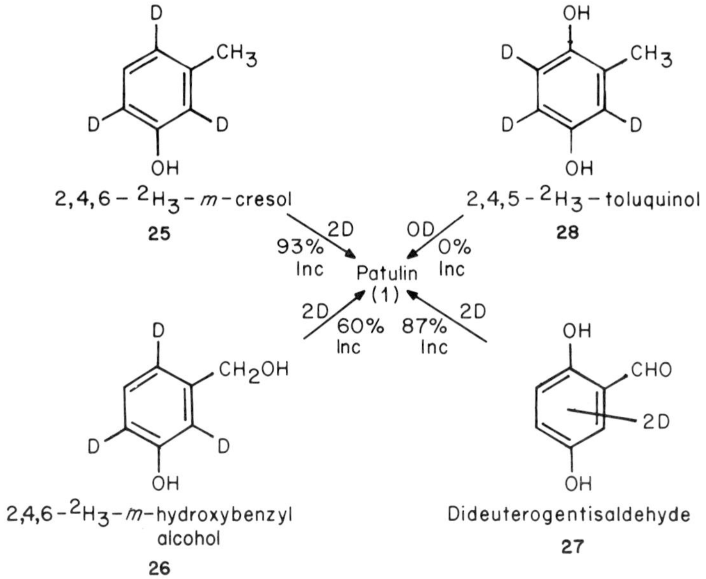

Fig. 21. Conversion of ring-deuterated aromatic metabolites into patulin. [From Zamir (1973) and Scott *et al.* (1973), with permission from the senior author and *Bioorg. Chem.*]

The study of the appearance of the metabolites has been extended by Forrester and Gaucher (1972a,b). These investigators have followed the disappearance of ^{14}C- and ^{3}H-labeled putative precursors and the formation of the intermediates with time. Transient intermediates could therefore be differentiated from end products, and a qualitative mechanism has been formulated. We have confirmed most of these results by *in vivo* experiments with ring-deuterated aromatic precursors (Scott and Yalpani, 1967; Zamir, 1973; Scott *et al.*, 1973). Our results are summarized in Fig. 21. $[2,4,6-^2H_3]$-*m*-Cresol (25) and $[2,4,6-^2H_3]$-*m*-hydroxybenzyl alcohol (26) are converted into dideuteropatulin with 93% and with 60% incorporations, respectively. The loss of one deuterium in these conversions implies that during the parahydroxylation to give the gentisaldehyde species, no NIH shift (Auret *et al.*, 1971) is observed (i.e., the deuterium is not retained by a shift to the carbon adjacent to the hydroxylation site). Dideuterogentis-aldehyde (ring deuterated) (27) has been converted *in vivo* into dideutero-patulin. In contrast, $[2,4,5-^2H_3]$toluquinol (28) has not been incorporated into patulin (Fig. 21).

A representative example of the mass spectrometry analysis is included in Table I.

TABLE I

Feeding of Ring-Deuterated *m*-Hydroxybenzyl Alcohol into Patulin[a]

Compound fed	$\% \, d_0$	$\% \, d_1$	$\% \, d_2$	$\% \, d_3$	$\% \, D$	NMR	$\%$ Incorporated
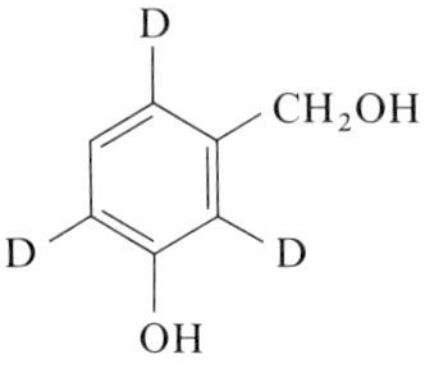 **26** Isolated (ring-deuterated *m*-hydroxybenzyl alcohol structure)	5.6	10.5	—	83.9	87.4	95	—
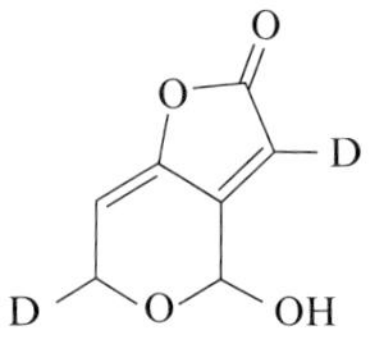 (deuterated patulin structure)	33.2	6.5	60.2	—	54.4	—	60
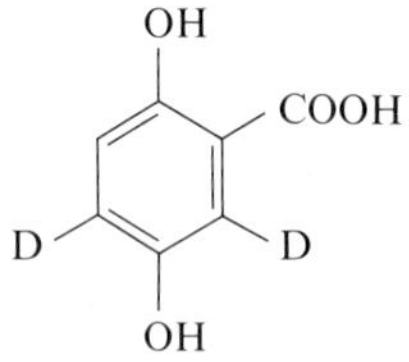 **10** (deuterated hydroxybenzoic acid structure)	27.1	10.1	58.6	—	66.4	—	73

[a] From L. Zamir (1973) and Scott *et al.* (1973), with permission from the senior author and *Bioorg. Chem.* $\%d_0$, d_1, d_2, and d_3 represent the percent enrichment in deuterium obtained from mass spectrometry at the molecular ion (M_0), at $M + 1$, $M + 2$, and $M + 3$, respectively, corrected for the natural abundances at $M + 1$, $M + 2$. $\%D \equiv \% \, ^2H$ mass spectrometry, and represents the total percent enrichment in deuterium relative to the exchangeable hydrogens; therefore, it can be compared to the $\% \, ^2H$ obtained from NMR: $\%$ Incorporated $= \% \, ^2H$ patulin/$\% \, ^2H$ precursor.

Patulin resulting from the feeding of $[2,4,6\text{-}^2H_3]$-*m*-cresol (**25**), $[2,4,6\text{-}^2H_3]$-*m*-hydroxybenzyl alcohol (**26**), and ring-deuterated dideuterogentisaldehyde (**27**) also has an unusual property: it is optically active (Fig. 22) (Scott and Yalpani, 1967; Scott, *et al.*, 1973; Zamir, 1973).

Patulin obtained from natural sources is racemic. The only new center which can become chiral by the introduction of deuterium is C(5) (Fig. 23). The absolute configuration of dideuteropatulin has not yet been determined.

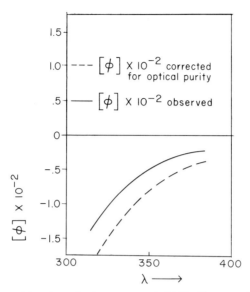

Fig. 22. Optical activity of patulin-d_2. From Zamir (1973). The curves in Fig. 25 show the observed molecular rotation and the mean value corrected for optical purity. The mean values obtained for deuterated patulin obtained from $[2,4,6\text{-}^2\mathrm{H}_3]$-$m$-hydroxybenzyl alcohol were as follows: $C = 0.0606$ gm/ 100ml, $[\phi]_{385} - 38°$, $[\phi]_{315} - 224°$. The $[\phi]_\lambda$ was calculated from: $[\phi]_\lambda = ([\phi]_{max} + [\phi]_{min})/2$, where $[\phi]_{max} = \phi$ observed $\times (100/\%\,d_2)$ and $[\phi]_{min} = \phi$ observed $\times [100/\% \, (d_1 + d_2)]$. The percentage deuterium content is shown in Table I. The molecular rotation of deuterated patulin was taken from this species, as it can be seen that the d_1 content was relatively small and gives a small range of values for the maximum and the minimum, thus giving the nearest possible approximation to the absolute molecular rotation for deuterated patulin.

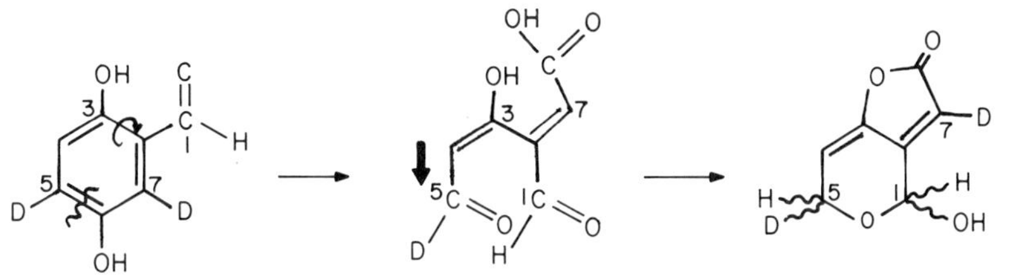

5,7–Dideuterogentisaldehyde   **29**   5,7–Dideuteropatulin

28   **30**

Fig. 23. Formation of dideuteropatulin. From Zamir (1973).

The last intermediate in the biosynthesis of patulin has been verified at the enzymatic level to be gentisaldehyde by Scott and Beadling (1974). $[2,4,6-^2H_3]$-m-Cresol (**25**) and $[2,4,6-^2H_3]$-m-hydroxybenzyl alcohol (**26**) will, therefore, eventually lead to $[5,7-^2H_2]$gentisaldehyde (**28**). $[5,7-^2H_2]$ Gentisaldehyde is cleaved by a dioxygenase to give the hypothetical intermediate (**29**) (Fig. 23). Stereospecific reduction at C(5) is followed by cyclization and lactonization to give $[5,7-^2H_2]$patulin (**30**). Toluquinol (**11**) is a cometabolite of patulin in *P. patulum*. The hydroxylase catalyzing the conversion of *m*-cresol to toluquinol has been partially purified and characterized (Murphy *et al.*, 1974). Toluquinol is not an intermediate in the patulin sequence. Indeed, $[2,4,5-^2H_3]$- and tritiated toluquinol (**28**) have not been incorporated into patulin (Scott and Yalpani, 1967; Scott *et al.*, 1973; Zamir, 1973; Forrester and Gaucher, 1972a,b) (Fig. 21). A new optically active compound has been obtained from that feeding (Scott and Yalpani, 1967; Scott, *et al.*, 1973; Zamir, 1973). A large-scale incubation of cold toluquinol has permitted the isolation of this derailment product. The structure and stereochemistry of this new epoxide that we named deoxyepoxidon are discussed in Section VII.

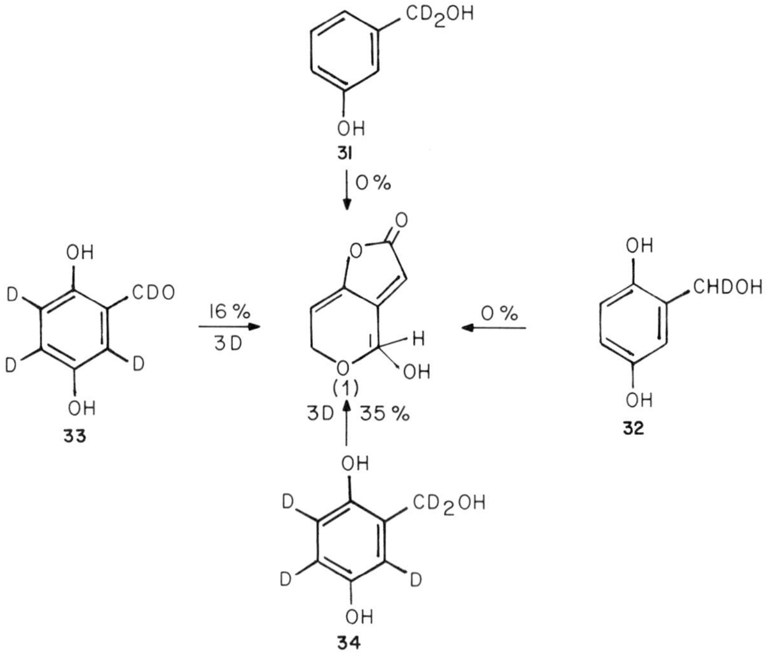

Fig. 24.   Conversion of side-chain-deuterated aromatic metabolites into patulin. [From Scott *et al.* (1973) with permission from the senior author and *Bioorg. Chem.*]

In order to obtain a complete picture of the detailed mechanism, we have analyzed the side-chain protons of the aromatic metabolites (Scott *et al.*, 1973; Zamir, 1973). $[1',1'-^2H_2]$-*m*-Hydroxybenzyl alcohol (**31**), $[1'-^2H]$ gentisyl-alcohol (**32**), $[2,4,5, (1')-^2H_4-]$gentisaldehyde (**33**), and $[2,4,5, (1',1')-^2H_5]$ gentisyl alcohol (**34**) have been fed to *P. patulum* (Fig. 24). The surprising result is that the side-chain-substituted deuteriums in the aromatic precursors are lost in the conversion to patulin (**1**) (Fig. 24). Ring-deuterated gentisaldehyde and gentisyl alcohol are positively incorporated, whereas the side-chain deuteriums are washed out. The side-chain protons have been shown not to be washed out during the work-up (Scott *et al.*, 1973; Zamir, 1973). Furthermore, the side-chain deuteriums are not lost at the aromatic stage before the conversion to patulin. Indeed, the feeding of $[1',1'-^2H_2]$-*m*-hydroxybenzyl alcohol (**31**) has enabled us to isolate dideuterogentisyl alcohol with the same enrichment in deuteriums. An attractive explanation for the loss of the side-chain deuteriums involves patulin lactone (**35**) (Scheme 1), a compound which has not yet been found in *P. patulum*. The assumption which has yet to be verified is that as soon as patulin is produced by the mold, it is in equilibrium with its oxidized from, patulin lactone.

The *in vivo* experiments using "whole cells" of *P. patulum* and tritiated or deuterated intermediates were verified at the enzymatic level. Scheme 1 represents the biosynthesis of patulin. The decarboxylation of 6-MSA (**4**) is the first step in the sequence. Indeed, isolation of 6-MSA decarboxylase (E_1) and its partial purification has verified this step *in vitro* (Light, 1969; Light and Vogel, 1975). The second step in the biosynthetic sequence is the hydroxylation of *m*-cresol (**6**) to *m*-hydroxybenzylalcohol (**7**). This second step has also been verified at the enzymatic level (E_2) (Murphy *et al.*, 1974). The oxygenase (E_4) involved in the bioconversion of *m*-hydroxybenzyl-alcohol (**7**) (Scheme 1) to gentisyl alcohol (**8**) has been characterized by Murphy and Lynen (1975). The dehydrogenase involved in the formation of gentisaldehyde (**9**) from gentisyl alcohol (**8**) has also been partially purified (Scott and Beadling, 1974). Forrester and Gaucher (1972a,b) found that ring-tritiated gentisyl alcohol was not incorporated into patulin. In our hands (Fig. 24), however, ring-deuterated gentisyl alcohol (**34**) was a precursor. As the last step involves gentisaldehyde (**9**) (Scott and Beadling, 1974), the positive incorporation of gentisyl alcohol must involve a dehydrogenation step. The enzymes involved in the synthesis of toluquinol (**11**) (E_3) (Murphy *et al.*, 1974), of *m*-hydroxybenzaldehyde (**13**) (E_5) (Scott and Beadling, 1974; Forrester and Gaucher, 1972a,b), and of *m*-hydroxybenzoic acid (E_6) (Murphy and Lynen, 1975) have also been characterized. The oxygenase (E_7) was purified and was shown to catalyze the conversion of gentisaldehyde to patulin in the presence of O_2 and NADPH (see Scheme 1) (Scott and Beadling, 1974).

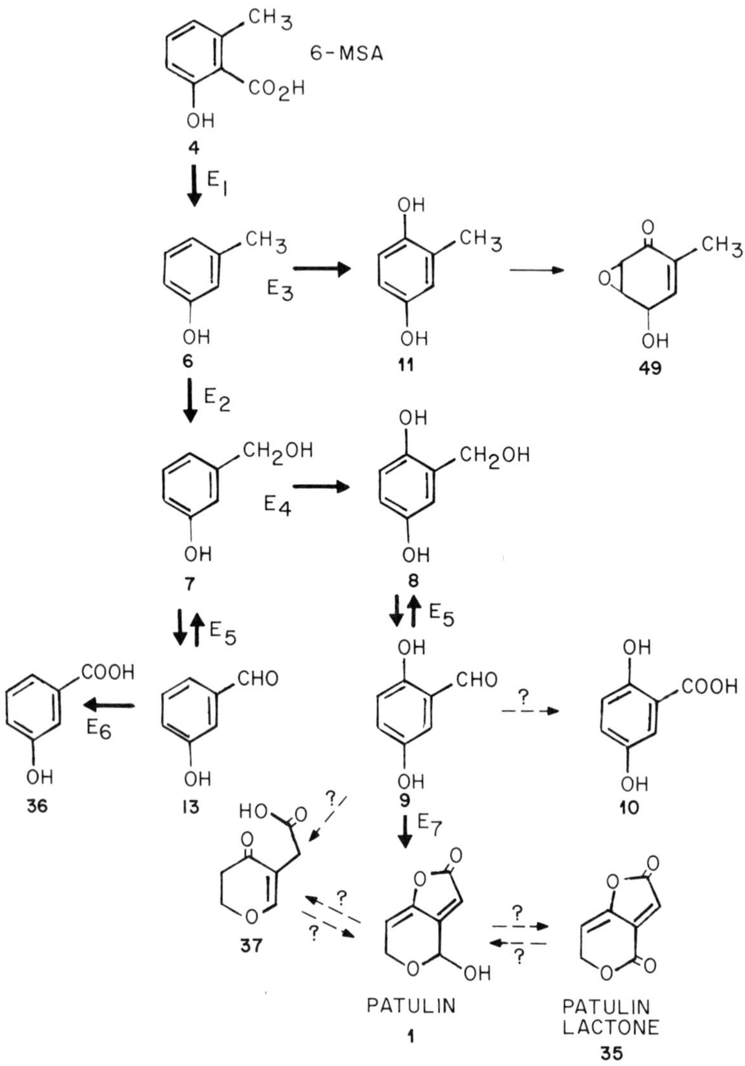

Scheme 1. Proposed pathway of patulin biosynthesis. This figure is modified after the various experimental results obtained from different research groups (Zamir, 1973; Scott *et al.*, 1973; Light, 1969; Light and Vogel, 1975; Murphy *et al.*, 1974; Scott and Beadling, 1974; Murphy and Lynen, 1975; Forrester and Gaucher, 1972).

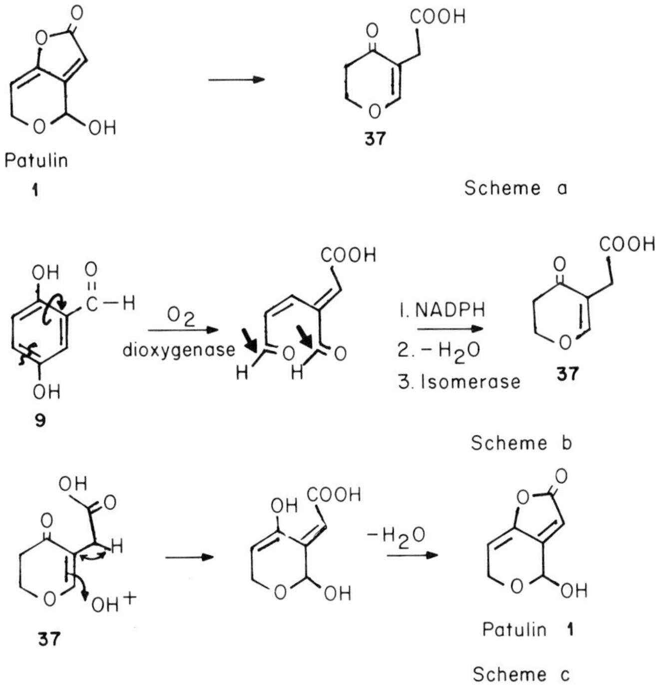

Fig. 25.   Postulated mechanisms for the intermediacy of deoxypatulinic acid.

Scheme 1 also includes deoxypatulinic acid (37) (Scheme 1), which has been shown to be a cometabolite of patulin in *P. patulum* (Scott *et al.*, 1972). The questions that arise are the following: Is it an end product of patulin (1) metabolism? Is it an end product of gentisaldehyde (9) metabolism? Or is it an intermediate between gentisaldehyde (9) and patulin (1)? These three biogenetic mechanisms are described in Fig. 25. Scheme a represents the metabolism of patulin (reduction). Scheme b would involve extensive reduction of the cleavage product of gentisaldehyde followed by dehydration and isomerization. Deoxypatulinic acid (37) either could be an end product or could be converted to patulin as outlined in scheme c.

B. Orsellinic Acid → Substituted Derivative

Several aromatic compounds have been postulated as plausible intermediates between orsellinic acid (17) and penicillic acid (2). Axberg and Gatenbeck (1975a,b) have provided experimental evidence involving intermediates beyond orsellinic acid. Putative precursors have been synthesized

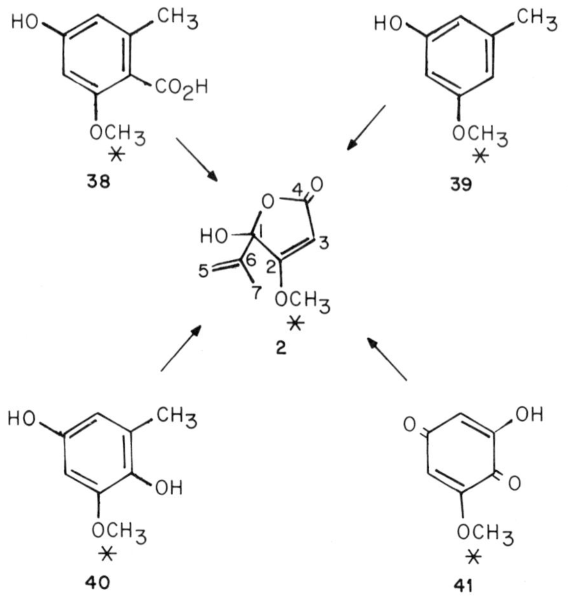

Fig. 26. Conversion of labeled six-membered ring putative precursors into penicillic acid, modified after Axberg and Gatenbeck (1975).

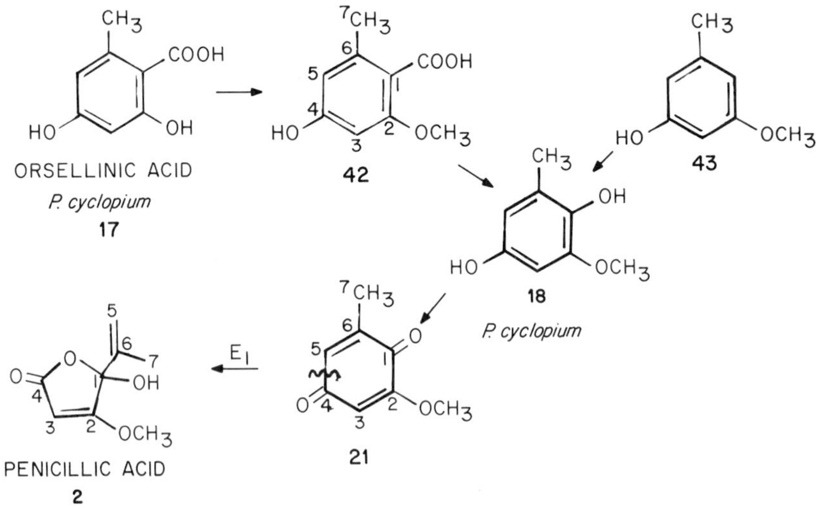

Fig. 27. Proposed pathway for penicillic acid formation, modified after Axberg and Gatenbeck (1975).

with a radioisotope on a specific carbon. The labeled aromatic compounds which are positively incorporated into penicillic acid are 2-O-[^{14}CH$_3$] orsellinic acid (**38**) (Fig. 26); 1-O-[^{14}CH$_3$]orcinol (**39**) (Fig. 26); 6-O-[^{14}CH$_3$]-2-CH$_3$-benzoquinone (1,4) (**40**) (Fig. 26); and 1,4-dihydroxy-6-O-[^{14}CH$_3$]-2-methylbenzene (**41**) (Fig. 26). Degradation of the resulting penicillic acid has located the radioisotope on the methoxy group at C(2). Radioactive dilution (Better and Gatenbeck, 1976) has demonstrated that compound (**18**) (Fig. 27) is a cometabolite of penicillic acid in *P. cyclopium*. Axberg and Gatenbeck (1975a,b) have partially purified a cell-free preparation which could convert 3-methoxytoluquinone (**21**) *in vitro* to penicillic acid in the presence of O$_2$ and NADPH.

The following pathway for the secondary transformations of orsellinic acid (**17**) has been postulated (Fig. 27): The first step is a selective methylation of one hydroxyl group to give **42**. Oxidative decarboxylation of **42** generates **18**. Compound **18** can also be formed from methoxyorcinol (**43**) (Fig. 27). Further oxidation of **18** yields compound **21**, which will be oxidatively cleaved to penicillic acid (**2**). The enzyme E$_1$ has been partially purified and has been shown to catalyze this reaction.

VI. CLEAVAGE OF THE AROMATIC PRECURSORS

A. Substrates

In vivo experiments with radioisotopes and deuterated intermediates have suggested that gentisaldehyde is the substrate for the oxidative cleavage which produces patulin (Scott *et al.*, 1973; Forrester and Gaucher, 1972a,b). Isolation of the enzyme catalyzing this conversion *in vitro* has confirmed the conclusions of this study (Scott and Beadling, 1974). This partially purified enzymatic preparation requires O$_2$, and NADPH, is stimulated by ATP, and is inhibited by Fe^{2+} chelators. In the biosynthesis of penicillic acid, 3-methoxytoluquinone (**21**) has been indicated to be the substrate for the oxidative cleavage (Axberg and Gatenbeck, 1975a,b; Better and Gatenbeck, 1976). Verification has involved the isolation of the enzyme complex that can catalyze the ring cleavage of 3-methoxytoluquinone and forms penicillic acid. As a typical oxygenase, this enzyme requires O$_2$, and NADPH and is stimulated by flavin mononucleotide (FMN) and Fe^{2+}.

B. Cleavage Site and Stereochemical Implications

The formation of patulin (**1**) from gentisaldehyde (**9**) is rationalized by cleavage at the site shown in Fig. 28 (⦂). Rotation around C(2)–C(3) yields intermediate **44**. We have seen that 5,7-dideuterogentisaldehyde (**28**) has generated optical activity in patulin (**30**) owing to a stereospecific reduction at C(5) (see Fig. 23). The absolute stereochemistry at C(5) in the dideuteropatulin (**30**) has not yet been determined. It would be interesting to synthesize a different diastereomer of patulin (**45**) by using the enzyme complex, O_2, $NADP^2H_2$, and ATP to catalyze the ring cleavage of cold gentisaldehyde (Fig. 28). ^2H NMR might be an important tool to help elucidate the absolute configuration of optically active deuterated patulin.

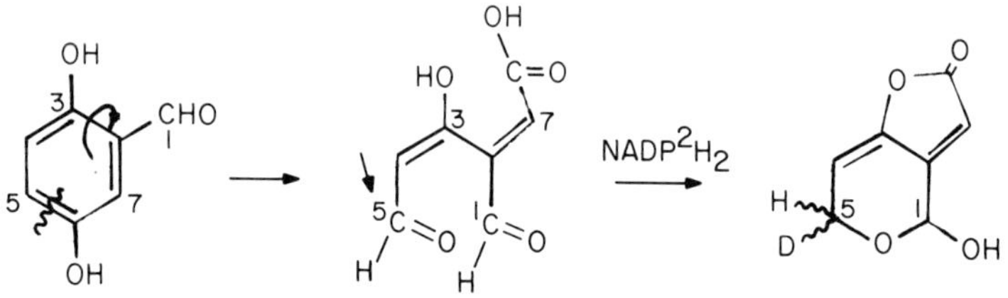

Fig. 28. Postulated formation of a different diastereomer of deuterated patulin.

The formation of penicillic acid can be explained mechanistically by cleavage at two different sites. The cleavage site has been demonstrated by Mosbach since 1960. Recently, this result has been confirmed by ^{13}C NMR studies (Seto *et al.*, 1974), as well as ^3H NMR investigations (Al-Rawi *et al.*, 1974; Elvidge *et al.*, 1977). Because additional mechanistic as well as stereochemical implications have been deduced, these results will be discussed in detail.

Seto *et al.* (1974) have employed their original technique based on ($^{13}C,^{13}C$) coupling (Seto *et al.*, 1973) in order to establish the "intact" acetate units. The enriched [^{13}C]penicillic acid resulting from the feeding of sodium [1,2-^{13}C]acetate is isolated and purified. The ^{13}C NMR spectrum of the enriched penicillic acid has shown ($^{13}C,^{13}C$)couplings between C(2) and C(3), as we as between C(6) and C(7). Therefore, C(2)–C(3), as well as C(6)–C(7), represent intact acetate units (heavy lines in Fig. 29). This result confirms that the cleavage site in the aromatic intermediate (orsellinic acid or, more probably 3-methoxytoluquinone) is between C(4) and C(5) (Fig. 29,). The ^{13}C NMR spectrum of the enriched penicillic acid also shows a slight coupling between C(5) and C(6). To explain this experimental result, the investigators (Seto *et al.*, 1974) have postulated the formation of two differently labeled penicillic acids (A and B) (**46**) and (**47**) (Fig. 29), where penicillic acid A is the predominant form. Penicillic acid B is assumed to originate from the A form by slight isomerization of the double bond at an undetermined step in the biosynthetic pathway.

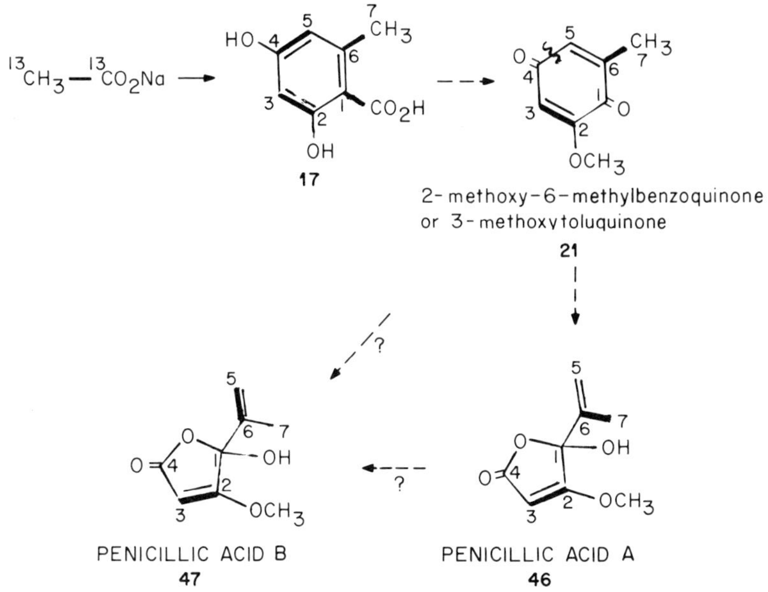

Fig. 29. Labeling distribution of ($^{13}CH_3$–$^{13}CO_2NA$)-derived penicillic acid, modified after Seto *et al.* (1974).

The ^3H NMR of the [^3H]acetate-derived penicillic acid (Al-Rawi *et al.*, 1974; Elvidge *et al.*, 1977) has shown ^3H incorporations at C(3), C(5), and C(7). This result also confirms that ring scission occurs at C(4)–C(5). Following the specific NMR assignments (Elvidge *et al.*, 1977) for H_a and H_b at C(5), the incorporation of ^3H has been shown to be entirely on H_b, i.e., *trans* to the methyl group. Some ^3H has also been found on H_a (Fig. 30). The predominance of the label on H_b is probably indicative of the stereospecificity of the dehydrogenase that is involved at a later stage in the sequence. The degradation of [^3H]malonate-derived penicillic acid has confirmed that penicillic acid is derived from one acetyl and three malonyl units (Elvidge *et al.*, 1977; Bentley and Keil, 1962).

Fig. 30. Structure of penicillic acid which shows the two distinct methine protons at C(5). [From Al-Rawi *et al.* (1974) and Elvidge *et al.* (1977), with permission from the senior authors and *J. Chem. Soc.*]

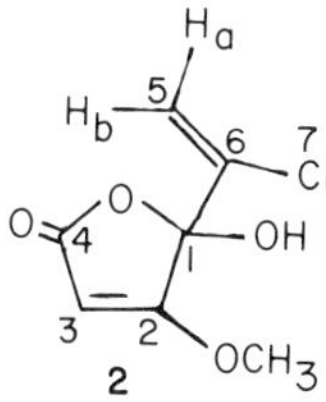

VII. DERAILMENT METABOLITES

The feeding of a putative precursor can sometimes result in the production of an unusual metabolite which otherwise is not a natural product. This metabolite does not represent the *in vivo* processes and is only a derailment product or "forced" metabolite. In the case of patulin and penicillic acid, these derailment products are 6-ethylsalicylic acid, homoorsellinic acid, and deoxyepoxidon.

A. Homoorsellinic Acid

Early studies of Mosbach (1964) have shown that addition of radioactive sodium propionate to *P. barnense* yields a new radioactive metabolite. Synthesis and chemical degradations show this compound to be the higher homologue of orsellinic acid (17). This compound, called homoorsellinic acid (47), is not a natural metabolite of *P. barnense* (Mosbach, 1964). It is a product of a "forced" feeding: propionyl-CoA has replaced acetyl-CoA as a starter unit (Fig. 31). Two possible explanations can be considered: Either sodium propionate has induced a new enzyme to form this homo acid, or its biosynthesis involves the same enzyme complex responsible for orsellinic acid formation.

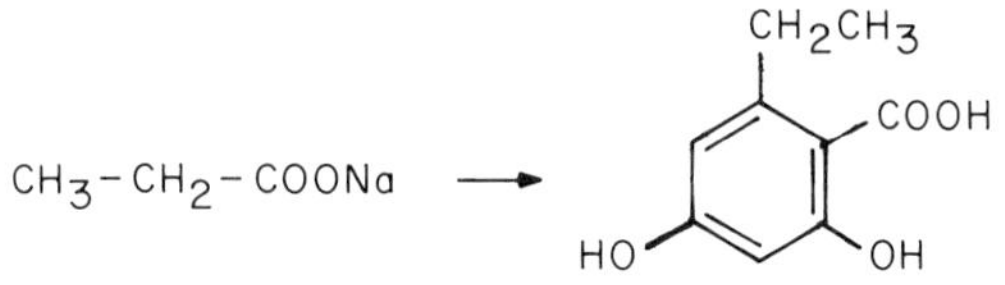

$$CH_3-CH_2-COONa \longrightarrow$$

HOMOORSELLINIC ACID
47

Fig. 31.   Formation of homoorsellinic acid, modified after Mosbach (1964).

B. 6-Ethylsalicylic Acid

Recently, Dimroth and co-workers (1976) have studied the specificity of the multienzyme 6-MSA synthetase for the starter unit: acetyl-CoA. Replacement of acetyl-CoA with the higher homologue propionyl-CoA has resulted in the formation of 6-ethylsalicylic acid (48) (Fig. 32) (6-ESA). This result is very similar to the homoorsellinic acid synthesis (Mosbach, 1964). Homoorsellinic acid (47) is, however, a result of *in vivo* experiments with sodium propionate, whereas 6-ESA (48) is formed *in vitro* with the purified 6-MSA synthetase. We can conclude, therefore, that derailment compounds must involve the same enzyme complex as the corresponding natural metabolites.

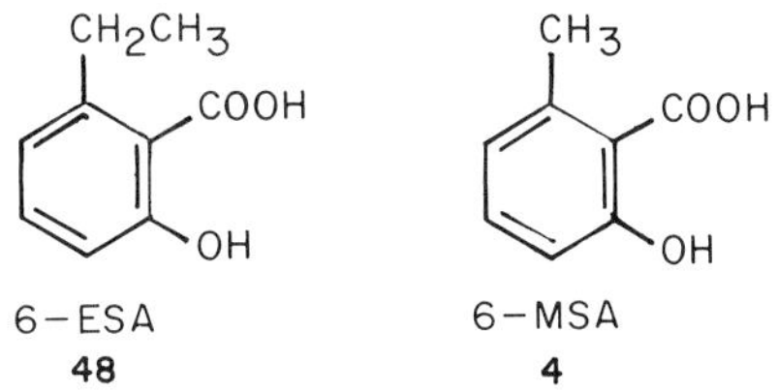

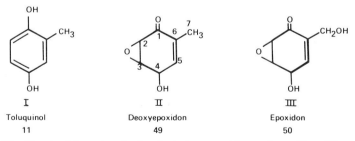

Fig. 32. Structural formulas of 6-ethylsalicylic acid and 6-methylsalicylic acid.

C. Deoxyepoxidon

Deuterotoluquinol is not incorporated into patulin (Scott *et al.*, 1973; Zamir, 1973), and an unknown optically active compound is produced. From the feeding of cold toluquinol we could isolate this new compound, which is not known as a metabolite of *P. patulum*. It must have been biosynthesized from the "forced" feeding of toluquinol. The structure of this derailment product is assigned as **49** (Fig. 33) on the basis of the following evidence. Mass spectrometry has established the exact molecular weight as $C_7H_8O_3$. In the infrared spectrum, the presence of hydroxyl (3410 cm^{-1}) and α,β-unsaturated ketone (1655 cm^{-1}) is inferred. This latter assignment is in accord with the ultraviolet spectrum: λ_{max} 242 nm (ε 4700). The 100 MHz ^{1}H NMR displays a methyl singlet at $\delta 1.8$, a doublet at $\delta 3.48$ H(2) coupled to H(3) which appears as a multiplet at $\delta 3.8$. H(4) is centered at $\delta 4.72$ and the vinyl H(5) at $\delta 6.46$, both appearing as multiplets. The NMR of this new metabolite has been compared with the NMR assignments for epoxidon (**50**) (Closse *et al.*, 1966) (see Fig. 33), a metabolite of *Phoma* S1019 which also shows H(2) as a doublet ($\delta 3.40$), H(3) at $\delta 3.77$, H(4) at $\delta 4.64$, and H(5) at $\delta 6.42$. The close similarity of these resonances indicates that the new metabolite is in fact deoxyepoxidon (**49**) (Fig. 33).

Deoxyepoxidon is optically active, and from optical rotatory dispersion and circular dichroism analogies of similar compounds we have assigned

Fig. 33. Structural formulas of toluquinol, deoxyepoxidon, and epoxidon. [From Zamir (1973) and Scott *et al.* (1973), with permission from the senior author and *Bioorg. Chem.*]

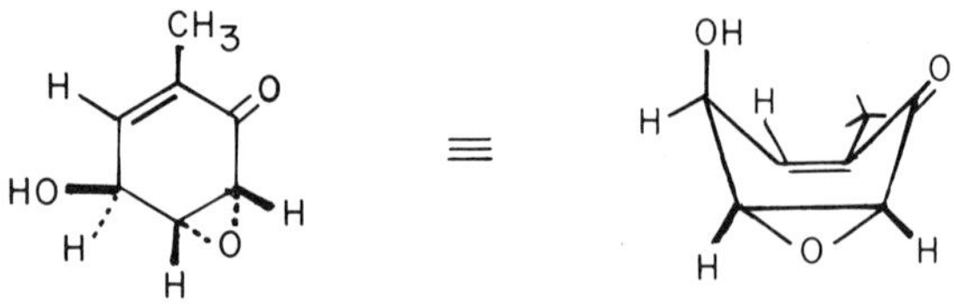

Deoxyepoxidon **49**

Fig. 34. Postulated absolute configuration of deoxyepoxidon. From Zamir (1973).

(Zamir, 1973; A. I. Scott and L. Zamir, unpublished results) the absolute configuration of deoxyepoxidon as shown in Fig. 34.

VIII. METABOLIC GRIDS AND CONCLUDING REMARKS

Patulin and penicillic acid are produced by different fungal species. However, their biosynthetic pathways are very similar. They both arise from enzymatic oxidative cleavage of an aromatic compound derived from one acetyl-CoA and three malonyl extending units. The polyketo chain is modified by a reduction and dehydration prior to internal aldol cyclization to give 6-MSA (**4**), the first aromatic compound in the sequence leading to patulin. The formation of orsellinic acid (**17**) does not involve any modification of the polyketide chain prior to the intramolecular aldol reaction. The 6-MSA synthetase has been extensively purified (190-fold) and investigated. The biosynthesis of 6-MSA is visualized by Lynen's elegant model. The different steps in this model have not yet been verified experimentally. In contrast, the orsellinic acid synthetase has been only partially purified (only 5-fold), and therefore its properties could not be investigated. The metabolic grid leading to patulin (**1**) is shown in Scheme 1.

Most of the steps in Scheme 1 have been established at the enzymatic level (heavy arrows; the enzymes detected are shown above these arrows). The unanswered questions in the biosynthesis of patulin are the following: (a) What is the absolute configuration of the optically active deuteropatulin generated from the feeding of ring-deuterated aromatic precursors? (b) Is deoxypatulinic acid (**37**) in Scheme 1 involved in patulin biosynthesis or in its metabolism? (c) Is patulin-lactone (**35**) a metabolite of *P. patulum*? If not, why are the side-chain deuteriums lost in the conversion of the aromatic precursors into patulin?

The metabolic grid leading to penicillic acid is shown in Fig. 27. Only the last step has been verified at the enzymatic level. The other conversions

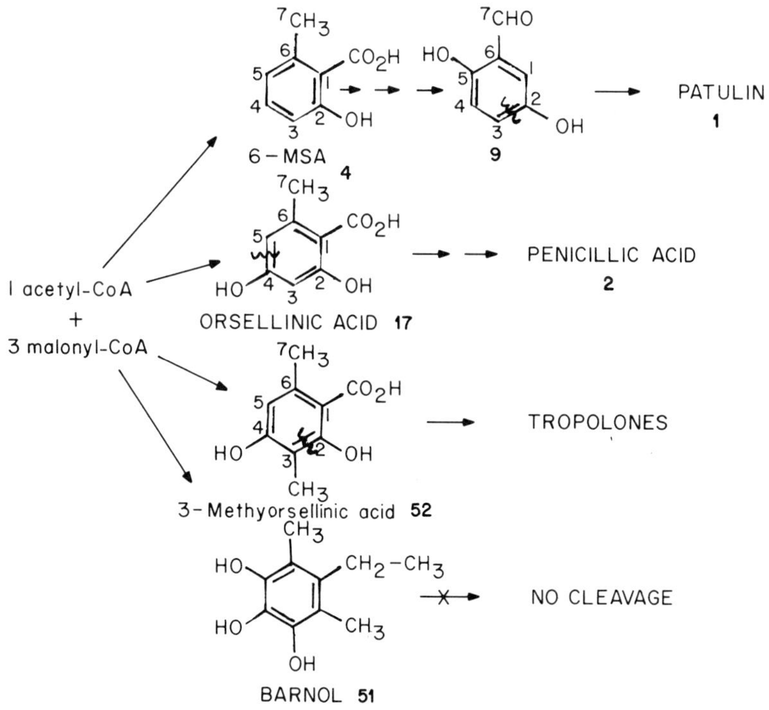

Fig. 35.   Cleavage sites of different aromatic metabolites.

are suggested from *in vivo* experiments with radioisotopic labeled precursors. The only metabolites which have been found at present in *P. cyclopium* are orsellinic acid (**17**), **18**, and penicillic acid (**2**).

Another mold, *P. barnense*, has been shown to produce orsellinic acid, 1,4-dihydroxy-2-methoxy-6-methylbenzene (**18**) (Fig. 27), penicillic acid (**2**), and another aromatic compound, barnol (**51**) (Fig. 35) (Axberg and Gatenbeck, 1975; Better and Gatenbeck, 1976; Mosback and Ljungcrantz, 1965). The amount of secondary metabolites produced has been shown to depend markedly on the culture media. Czapek–Dox produces large amounts of penicillic acid and orsellinic acid and only traces of barnol, whereas Raulin Thom generates mainly barnol. 1,4-Dihydroxy-2-methoxy-6-methylbenzene (**18**) (Fig. 27) is always present, regardless of the medium. Labeling experiments (Ljungcrantz and Mosbach, 1964; Better and Gatenbeck, 1977) have shown that **18** and orsellinic acid (**17**) are not involved in the biosynthesis of barnol. The biosynthesis of penicillic acid (**2**) via orsellinic acid (**17**) in *P. barnense* is unrelated to barnol formation. The only link between these two pathways is the early tetraketide intermediate, which is subjected to various

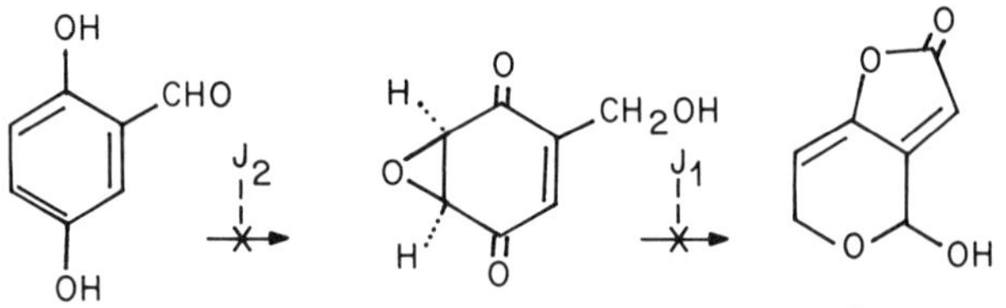

9   53   1
Gentisaldehyde   Phyllostine   PATULIN

Fig. 36. Intermediacy of phyllostine in patulin biosynthesis, modified after Sekiguchi and Gaucher (1978).

secondary reactions prior to aromatization. 2,4-Dihydroxy-6-ethyl-5-methylbenzaldehyde has been shown *in vivo* to be the aromatic precursor to barnol (**51**) (Fig. 35).

The specificity of the oxygenases which cleave aromatic compounds is shown in Fig. 35. Orsellinic acid (**17**) via 3-methoxytoluquinone (**21**) is cleaved at C(4)–C(5) to give penicillic acid (**2**). On the other hand, 3-methylorsellinic acid (**52**) in a different fungus is cleaved at C(2)–C(3) to yield tropolones (Scott and Wiesner, 1972). The methyl group on the aromatic ring, therefore, determines the different cleavage site. If we use the same nomenclature in *P. patulum*, the cleavage is at C(2)–C(3); here, the substrate is gentisaldehyde (**9**). I would not be surprised if the corresponding quinone will be found to be a better substrate for the cleavage enzyme.

More recently, Sekiguchi and Gaucher (1978) isolated from a patulin negative mutant (Pat⁻, J₁) the epoxyquinone (−)-phyllostine (**53**) (Fig. 36). This compound (**53**) was efficiently incorporated into patulin. The authors of this recent paper found a second patulin-negative mutant (J₂) (Fig. 36) which accumulated gentisaldehyde, but no (−)-phyllostine. Addition of cold (−)-phyllostine to this (Pat⁻, J₂) mutant led to the production of patulin. (−)-Phyllostine is, therefore, very probably formed after gentisaldehyde in patulin biosynthesis.

These basic findings lead to interesting mechanistic speculations. Sekiguchi and Gaucher (1978) postulate that phyllostine (**53**) arises from gentisaldehyde (**9**) via an internal oxidation–reduction reaction mediated by a monooxygenase and NADPH (Fig. 37). They then assume that phyllostine is converted by a "simple rearrangement" to a seven-membered ring lactone (**54**) (Fig. 37). Hydrolysis will yield the open form of patulin (**55**) (Fig. 37), which will close to patulin (**1**) by dehydration and hemiacetal formation. They do not elaborate on that simple rearrangement.

The questions that come to mind are: (a) Is phyllostine formed by the same pathway as the forced metabolite deoxyepoxidon? (b) How does this rearrangement occur? (c) Can it adequately explain the experimental results

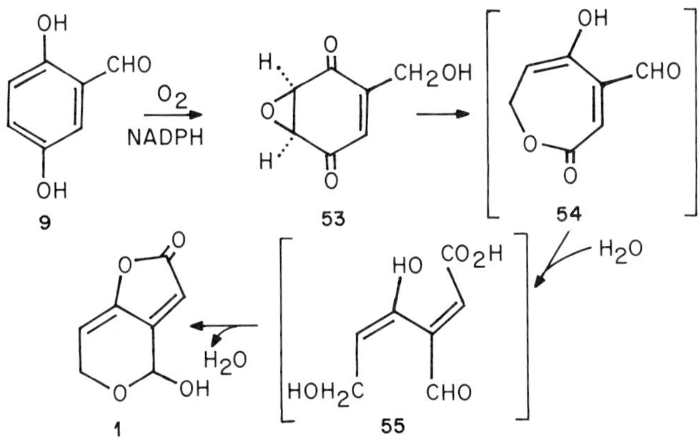

Fig. 37. Postulated mechanism of the conversion of gentisaldehyde to patulin, modified after Sekiguchi and Gaucher (1978).

that ring-deuterated aromatic precursors led to optically active patulin? (d) Can it determine why the aromatic side-chain deuteriums are lost? (e) Could patulin lactone, a postulated intermediate, still be involved? (f) Where does deoxypatulinic acid fit into that suggested biosynthetic scheme?

I will, therefore, suggest a hypothetical scheme describing the conversion of gentisaldehyde (9) into patulin (1), with an attempt to answer these six questions (see Figs. 38–40). I tend to believe that most pathways are complex metabolic grids, and that the patulin biosynthesis is a typical example. By analogy to penicillic acid biosynthesis, where 3-methoxytoluquinone is produced after orsellinic acid, I would first postulate the oxidation of gentisaldehyde (9) to the quinone 56 (Fig. 38). The hypothetical enzyme (E_8) catalyzing this reaction might also be responsible for the oxidation of gentisyl alcohol (8) to the quinone (57) (Fig. 38). The dehydrogenase involved in the reversible conversion of compounds 56 and 57 could be E_5 or a different enzyme. An epoxidase (E_9) could then convert 56 to 58 and 57 to (−)-phyllostine (53). This epoxidase (E_9) could also have been involved in the biosynthesis of the forced metabolite deoxyepoxidon (49) (see Scheme 1). If the dehydrogenase (E_5) is not very specific, then it would also be responsible for the reversible reaction from 58 to phyllostine (53) (Fig. 38).

Specific reduction of the epoxide (58) at position 4 mediated by a dehydrogenase E_{10} and the coenzyme NADPH generates the intermediate 59 (Fig. 39). H_3O^+ will generate the seven-membered ring lactone, 60. This reaction has to be catalyzed by an enzyme, for this prototropy has to be very specific to explain the optical activity of patulin derived from ring-deuterated gentisaldehyde. Reduction of the seven-membered ring lactone 60 in the presence

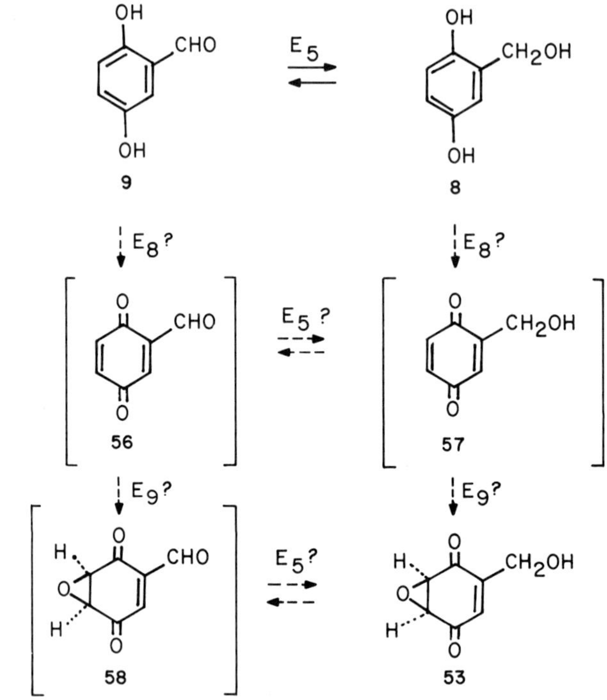

262

Lolita O. Zamir

Fig. 38. Postulated mechanism of the conversion of gentisaldehyde to (−)-phyllostine.

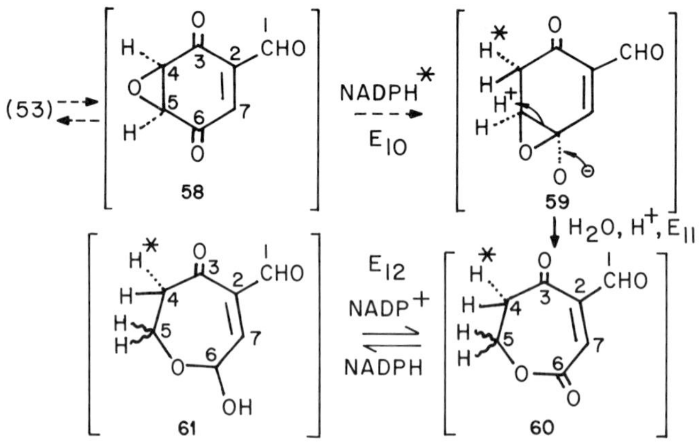

Fig. 39. Postulated mechanism of the conversion of (−)-phyllostine to a seven-membered ring hemiacetal.

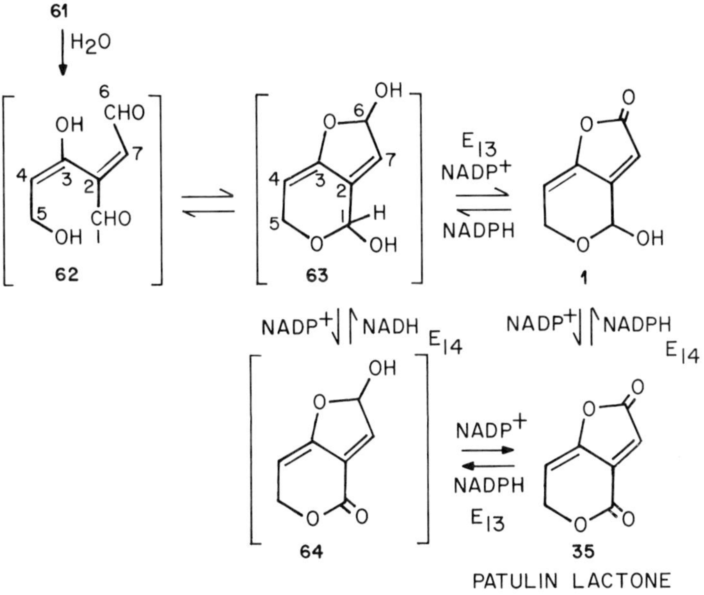

Fig. 40. Postulated mechanism of the conversion of the seven-membered ring hemiacetal to patulin.

of E_{12} will give the seven-membered ring hemiacetal, **61** (Fig. 39). Hydrolysis of **61** and rotation around the C(2)–C(3) bond will give the open form (**62**), which will readily cyclize the hemiacetal (**63**) (Fig. 40). Oxidation of the —OH group at C(1) with the dehydrogenase E_{14} and NADP$^+$ will give compound **64**. Further oxidation, mediated by a different enzyme (E_{13}), will give patulin lactone (**35**) (Fig. 40). A dehydrogenase (E_{14}) will then yield patulin (**1**). Compound (**63**) can also give patulin with the same dehydrogenase E_{13} which would be specific to C(6). According to this scheme, E_{14} is specific to oxidation reduction of C(1) (Fig. 40). End products unrelated to patulin biosynthesis such as desoxypatulinic acid (*P. patulum*) or ascladiol (*Aspergillus clavatus*) (Suzuki *et al.*, 1971) could be derived from compound **60** (Fig. 41). Hydrolysis of **60** and rotation around C(2)–C(3) will give the open-chain compound **65**. Reduction at C(1) and cyclization would yield ascladiol (**66**). Reduction at C(1) of compound **65**, elimination of water from C(1) and C(5), as well as isomerization of the double bond from C(2)–C(7) to C(1)–C(2) will yield deoxypatulinic acid (Fig. 41).

In conclusion, the proposed scheme answers the various questions: (a) Phyllostine might have been biosynthesized by the same monooxygenase which produced deoxyepoxidon (Fig. 38). (b) The rearrangement between phyllostine (**53**) and the seven-membered ring lactone (**60**) is shown in Fig. 30.

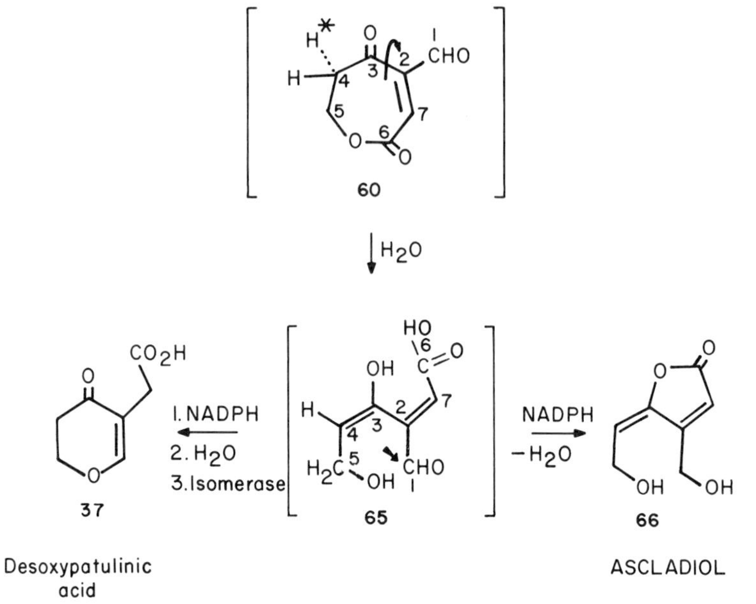

Fig. 41. Postulated biosynthesis of ascladiol and deoxypatulinic acid.

(c) The optically active deuteropatulin is generated from deuterium at position C(5) (Fig. 30). The addition of H^+ being enzyme mediated could be stereospecific and therefore will generate a chiral carbon at C(5). There are various possible push–pull arrow mechanisms which can explain the conversion of 59 to 60. All of them would imply stereospecific additions of H^+ at C(5) and would explain optically active deuteropatulin. (d) The patulin lactone involvement in Fig. 40: Scott et al. (1973) and Zamir (1973) found that the side-chain deuteriums of the aromatic precursors are lost on the way to patulin. The side-chain deuteriums would end up at C(1) of patulin. The only plausible explanation would be oxidation of the C(1)–OH. This could occur either after patulin formation (Fig. 40) or prior to its formation. Therefore, this postulated scheme is in accord with these experimental results. (e) Figure 41 shows a plausible biosynthetic scheme for deoxypatulinic acid or ascladiol.

The finding of phyllostine as a precursor to patulin induces the prediction of a similar intermediate in penicillic acid biosynthesis (Fig. 42). Therefore, I would predict that a plausible intermediate after the 3-methoxytoluquinone step would be the epoxyquinone 67 (Fig. 42). Specific reduction at C(6) catalyzed by a dehydrogenase and NADPH would rearrange the epoxide 68 (Fig. 42). Hydrolysis of 68 will yield the seven-membered ring lactone, 69. This lactone (69) (Fig. 42) differs from the one proposed (22) (Fig. 14) as it

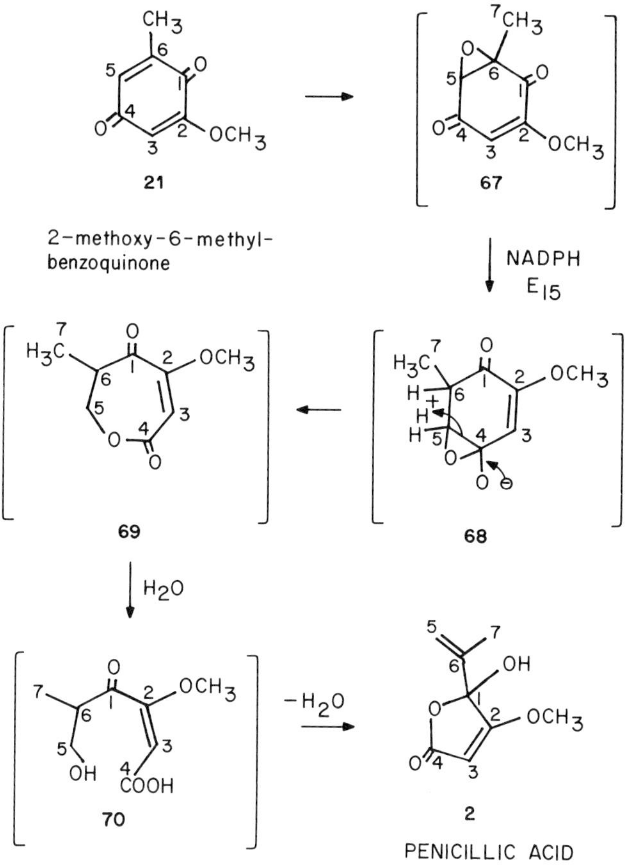

Fig. 42. Postulated mechanism for the steps beyond 2-methoxy-6-methylbenzoquinone in penicillic acid biosynthesis.

has no double bond at C(5)–C(6). Hydrolysis of **69** (Fig. 42) will yield the open chain compound **70**, which, on dehydration and lactolization, produces penicillic acid. This hypothetical scheme (Fig. 42) has to be validated with penicillic acid-negative mutants which would accumulate one of these putative intermediates.

Since this chapter was written, a new epoxide, isoepoxydon, was isolated (Sekiguchi and Gaucher, 1979 a,b; Gaucher, 1979). Its structure was characterized as a partially reduced derivative of (–)-phyllostine, and its stereochemistry was elucidated. Isoepoxydon was successfully converted into patulin by a cell-free preparation from *Penicillium urticae*. Isoepoxydon and phyllostine are interconvertible by an NADPH-dependent dehydrogenase.

It is still uncertain whether phyllostine, isoepoxydon, or both are obligatory intermediates to patulin. The possible role of isoepoxydon *in vivo* can easily be accommodated with the mechanisms postulated elsewhere in this text. We have assumed that dioxygenases are involved in the case of patulin and of penicillic acid, but in fact it is still unknown if monooxygenases or dioxygenases are involved. It is obvious that advances in the purification methods for enzymes will be of great importance in biosynthesis. Availability of a pure enzyme can lead to a detailed investigation of its properties and, therefore, its mode of action. It would be extremely important for detoxification studies to be able to understand and predict the cleavage sites of oxygenases.

REFERENCES

Alperden, I., Mintzlaff, H. J., Tauchmann, F., and Leistner, L. (1973). *Fleischwirtschaft*, **53**, 566.
Al-Rawi, J. M. A., Elvidge, J. A., Jaiswal, D. K., Jones, J. R., and Thomas, R. (1974). *J. Chem. Soc. Chem. Commun.*, p. 220.
Alsberg, C. L., and Black, O. F. (1913). *U.S. Dept. Agric. Bur. Plant. Ind. Bull.*, p. 270.
Auret, B. J., Boyd, D. R., Robinson, P. M., Watson, C. G., Daly, J. W., and Jerina, D. M. (1971). *J. Chem. Soc., Chem. Commun.*, p. 1585.
Axberg, K., and Gatenbeck, S. (1975a). *Acta Chem. Scand. Ser. B.* **29**, 749.
Axberg, K., and Gatenbeck, S. (1975b). *FEBS Lett.* **54**, 18.
Bassett, E. W., and Tanenbaum, S. W. (1960). *Biochim. Biophys. Acta.* **40**, 535.
Bentley, R., and Keil, J. G. (1961). *Proc. Chem. Soc. London*, p. 111.
Bentley, R., and Keil, J. G. (1962). *J. Biol. Chem.* **237**, 867.
Better, J., and Gatenbeck, S. (1976). *Acta Chem. Scand. Ser. B.* **30**, 368.
Better, J., and Gatenbeck, S. (1977). *Acta Chem. Scand. Ser. B.* **31**, 391.
Birch, A. J., Massy-Westrop, R. A., and Moye, C. J. (1955). *Aust. J. Chem.* **8**, 539.
Birch, A. J., Blance, G. E., and Smith, H. (1958). *J. Chem. Soc.*, p. 4582.
Birkinshaw, J. H., and Raistrick, H. (1942). *Biochem. J.* **26**, 441.
Birkinshaw, J. H., Oxford, A. E., and Raistrick, H. (1936). *Biochem. J.* **30**, 394.
Birkinshaw, J. H., Bracken, A., Michael, S. E., and Raistrick, H. (1943). *Lancet* **245**, 625.
Birkinshaw, J. H., and Gowland, A. (1962). *Biochem. J.* **84**, 342.
Bloxsidge, J., Elvidge, J. A., Jones, J. R., and Evans, E. A. (1971). *Org. Magn. Reson.* **3**, 127.
Boyd, E. M. (1944). *Can. Med. Assoc. J.* **50**, 159.
Brock, D. J. H., and Bloch, K. (1966). *Biochem. Biophys. Res. Commun.* **23**, 775.
Bu'lock, J. D., and Ryan, A. J. (1958). *Proc. Chem. Soc. London*, p. 222.
Bu'lock, J. D., Smalley, H. M., and Smith, G. N. (1962). *J. Biol. Chem.* **237**, 1778.
Bu'lock, J. D., Hamilton, D., Hulme, M. A., Powell, A. J., Smalley, H. M., Shepherd D., and Smith, G. N. (1965). *Can. J. Microbiol.* **11**, 765.
Capitaine, R., and Balouet, G. (1974). *Mycopathol. Mycol. Appl.* **54**, 361.
Ciegler, A., Beckwith, A. C., and Jackson, L. K. (1976). *Appl. Environ. Microbiol.* **31**, 664.
Ciegler, A., Vesonder, R. F., and Jackson, L. K. (1977). *Appl. Environ Microbiol.* **33**, 1004.
Closse, A., Mauli, R., and Sigg, H. P. (1966). *Helv. Chim. Acta* **49**, 204.
Dailey, R. E., Brouwer, E., Blaschka, A. M., Reynalds, E. F., Green, S., Monlux, W. S., and Ruggles, D. I. (1977). *Toxicol. Environ. Health* **2**, 713.

Dickens, F. (1967). *In* "Carcinogenesis: A Broad Critique," p, 447. Williams & Wilkins, Baltimore.

Dickens, F., and Jones, H. E. H. (1961). *Brit. J. Cancer* **15**, 85.

Dimroth, P., Walter, H., and Lynen, F. (1970). *Eur. J. Biochem.* **13**, 98.

Dimroth, P., Greull, G., Seyffert, R., and Lynen, R. (1972). *Hoppe-Seyler's Z. Physiol. Chem.* **353**, 126.

Dimroth, P., Ringelmann, E., and Lynen, F. (1976). *Eur. J. Biochem.* **68**, 591.

Ehrensvard, G. (1955). *Exp. Cell Res. Suppl.* **3**, 102.

Elvidge, J. A., Jaiswal, D. K., Jones, J. R., and Thomas, R. (1977). *J. Chem. Soc. Perkin Trans. 1*, p. 1080.

Florey, H. W. E., Heatley, N. G., Jennings, M., Sanders, A. G., Abraham, E. P., and Flory, M. E. (1949). *In* "Antibiotics," Vol. II, p. 1774. Oxford Univ. Press, London and New York.

Forrester, P. I., and Gaucher, G. M. (1972a). *Biochemistry* **11**, 1102.

Forrester, P. I., and Gaucher, G. M. (1972b). *Biochemistry* **11**, 1108.

Gatenbeck, S., and Mosbach, K. (1959). *Acta Chem. Scand.* **13**, 1561.

Gaucher, G. M., and Shepherd, M. G. (1968). *Biochem. Biophys. Res. Commun.* **32**, 664.

Gaucher, G. M. (1979). *J. of Food Protection* **42**, 810.

Holtermüller, K. H., Ringelmann, E., and Lynen, F. (1970). *Hoppe-Seyler's Z. Physiol. Chem.* **351**, 1411.

Hubbard, C. R., Mitchell, A. D., and Ware, G. M. (1977). *Acta Crystallogr. Sect. B.* **33**, 928.

Light, R. J. (1967). *J. Biol. Chem.* **242**, 1880.

Light, R. J. (1969). *Biochim. Biophys. Acta* **191**, 430.

Light, R. J., and Hager, L. P. (1968). *Arch. Biochem. Biophys.* **125**, 326.

Light, R. J., and Vogel, G. (1975). *Methods Enzymol.* **42**, 530.

Ljungcrantz, I., and Mosbach, K. (1964). *Biochim. Biophys. Acta* **86**, 203.

Lynen, F. (1967a). *Pure Appl. Chem.* **14**, 137 (1967).

Lynen, F. (1967b). *In* "Organizational Biosynthesis" (H. J. Vogel, J. O. Lampen, and V. Bryson, eds.), p. 243. Academic Press, New York.

Lynen F., and Tada, M. (1961). *Angew. Chem.* **73**, 513.

Lynen, F., Oesterhelt, D., Schweizer, E., and Willecke, K. (1968). *In* "Cellular Compartmentalization and Control of Fatty Acid Metabolism," p. 1. Universitetsforlaget, Oslo.

Mosbach, K., (1959). *Z. Naturforsch.* **146**, 69.

Mosbach, K. (1960). *Acta Chem. Scand.* **14**, 457.

Mosbach, K. (1961). *Naturwissenschaften* **48**, 525.

Mosbach, K. (1964). *Acta Chem. Scand.* **18**, 1591.

Mosbach, K., and Ljungcrantz, I. (1965). *Physiol. Plant.* **18**, 1.

Murphy, G., and Lynen, F. (1975). *Eur. J. Biochem.* **58**, 467.

Murphy, G., Vogel, G., Grippahl, G., and Lynen, F. (1974). *Eur. J. Biochem.* **49**, 443.

Raphael, R. A. (1947). *J. Chem. Soc.*, p. 805.

Raphael, R. A. (1948). *J. Chem. Soc.*, p. 1508.

Raphael, R. A. (1950). *R. Inst. Chem. Lect. Monogr. Rep.* **3**, 18.

Reiss, J. (1972). *Naturwissenschaften* **59**, 37.

Reiss, J. (1973). *Chem. Mikrobiol. Technol. Lebensm.* **2**, 171.

Sansing, G. A., Lillehoj, E. B., and Detroy, R. W. (1976) *Toxicon* **14**, 213.

Scott, A. I., and Beadling, L. (1974). *Bioorg. Chem.* **3**, 281.

Scott, A. I., and Wiesner, K. J. (1972). *J. Chem. Soc. Commun.*, p. 1075.

Scott, A. I., and Yalpani, M. (1967). *J. Chem. Soc. Chem. Commun.*, p. 945.

Scott, A. I., Phillips, G. T., and Kircheis, U. (1971). *Bioorg. Chem.* **1**, 380.

Scott, A. I., Zamir, L., Phillips, G. T., and Yalpani, M. (1973). *Bioorg. Chem.* **2**, 124.

Scott, A. I., Beadling, L. C., Georgopapadakou, N. H., and Subbarayan, C. R. (1974). *Bioorg. Chem.* **3**, 238.

Scott, P. M. (1974). *In* "Mycotoxins" (I. F. H. Purchase, ed.), p. 384. Elsevier, New York.
Scott, P. M., Kennedy, B., and Van Walbeck, W. (1972). *Experientia* **28**, 1252.
Scott, P. M., Fuleki, T., and Harwig. J. (1977). *J. Agric. Food Chem.* **25**, 434.
Sekiguchi, J., and Gaucher, G. M. (1978). *Biochemistry* **17**, 1787.
Sekiguchi, J., and Gaucher, G. M. (1979a). *Biochem. J.*, 445.
Sekiguchi, J., and Gaucher, G. M. (1979b). *Can. J. Microbiol.* **25**, 881.
Serratosa, F. (1961). *Tetrahedron* **16**, 185.
Seto, H., Cary, L. W., and Tanabe, M. (1973). *J. Chem. Soc. Chem. Commun.*, p. 867.
Seto, H., Cary, L. W., and Tanabe, M. (1974). *J. Antibiot.* **27**, 558.
Simpson, T. J., and Holker, J. S. E. (1977). *Biochemistry* **16**, 229.
Singh, J. (1967). *In* "Antibiotics" (D. Gottlieb and P. D. Shaw, eds.), Vol. I p. 621. Springer-Verlag, Berlin and New York.
Snow, J. P., Lucas, G. B., Harvan, D., Pero, R. W., and Owens, R. G. (1972). *Appl. Microbiol.* **24**, 34.
Stansfield, J. M., Francis, A. E., Stuart-Harris, C. H. (1944). *Lancet* **2**, 370.
Stoloff, L. (1976). *N.Y. State Agric. Exp. Stn. Geneva, Spec, Rep.* **19**, 51.
Suzuki, T., Takeda, M., and Tanabe, H. (1971). *Chem. Pharm. Bull.* **19**, 1786.
Tanenbaum, S. W., and Bassett, E. W. (1958). *Biochim. Biophys. Acta* **28**, 21.
Tanenbaum, S. W., and Bassett, E. W. (1959). *J. Biol. Chem.* **234**, 1861.
Thorpe, C. W., Johnson, R. L. (1974). *J. Assoc. Off. Anal. Chem.* **57**, 861.
Ukai, T., Yamamoto, Y., and Yamamoto, T. (1954). *J. Pharm. Soc. (Japan)* **74**, 450.
Wikholm, R. J., and Moore, H. W. (1972). *J. Am. Chem. Soc.* **94**, 6152.
Wilson, D. M. (1976). *In* "Mycotoxins and Other Fungal Related Food Problems" (J. V. Rodricks, ed.), p. 90. Am. Chem. Soc., Washington, D.C.
Wilson, B. J., and Hayes, A. W. (1973). *In* "Toxicants Occurring Naturally in Foods," p. 372. Nat. Acad. Sci., Washington, D.C.
Woodward, R. B., and Singh, G. (1949). *J. Am. Chem. Soc.*, **71**, 758.
Woodward, R. B., and Singh, G. (1950). *J. Am. Chem. Soc.*, **72**, 1428.
Zamir, L. O. (1973). Ph.D. Thesis, Yale University, New Haven, Connecticut.

8

The Biosynthesis of the Cytochalasans

CH. TAMM

I. INTRODUCTION

The discovery of the cytochalasans resulted from the observation that culture filtrates of certain microorganisms produced morphological changes in the hyphae of test fungi and unusual effects in mammalian cells in tissue cultures (Rothweiler and Tamm, 1966; Carter 1967, 1972). The isolation of the first two compounds of this class and the determination of their structures were achieved about at the same time, and independently of each other, by Rothweiler and Tamm (1966) and Aldridge *et al.* (1967a). The substances isolated from culture filtrates of *Phoma exigua* were named phomin and dehydrophomin, while those obtained from culture filtrates of *Helminthosporium dematioideum* were called cytochalasins A and B. Cytochalasin A proved to be identical with dehydrophomin, and cytochalasin B with phomin.

Soon afterward, a Japanese group (Hayakawa *et al.*, 1968) isolated zygosporin A from cultures of *Zygosporium masonii*, and Aldridge and Turner (1969a) isolated cytochalasins C and D from *Metarrhizium anisopliae*. Zygosporin A was found to be identical with cytochalasin D (Aldridge and Turner, 1969b; Minato and Matsumoto, 1970). One year later, Minato and Katayama (1970) reported the isolation of the zygosporins D, E, F, and

269

The Biosynthesis of Mycotoxins
Copyright © 1980 by Academic Press, Inc.
All rights of reproduction in any form reserved.
ISBN 0-12-670650-6.

G as further metabolites of *Z. masonii*. In 1972, the British group (Aldridge *et al.*, 1972) published the structure of cytochalasins F and E, metabolites of *H. dematioideum* and *Rosellinia necatrix*, respectively. The chemistry of these cytochalasans has been reviewed in 1973 (Binder and Tamm, 1973a,b). Binder and Tamm (1973c,d) isolated deoxaphomin, protophomin, and proxiphomin as minor metabolites of *P. exigua*. In the same year, Sekita *et al.* (1973) discovered the chaetoglobosins A and B in *Chaetomium globosum*. They were followed by the chaetoglobosins C, D, E, and F (Umeda *et al.*, 1975) and, recently, by chaetoglobosins G and J (Sekita *et al.*, 1977). The chaetoglobosins contain an indolyl group in the place of the phenyl group. The same structural element is also present in cytochalasin G, which is produced by an unidentified *Nigrosabulum sp.* (Cameron *et al.*, 1974). Finally, two substances were isolated in India from *Phomopsis paspali*, a pathogen kodo millet, named paspalin P-1 and P-2. They were identical with kodo-cytochalasin-1 and -2, respectively (Patwardhan *et al.*, 1974), and renamed cytochalasins H and J, respectively.

The compounds which have been isolated are listed in Table I. They have been named either according to their origin or on the basis of their biological activity. Because some of these trivial names overlapped and the numbering of the basic skeletons differed, a systematic nomenclature was introduced by Binder *et al.* (1973), which now is accepted. The systematic names of the metabolites are given in Table I with the trivial names, as well as the molecular formulas and the microorganisms from whose cultures they were isolated. So far, 24 natural cytochalasans are known.

A multitude of reports on the physiological activity of the cytochalasans have appeared. All cytochalasans inhibit cytoplasmic cleavage in mammalian cell cultures, but differ in the intensity of their action. In the presence of cytochalasin B, normal mitosis occurs in mammalian cells, but cytokinesis, i.e., the cleavage of the cell plasma, is blocked (Carter, 1967; Krishan, 1971). Prolonged contact with cytochalasin B leads to the formation of large multinucleate cells, but instead of doubling the number of nuclei per cell, each mitosis gives only one new nucleus. High concentrations, 10 to 20 times the quantity required for the inhibition of cytokinesis, causes ejection of the cell nucleus. These processes are reversible.

Another striking characteristic of cytochalasans is the inhibition of cell movement (Holzer *et al.*, 1975). This effect has been used to separate viable nuclei (karyoplasts) from their cytoplasm (Shay *et al.*, 1974; Ege *et al.*, 1974). Some cytochalasans affect fungal growth (Betina *et al.*, 1972; Larpent, 1974), phagocytosis (Davies *et al.*, 1971; Allison *et al.*, 1971; Nakagawara *et al.*, 1974; Ichikawa *et al.*, 1975), platelet aggregation and clot retraction (White, 1971; Haslam, 1972; Partridge *et al.*, 1975; Haslam *et al.*, 1975), glucose transport (Mak *et al.*, 1974), and parathyroid secretion (Williams and Wolff,

TABLE I

List of Natural Cytochalasins

Trivial name	Systematic name	Molecular formula	Structural formula	Microorganism	References
[11]Cytochalasans Cytochalasin C	(7S,16S,18R,21R)-21-Acetoxy-7,18-dihydroxy-16,18-dimethyl-10-phenyl-[11]cytochalasa-5(6),13(E),19(E)-triene-1,17-dione	$C_{30}H_{37}NO_6$	5	*Metarrhizium anisopliae*	Aldridge and Turner (1969a)
Cytochalasin D = zygosporin A	(7S,16S,18R,21R)-21-Acetoxy-7,18-dihydroxy-16,18-dimethyl-10-phenyl-[11]cytochalasa-6(12),13(E),19(E)-triene-1,17-dione	$C_{30}H_{37}NO_6$	6	*M. anisopliae, Zygosporium masonii*	Hayakawa et al. (1968) Aldridge and Turner (1969a,b) Tsukuda et al. (1969) Minato and Matsumoto (1970) Tsukuda and Koyama (1972)
Cytochalasin G	(6S,7S,16S)-6,7-Epoxy-10-(indol-3-yl)-16-methyl-[11]cytochalasa-13(E)-ene-1,18,21-trione	$C_{29}H_{34}N_2O_4$	7	*Nigrosabulum* sp.	Cameron et al. (1974)
Cytochalasin H = paspalin P-1 = kodo-cytochalasin-1	(7S,16S,18S,21R)-21-Acetoxy-7,18-dihydroxy-16,18-dimethyl-10-phenyl-[11]cytochalasa-6(12),13(E),19(E)-trien-1-one	$C_{30}H_{39}NO_5$	8	*Phomopsis paspali*	Pendse (1974) Patwardhan et al. (1974) Beno and Christoph (1976) Beno et al. (1977) McMillan et al. (1977)
Cytochalasin J = paspalin P-2 = kodo-cytochalasin-2	(7S,16S,18S,21R)-7,18,21-Trihydroxy-16,18-dimethyl-10-phenyl-[11]cytochalasa-6(12), 13(E), 19(E)-trien-1-one	$C_{28}H_{37}NO_4$	9	*P. paspali*	Pendse (1974) Patwardhan et al. (1974)
Zygosporin D	(7S,16S,18R,21R)-7,18,21-Trihydroxy-16,18-dimethyl-10-phenyl-[11]cytochalasa-6(12),13(E),19(E)-triene-1,17-dione	$C_{28}H_{35}NO_5$	10	*Zygosporium masonii*	Minato and Katayama (1970)
Zygosporin E	(7S,16S,18R)-21-Acetoxy-7-hydroxy-16,18-dimethyl-10-phenyl-[11]cytochalasa-6(12),13(E),19(E)-triene-1,17-dione	$C_{30}H_{37}NO_5$	11	*Z. masonii*	Minato and Katayama (1970)

(continued)

TABLE I (*continued*)

Trivial name	Systematic name	Molecular formula	Structural formula	Microorganism	References
Zygosporin F	(7S,16S,18R,21R)-7,21-Diacetoxy-18-hydroxy-16,18-dimethyl-10-phenyl-[11]cytochalasa-6(12), 13(E), 19(E)-triene-1, 17-dione	$C_{32}H_{39}NO_7$	12	*Z. masonii*	Minato and Katayama (1970)
Zygosporin G	(16S,18R,21R)-21-Acetoxy-18-hydroxy-16,18-dimethyl-10-phenyl-[11]cytochalasa-6(7),13(E),19(E)-triene-1,17-dione	$C_{30}H_{37}NO_5$	13	*Z. masonii*	Minato and Katayama (1970)
[13]Cytochalasans Deoxaphomin	(7S,16R,20R)-7,20-Dihydroxy-16-methyl-10-phenyl-[13]cytochalasa-6(12),13(E),21(E)-triene-1,23-dione	$C_{29}H_{37}NO_4$	14	*Phoma* (S 298)	Binder and Tamm (1973c)
Proxiphomin	16-Methyl-10-phenyl-[13]cytochalasa-6(7),13(E),21(E)-triene-1,23-dione	$C_{29}H_{37}NO_2$	15	*Phoma* (S 298)	Binder and Tamm (1973d)
Protophomin	16-Methyl-10-phenyl-[13]cytochalasa-5(6),13(E),21(E)-triene-1,7,23-trione	$C_{29}H_{35}NO_3$	16	*Phoma* (S 298)	Binder and Tamm (1973d)
Chaetoglobosin A	(6S,7S,16S,19R)-6,7-Epoxy-10-(indol-3-yl)-19-hydroxy-16,18-dimethyl-[13]cytochalasa-13(E),17(E),21(E)-triene-1,20,23-trione	$C_{32}H_{36}N_2O_5$	17	*Chaetomium globosum*	Sekita *et al.* (1973) Silverton *et al.* (1976)
Chaetoglobosin B	(7S,16R,19R)-10-(Indol-3-yl)-7,19-dihydroxy-16,18-dimethyl-[13]cytochalasa-5(6),13(E),17(E),21(E)-tetraene-1,20,23-trione	$C_{32}H_{36}N_2O_5$	18	*C. globosum*	Sekita *et al.* (1973)
Chaetoglobosin C	(6S,7S,16S)-6,7-Epoxy-10-(indol-3-yl)-16,18-dimethyl-[13]cytochalasa-13(E),17(E)-diene-1,19,20,23-tetraone	$C_{32}H_{36}N_2O_5$	19	*C. globosum*, *Penicillium aurantio-virens*	Sekita *et al.* (1973) Sekita *et al.* (1976) Springer *et al.* (1976)
Chaetoglobosin D	(7S,16R,19R)-7,19-Dihydroxy-10-(indol-3-yl)-16,18-dimethyl-[13]cytochalasa-6(12),13(E),17(E),21(E)-tetraene-1,20,23-trione	$C_{32}H_{36}N_2O_5$	20	*C. globosum*	Umeda *et al.* (1975) Sekita *et al.* (1976)

Name	Description	No.	Formula	Organism	Reference
Chaetoglobosin E	(7S,16R)-7,20-Dihydroxy-10-(indol-3-yl)-16,18-dimethyl-[13]cytochalasa-5(6),13(E),17(E)-triene-1,19,23-trione	21	$C_{32}H_{38}N_2O_5$	C. globosum	Umeda et al. (1975), Sekita et al. (1976)
Chaetoglobosin F	(6S,7S,16R)-6,7-Epoxy-20-hydroxy-10-(indol-3-yl)-16,18-dimethyl-[13]cytochalasa-13(E),17(E)-diene-1,19,23-trione	22	$C_{32}H_{38}N_2O_5$	C. globosum	Umeda et al. (1975), Sekita et al. (1976)
Chaetoglobosin G	(7S,16R)-7-Hydroxy-10-(indol-3-yl)-16,18-dimethyl-[13]cytochalasa-5(6),13(E),17(E)-triene-1,19,20,23-tetraone	23	$C_{32}H_{36}N_2O_5$	C. globosum	Sekita et al. (1977)
Chaetoglobosin J	(16R,19R)-19-Hydroxy-10-(indol-3-yl)-16,18-dimethyl-[13]cytochalasa-6(7),13(E),17(E),21(E)-tetraene-1,20,23-trione	24	$C_{32}H_{36}N_2O_4$	C. globosum	Sekita et al. (1977)
24-Oxa-[14]cytochalasans					
Cytochalasin A = 20-dehydrophomin	(7S,16R)-7-Hydroxy-16-methyl-10-phenyl-24-oxa-[14]cytochalasa-6(12),13(E),21(E)-triene-1,20,23-trione	25	$C_{29}H_{35}NO_5$	Phoma exigua var. exigua, Helminthosporium dematioideum	Rothweiler and Tamm (1966, 1970), Aldridge et al. (1967a,b), McLaughlin et al. (1970), Scott et al. (1975), Pribela et al. (1975)
Cytochalasin B = phomin	(7S,16R,20R)-7,20-Dihydroxy-16-methyl-10-phenyl-24-oxa-[14]cytochalasa-6(12),13(E),21(E)-triene-1,23-dione	26	$C_{29}H_{37}NO_5$	Phoma exigua var. exigua, H. dematioideum, Hormiscium	Rothweiler and Tamm (1966, 1970), Aldridge et al. (1967a; 1967b), Scott et al. (1975), Pribela et al. (1975)
Cytochalasin F	(6S,7S,16R,20R)-6,7-Epoxy-20-hydroxy-16-methyl-10-phenyl-24-oxa-[14]cytochalasa-13(E),21(E)-diene-1,23-dione	27	$C_{29}H_{37}NO_5$	H. dematioideum	Aldridge et al. (1972, 1973)
21,23-Dioxa-[13]cytochalasans					
Cytochalasin E	(6S,7S,16R,18R)-6,7-Epoxy-18-hydroxy-methyl-10-phenyl-21,23-dioxa-[13]cytochalasa-13(E),19(E)-diene-1,17,22-trione	28	$C_{28}H_{33}NO_7$	Rosellinia necatrix, Aspergillus clavatus	Aldridge et al. (1972, 1973), Büchi et al. (1973)

1971; Chertow *et al.*, 1974). Other processes affected include production of cytoplasmic streaming (Wessels *et al.*, 1971), tail resorption in lunicate larvae (Lash *et al.*, 1970), contraction of myocardium (Wessels *et al.*, 1971), and release of growth hormones (Schofield, 1971).

So far, only cytochalasins A, B, D, and E have been studied biologically in detail. Japanese workers have tested structure–activity relationships of cytochalasin D and its derivatives in an attempt to lower toxicity without losing its strong tumor-inhibiting properties (Minato *et al.*, 1973). Cytological studies with chaetoglobosins indicated high activity despite replacement of the usual phenyl group with an indolyl moiety (Umeda *et al.*, 1975).

II. STRUCTURE

Chemically, the cytochalasans are characterized by a highly substituted perhydroisoindolone group, to which is fused a macrocyclic ring which is either carbocyclic, a lactone, or a cyclic carbonate. Four types of naturally occurring basic skeletons are known (see Fig. 1): (1) [11]cytochalasans; (2) [13]cytochalasans; (3) 24-Oxa-[14]cytochalasans; and (4) 21,23-Dioxa-[13]cytochalasans. In the majority of the metabolites, in 20 compounds, the macrocyclic ring contains only carbon atoms. Three cytochalasans are macrolides (24-oxa-[14]cytochalasans), and only one is a diester of carbonic

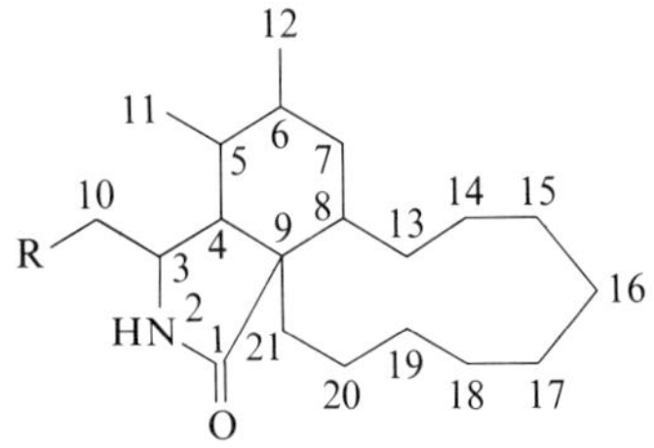

1 R = phenyl, indol-3-yl 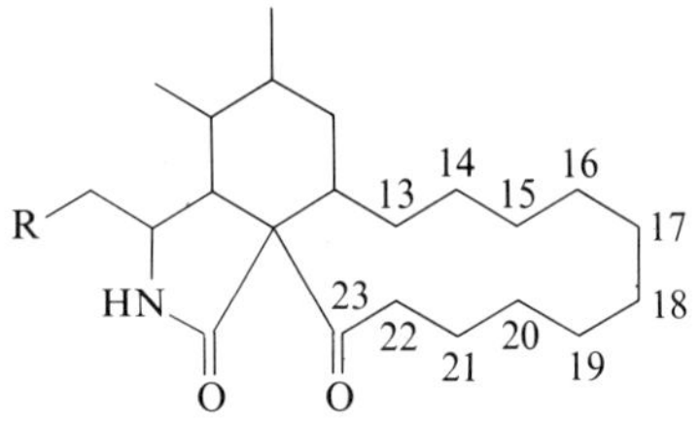   2 R = phenyl, indol-3-yl

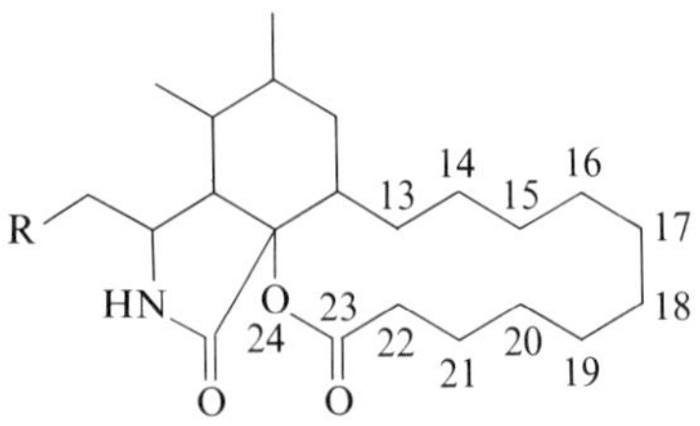

3 R = phenyl 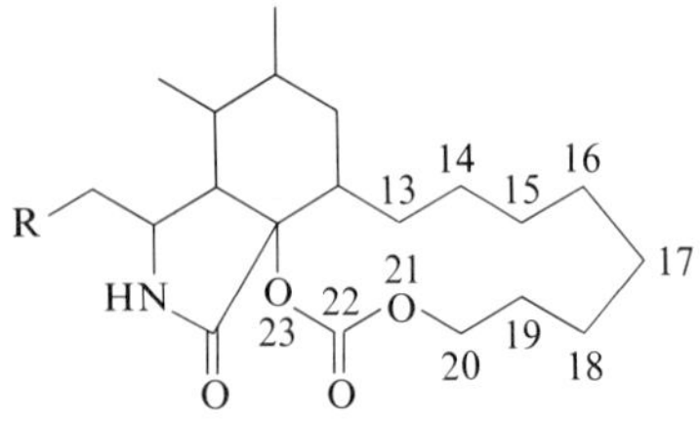   4 R = phenyl

Fig. 1.   The basic skeletons of the cytochalasans.

acid (21,23-dioxa-[13]cytochalasan). The 20 carbocyclic compounds contain either an 11-membered or a 13-membered ring system ([11]cytochalasans and [13]cytochalasans, respectively), whereby the number of both groups is nearly equal.

The structures of the natural cytochalasans are represented in Figs. 2–5. References to the corresponding literature are included in Table I.

The structures of the cytochalasans have been determined by chemical and spectral methods. The first metabolites whose structure elucidations were completed were cytochalasins A, B, and D. The absolute configurations

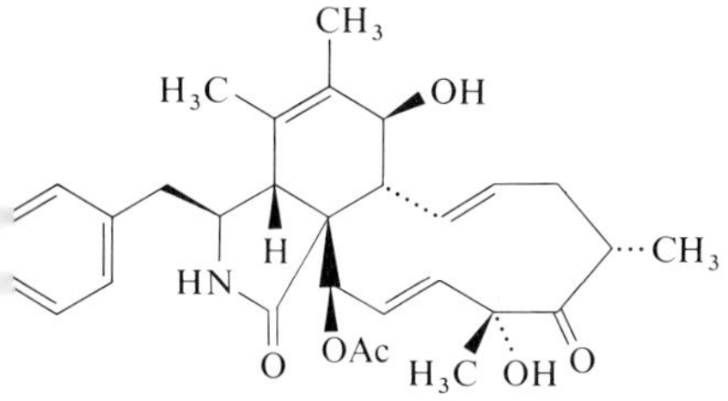

5 Cytochalasin C

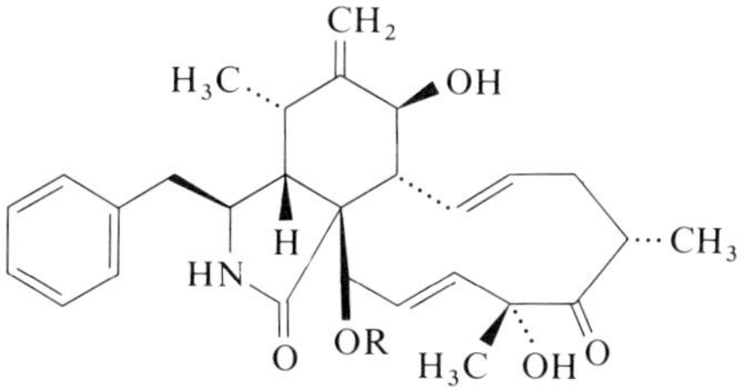

6 R = Ac: Cytochalasin D
   (Zygosporin A)
10 R = H: Zygosporin D

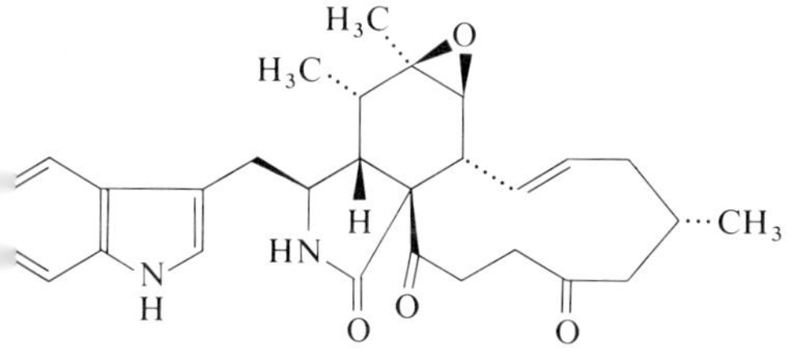

7 Cytochalasin G

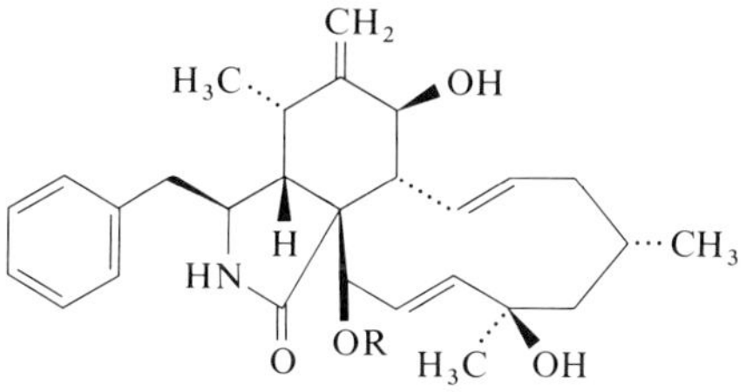

8 R = Ac: Cytochalasin H
9 R = H: Cytochalasin J

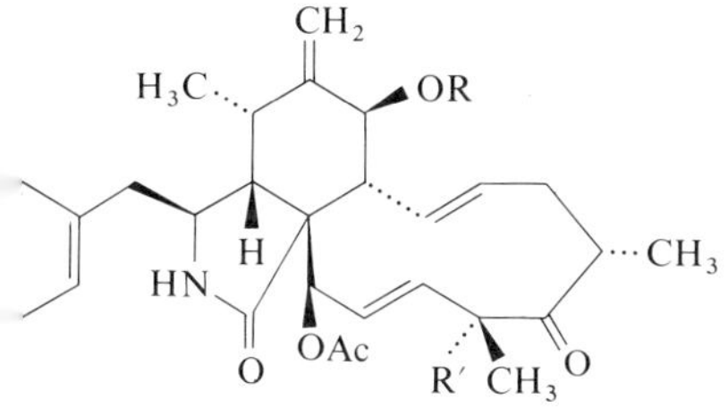

11 R = R′ = H: Zygosporin E
12 R = Ac; R′ = OH: Zygosporin F

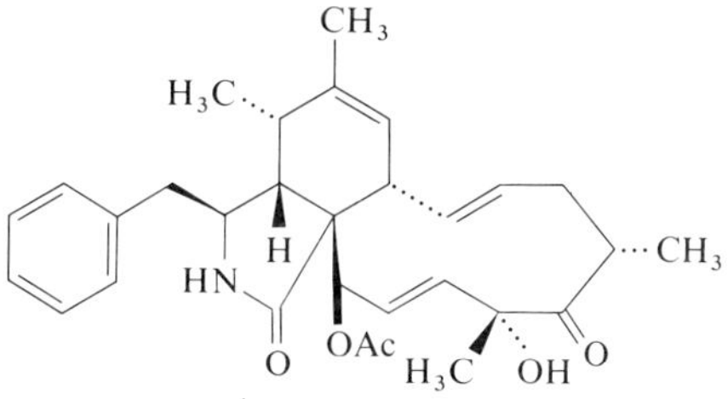

13 Zygosporin G

Fig. 2.   Structural formulas of the [11]cytochalasans.

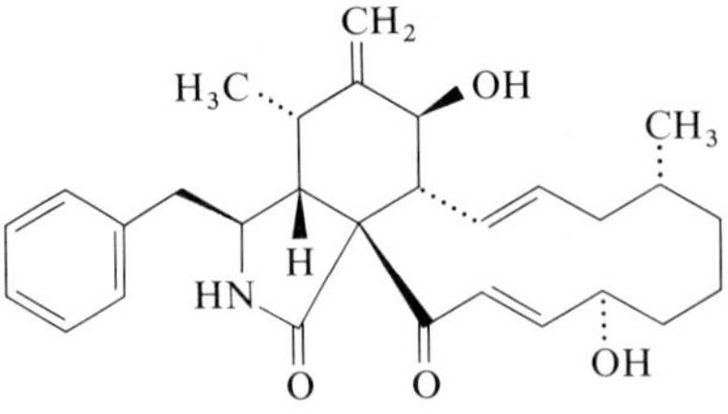

14 Deoxaphomin

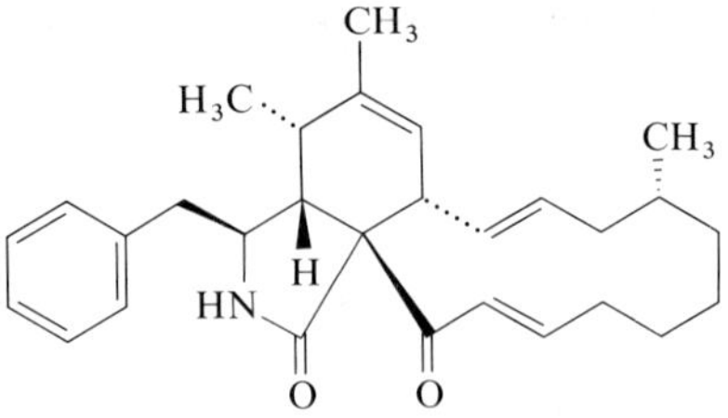

15 Proxiphomin

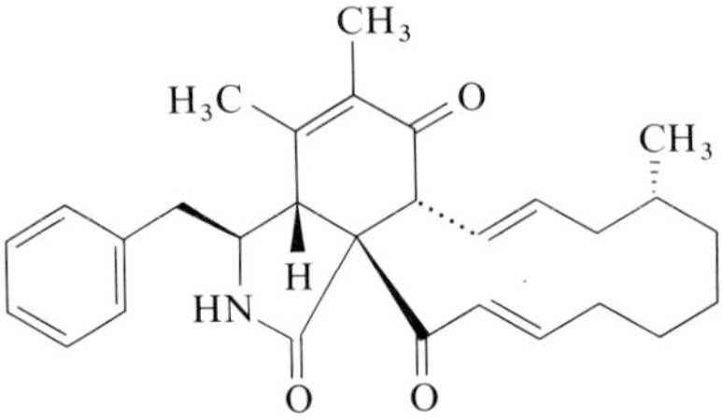

16 Protophomin

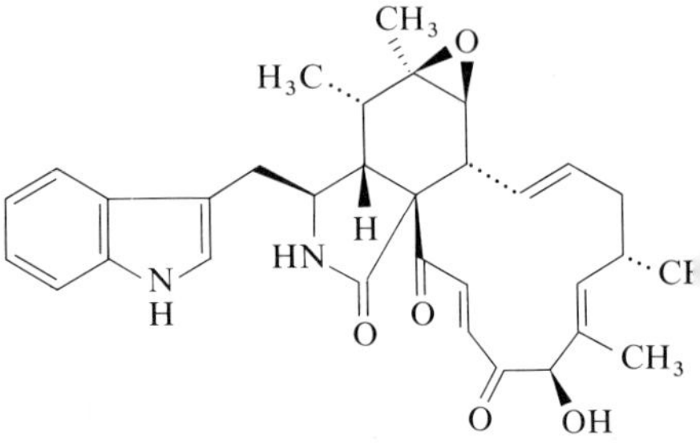

17 Chaetoglobosin A

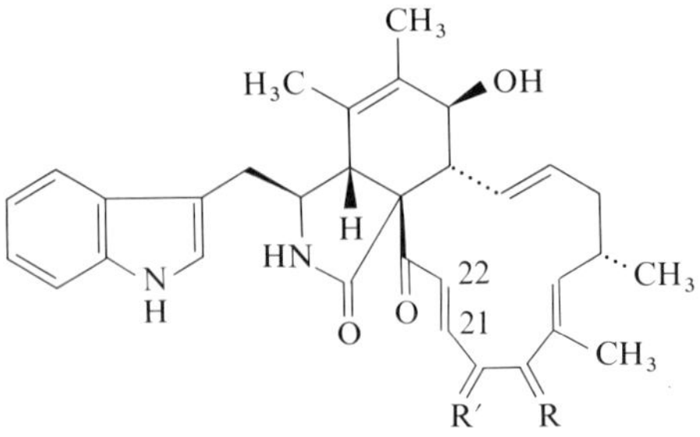

18 R = $\overset{H}{\underset{OH}{\diagdown}}$; R′ = O: Chaetoglobosin B

21 R = O; R′ = $\overset{H}{\underset{OH}{\diagdown}}$: 21,22-Dihydro: Chaetoglobosin E

23 R = R′ = O: 21,22-Dihydro: Chaetoglobosin G

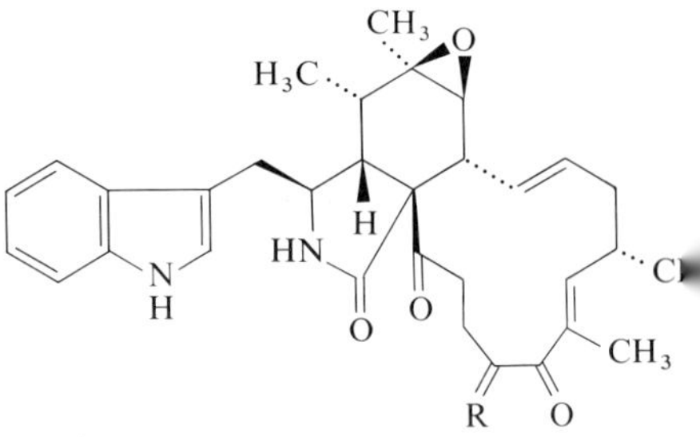

19 R = O: Chaetoglobosin C

22 R = $\overset{H}{\underset{OH}{\diagdown}}$: Chaetoglobosin F

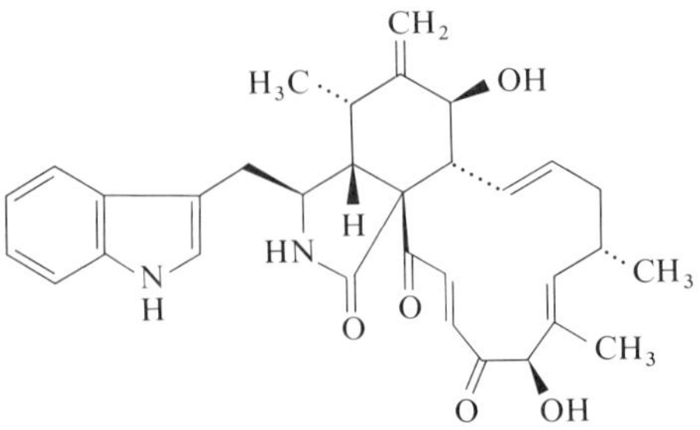

20 Chaetoglobosin D

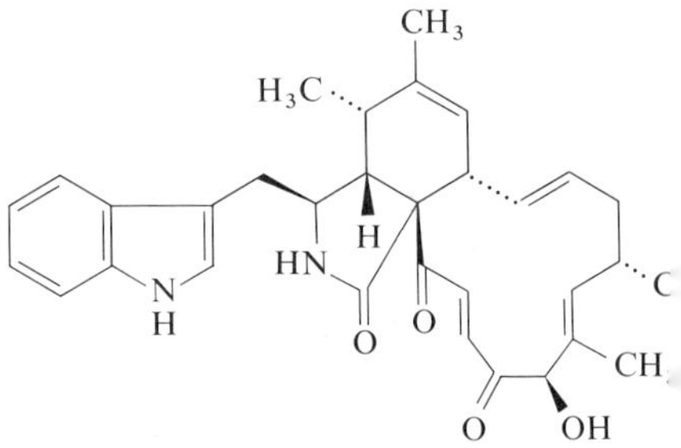

24 Chaetoglobosin J

Fig. 3. Structural formulas of the [13]cytochalasans.

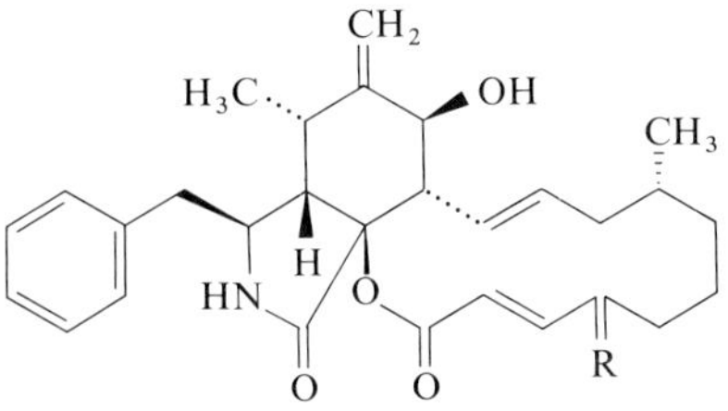

25 R = O: Cytochalasin A
(Dehydrophomin)

26 R = H, OH : Cytochalasin B
(Phomin)

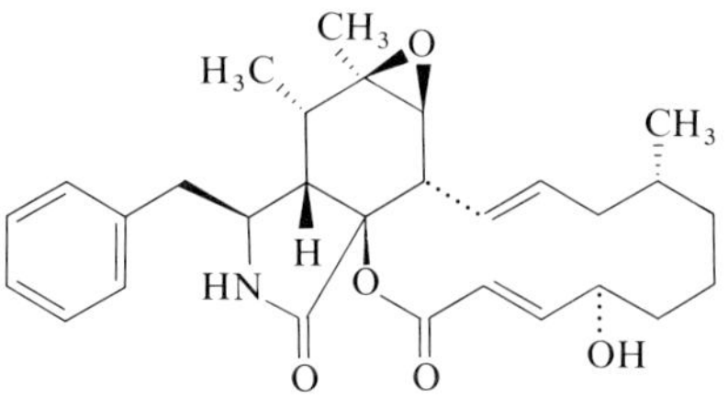

27 Cytochalasin F

Fig. 4.   Structural formulas of the 24-oxa-[14]cytochalasans.

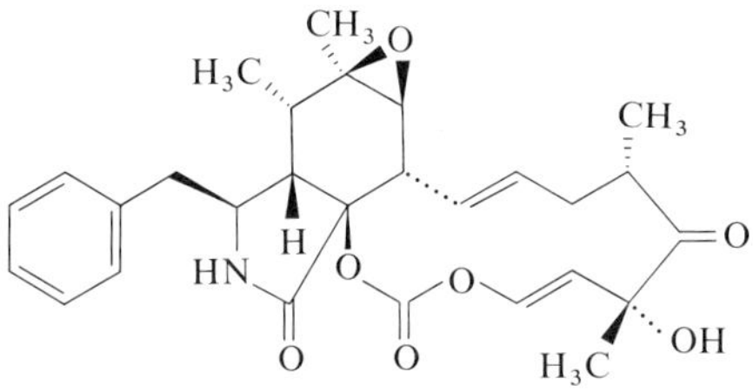

28 Cytochalasin E

Fig. 5.   Structural formula of the 21,23-dioxa-[13]cytochalasan.

of the two latter compounds were established by X-ray analysis (McLaughlin *et. al.*, 1970; Tsukuda *et al.*, 1969; Tsukuda and Koyama, 1972, respectively). Most of the subsequent metabolites were structurally correlated with them. Crystal X-ray diffraction analyses have also been carried out for cytochalasin E (Binder *et al.*, 1973); cytochalasin G (Cameron *et al.*, 1974); chaetoglobosins A (Silverton *et al.*, 1976) and C (Springer *et al.*, 1976); and, finally, cytochalasin H (Beno and Christoph, 1976; Beno *et al.*, 1977; McMillan *et al.*, 1977).

The configuration of the isoindolole part of all cytochalasans is identical. This is also true for those sections of the macrocyclic system which possess identical structures. There are only two exceptions. The stereochemistry at C(18) of cytochalasin H and J is different from that established for the same functionality in other closely related cytochalasins, e.g., cytochalasin D.

III. BIOSYNTHESIS

After the elucidation of the structural formulas and the establishment of the identity of the absolute configuration of the cytochalasins A, B, and

D, the investigation of the biosynthesis of the latter two metabolites was initiated in our laboratory in 1970. The biosynthetic studies are carried out as *in vitro* experiments. A synthetic medium serves for the cultivation of the microorganisms. The culture is incubated with potential biogenetic precursors radioactively labeled (^{3}H, ^{14}C) or labeled with the radioinactive isotopes ^{13}C or ^{15}N. If possible, the precursors are added to the culture when the cytochalasin production begins. For this purpose, the rate of formation of the secondary metabolite must be determined. The cytochalasins are isolated in the usual fashion. To localize the radioactive atoms incorporated into the molecule, the specimen is subjected to a specific chemical degradation. In the experiments with ^{13}C-labeled precursors, carbon-13 nuclear magnetic resonance (^{13}C NMR) is used. Mass spectrometry serves for the determination of nitrogen-15.

Experimental data on the biosynthesis of cytochalasans are available at present only for cytochalasin B (**26**), cytochalasin D (**6**), and deoxaphomin (**14**). The first experiments were carried out with cytochalasin B.

A. Cytochalasin B

Binder *et al.* (1970) administered a number of ^{14}C- and ^{3}H-labeled potential precursors to growing cultures of *P. exigua* var. *exigua* (Strain S 298). The degradation of the radioactive specimen initially involved reactions that have been carried out in the determination of the structure of cytochalasin B (**26**); it was later confined to methods, such as cleavage with periodate, Kuhn–Roth oxidation, Schmidt degradation of acids, that proceed specifically in high yields (see Figs. 6 and 7).

Dodecahydrocytochalasin B, which resulted from the catalytic hydrogenation of cytochalasin B (**26**) with platinum oxide in glacial acetic acid, was oxidized by chromium trioxide in sulfuric acid (Kuhn–Roth oxidation) to give three equivalents of acetic acid [C(5) and C(11), C(6) and C(12), C(16) and 16-methyl]. Acetic acid was degraded further with sodium azide in polyphosphoric acid (Schmidt procedure) to carbon dioxide (isolated as barium carbonate) and methylamine (isolated as picrate). After treatment of di-*O*-acetylcytochalasin B with ozone and catalytic hydrogenation with palladium of the ozonide, formaldehyde was obtained (isolated as formaldimedone) [C(12)]. Ozonolysis of cytochalasin B (**26**) and subsequent treatment of the products with sodium borohydride yielded the γ-lactams I (**30**) and II (**31**), and 3-methyloctane-1,7,8-triol (**32**). Kuhn–Roth oxidation of γ-lactam II (**31**) using a modified procedure allowed the isolation of one equivalent each of acetic acid [C(5) and C(11)] and benzoic acid [C(10) and 10-phenyl]. Catalytic hydrogenation of γ-lactam **31** led to the hexahydro derivative, **31a**. Kuhn–Roth oxidation of the latter gave one

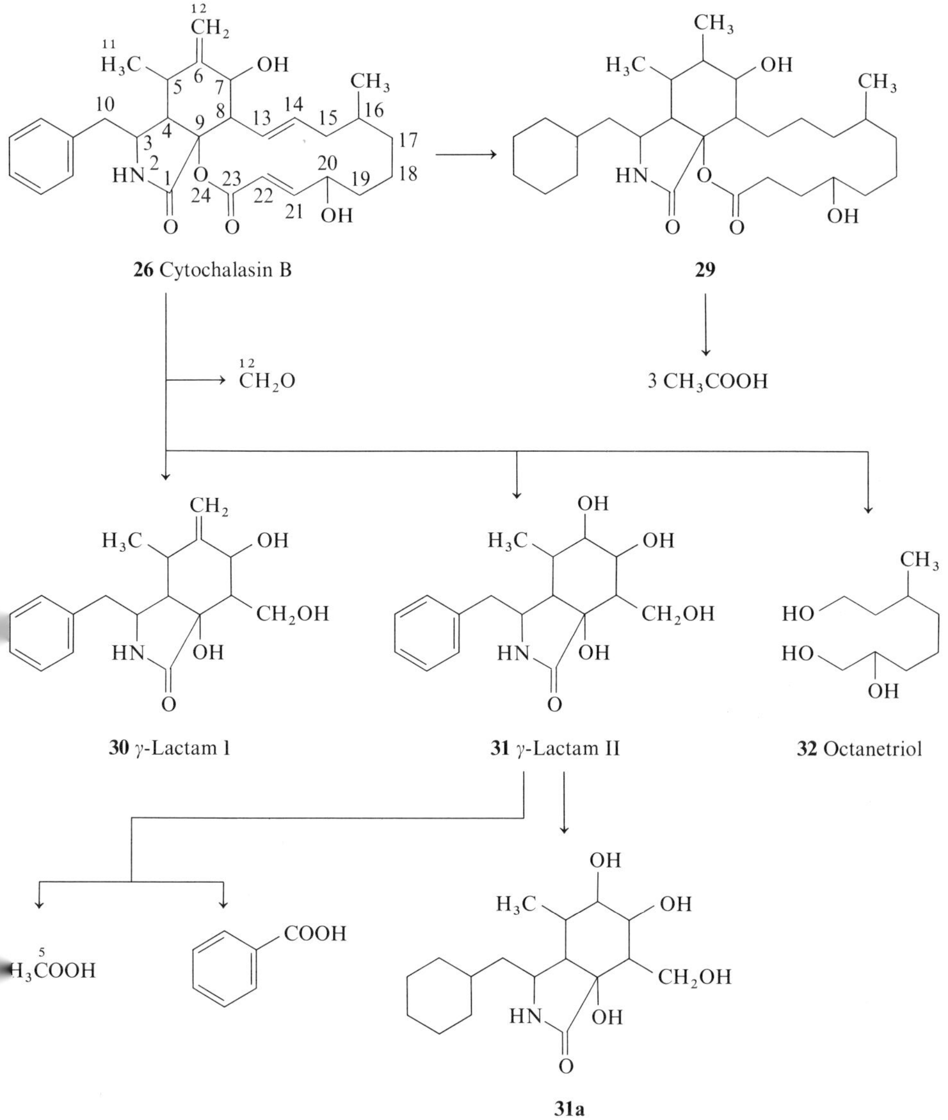

Fig. 6.   Degradation of cytochalasin B.

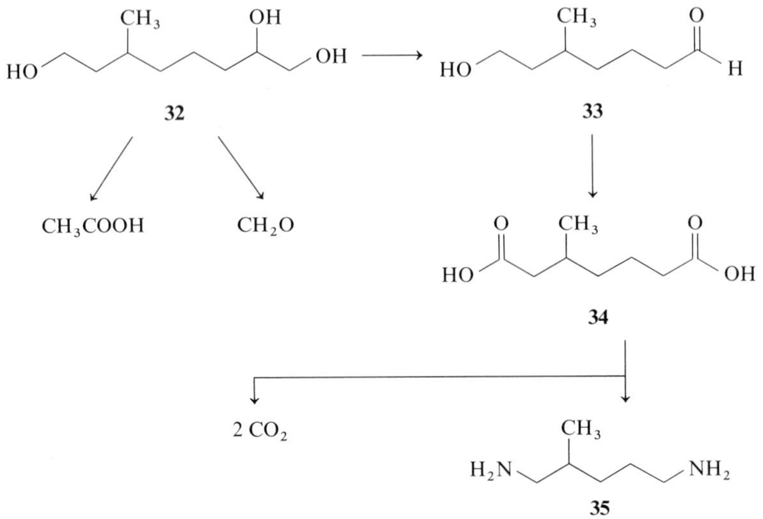

Fig. 7. Degradation of 3-methyloctane-1,7,8-triol.

equivalent of acetic acid [C(5) and C(11)], which again was degraded to carbon dioxide and methylamine.

On treatment with periodate, the third ozonolysis product, 3-methyloctane-1,7,8-triol (32), yielded formaldehyde [(21)] and 5-methyl-7-hydroxyheptanal (33). The hydroxyaldehyde 33 was oxidized by chromium trioxide to 3-methylpimelic acid (34). Schmidt degradation of the latter gave carbon dioxide [C(14) and C(20)] and 1,5-diamino-2-methylpentane (35) (isolated as dipicrate). Kuhn–Roth oxidation of octanetriol (32) yielded one equivalent of acetic acid [C(16) and 16-methyl].

High absolute rates of incorporation were observed for DL-phenylalanine [4.9% if labeled at C(1) and 6.7% for labeling at C(2)]. An experiment with L-[U-^{14}C,4'-^{3}H]phenylalanine proved that the amino acid is incorporated including the carboxy group. Modified Kuhn–Roth oxidation yielded one equivalent of benzoic acid, isolated as p-bromophenacyl ester, whose ^{14}C activity was 79% of the total activity. This value corresponds to seven-ninths of the activity of cytochalasin B (seven of the nine carbon atoms of phenylalanine). The tritium activity was retained to 100% at the same time.

The incorporation of sodium [1-^{14}C]acetate was low, but the radioactivity showed an alternating distribution in cytochalasin B. The ratio of 4:4:1 of the distribution in γ-lactam I (30), octanetriol (32), and glycol (not isolated) corresponds to the incorporation of nine acetate units. The same result was found for the distribution of radioactivity after the incorporation of sodium [1-^{14}C]malonate, which acts as chain propagator. The rate of incorporation of sodium [2-^{14}C]malonate was twice as high as that of sodium [1-^{14}C]malonate. The latter loses half its activity because of decarboxylation. Alternating distribution of radioactivity was also found for the incorporated malonates. Sodium [2-^{14}C]propionate was incorporated as a C$_2$ unit wherein C(2) of propionic acid corresponds to the carboxy group of acetic acid. After the incorporation of sodium [1-^{14}C]propionate, the radioactivity was concentrated exclusively in the β-lactam moiety of the molecule. An interpretation of this result will be offered below.

L-[CH$_3$-^{14}C]Methionine showed a high rate of absolute incorporation (2%). The radioactivity was localized at C(12) and at 16-methyl. The methyl group attached to C(5) was devoid of activity.

Although the position of incorporation of radioactive phenylalanine and methionine could be completely determined by degradation experiments, the mode of utilization of sodium [^{14}C]acetate was only partially accessible (see Fig. 8). Of special interest were carbon atoms C(1) and C(9) in the lactam ring, for they occur at the juncture of amino acid and the anticipated polyketide biogenetic paths, and were inaccessible by degradation. The ^{13}C NMR studies carried out by Graf et al. (1974) demonstrated the usefulness of single-frequency decoupling and partially relaxed Fourier transform (PRFT) in making assignments of ^{13}C NMR signals for cytochalasin B (26), and corroborate the biosynthetic proposals for the origin

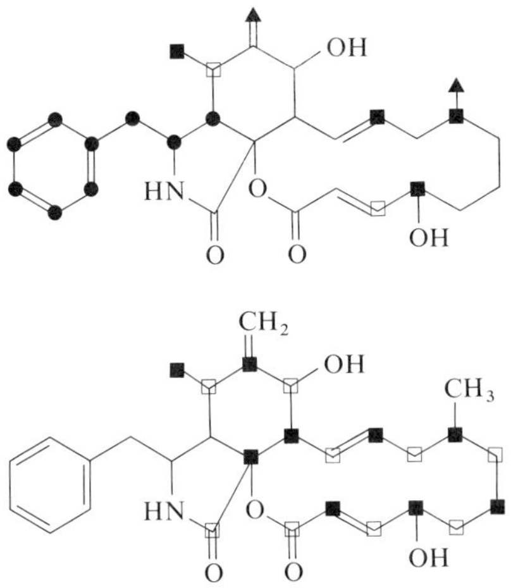

Fig. 8. Atoms in cytochalasin B (26) detected by degradation of ^{14}C- and ^{3}H-labeled specimens and by PRFT ^{13}C NMR spectroscopy. Upper structure: □ = [1-^{14}C]acetate, [2-^{14}C]propionate; ■ = [2-^{14}C]malonate; ▲ = L-[CH$_3$-^{14}C]Methionine; ● = DL-[1-^{14}C]-, DL-[2-^{14}C]phenylalanine, L-[4′-^{3}H, U-^{14}C]phenylalanine. Lower structure: □ = [1-^{13}C]acetate; ■ = [2-^{13}C]acetate; □—■ = [1,2-^{13}C]acetate.

of the metabolite. The absolute incorporation rate and the expected average enhancement of the ^{13}C NMR integral per labeled atom were determined by comparison of the mass spectra of labeled and unlabeled material. The results obtained after incorporation of sodium $[1\text{-}^{13}\text{C}]$- and $[2\text{-}^{13}\text{C}]$acetates (Graf et al. (1974) and sodium $[1,2\text{-}^{13}\text{C}]$acetate (Robert and Tamm, unpublished results), which are summarized in Fig. 8, confirmed the labeling pattern derived from experiments with sodium $[^{14}\text{C}]$acetate. Because C(1) and C(9), respectively, were ^{13}C-labeled, it was assumed that these carbon atoms are the terminus of a C_{18}-polyketide intermediate. It is interesting to note that sodium $[1\text{-}^{14}\text{C}]$butyrate was incorporated into cytochalasin B (26). The distribution of radioactivity has not yet been determined. On the other hand, neither glycerol tripalmitate nor stearate was incorporated.

The isolation of deoxaphomin (14), proxiphomin (15), and protophomin (16) had suggested that a carbocyclic [13]cytochalasan could generate the macrolide system of cytochalasin B (26) by an enzymatic Baeyer–Villiger-type oxygen insertion between C(9) and C(23) (Binder and Tamm, 1973c, 1973d). This hypothesis was tested by feeding of L-$[4'\text{-}^3\text{H}, U\text{-}^{14}\text{C}]$phenylalanine to growing cultures of P. exigua (Robert and Tamm, 1975). After fermentation was complete, deoxaphomin (14) and cytochalasin B (26) were separated by careful crystallization and preparative thin layer chromatography. The purity of isolated deoxaphomin (14) was checked by dilution with inactive cytochalasin B (26), repetition of the separation process, and measurement of the radioactivity of both substances. In this way it was shown that active deoxaphomin (14) contained no more than 1.4% of active cytochalasin B (26). The radioactive deoxaphomin (14) was administered to cultures of the same microorganism. It was well incorporated into cytochalasin B (26), the absolute rates of incorporation being 7.0–8.8%. The constant $^3\text{H}:^{14}\text{C}$ ratio and the $^3\text{H}:^{14}\text{C}$ ratio of benzoic acid obtained by a modified Kuhn–Roth oxidation of cytochalasin B (26) gave evidence of significant and intact incorporation. They demonstrate that deoxaphomin (14) can act as an immediate biogenetic precursor of cytochalasin B (26) in P. exigua (Robert and Tamm, 1975).

B. Cytochalasin D

The great structural similarity of the carbocyclic cytochalasin D (6) and the macrolide cytochalasin B (26), and the fact that their relative and absolute configurations are identical in the region of identical structural elements, suggested similar biogenetic pathways. Biosynthetic experiments with cytochalasin D (6) using growing cultures of Z. masonii have shown that the same precursors are incorporated to a similar degree as in cytochalasin B

(26). Lebet and Tamm (1974) determined the distribution of the radioactivity originating from incorporated L-[4'-^{3}H,U-^{14}C] phenylalanine and L-[CH$_3$-^{14}C] methionine by careful chemical degradation of [^{14}C]- and [^{3}H-^{14}C]cytochalasin D (6). The degradation of radioactive cytochalasin D after the incorporation of sodium [1-^{14}C]- and [2-^{14}C]acetates and of [2-^{14}C]propionate was carried out by Vederas *et al.* (1975) (see Fig. 9).

Kuhn–Roth oxidation of dodecahydrocytochalasin D (36), obtained from cytochalasin D (6) by catalytic hydrogenation with platinum oxide in glacial acetic acid, yielded four equivalents of acetic acid [C(5) and C(11), C(6) and C(12), C(16) and 16-methyl, C(18) and 18-methyl]. Acetic acid was degraded to methylamine and carbon dioxide by the Schmidt procedure. Kuhn–Roth oxidation of deacetylcytochalasin D (zygosporin D) (10) under special conditions gave one equivalent of benzoic acid and three equivalents of acetic acid [C(5) and C(11), C(16) and 16-methyl, C(18) and 18-methyl]. Ozonolysis of cytochalasin D (6), reductive cleavage of the ozonide by sodium borohydride, and acetylation yielded 1,6-diacetoxy-2,4-dimethylhexane-2,3-diol (42); 1,3,6-triacetoxy-2,4-dimethylhexan-2-ol (43); and the γ-lactams 39 and 40. This sequence of reactions allows the determination of the methyl groups at C(16) and C(18) together and of the 11-methyl group separately. By combination of various values, C(12) is determined again. Use was also made of the acid 44. The base-catalyzed hydrolysis of cytochalasin D (6) led to a thermodynamically controlled mixture of the two epimeric acids 44a and 44b, which were separated via the methyl esters. The configuration of C(9) was assigned on the basis of the spectral data. It is assumed that cytochalasin D (6) is first deacetylated to give zygosporin D (10), which is cleaved between C(9) and C(21) by a retro-aldol reaction. The enol form of the five-membered ring allows isomerization at C(9). By the attack of base at C(17) of the vinylogous 1,3-dicarbonyl system, the epimeric acids 44 and levulinic aldehyde are produced. By these reactions the 11-methyl, the 12-methylene, and the methyl group at C(16) are determined. The radioactivity of the single carbon atoms C(16) and C(18) can be calculated from the various data by forming the differences of activities.

Schmidt degradation of the acid 44 and fixation of the evolved carbon dioxide with barium hydroxide localized the label at C(17). Kuhn–Roth oxidation of 44 and Schmidt cleavage of the resulting two equivalents of acetic acid yielded the activities of both C(16) and its methyl substituent by comparison of the same sequence on the deacetylated γ-lactams 39 and 40, respectively. Ozonolysis of acid 44 followed by reduction gave the epimeric lactam triols 45a and 45b, respectively. The usual Kuhn–Roth and Schmidt route offered independent determinations of C(11) and C(5). A combined value for C(14) and C(15) could be calculated from the activity

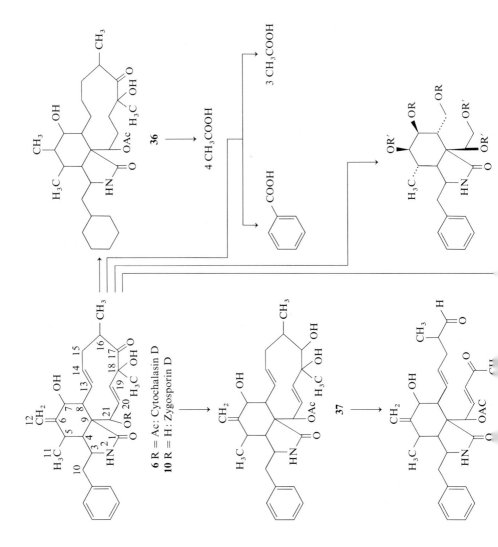

6 R = Ac: Cytochalasin D
10 R = H: Zygosporin D

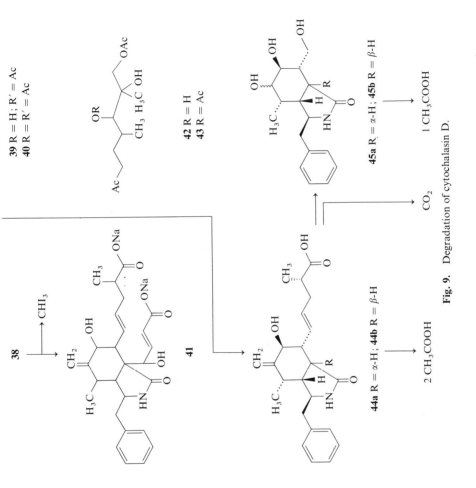

Fig. 9. Degradation of cytochalasin D.

285

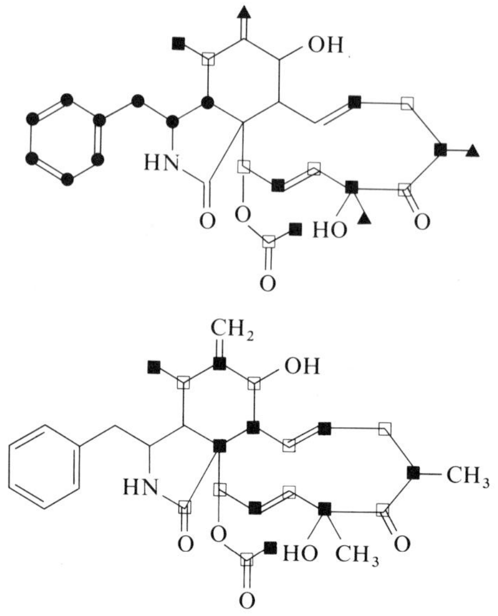

Fig. 10. Atoms in cytochalasin D (**6**) detected by degradation of ^{14}C- and ^{3}H-labeled specimens and by PRFT ^{13}C NMR spectroscopy. Upper structure: □ = [1-^{14}C]acetate, [2-^{14}C]propionate; ■ = [2-^{14}C]acetate, [2-^{14}C]diethyl malonate; ▲ = L-[CH$_3$-^{14}C]methionine; ● = L-[4′-^{3}H][U-^{3}H]phenylalanine. Lower structure: □ = [1-^{13}C]acetate; ■ = [2-^{13}C]acetate; □—■ = [1,2-^{13}C]acetate.

difference between lactams **44** and **45** because labeling at C(17), C(16), and 16-methyl had been previously elucidated.

The determination of the methyl group at C(18) required a special degradation sequence. Dihydrocytochalasin D (**37**), which is obtained from cytochalasin D (**6**) by reduction with sodium borohydride, was cleaved with periodate to give the 17,18-secoaldehyde **38**. Treatment of the product (**38**) with iodine and sodium hydroxide yielded the sodium salt **41** and iodoform, which originates from the methyl group at C(18). The results, summarized in Fig. 10, demonstrate that the building blocks are one unit of phenylalanine, three units of methionine, and acetate units. The polyketide labeling pattern was elucidated by completion of the incorporation of sodium [1-^{14}C]- and [2-^{14}C]acetates and the determination of the distribution of radioactivity by chemical degradation, as outlined in the preceding paragraph. Subsequent feeding of the corresponding ^{13}C-labeled acetates confirmed the results and established the alternating pattern of labeling in the C_{16}-polyketide moiety. The mode of incorporation of doubly labeled sodium [1,2-^{13}C]acetate, as elucidated by PRFT ^{13}C NMR spectroscopy, suggested coupling of acetate in head-to-tail fashion to form the nonbranched C_{16}-polyketide moiety (Graf *et al.*, 1974; Vederas *et al.*, 1975).

The assignments of ^{13}C NMR signals for cytochalasin D (6) were made by single-frequency decoupling and PRFT, as for cytochalasin B (26) (Graf *et al.*, 1974).

Other common carboxylic acids—e.g., propionic, butyric, myristic, and palmitic acids—were also found to be incorporated into cytochalasin D (6) (Vederas *et al.*, 1975). Feeding of sodium [1-^{13}C]propionate produced an enhancement at C(4) in the ^{13}C NMR spectrum, indicating the production of phenylalanine labeled at C(1) via the shikimate pathway. However, this pathway seems to be of secondary importance. The other even-numbered saturated acids underwent β-oxidation to yield C(1)-labeled acetate, which was incorporated in the usual manner. It is concluded that neither saturated nor unsaturated fatty acids are biogenetic intermediates of the cytochalasins.

The mode of incorporation of phenylalanine into cytochalasin D (6) was examined in detail by Vederas and Tamm (1976) because L-phenylalanine (2*S* configuration) and the DL- and L-amino acids appeared to be equally good precursors, although cytochalasin D (6) possesses the *S*- configuration at the corresponding C(3). Both enantiomers of phenylalanine (46) stereo-specifically labeled with tritium at C(2) and C(3) and with ^{14}C (as internal standard) were administered to cultures of *Z. masonii* in the usual fashion. The results indicated transamination of the phenylalanines, with almost complete hydrogen loss at the α position and extensive loss at the β position. Incorporation of racemized precursor, (2*RS*,3*R*)- and (2*RS*,3*S*)-[3-^{3}H]-phenylalanine, demonstrated that the loss of hydrogen had actually occurred at position 3, and that the large decrease in the ^{3}H : ^{14}C ratio was not due solely to an isotope effect at C(2). Conversion of phenylalanine (46) into derivatives of dehydrophenylalanine (47), cinnamic acid (48), or phenyl-pyruvic acid (49) could explain the loss of tritium and the equal incorporation rates of both enantiomers. However, the loss of 98% of ^{15}N label from [^{15}N]phenylalanine excluded the sole intermediacy of dehydrophenylalanine (47).

Cinnamic acid (48) is synthesized universally in higher plants and widely in fungi from (2*S*)-phenylalanine by phenylalanine ammonium lyase. This process is a *trans* elimination of the elements of ammonia, with stereospecific loss of the 3-*pro*(*S*) proton of phenylalanine (46). Phenylpyruvic acid (49) (shown in its enol form) is the normal biogenetic precursor of phenylalanine, and is in equilibrium with it by means of the action of aminotransferases and amino acid oxidases (see Fig. 11). To distinguish between the partici-pation of cinnamic acid (48) and phenylpyruvic acid (49) and to clarify the mechanism involved in the proton losses, (2*R*,3*S*)-[3-^{3}H]-, (2*S*,3*R*)-[3-^{3}H], and (2*S*)-[*U*-^{14}C]phenylalanines were administered to the cultures. The incorporations resulted in the removal of 57% and 76%, respectively, of the labeled hydrogen.

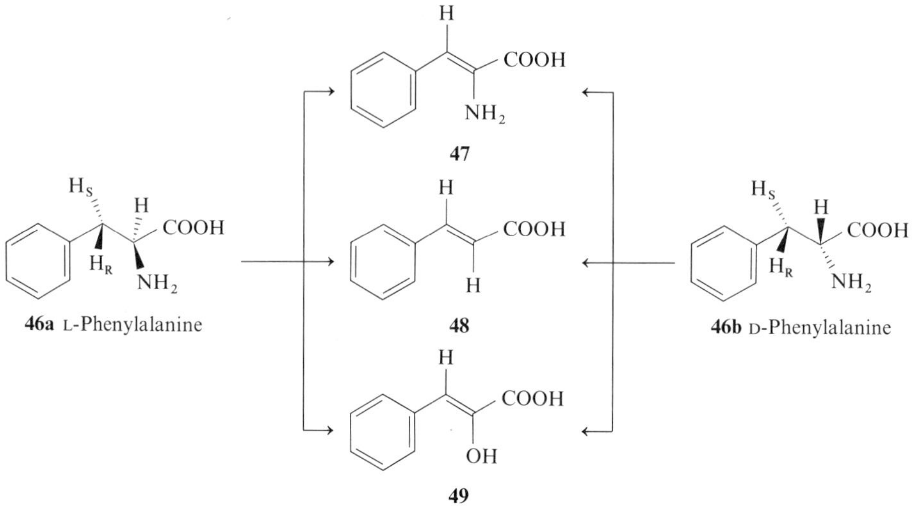

Fig. 11. Interconversion of L- and D-phenylalanine.

The low incorporation of [3-^{14}C]cinnamic acid (**48**) and the loss of both 3-*pro*(R) and 3-*pro*(S) protons from phenylalanine supported the participation of phenylpyruvic acid (**49**) in a transamination process. In addition, intermediates involving enzymatic hydroxylation at C(3) of a phenylalanine derivative were disfavored, because this type of reaction generally occurs with retention of configuration. This conclusion was confirmed by the intact incorporation of radioactive phenylpyruvic acid (**49**), prepared by aerobic enzymatic oxidation of (2S)-[4'-^{3}H, U-^{14}C]phenylalanine with L-amino acid oxidase from *Crotalus atrox* venom and catalase from bovine liver into cytochalasin D (**6**). The absolute incorporation rate of 6.5% of phenylpyruvic acid (**49**) was similar to that obtained with phenylalanine (**46**).

Reversible transamination occurs in many antibiotic biosyntheses. In contrast to the observations with cytochalasin D (**6**), the naturally abundant L-amino acids are often more efficiently incorporated than their antipodes, even in cases where the end product possesses the configuration corresponding to the D-amino acid. This may be due to improved transport across the cell membrane by permeases, or to racemization after biochemical elaboration.

The flavoprotein D-amino acid oxidases ordinarily do not exchange the β-hydrogens of their substrates. In transaminations, the exact mechanism of β-proton loss remains less clear. Initial aldimine (**50**) formation with pyridoxal phosphate is very rapid, even in the absence of enzyme (see Fig. 12).

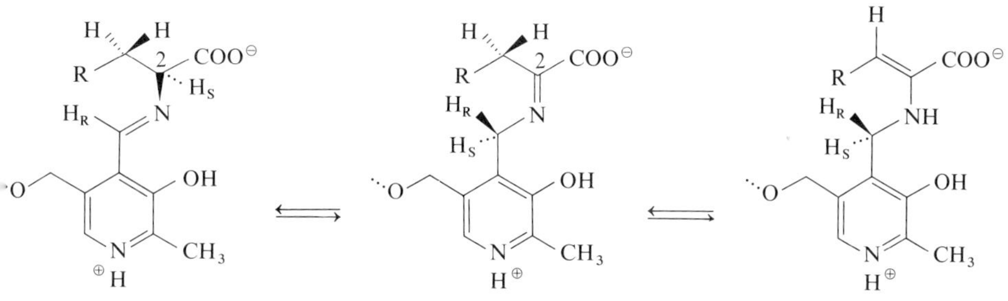

Fig. 12. Reversible transamination with pyridoxal phosphate.

The biological process is probably a transamination with pyridoxal phosphate, which is bound in imine form by an amino group of the protein. Tautomerization of the ketimine (**51**) is the rate-determining step. With L-amino acids, the same protein amino group reversibly transfers hydrogen (H_S in Fig. 12) from position 2 to C(4') of the coenzyme complex in *cis* fashion across the *si* face. D-Amino acids also add the *pro(S)* proton to C(4'), although their transamination requires different enzymes. Ketimine (**51**) may reversibly isomerize to the enamine **52** in an enzyme-assisted process, thereby effecting β-proton exchange, or it may hydrolyze directly to the keto acid. Because inductive and steric effects combine to make phenylalanine (**46**) one of the most rapidly transaminating acids without an acid–base side chain, and because the derived enamine **52** is stabilized by additional conjugation, the β-hydrogen atoms should be especially labile in biological systems.

Experiments with (2*S*,3*R*)- and (2*R*,3*S*)-[3-^{3}H]phenylalanines gave tritium retentions of 44% and 24%, respectively (Vederas and Tamm, 1976). Simultaneous incorporation of equal amounts of both enantiomers led to the expected 34% retention of hydrogen label. Transamination occurs stereospecifically at position 2 of the amino acid; therefore, the participation of at least two enzymes with different stereochemical requirements at the 3 position is reasonable. Two biosynthetic pathways are consistent with the data available (see Fig. 13). Path A in Fig. 13 depicts (2*S*)-phenylalanine as the actual precursor which is in rapid equilibrium with its enantiomer; in path B phenylpyruvic acid (**49**), derived directly from shikimic acid, is the primary precursor. Considerable suppression of the incorporation of D-amino acid by phenylpyruvic acid (**49**) indicated that the naturally abundant L-enantiomer is the actual primary precursor, thus demonstrating that path A (Fig. 13) is probably the main biosynthetic route. Both enantiomers are in rapid equilibrium with phenylpyruvic acid (**49**) via the action of aminotransferases or amino acid oxidases. The stereochemistry of hydrogen loss

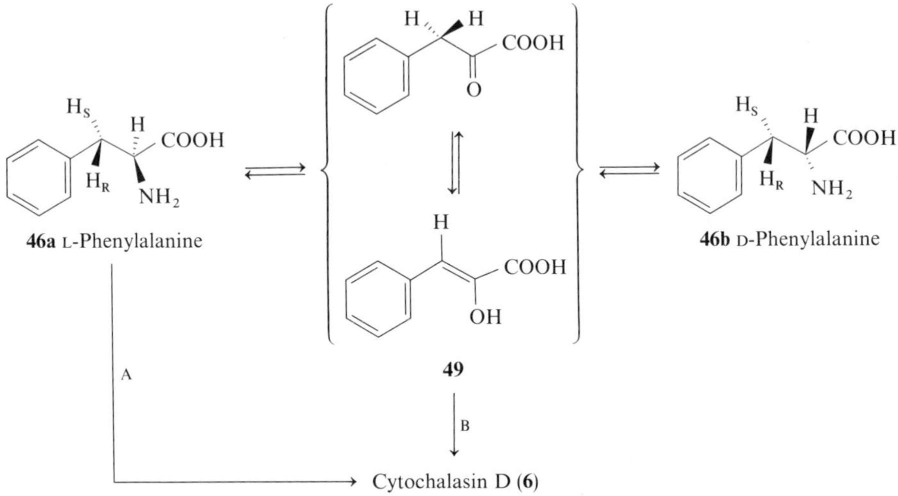

Fig. 13. Incorporation of phenylalanine (**46**) into cytochalasin D (**6**).

from C(2) and C(3) phenylalanines indicated that at least two different enzyme-dependent mechanisms are involved.

IV. BIOSYNTHETIC SCHEME

The structures of cytochalasins B (**26**) and D (**6**), and the results of the corresponding incorporation experiments, clearly demonstrate closely related biogenetic pathways from a polyketide-derived chain with, respectively, two and three introduced C_1 units, which is combined with phenylalanine. The assembly of the pieces poses a problem because it involves two chemically difficult condensations—methylene-to-methylene to form the bond between C(8) and C(9), and carbonyl-to-carbonyl to form the bond between C(4) and C(5)—rather than the preferred methylene-to-carbonyl condensations.

In the proposed scheme of the biosynthesis of cytochalasins A (**25**) and B (**26**), outlined in Fig. 14, the amide linkage of the nonaketide **53** to phenylalanine (**46**) may be regarded as the initial step. The subsequent condensation of the amide **54** leads to the five-membered ring of the γ-lactam **55**, which is a derivative of tetramic acid. One of the carbonyl groups of γ-lactam **55** reacts with the penultimate carbon atom of the ketide after reduction to the intermediate **56**, with formation of the bond between C(4) and C(5). Partial reductions and water eliminations yield the bicyclic intermediate **58**, in which the bond between C(8) and C(9) is transformed by condensation. By an

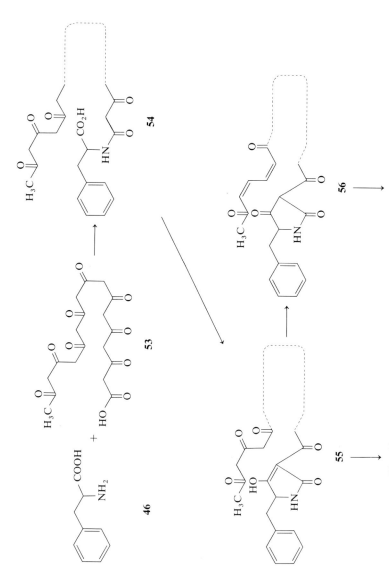

Fig. 14. Biosynthesis of cytochalasin A (**25**) and B (**26**). Hypothetical scheme.

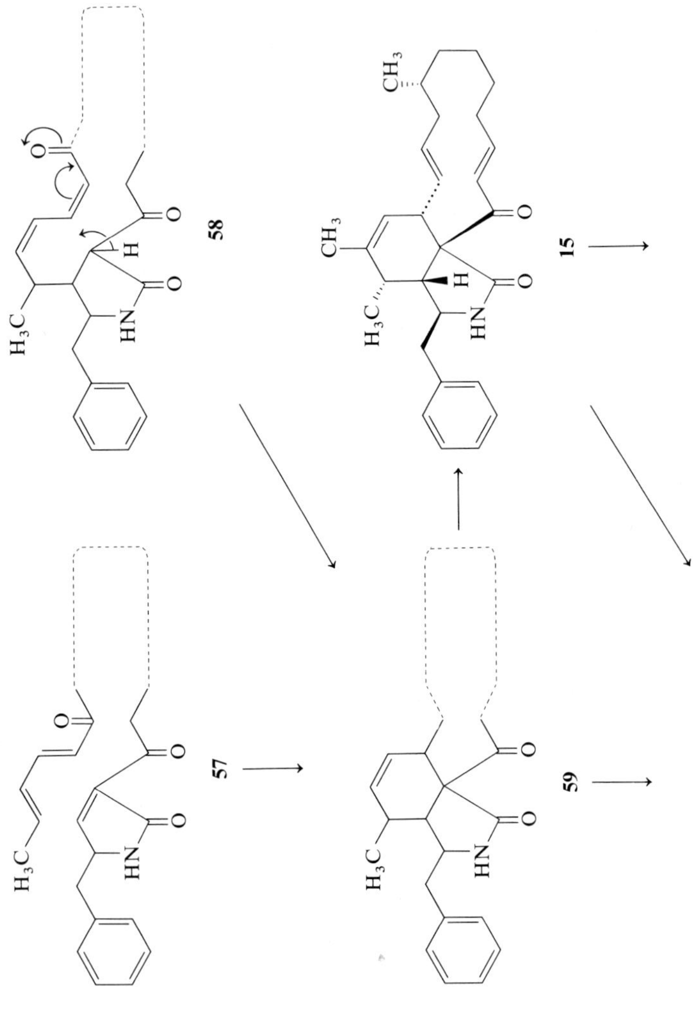

57 →

58

59 →

15 →

292

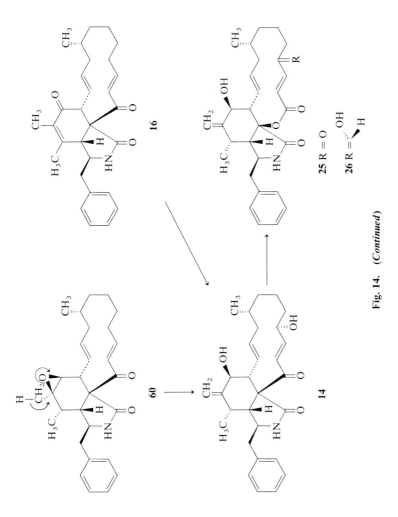

16

60 → **14**

25 R = O

26 R = ⟨OH / H⟩

Fig. 14. (*Continued*)

293

R = phenyl, 3'-indolyl

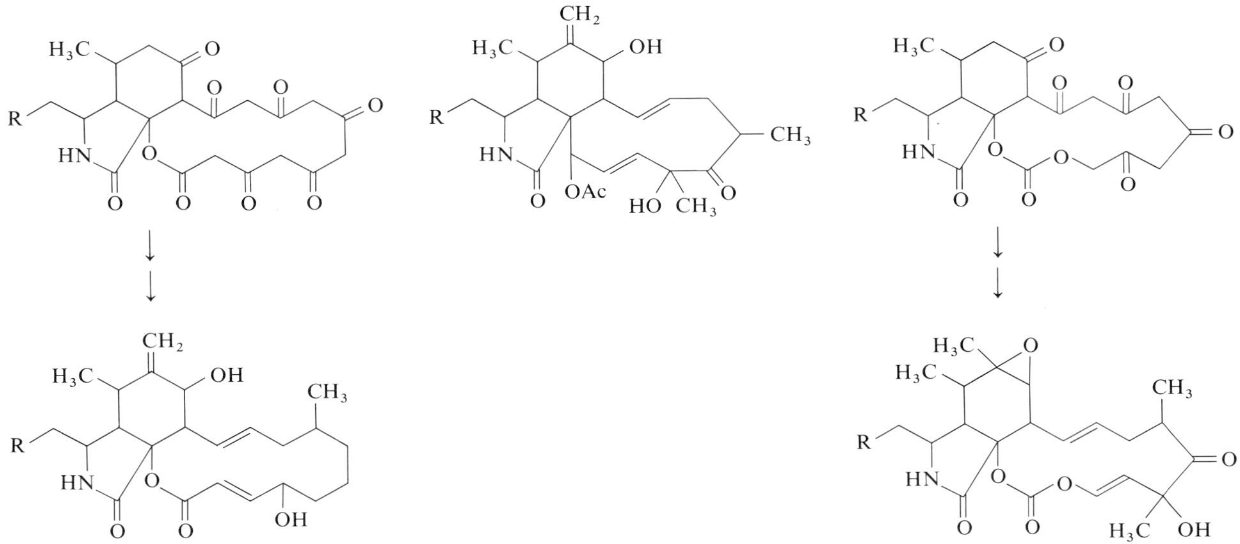

Fig. 15. General biosynthetic scheme for the cytochalasans.

295

alternative stereochemically more attractive, sequence of reactions, γ-lactam 55 is transformed to intermediate 57 by reduction and dehydration. The latter can undergo an internal Diels–Alder-type cyclization to form the tetracyclic system 59, possessing the required relative stereochemistry at four positions, namely C(4), C(5), C(8), and C(9). This can also be formed by an alternative sequence of reactions with a modified polyketide chain. The next steps are the two methylations at C(6) and C(16), and suitable modification by reductions and eliminations of the macrocycle. The product formed is identical with proxiphomin (15). Subsequent isomerization and allylic oxidation of the cyclohexane ring lead to protophomin (16), which is transformed readily to deoxaphomin (14). An alternative reaction of proxiphomin (15) is the epoxidation of the cyclohexene ring. It yields the ring system 60, which is found in some cytochalasins. Such epoxides might be the actual biogenetic precursors of the unsaturated alcohol system present in several cytochalasins. Opening of the epoxy group, as indicated in structure 60, leads to deoxaphomin (14). Finally, the Baeyer–Villiger-type oxidation converts the carbocyclic to the lactone system by insertion of an oxygen atom between C(23) and C(9). Allylic oxidation at C(20) yields cytochalasins A (25) and B (26). The individual steps, some of which are interchangeable in their order, all correspond to known reactions.

In the biosynthesis of cytochalasin D (6), an octaketide combines with phenylalanine in the same fashion to form the carbocyclic [11]cytochalasan system. Three instead of two methylations on C(6), C(16), and C(18) with S-adenosylmethionine are required.

The third type of large ring, a cyclic alkyl carbonate grouping, as represented by cytochalasin E (28), might also arise from carbocyclic precursors. The carbonate group results from a second Baeyer–Villiger-type insertion of oxygen into a lactone ring. The carbonate atom C(22) would thus be derived from the carboxy group of acetate.

Chaetoglobosins A–J and cytochalasin G, which contain an indole ring system in place of the phenyl ring, appear to be biosynthesized from tryptophan, rather than from phenylalanine, and a polyketide. But no experimental proof is available at present.

The great structural similarity among the four basic types of cytochalasans known as present, i.e., the [11]cytochalasans, [13]cytochalasans, 24-oxa-[14]cytochalasans, and 21,23-dioxa-[13]cytochalasans, and the experimental evidence available, permit one to postulate a common biogenetic scheme for all cytochalasans. Such a scheme is shown in Fig. 15. The tricyclic systems, which result from the combination of the amino acid with a C_{16}- or C_{18}-polyketide or a biogenetic equivalent, may be structures of a lower oxidation state. It also is unknown at what stage of the biogenetic sequence the introduction of the additional C_1 units takes place.

It is evident that the final validity of this general biogenetic scheme requires additional experimental data, e.g., incorporation of tryptophan into the chaetoglobosins and cytochalasin G, isolation of intermediates of the biogenetic sequence, and discovery of new cytochalasans, possibly with the as yet unknown basic skeletons and structural elements derived from other natural amino acids.

ADDENDUM

Very recently Keller-Schierlein and Kupfer (1979) reported the isolation and structure of four new metabolites of *Aspergillus microcysticus*, the aspochalasins A (10-isopropyl-14-methyl-[11]cytochalasa-6,13-diene-1,17,18,21-tetrone), B (17-hydroxy-10-isopropyl-14-methyl-[11]cytochalasa-6,13,19-triene-1,18,21-trione), C (17,18-dihydroxy-10-isopropyl-14-methyl-[11]cytochalasa-6,13,19-triene-1,21-dione), and D. The latter is a diastereomer of aspochalasin C. The aspochalasins contain an isopropyl group at C-10 indicating leucin being a biogenetic precursor. The isolation of the aspochalasins has raised the number of natural cytochalasans from 24 to 28.

REFERENCES

Aldridge, D. C., and Turner, W. B. (1969a). *J. Chem. Soc. C*, pp. 923–928.
Aldridge, D. C., and Turner, W. B. (1969b). *J. Antibiot. (Tokyo)* 22, 170.
Aldridge, D. C., Armstrong, J. J., Speake, R. N., and Turner, W. B. (1967a). *Chem. Commun.*, pp. 26–27.
Aldridge, D. C., Armstrong, J. J., Speake, R. N., and Turner, W. B. (1967b). *J. Chem. Soc. C*, pp. 1667–1676.
Aldridge, D. C., Burrows, B. F., and Turner, W. B. (1972). *J. Chem. Soc. Chem. Commun.*, pp. 148–149.
Aldridge, D. C., Greatbanks, D., and Turner, W. B. (1973). *J. Chem. Soc. Chem. Commun.*, pp. 551–552.
Allison, C. A., Davies, P. and De Petries, S. (1971). *Nature New Biol.* 232, 153.
Beno, M. A., and Christoph, G. G. (1976). *J. Chem. Soc. Chem. Commun.*, pp. 334–345.
Beno, M. A., Cox, R. H., Wells, J. M., Cole, J. R., Kirksey, J. W., and Christoph, G. G. (1977). *J. Am. Chem. Soc.* 99, 4123–4130.
Betina, V., Micekova, D., and Nemec, P. (1972). *J. Gen. Microbiol.* 71, 343.
Binder, M., and Tamm, Ch. (1973a). *Angew. Chem.* 85, 369–381.
Binder, M., and Tamm, Ch. (1973b). *Angew. Chem. Int. Ed.* 12, 370–380.
Binder, M., and Tamm, Ch. (1973c). *Helv. Chim. Acta* 56, 966–976.
Binder, M., and Tamm, Ch. (1973d). *Helv. Chim. Acta* 56, 2387–2396.
Binder, M., Kiechel, J.-R., and Tamm, Ch. (1970). *Helv. Chim. Acta* 53, 1797–1812.
Binder, M., Tamm, Ch., Turner, W. B., and Minato, H. (1973). *J. Chem. Soc. Perkin Trans. 1*, pp. 1146–1147.
Büchi, G., Kitaura, Y., Yuan, S.-S., Wright, H. E., Clardy, J., Demain, A. L., Glinsukar, T., Hunt, N., and Wogan, G. N. (1973). *J. Am. Chem. Soc.* 95, 5423–5425.
Cameron, A. F., Freer, A. A., Hesp, B., and Strawson, S. J. (1974). *J. Chem. Soc. Perkin Trans. 2*, pp. 1741–1744.
Carter, S. B. (1967). *Nature (London)* 213, 261–264.

298   Ch. Tamm

Carter, S. B. (1972). *Endeavour* **31**, 77–82.
Chertow, B. S., Williams, G. A., Norris, R. M., Baker, G. R., Surbaugh, R. D., and Hargis, G. K. (1974). *Clin. Res.* **22**, 337A.
Davies, A. T., Estensen, R. D., and Quie, P. G. (1971). *Proc. Soc. Exp. Biol. Med.* **137**, 161–164.
Ege, T., Hamberg, H., Krondahl, U., Ericsson, J., and Ringertz, N. R. (1974). *Exp. Cell Res.* **87**, 365–377.
Graf, W., Robert, J.-L., Vederas, J. C., Tamm, Ch., Solomon, P. H., Miura, I., and Nakanishi, K. (1974). *Helv. Chim. Acta* **57**, 1801–1815.
Haslam R. J. (1972). *Biochem. J.* **127**, 34.
Haslam, R. J., Davidson, M. M. L., and McClenaghan, M. D. (1975). *Nature (London)* **253**, 455–457.
Hayakawa, S., Matsushima, T., Kimura, T., Minato, H., and Katagiri, K. (1968). *J. Antibiotics (Tokyo)* **21**, 523–524.
Holzer, H., Croop, J., Dienstman, S., Ishikawa, H., and Somlys, A. P. (1975). *Proc. Natl. Acad. Sci. U.S.A.* **72**, 513.
Ichikawa, Y., Maeda, M., and Horiuchi, M. (1975). *Exp. Cell Res.* **90**, 20–30.
Keller-Schierlein, W., and Kupfer, E. (1979). *Helv. Chim.* Acta **62**, 1501–1524.
Krishan, A. (1971). *J. Ultrastruct. Res.* **36**, 191–204.
Larpent, J. P. (1974). *Biol. Plant* **16**, 250–254.
Lash, J., Cloney, R. A., and Minor, R. R. (1970). *Biol. Bull.* **139**, 427.
Lebet, C. R., and Tamm, Ch. (1974). *Helv. Chim. Acta* **57**, 1785–1801.
McLaughlin, G. M., Sim, G. A., Kiechel, J.-R., and Tamm, Ch. (1970). *Chem. Commun.*, pp. 1398–1399.
McMillan, J. A., Chiang, C. C., Greensley, M. K., Paul, I. C., Patwardhan, S. A., Dev, S., Beno, M. A., and Christoph, G. G. (1977). *J. Chem. Soc. Chem. Commun.*, pp. 105–106.
Mak, K. M., Trier, J. S., Serfilippi, D., and Donaldson, R. M., Jr. (1974). *Exp. Cell Res.* **86**, 325–332.
Minato, H., and Katayama, T. (1970). *J. Chem. Soc. C*, pp. 45–47.
Minato, H., and Matsumoto, M. (1970). *J. Chem. Soc. C*, pp. 38–45.
Minato, H., Katayama, T., Matsumoto, M., Katagiri, K., Matsuura, S., Sunagawa, N., Hori, K., Harada, M., and Takeuchi, M. (1973). *Chem. Pharm. Bull.* **21**, 2268–2277.
Nakagawara, A., Takeshige, K., and Minakami, S. (1974). *Exp. Cell Res.* **87**, 392–394.
Partridge, T., Jones, G. E., and Gillett, R. (1975). *Nature (London)* **253**, 632–634.
Patwardhan, S. A., Pandey, R. C., Dev, S., and Pendse, G. S. (1974). *Phytochemistry* **13**, 1985–1988.
Pendse, G. S. (1974). *Experientia* **30**, 107–108.
Príbela, A., Tomko, J., and Dolejš, L. (1975). *Phytochemistry* **14**, 285.
Robert, J.-L., and Tamm, Ch. (1975). *Helv. Chim. Acta* **58**, 2501–2504.
Rothweiler, W., and Tamm, Ch. (1966). *Experientia* **22**, 750–752.
Rothweiler, W., and Tamm, Ch. (1970). *Helv. Chim. Acta* **54**, 696–724.
Schofield, J. G. (1971). *Nature New Biol.* **234**, 215–216.
Scott, P. M., Harwig, J., Chen, Y.-K., and Kennedy, B. P. C. (1975). *J. Gen. Microbiol.* **87**, 177–180.
Sekita, S., Yoshihira, K., Natori, S., and Kuwano, H. (1973). *Tetrahedron Lett.*, pp. 2109–2112.
Sekita, S., Yoshihira, K., Natori, S., and Kuwano, H. (1976). *Tetrahedron Lett.*, pp. 1351–1354.
Sekita, S., Yoshihira, K., and Natori, S. (1977). *Tetrahedron Lett.*, pp. 2771–2774.
Shay, J. W., Porter, K. R., and Prescott, D. M. (1974). *Proc. Natl. Acad. Sci. U.S.A.* **71**, 3059.
Silverton, J. V., Akiyama, T., Kabuto, C., Sekita, S., Yoshihira, K., and Natori, S. (1976). *Tetrahedron Lett.*, pp. 1349–1350.
Springer, J. P., Clardy, J., Wells, J. M., Cole, R. J., Kirksey, J. W., Macfarlane, R. D., and Torgerson, D. F. (1976). *Tetrahedron Lett.*, pp. 1355–1358.

Tsukuda, Y., and Koyama, H. (1972). *J. Chem. Soc. Perkin Trans. 2*, pp. 739–744.

Tsukuda, Y., Matsumoto, M., Minato, H., and Koyama, H. (1969). *Chem. Commun.*, p. 41.

Umeda, M., Ohtsubo, K., Saito, M., Sekita, S., Yoshihira, K., Natori, S., Udagawa, S., Sakabe, F., and Kurata, H. (1975). *Experientia* **31**, 435–438.

Vederas, J. C., and Tamm, Ch. (1976). *Helv. Chim. Acta* **59**, 558–566.

Vederas, J. C., Graf, W., David, L., and Tamm, Ch. (1975). *Helv. Chim. Acta* **58**, 1886–1898.

Wessells, N. K., Spooner, B. S., Ash, J. F., Bradley, M. O., Luduena, M. A., Taylor, E. L., Wrenn, J. T., and Yamada, K. M. (1971). *Science* **171**, 135–143.

White, G. J. (1971). *Roussel Conference on Platelet Aggregation*, March 4, 1971. Masson, Paris.

Williams, J. A., and Wolff, J. (1971). *Biochem. Biophys. Res. Commun.* **44**, 422–425.

9

The Biosynthesis of Gliotoxin
and Related Epipolythiodioxopiperazines

G. W. KIRBY AND D. J. ROBINS

I. INTRODUCTION

The epipolythiodioxopiperazines constitute a group of toxic, fungal metabolites exemplified by the first known member, gliotoxin (**1**). Reviews have appeared on the structure, chemistry, biosynthesis, and biological activity of these metabolites (Hardy and Ridge, 1973; Johne and Gröger, 1977; Leigh and Taylor, 1976; Sammes, 1975; Taylor, 1971). In this chapter

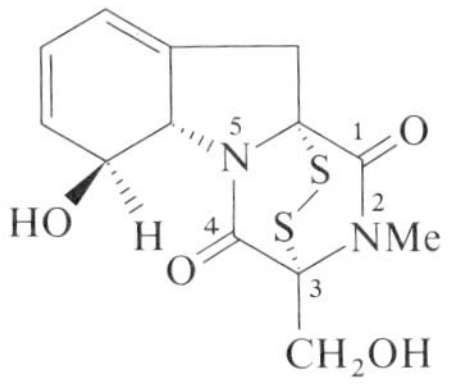

1

The Biosynthesis of Mycotoxins
Copyright © 1980 by Academic Press, Inc.
All rights of reproduction in any form reserved.
ISBN 0-12-670650-6.

we shall survey the biosynthesis of epipolythiodioxopiperazines and the related di(methylthio) derivatives, with emphasis on pathways which have received experimental attention.

II. SURVEY OF STRUCTURAL TYPES

Tables I–III provide a comprehensive list of known structures, all of which may be represented by the general formulas **2** and **3**. In all compounds, one

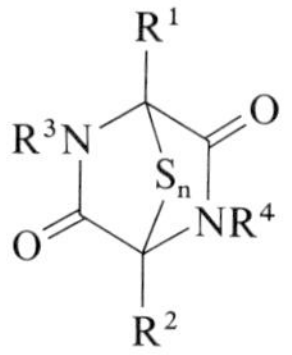

$$R^3N \diagdown \overset{R^1}{\underset{S_n}{\diagup}} \diagup \overset{O}{\diagdown} NR^4 \quad ; \quad R^2$$

2 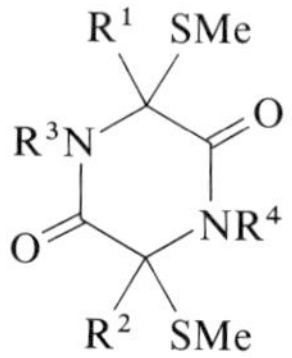   **3**

or both of the residues R^1 and R^2 appear, either by inspection of structures or from feeding experiments, to be derived from the aromatic amino acids, phenylalanine (**4**; R = H), tryptophan (**5**), or tyrosine (**4**; R = OH). The other residue may be derived from alanine (**6**; R = H), serine (**6**; R = OH), or,

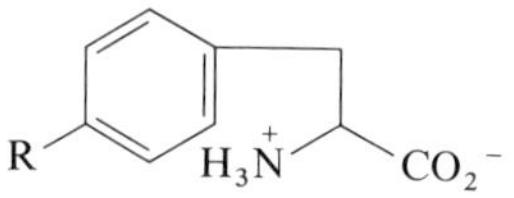

4 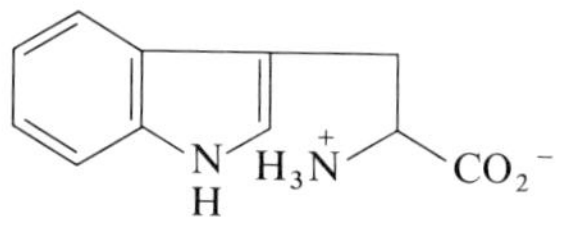   **5**

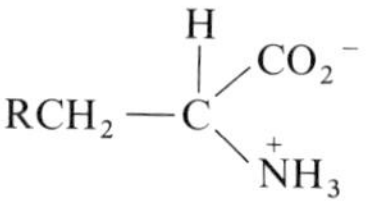

$$RCH_2 - \overset{H}{\underset{\overset{+}{N}H_3}{C}} \diagup \overset{CO_2^-}{}$$

6

for antibiotic A30641 (Table III), glycine. To date, residues of other amino acids, such as leucine and proline, which appear in many naturally occurring dioxopiperazines lacking sulfur (e.g., Johne and Gröger, 1977; Sammes, 1975; Turner, 1971), have not been found in the series **2** and **3**. With one exception, antibiotic A30641 (Table III), the metabolites **2** and **3** are alkylated on both nitrogen atoms, either by methylation or by cyclization, onto an oxidatively modified, aromatic amino acid residue. The sulfur bridge of the epipolythio derivatives (**2**) may vary in length ($n = 2$, 3, or 4), and, occasionally, all three members of a particular series have been isolated from cultures of a single organism. The di(methylthio) compounds (**3**) often occur together

TABLE I

Metabolites Derived from Phenylalanine

Compound	Structure	References[a]
Hyalodendrin $n = 2$		1
$n = 4$		2
$n = 2$		3
$n = 4$		3
	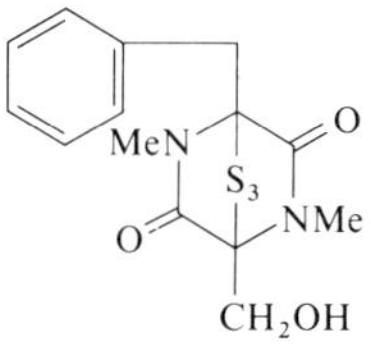	4
Gliovictin	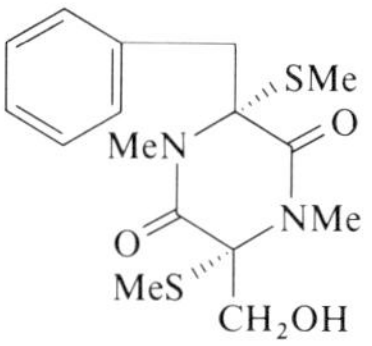	3, 5
Gliotoxin (R = H)		6
Gliotoxin acetate (R = Ac)		7
Dehydrogliotoxin	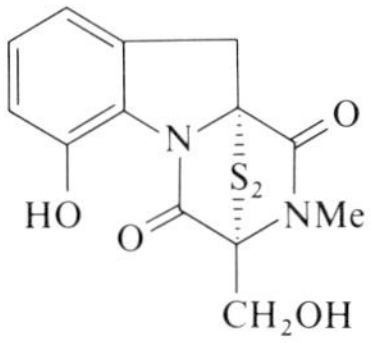	8
Isodehydrogliotoxin	As dehydrogliotoxin, but different position of phenolic group	9
Bisdethiodi(methylthio)gliotoxin	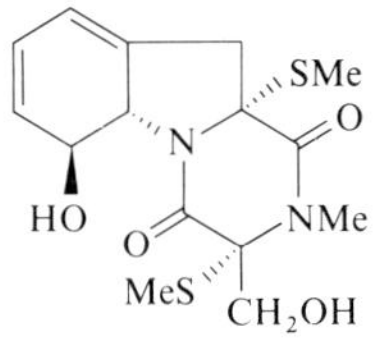	10

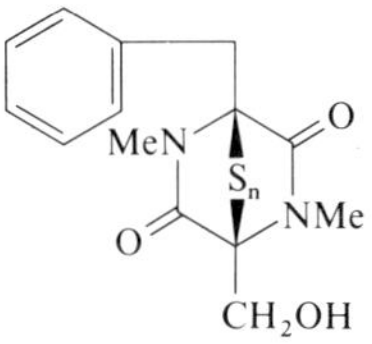

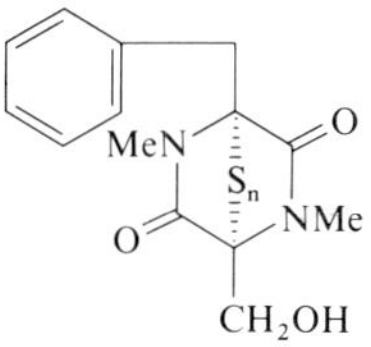

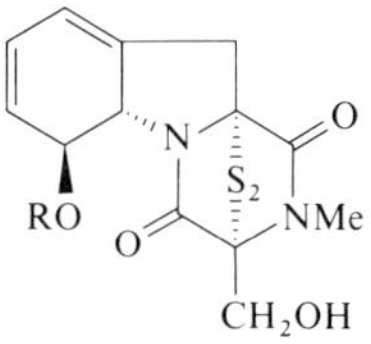

(*continued*)

TABLE I (*continued*)

Compound	Structure	References[a]
Aranotin (R = H) O-Acetylaranotin (R = Ac)		11, 12 11, 13
Apoaranotin	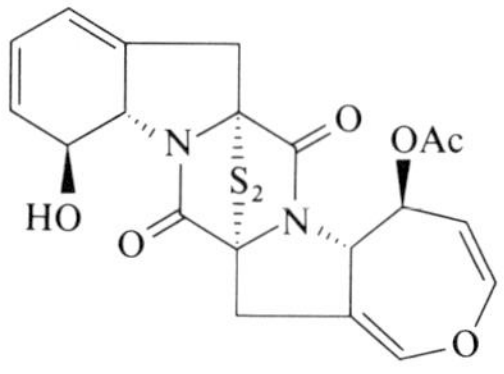	14
Bisdethiodi(methylthio)acetylaranotin	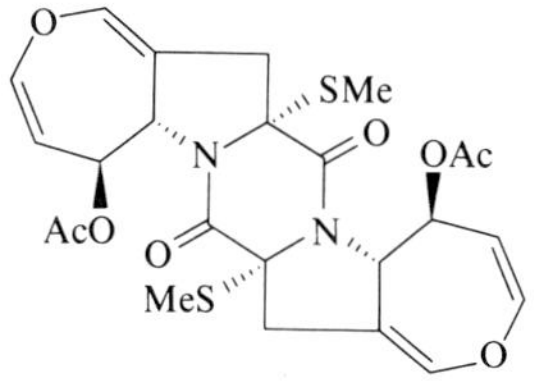	11, 12
Bisdethiodi(methylthio)acetylapoaranotin	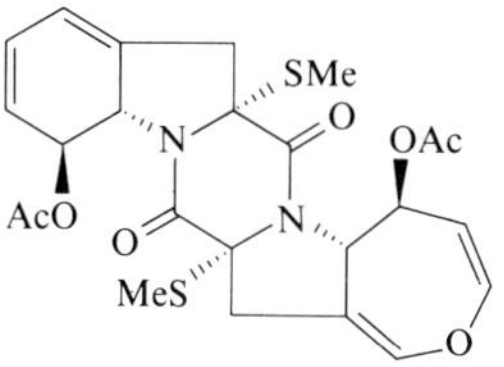	14
Epicorazine A	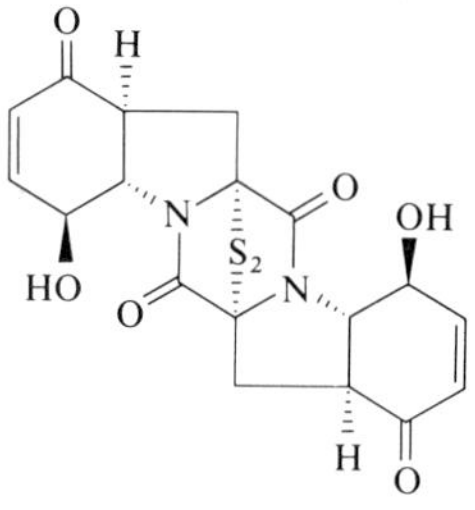 or antipode	15

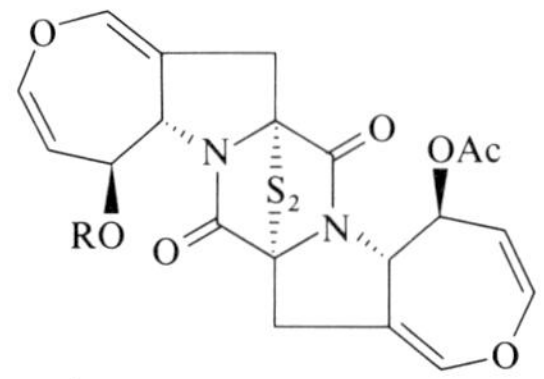

[a] References: (1) Strunz *et al.* (1973). (2) Strunz *et al.* (1975). (3) Michel *et al.* (1974). (4) DeVault and Rosenbrook (1973). (5) Dorn and Arigoni (1974). (6) Bell *et al.* (1958); Beecham *et al.* (1966). (7) Johnson *et al.* (1953). (8) Lowe *et al.* (1966). (9) Unpublished, cited in Taylor (1967). (10) Kirby *et al.* (1977, unpublished results). (11) Moncrief (1968). (12) Nagarajan *et al.* (1968a). (13) Nagarajan *et al.* (1968b); Cosulich *et al.* (1968). (14) Neuss *et al.* (1968b). (15) Baute *et al.* (1976); Deffieux *et al.* (1977).

TABLE II

Metabolites Derived from Tryptophan

Compound	Structure	References[a]
Sporidesmin ($n = 2$)	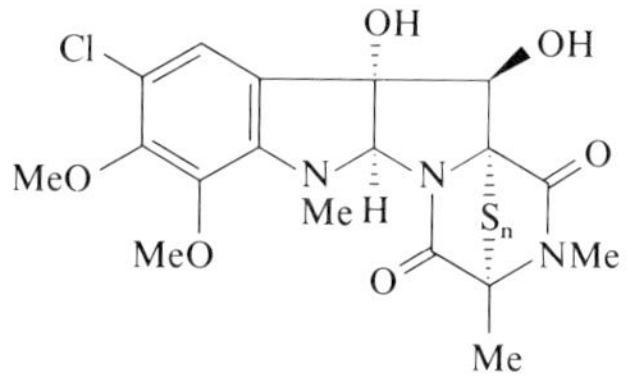	1, 2
Sporidesmin B	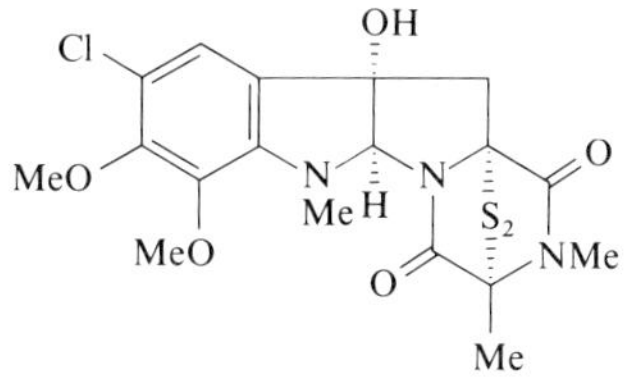	1
Sporidesmin C	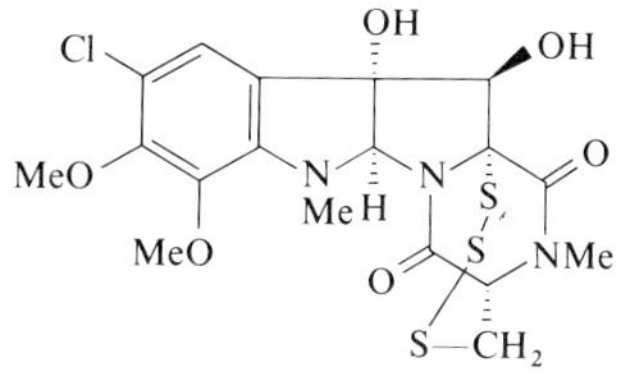	3
Sporidesmin D	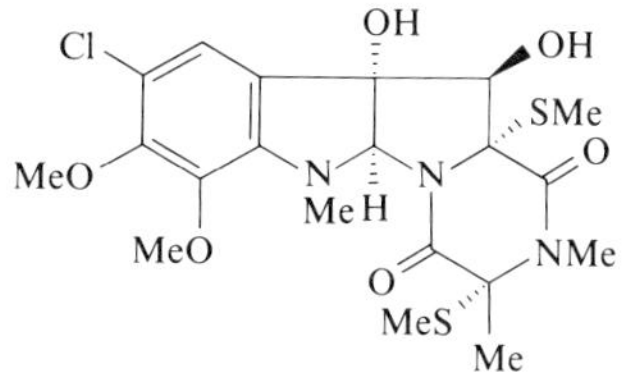	4
Sporidesmin E	As sporidesmin, but $n = 3$	5
Sporidesmin F	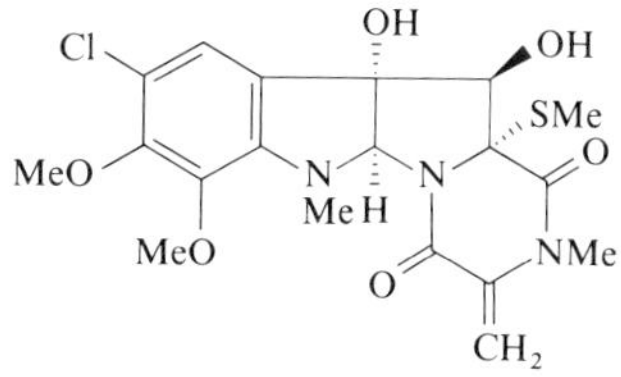	4
Sporidesmin G	As sporidesmin, but $n = 4$	6
Sporidesmin H	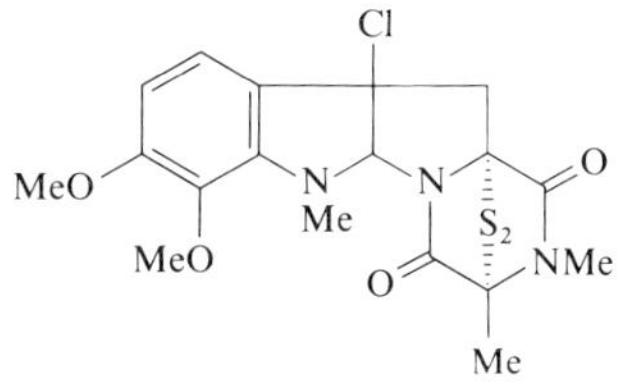	7

(continued)

TABLE II (*continued*)

Compound	Structure	References[a]
Chaetocin (R = H)		8
Dihydroxychaetocin (R = OH)		9
Verticillin A		10
Verticillin B		10
Verticillin C	As verticillin B, but with S₂ and S₃ bridges	10
Chetomin		11

[a] References: (1) Ronaldson *et al.* (1963). (2) Beecham *et al.* (1966). (3) Hodges and Shannon (1966). (4) Jamieson *et al.* (1969). (5) Rahman *et al.* (1969). (6) Francis *et al.* (1972); Przybylska *et al.* (1973). (7) Cited in Siuda and DeBernadis (1973). (8) Hauser *et al.* (1970); Weber (1972). (9) Hauser *et al.* (1972). (10) Minato *et al.* (1973). (11) McInnes *et al.* (1976); Brewer *et al.* (1972).

TABLE III

Metabolites Derived from Tyrosine (Tentative Assignments)

Compound	Structure	References[a]
Sirodesmin A ($n = 2$)	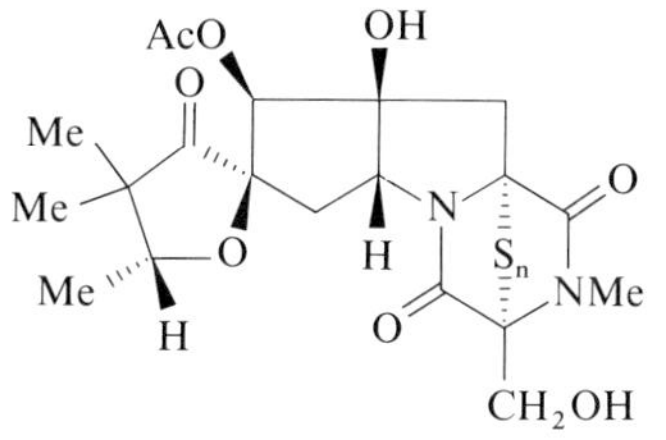	1
Sirodesmin B ($n = 4$)		1
Sirodesmin C ($n = 3$)		1
Sirodesmin G	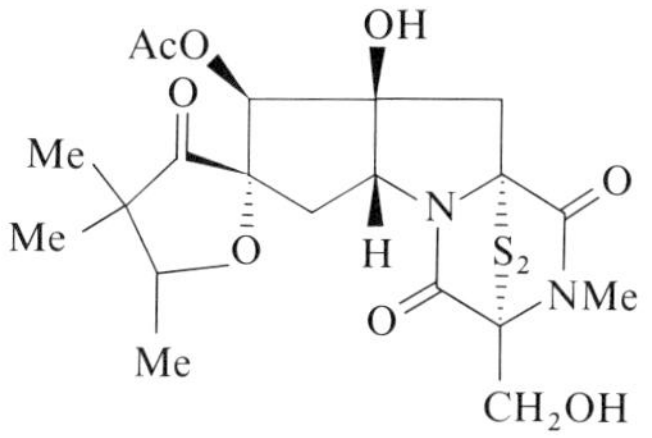	1
Antibiotic A30641	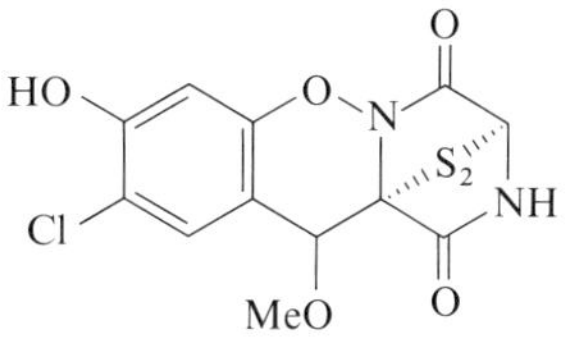	2

[a] References: (1) Curtis *et al.* (1977). (2) Berg *et al.* (1976, 1977).

with the corresponding bridged sulfides; a close biosynthetic relationship is clearly indicated but not yet proven.

For convenience of discussion, the metabolites have been classified according to their biosynthetic derivation, either established' by experiment or implied by structure, from phenylalanine (Table I), tryptophan (Table II), and tyrosine (Table III). Table IV lists metabolites of unknown structure.

TABLE IV

Metabolites of Unknown Structure

Compound	References[a]
Melinacidins II, III, and IV	1
Oryzachlorin	2

[a] References: (1) Argoudelis (1972); (2) Kato *et al.* (1969).

We shall begin with an account of the biosynthesis of gliotoxin (**1**), a representative of the phenylalanine group of epidisulfides.

III. THE BIOSYNTHESIS OF GLIOTOXIN

A. Incorporation of Phenylalanine and Serine

Suhadolnik and Chenoweth (1958) were the first to demonstrate that phenylalanine (**4**; R = H), rather than tryptophan (**5**), provides the reduced indole nucleus of gliotoxin (**1**). Both DL-[1-^{14}C]- and DL-[2-^{14}C]phenylalanine were incorporated efficiently (4–12%) into gliotoxin in cultures of *Trichoderma viride*. In contrast, no incorporation of DL-[7a-^{14}C]tryptophan was observed, although this amino acid was taken up from the culture medium and radioactivity appeared in the mycelium. Degradation (Fig. 1) of gliotoxin derived from DL-[1-^{14}C]phenylalanine showed that radioactivity resided largely (82%) at position 1, suggesting that the carbon skeleton of the amino acid had been incorporated intact; this conclusion has been amply confirmed by later work (see below).

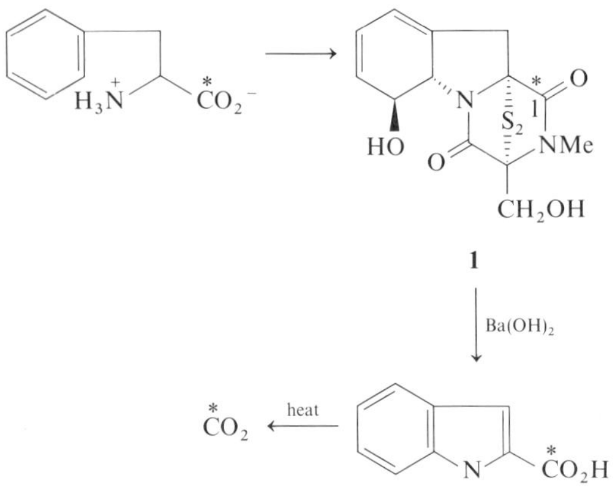

Fig. 1.   Degradation of gliotoxin (**1**) derived from DL-[1-^{14}C]phenylalanine.

Feeding experiments with serine (**6**; R = OH) (Winstead and Suhadolnik, 1960) were complicated by metabolic transfer of the methylene group [C(3)] into the C_1 pool of the organism. Thus, DL-[3-^{14}C]serine gave gliotoxin containing 25% of its activity in the *N*-methyl group, as shown by hydrolysis to liberate methylamine. As expected, DL-[*S*-methyl-^{14}C]methionine was a more efficient source of this group. However, the incorporation of DL-[1-^{14}C]serine was more easily interpreted (Fig. 2). No ^{14}C activity was found

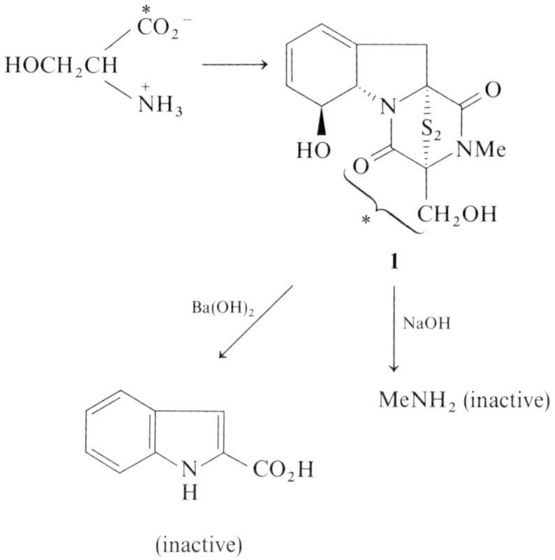

Fig. 2. Degradation of gliotoxin (1) derived from DL-[1-^{14}C]serine.

in either the N-methyl group of gliotoxin or the derived indole-2-carboxylic acid, a result consistent with incorporation of serine into the lower portion of the dioxopiperazine ring.

Metabolic studies (Bose et al., 1968a,b) using the stable isotopes ^{15}N and ^{13}C, provided further insight into the construction of the gliotoxin skeleton from simple amino acids. Isotopic enrichments were determined by mass spectrometry; the derivative 7, formed from gliotoxin by treatment with

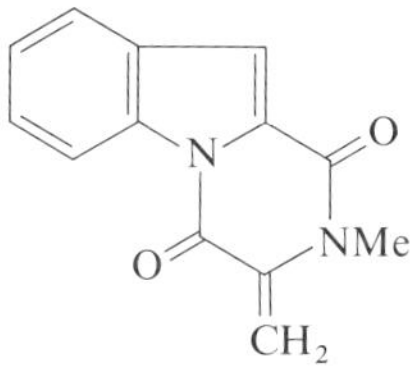

7

activated alumina, was especially suitable for this purpose. Glycine, aspartic acid, and glutamic acid provided, presumably by the familiar transamination processes, both nitrogen atoms of gliotoxin even in a culture medium rich in NH_4^+. [^{15}N]Phenylalanine gave gliotoxin labeled primarily in N(5) [as in (1)], but an experiment (Bose et al., 1968b) with the doubly labeled precursor, [1-^{14}C,^{15}N]phenylalanine, showed greater isotopic dilution of ^{15}N than ^{14}C. Thus, extensive deamination and reamination must have occurred; this conclusion is supported by the finding that L-[1-^{14}C]- and

D-[1-^{14}C]phenylalanines were incorporated into gliotoxin with similar efficiency. Finally, the observation that [1-^{13}C]- and [3-^{14}C]phenylalanines were incorporated with the same isotopic dilution provided further proof that the amino acid side chain [C(1) to C(3)] remained intact during formation of gliotoxin.

B. Formation of the Cyclohexadienol Ring

In their pioneering studies with *T. viride*, Winstead and Suhadolnik (1960) considered whether *m*-tyrosine (**8**) might be an intermediate in gliotoxin

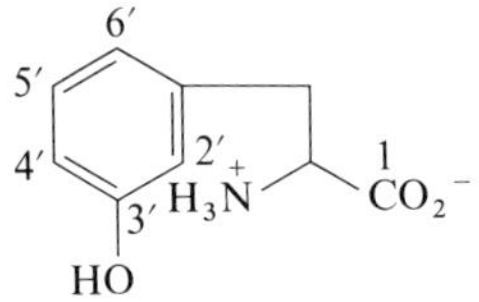

8

biosynthesis. Indeed, they reported high incorporation (30–44%) of tritium into gliotoxin when generally tritiated DL-*m*-tyrosine was fed to the organism. However, subsequent attempts, by three independent research groups, to reproduce this observation have failed. It now appears clear, from the following investigations, that neither *m*-tyrosine nor any other hydroxybenzene derivative is involved as an obligatory intermediate in gliotoxin biosynthesis, at least in *T. viride*.

Bu'Lock and Ryles (1970) fed DL-[1-^{14}C]phenylalanine and DL-[1-^{14}C]-*m*-tyrosine in parallel to *T. viride* under carefully matched conditions. The former amino acid was converted (5.4% incorporation, × 33 isotopic dilution), as expected, into gliotoxin; the latter gave gliotoxin with an activity [0.053% incorporation, × (7.7 × 10^3) isotopic dilution] judged to be insignificant. A similar negative result was obtained with DL-[4′,5′,6′-^{3}H]-2′,3′-dihydroxyphenylalanine and DL-[3′,5′-^{3}H]-*o*-tyrosine. More compellingly, incorporation of DL-[2′,3′,4′,5′,6′-^{2}H$_5$]phenylalanine into gliotoxin was shown by mass spectrometry to proceed without appreciable loss of deuterium. It follows that *m*-tyrosine (**8**), even if poorly metabolized when fed externally to the organism, cannot be an obligatory intermediate between phenylalanine and gliotoxin.

Johns and Kirby (1971) reached the same conclusions using somewhat different methods. DL-[2′,4′,6′-^{3}H]-*m*-Tyrosine and DL-[1-^{14}C]phenylalanine were fed as a mixture to *T. viride* to facilitate comparison of their relative incorporations. The ^{14}C:^{3}H ratio of the derived gliotoxin showed that phenylalanine was incorporated at least 100 times more efficiently than *m*-tyrosine. The fate of the aryl hydrogens of phenylalanine was then explored using tritium labeling. m-Tritiated phenylalanine carrying a reference ^{14}C label at C(1) (Fig. 3) was incorporated into gliotoxin with full retention of tritium. Dehydration and desulfuration of the gliotoxin afforded 7 without tritium loss, whereas dehydrogenation to give 9 occurred with ca. 50% loss of tritium. Thus, tritium at the *meta* position of phenylalanine is retained during biosynthesis, and ca. 50% appears at C(6) in gliotoxin (Fig. 3). This finding does not rigorously exclude m-tyrosine as an intermediate. Conceivably, m-hydroxylation of phenylalanine might proceed with migration of tritium to a neighboring (*ortho* or *para*) position followed by loss of hydrogen.

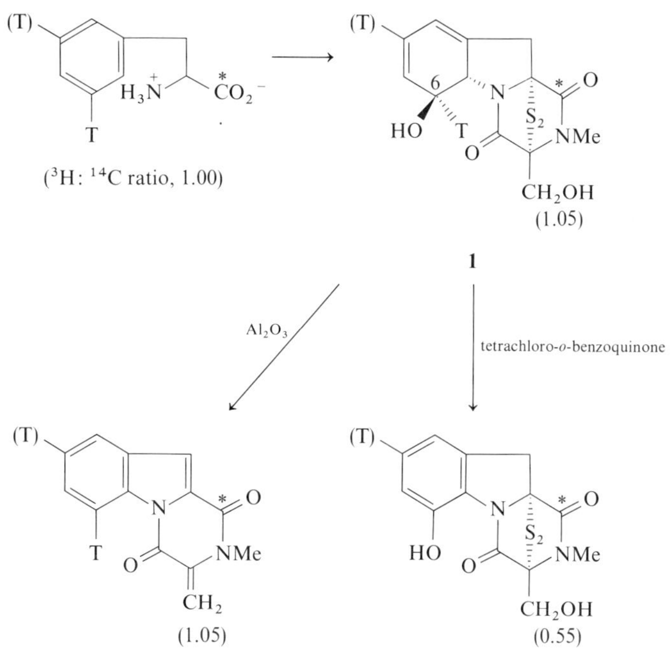

Fig. 3.   Incorporation of DL-[1-^{14}C; 3', 5'-^{3}H]phenylalanine into gliotoxin. Tritium was used in tracer amounts; (T) indicates alternative sites for the label arising from the symmetry of the precursor. Relative ^{3}H:^{14}C ratios are given in parentheses.

A reverse migration during closure of the nitrogen ring might then replace tritium at its original site. This possibility was discounted by complementary feeding experiments with o- and p-tritiated precursors. Both DL-[1-^{14}C,2',6'-^{3}H]- and DL-[1-^{14}C,4'-^{3}H]phenylalanines were incorporated into gliotoxin with full retention of tritium. Degradation of gliotoxin (as in Fig. 3) from the former feeding gave 7 and 9, both with loss of half the tritium. Gliotoxin derived from p-tritiated phenylalanine retained, as expected, all its tritium on conversion into **7** and **9**. It is clear, therefore, that neither loss nor migration of tritium (and, by implication, of hydrogen) occurs during biosynthesis.

Finally, independent studies by Brannon *et al.* (1971) gave results fully in accord with the foregoing findings. They found that DL-$[3-^{14}C]$phenylalanine was incorporated into gliotoxin with consistently greater efficiency than DL-$[2-^{14}C]$-*m*-tyrosine in both *T. viride* and *Penicillium terlikowskii*.

At present, the formation of the cyclohexadienol ring of gliotoxin (Fig. 4) is thought to involve, at some undetermined point in the biosynthetic pathway, an arene oxide intermediate of the type **10** invoked (Neuss *et al.*, 1968a, b) to explain the oxepin ring of the aranotins (see below). The isomeric oxide **11** is also mechanistically acceptable but could not serve directly as a precursor for the aranotin ring system. The formation and cyclization of an arene oxide need not, of course, disturb the hydrogens attached to the original phenyl group of phenylalanine. This scheme accommodates the results of all feeding experiments with the exception of the reported [cited in (Leigh and Taylor, 1976)] incorporation of phenolic precursors, e.g., **9**, into gliotoxin. However, although compounds of this type are excluded as obligatory intermediates, they might, in principle, be involved in alternative, minor pathways.

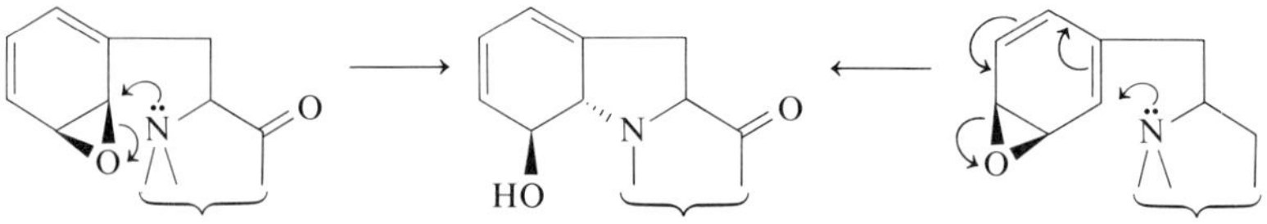

10   **11**

Fig. 4.   Arene oxides as intermediates in the biosynthesis of gliotoxin.

C. Status of *cyclo*(L-Phenylalanyl-L-seryl) as an Intermediate

Curiously, nearly 20 years separate the original feeding experiments with phenylalanine (Suhadolnik and Chenoweth, 1958) and the first clear identification of an intermediate on the pathway to gliotoxin. *cyclo*(L-Phenylalanyl-L-seryl) (**12**) is, *a priori*, an attractive candidate as an intermediate,

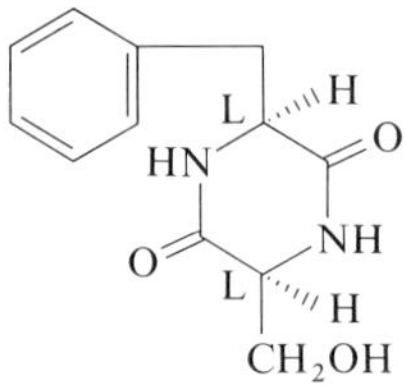

12

because it combines in a simple way the two recognized amino acid precursors. Accordingly, MacDonald and Slater (1975) fed $cyclo$(L-[1-^{14}C]-phenylalany-L-seryl) to $P.$ $terlikowskii$, but observed only a low incorporation into gliotoxin despite efficient uptake of the cyclodipeptide into the mycelium. They concluded that 12 could not be a free intermediate. In contrast, Bu'Lock and Leigh (1975), using $T.$ $viride$ (probably a $Gliocladium$ sp.), observed a high incorporation (21%) of activity into gliotoxin from a mixture of $cyclo$(L-phenylalanyl-L-seryl) and $cyclo$(L-phenylalanyl-D-seryl). Their precursor mixture was prepared from L-[Ar-^{3}H]phenylalanine and DL-[1-^{14}C]serine, and, significantly, the isotope ratios in the precursor and metabolite were identical within experimental error. It appeared, therefore, that 12, or its LD-diastereoisomer, was incorporated intact into gliotoxin. They considered that the high levels of 12 administered to cultures by the Canadian group (MacDonald and Slater, 1975) could well explain the poor incorporation, although they noted that different organisms had been employed in the two studies.

More recent work with $T.$ $viride$ ($Gliocladium$ $deliquescens$) (Kirby et al., 1978) has confirmed and extended Bu'Lock and Leigh's observations. ^{14}C-Labeled samples of all four stereoisomers of $cyclo$(phenylalanylseryl) were fed to cultures growing under standard conditions. The LL-isomer was incorporated efficiently (up to 50%) into gliotoxin, whereas none of the other stereoisomers was incorporated to any significant extent. Moreover, $cyclo$(L-[4-^{3}H]phenylalanyl-L-[3-^{14}C]seryl) gave gliotoxin with essentially the same isotope ratio, and hydrolysis of this gliotoxin yielded inactive methylamine. These last two observations strongly support the belief that 12, or a corresponding, open dipeptide, is incorporated intact into gliotoxin. Complete cleavage of 12 would almost certainly have led to differential dilution of the constituent amino acids by endogenous material, with a consequent change in the isotope ratio. Also, some activity from the liberated L-[3-^{14}C]serine should have passed into the N-methyl group of gliotoxin (Winstead and Suhadolnik, 1960).

The same group (Kirby et al., 1978) tested the status of 12 as a free intermediate in $T.$ $viride$ by an "intermediate-trapping" experiment. Nonradioactive 12 was incubated with the organism and, 2 hr later, L-[U-^{14}C]-phenylalanine was added to the medium. The culture filtrate was extracted with chloroform to remove gliotoxin and then with ethyl acetate to remove the cyclodipeptide (12). This was diluted with pure, inactive 12, and the mixture crystallized to constant ^{14}C activity. The residual activity corresponded to 1.3% of that administered as L-[U-^{14}C]phenylalanine. Thus, 12 had been formed from phenylalanine and is presumably present in the organism under normal conditions of growth. It remains to be seen whether the metabolism of *P. terlikowskii* differs in any significant way from that of *T. viride*.

D. Formation of 3*a*-Deoxygliotoxin, an Unnatural Metabolite of *Trichoderma viride*

The efficient biosynthetic transformation of **12** into gliotoxin prompted Kirby and Robins (1976) to explore the metabolism of structurally modified analogues in *T. viride*. Providing that the enzymes catalyzing the elaboration of **12** do not have high substrate specificities, then analogues of **12** might be converted into new, unnatural derivatives of gliotoxin. This was found to be true for *cyclo*(L-alanyl-L-phenylalanyl) (**13**) (Fig. 5).

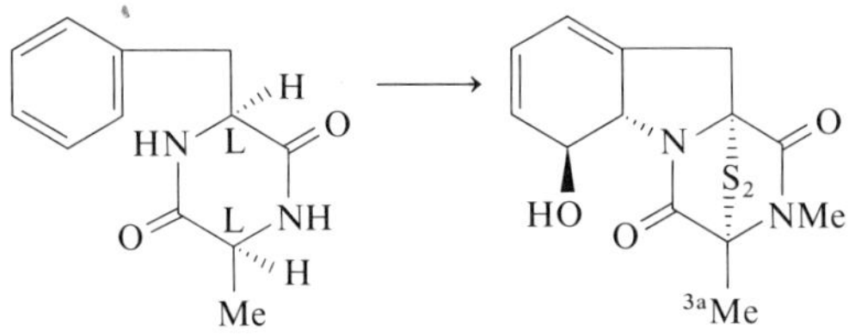

13   **14**

Fig. 5. Formation of 3*a*-deoxygliotoxin in *Trichoderma viride* (*Gliocladium deliquescens*).

The cyclodipeptide **13**, labeled uniformly with ^{14}C in the phenylalanyl unit, was administered (1.0–8.0 mg per 100 ml culture medium) to cultures of *T. viride* (*G. deliquescens*). Dimethyl sulfoxide was used to dissolve the precursor. After the usual period of incubation, the chloroform-soluble products were examined by autoradiography and radioscanning of thin layer chromatographic plates. A new metabolite was detected and fully characterized spectroscopically as 3*a*-deoxygliotoxin (**14**) after chromatographic separation and crystallization. No detectable amounts of the new substance (**14**) were formed when the organism was grown in the absence of **13**. Furthermore, the specific activities of **13** and **14** were identical within experimental error, showing that appreciable dilution of **14** with endogenous material had not occurred. Therefore, 3*a*-deoxygliotoxin had been formed in response to administration of the precursor **13**.

The "unnatural" transformation **13** → **14**, proceeded about as efficiently (up to 40% conversion) as the natural process (see Section III,C) despite a structural change, OH → H, close to the site of two later enzymatic processes, *N*-methylation and sulfur insertion. Experiments with other analogues of *cyclo*(L-phenylalanyl-L-seryl) may delineate the substrate specificities of the late-stage enzymes and lead to the detection of analogues of natural, transient intermediates.

E. Late-Stage Processes

Three processes at least are required to transform $cyclo$(L-phenylalanyl-
L-seryl) (12) into gliotoxin (1), namely, N-methylation, oxidative cyclization
onto the phenyl ring, and introduction of the sulfur bridge. Nothing is known
of the order of these processes, nor does any clear pattern emerge from inspection of the structures of other sulfur-bridged dioxopiperazines. Also, it
cannot be assumed that a unique sequence of transformations obtains even
in a single organism. N-Methylation is likely to involve transmethylation
from methionine, and the problem of oxidative cyclization has been discussed
earlier (Section III,B). In the remainder of this section we shall consider the
origin of the disulfide bridge.

The biosynthetic introduction of sulfur into gliotoxin has been the subject
of some discussion (Sammes, 1975; Taylor, 1971) and a little experimentation
but, so far, no firm conclusions have been reached. Sulfur enters the gliotoxin
molecule carrying with it no structural clue to its metabolic origin. Also, the
interpretation of feeding experiments with ^{35}S-labeled precursors is necessarily complicated by the possibility of sulfur transfer among various,
plausible sulfur donors. Some interesting, preliminary results have, nevertheless, appeared. Neuss et $al.$ (1968a) observed good incorporation of
radioactivity from L-^{35}S]methionine (15) into gliotoxin in cultures of $P.$
$terlikowskii$ (10.2% incorporation) and $T.$ $viride$ (3.3%). They also studied,
using $T.$ $viride$, the effect of various radioinactive diluents, added in 1000-
fold excess, on gliotoxin production and the incorporation of ^{35}S from 15.
Most significantly, L-cysteine (16) caused an increase (2.3-fold) in the yield of

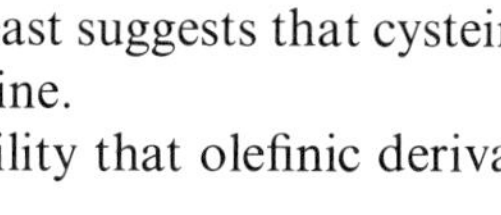

$$\overset{*}{Me}SCH_2CH_2CH \overset{\displaystyle CO_2^-}{\underset{\displaystyle \overset{+}{N}H_3}{\diagdown}} \qquad HSCH_2CH \overset{\displaystyle CO_2^-}{\underset{\displaystyle \overset{+}{N}H_3}{\diagdown}}$$

$$\textbf{15} \qquad\qquad\qquad \textbf{16}$$

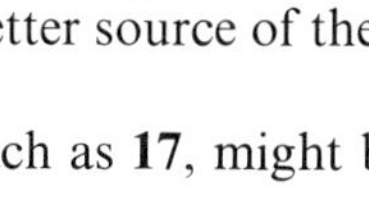

gliotoxin together with a marked reduction (to 0.1%) in the incorporation of
[35]S. This at least suggests that cysteine is a better source of the sulfur bridge
than methionine.

The possibility that olefinic derivatives, such as 17, might be involved in

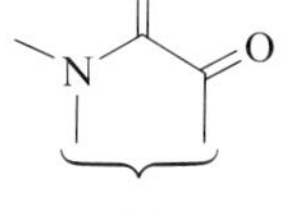

$$\textbf{17}$$

316   G. W. Kirby and D. J. Robins

the introduction of sulfur has also been explored. To this end, $[3\text{-}^2\text{H}_2]$-phenylalanine (**18**) (Fig. 6) was fed to *T. viride* (*G. deliquescens*) (Johns *et al.*, 1975). The derived gliotoxin was shown by mass spectrometry to consist largely of a monodeuterated species mixed, of course, with unlabeled material. The NMR spectrum showed, within the sensitivity limits of the method, that the product was stereospecifically deuterated, and a tentative assignment of the stereochemistry (as in **19**) was made. Separate feedings of stereoselectively deuterated and tritiated (3*R*)- and (3*S*)-phenylalanines established that hydrogen loss from the methylene group was also stereospecific and occurred with retention of configuration at this center (Fig. 6).

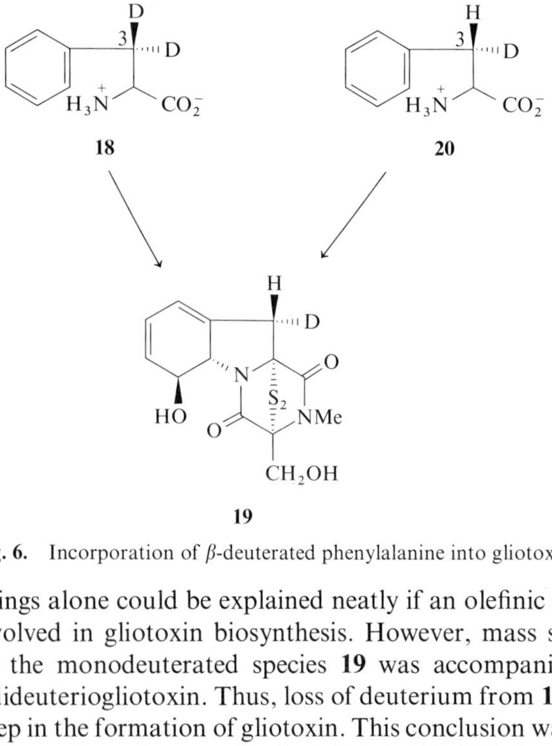

Fig. 6.   Incorporation of β-deuterated phenylalanine into gliotoxin.

These findings alone could be explained neatly if an olefinic intermediate (**17**) were involved in gliotoxin biosynthesis. However, mass spectrometry showed that the monodeuterated species **19** was accompanied by small amounts of dideuteriogliotoxin. Thus, loss of deuterium from **18** was not an obligatory step in the formation of gliotoxin. This conclusion was reinforced when the incorporation of stereoselectively labeled $[3\text{-}^3\text{H}]$phenylalanine into mycelial protein was examined. Hydrolysis of the washed mycelium yielded phenylalanine, which was purified and assayed for both tritium content and tritium configuration. In this way, it was shown that passage of $[3\text{-}^3\text{H}]$phenylalanine into the protein involved extensive loss of tritium from the (3*R*) form and retention of tritium from the (3*S*) form (configuration as in **20**). Furthermore, it was concluded that hydrogen removal and replacement in the methylene group of phenylalanine had occurred with retention of

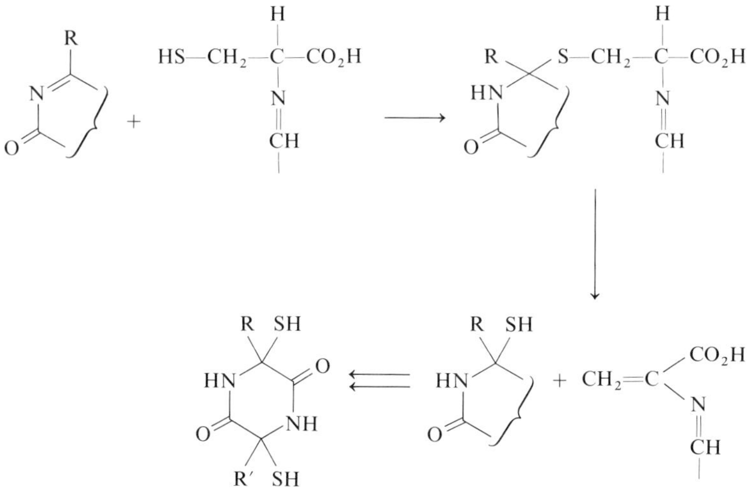

Fig. 7.   A possible pathway for the introduction of sulfur into a dioxopiperazine.

configuration. These stereochemical results matched those for the incorporation of deuterium and tritium into gliotoxin. It appeared, therefore, that, in *T. viride*, stereospecific exchange of one of the methylene hydrogens of phenylalanine takes place and proceeds faster than incorporation of the amino acid into either protein or gliotoxin.

A proper understanding of the mechanism for the introduction of sulfur into gliotoxin, and other epipolythiodioxopiperazines, requires identification of (a) the first-formed sulfur derivative, (b) its immediate precursor, and (c) the sulfur donor. Suitable candidates for (a) and (b) might profitably be synthesized and tested for incorporation into gliotoxin, but (c) is likely to prove elusive unless active cell-free systems can be obtained. At present, the reaction scheme shown in Fig. 7 accommodates what little is known experimentally. Cysteine, possibly in combination with pyridoxal, is suggested for the sulfur donor, and a dehydrodioxopiperazine is suggested for the sulfur acceptor. Consecutive introduction of two thiol groups would give **21** suitable for oxidative cyclization to an epidisulfide or methylation to a di(methylthio) compound.

IV. THE BIOSYNTHESIS OF THE ARANOTINS

The aranotin (**22**; R = H) group of metabolites, first studied at the Lilly and Lederle laboratories, show an interesting and informative structural resemblance to gliotoxin.

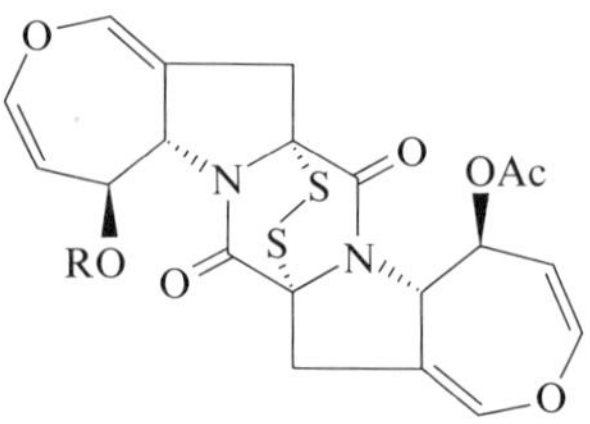

22

Preliminary biosynthetic studies (Neuss *et al.*, 1968a) were conducted on the formation of bisdethiodi(methylthio)acetylaranotin (**23**) (BDA) in *Ara-*

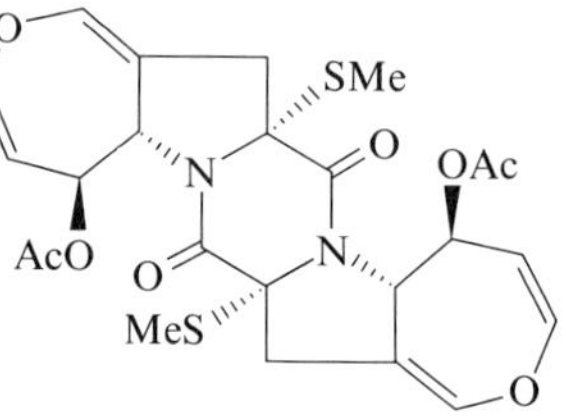

23

chniotus aureus. Activity from L-[*methyl*-^{14}C]methionine, DL-[3-^{14}C]serine, and DL-[2-^{14}C]tryptophan was incorporated quite efficiently into BDA. In each case, Zeisel degradation of the metabolite gave methyl iodide, derived from the S-methyl groups, which contained most of the activity. As expected, methionine was found to be the most efficient (6.46% incorporation) and specific (96% in the S-methyl groups) source of the S-methyl carbon. However, the same amino acid was also an effective sulfur donor. When a mixture of L-[^{35}S]methionine and L-[*methyl*-^{3}H]methionine was fed to *A. aureus*, the derived BDA contained both ^{35}S (2.77% incorporation) and ^{3}H (11.3%). The substantially higher incorporation of ^{3}H than ^{35}S indicated that an intact S-methyl group was probably not transferred to the dioxo-piperazine ring system. Both L- and D-[1-^{14}C]phenylalanines were incorporated into BDA with similar efficiency (3.15% and 2.42%, respectively) but the metabolite was not degraded to locate the label.

In a later investigation (Brannon *et al.*, 1971), DL-[3-^{14}C]phenylalanine was shown to be a much more efficient precursor than DL-[2-^{14}C]-*m*-tyrosine and DL-3′,5′-[2-^{14}C]dihydroxyphenylalanine for BDA in *A. aureus*. This finding matches that discussed earlier (Section III,B) for the biosynthesis of gliotoxin. When a mixture of DL-[3-^{14}C]phenylalanine and DL-[2′-^{3}H]-phenylalanine was fed, incorporations of both ^{14}C (7.04%) and ^{3}H (5.67%) were observed, showing that tritium in the *ortho* position of the phenyl ring was largely retained in BDA. A more comprehensive study of the metabolic fate of hydrogen in phenylalanine was made using *Aspergillus terreus*, a good source of acetylaranotin (**22**; R = Ac). Fully C-deuterated ($^2H_8$) DL-phenylalanine was used as the precursor, and the deuterium content of the derived acetylaranotin was determined mass spectrometrically from the proportions of the dominant (M^+-2S) ions. The acetylaranotin was found to contain large amounts of $[^2H_{14}]$ and $[^2H_7]$ species. It appeared, therefore, that the $[^2H_8]$phenylalanine had contributed to both halves of the symmetrical structure (**22**; R = Ac), and, in doing so, had lost only one deuterium atom, presumably from the α-position. The formation of $[^2H_7]$acetylaranotin is the expected consequence of concurrent incorporation of the deuterated precursor and undeuterated, endogenous phenylalanine. Again, the results are in close correspondence with those for gliotoxin, and it is clear that hydrogen loss from neither the phenyl nor the methylene group of phenylalanine is an obligatory process in the biosynthesis of acetylaranotin. There appears to be partial loss (Johns *et al.*, 1975) of methylene hydrogen, but his may simply result from an exchange process akin to that observed in *r. viride*.

The presence of oxepin rings in the aranotin structures is best explained Neuss *et al.*, 1968a,b) by the intervention of an arene oxide (Fig. 8) capable ` rapid valence tautomerism (see also Section III,B). The close biosynthetic lationship between the aranotin and gliotoxin ring systems is conveniently splayed in the structure of apoaranotin (**24**), a metabolite of *A. aureus*.

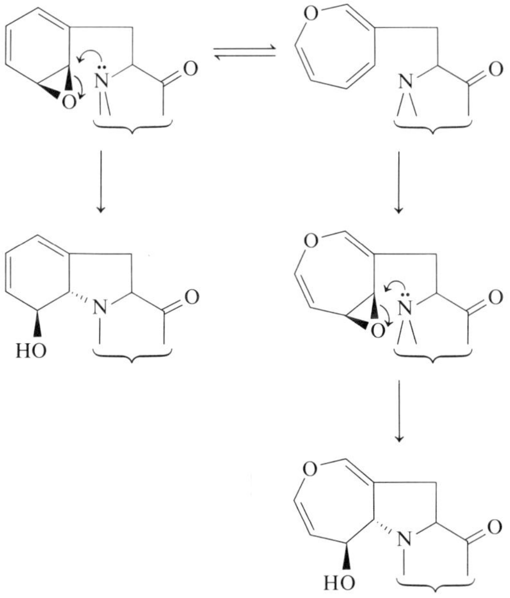

Fig. 8. Biosynthetic derivative of the aranotin and gliotoxin ring systems from a common arene oxide intermediate.

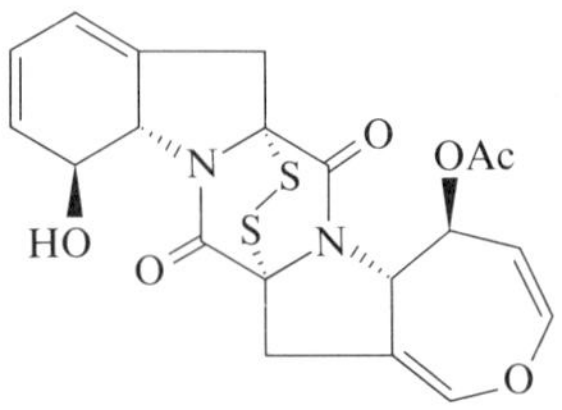

24

If the analogy with gliotoxin biosynthesis is extended, *cyclo*(L-phenylalanyl-L-phenylalanyl) should be a precursor for all members of the aranotin group, but, so far, this point has not been tested experimentally.

V. THE BIOSYNTHESIS OF SPORIDESMIN

Consideration of the structures of sporidesmin (**25**) and its cometabolites suggests a biosynthetic derivation from tryptophan and alanine, although, clearly, an extensive series of peripheral changes to the carbon skeleton must take place.

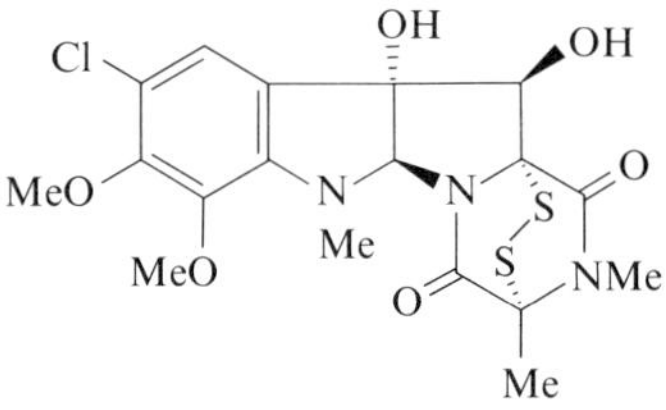

25

Towers and Wright (1969) tested a range of simple amino acids as precursors for sporidesmin using cultures of *Pithomyces chartarum* grown on seed test papers. Activity from DL-[3-^{14}C]tryptophan, L-[U-^{14}C]alanine, L-[U-^{14}C]- and DL-[1-^{14}C]serines, [U-^{14}C]- and [1-^{14}C]glycines, and L-[*methyl*-^{14}C]-methionine was incorporated into sporidesmin. No incorporation was observed with DL-[3-^{14}C]cysteine or L-[U-^{14}C]phenylalanine. The highest specific activities in sporidesmin were obtained with tryptophan and serine, but no degradations were performed to locate the sites of labeling. L-[^{35}S]-Cysteine, L-[^{35}S]methionine, and sodium [^{35}S]sulfate were all effective sources of sulfur, with L-cysteine giving the highest specific activity in sporidesmin.

Kirby and Varley (1974) studied the stereochemistry of hydrogen loss involved in the hydroxylation of the sporidesmin skeleton at C(3) (tryptophan numbering is used for clarity). Samples of DL-tryptophan, stereoselectively tritiated in the methylene group, were mixed with DL-[1-^{14}C]tryptophan to provide a reference label, and fed to *P. chartarum*. Acceptable incorporations of ^{14}C (0.37–1.1%) into sporidesmin were observed. Essentially complete retention of tritium from (3S)-[3-^{3}H]tryptophan and complete loss of tritium from (3R)-[3-^{3}H]tryptophan took place. This result is consistent with a hydroxylation reaction, of the familiar monooxygenase type, taking place with retention of configuration at the site of attack. However, hydroxylation via hydration of a 2,3 double bond or reductive opening of a 2,3 epoxide cannot be discounted. Because no satisfactory methods were available for the degradation of small quantities of sporidesmin, evidence for intact incorporation of tryptophan was sought with tactical use of ^{3}H and ^{14}C in various combinations. The same retention of tritium was observed when (3S)-[3-^{3}H]tryptophan was fed in admixture with [^{14}C]tryptophan labeled in either the side chain [C(1) or C(3)] or the nucleus [C(2′)]. There can be little doubt, therefore, that tryptophan contributes an intact indolyl-C$_3$ unit to the sporidesmin structure. Furthermore, DL-[2′-^{3}H,3-^{14}C]tryptophan was incorporated into sporidesmin without tritium loss. These results are summarized, in condensed form, in Fig. 9.

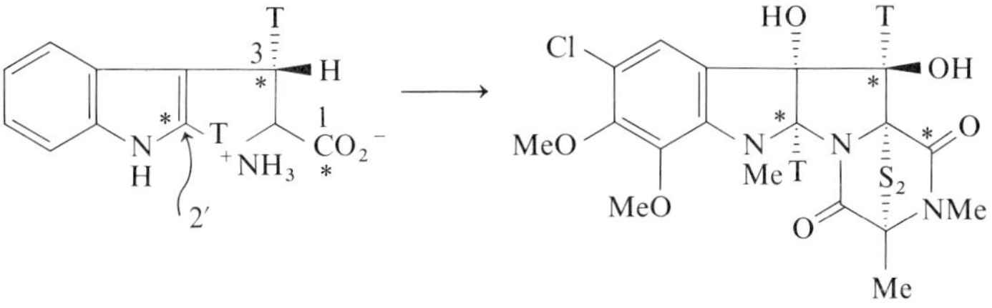

25

Fig. 9.   Incorporation of tritiated (T) and ^{14}C-labeled (*) tryptophan into sporidesmin (**25**). The results of four separate double-labeling experiments are superimposed.

The metabolic steps leading from tryptophan to sporidesmin have not been investigated in any detail, although one might expect a close correspondence with gliotoxin biosynthesis. For example, formation of the fused pyrrolidine system could involve an intermediate epoxide (**26**) analogous to

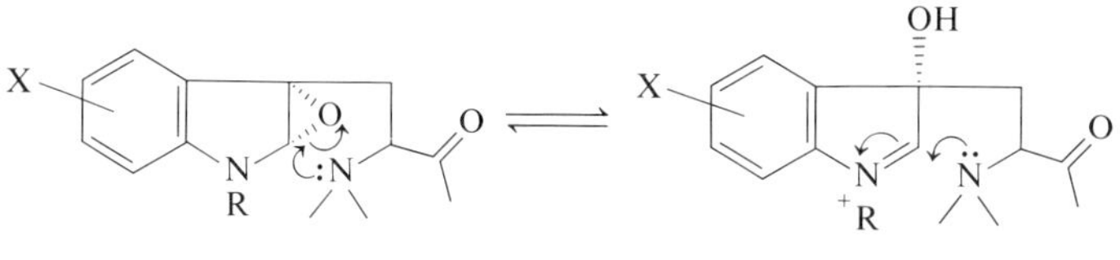

26

the benzene oxide derived from phenylalanine. Kirby and Varley (1974) studied the metabolism in *P. chartarum* of *cyclo*(L-alanyl-L-tryptophyl) (**27**),

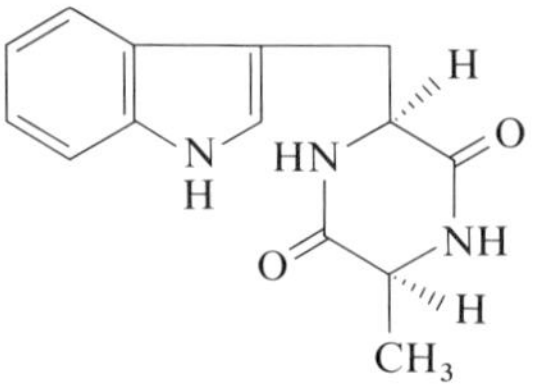

27

a known (Slater *et al.*, 1970) precursor of echinulin, a sulfur-free dioxopiperazine. Good incorporation (2.05%, based on ^{14}C) of *cyclo*(L-[3-^{3}H]alanyl-L-[3-^{14}C]tryptophyl) into sporidesmin was observed, but the ^{3}H:^{14}C ratio of the product was only 51% that of the precursor. This fall in isotope ratio may have arisen from partial or complete cleavage of **27** into its constituent amino acids followed by their separate incorporation. Alternatively, loss of tritium from the methyl group of the alanyl unit may have occurred via reversible formation of a dehydroalanyl derivative at some point in the biosynthetic pathway. Clearly, further studies are needed to settle the role of **27** in sporidesmin biosynthesis.

VI. CONCLUSIONS

So far, discussion has been confined to those metabolites whose biosynthesis has been investigated experimentally. Several important groups remain to be studied.

Hyalodendrin and related compounds of the phenylalanine group (see Table I), although simple in structure, contain the fundamental sulfur-bridged system and lack the complications of late-stage oxidation. Importantly, within this series the sulfur bridge is displayed in both possible absolute configurations. Comparative feeding experiments with the LL- and DD-forms of *cyclo*(phenylalanylseryl) would be especially interesting. Epicorazine A, tentatively assigned to the phenylalanine group, is isomeric with deacetyl-aranotin. The close correspondence between these structures is interesting in that the formation of both might involve two consecutive epoxidations of a phenyl ring.

The chaetocins and verticillins constitute an extensive series of tryptophan metabolites (see Table II) having a close structural relationship with the sporidesmins. However, two indole rings have been linked oxidatively, and this process, rather than epoxidation, is presumably responsible for closure of the pyrrolidine ring; there is precedence for this in the biosynthesis of, for example, chimonanthine (e.g., Kirby *et al.*, 1969). Chetomin shows an interesting variation in that one indole nucleus is attached via nitrogen and, consequently, cyclization onto this unit has not taken place.

In the sirodesmins (see Table III), the structure of the aromatic amino acid precursor has been obscured by prenylation, hydroxylation, and ring

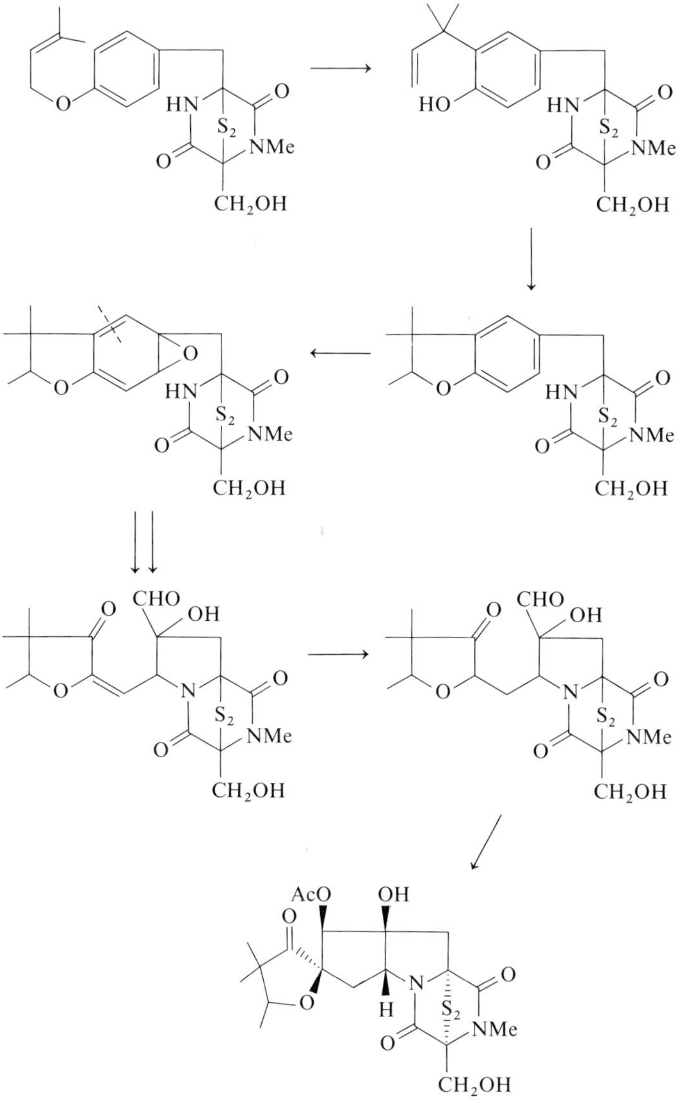

Fig. 10.   A possible biosynthetic pathway to sirodesmin A.

contraction. Curtis *et al.* (1977) suggest, very reasonably, a biosynthetic derivation from tyrosine, and recent, preliminary feeding experiments support this hypothesis (Bu'Lock, 1977). One possible scheme (Curtis *et al.*, 1977) for the conversion of a *cyclo*(seryltyrosyl) derivative into sirodesmin is shown in Fig. 10. The sirodesmins should provide a profitable area for biosynthetic inquiry, especially if sulfur-free dioxopiperazines, for example, *cyclo*(seryltyrosyl) and its prenyl derivatives, are involved as free intermediates.

ADDENDUM

The following papers relating to the structure and biosynthesis of epipolythiodioxopiperazines have appeared since submission of the original manuscript. They are listed, with their titles, under the most appropriate section headings.

Section I

Kirby, G. W. (1979). The biosynthesis of epipolythiodioxopiperazines. *Pure and Appl. Chem.* **51**, 705.

Section II (*Table I*)

Baute, M.-A., Deffieux, G., Baute, R., and Neveu, A. (1978). New antibiotics from the fungus *Epicoccum nigrum*. I. Fermentation, isolation and antibacterial properties. *J. Antibiot.* **31**, 1099.

Deffieux, G., Baute, M.-A., Baute, R., and Filleau, M.-J. (1978). New antibiotics from the fungus *Epicoccum nigrum*. II. Epicorazine A: Structure elucidation and absolute configuration. *J. Antibiot.* **31**, 1102.

Deffieux, G., Filleau, M.-J., and Baute, R. (1978). New antibiotics from the fungus *Epicoccum nigrum*. III. Epicorazine B: Structure elucidation and absolute configuration. *J. Antibiot.* **31**, 1106.

Deffieux, G., Gadret, M., Leger, J. M., and Carpy, A. (1979). Crystal structure of a new fungal metabolite of the epidithio-3,6-dioxo-2,5-piperazine group: Epicorazine B $(C_{18}H_{16}N_2O_6S_2 \cdot \frac{1}{2}C_2H_5OH)$. *Acta Crystallogr. Sect. B.* **35**, 2358.

Section II (*Table II*)

Rahman, R., Safe, S., and Taylor, A. (1978). Sporidesmins. Part 17. Isolation of sporidesmin H and sporidesmin J. *J. Chem. Soc. Perkin Trans. 1*, p. 1476.

Brewer, D., McInnes, A. G., Smith, D. G., Taylor, A., Walker, J. A., Loosli, H. R., and Kis, Z. L. (1978). Sporidesmins. Part 16. The structure of chetomin, a toxic metabolite of *Chaetomium cochliodes*, by nitrogen-15 and carbon-13 nuclear magnetic resonance spectroscopy. *J. Chem. Soc. Perkin Trans. 1*, p. 1248.

Section III (*Table I*)

Kirby, G. W., Robins, D. J., Sefton, M. A., and Talekar, R. R. (1980). Biosynthesis of bisdethiobis(methylthio)gliotoxin, a new metabolite of *gliocladium deliquescens*. *J. Chem. Soc. Perkin Trans. 1*, p. 119.

REFERENCES

Argoudelis, A. D. (1972). *J. Antibiot.* **25**, 171.

Baute, R., Deffieux, G., Baute, M.-A., Filleau, M.-J., and Neveu, A. (1976). *Tetrahedron Lett.*, p. 3943.

Beecham, A. F., Fridrichsons, J., and Mathieson, A. M. (1966). *Tetrahedron Lett.* p. 3131.

Bell, M. R., Johnson, J. R., Wildi, B. S., and Woodward, R. B. (1958). *J. Am. Chem. Soc.* **80**, 1001.

Berg, D. H., Massing R. P., Hoehn, M. M., Boeck, L. D., and Hamill, R. L. (1976). *J. Antibiot.* **29**, 394.

Berg, D. H., Hamill, R. L., and Hoehn, M. M. (1977). U.S. Patent 4 001 086 (*Chem. Abs.* **86**, 87 671).

Bose, A. K., Das, K. G., Funke, P. T., Kugajevsky, I., Shukla, O. P., Khanchandani, K. S., and Suhadolnik, R. J. (1968a). *J. Am. Chem. Soc.* **90**, 1038.

Bose, A. K., Khanchandani, K. S., Tavares, R., and Funke, P. T. (1968b). *J. Am. Chem. Soc.* **90**, 3593.

Brannon, D. R., Mabe, J. A., Molloy, B. B., and Day, W. A. (1971). *Biochem. Biophys. Res. Commun.*, p. 588.

Brewer, D., Duncan, J. M., Jerram, W. A., Leach, C. K., Safe, S., Taylor, A., Vining, L. C., Archibald, R. M., Stevenson, R. G., Mirocha, C. J., and Christensen, C. M. (1972). *Can. J. Microbiol.* **18**, 1129.

Bu'Lock, J. D. (1977). Chemical Society Autumn Meeting, September 20th, 1977, Aberdeen, Scotland.

Bu'Lock, J. D., and Leigh, C. (1975). *J. Chem. Soc. Chem. Commun.*, p. 628.

Bu'Lock, J. D., and Ryles, A. P. (1970). *Chem. Commun.*, p. 1404.

Cosulich, D. B., Nelson, N. R., and van den Hende, J. H. (1968). *J. Am. Chem. Soc.* **90**, 6519.

Curtis, P. J., Greatbanks, D., Hesp. B., Cameron, A. F., and Freer, A. A. (1977). *J. Chem. Soc. Perkin Trans. 1*, p. 180.

Deffieux, G., Gadret, M., and Leger, J. M. (1977). *Acta Crystallogr. Sect. B.* **33**, 1474.

DeVault, R. L., and Rosenbrook, W. (1973). *J. Antibiot.* **26**, 532.

Dorn, F., and Arigoni, D. (1974). *Experientia* **30**, 134.

Francis, E., Rahman, R., Safe, S., and Taylor, A. (1972). *J. Chem. Soc. Perkin Trans 1*, p. 470.

Hardy, P. M., and Ridge, B. (1973). *In* "Progress in Organic Chemistry" (W. Carruthers and J. K. Sutherland, eds.), Vol. VIII, p. 129. Butterworth, London.

Hauser, D. Weber, H. P., and Sigg, H. P. (1970). *Helv. Chim. Acta* **53**, 1061.

Hauser, D. Loosli, H. R., and Niklaus, P. (1972). *Helv. Chim. Acta* **55**, 2182.

Hodges, R., and Shannon, J. S. (1966). *Aust. J. Chem.* **19**, 1059.

Jamieson, W. D., Rahman, R., and Taylor, A. (1969). *J. Chem. Soc. C*, p. 1564

Johne, S., and Gröger, D. (1977). *Pharmazie* **32**, 1.

Johns, N., and Kirby, G. W. (1971). *Chem. Commun.*, p. 163; Johns, N. (1972). Ph.D. thesis, Loughborough University of Technology, Loughborough, England.

Johns, N., Kirby, G. W., Bu'Lock, J. D., and Ryles, A. P. (1975). *J. Chem. Soc. Perkin Trans. 1*, p. 383.

Johnson, J. R., Kidwai, A. R., and Warner, J. S. (1953). *J. Am. Chem. Soc.* **75**, 2110.

Kato, A. Saeki, T., Suzuki, S., Ando, K., Tamura, G., and Arima, K. (1969). *J. Antibiot.* **22**, 322.

Kirby, G. W., and Robins, D. J. (1976). *J. Chem. Soc. Chem. Commun.*, p. 354.

Kirby, G. W., and Varley, M. J. (1974). *J. Chem. Soc. Chem. Commun.*, p. 833. Varley, M. J. (1975). Ph. D. thesis, Loughborough University of Technology, Loughborough, England.

Kirby, G. W., Shah, S. W., and Herbert, E. J. (1969). *J. Chem. Soc. C*, p. 1916.

Kirby, G. W., Patrick, G. L., and Robins, D. J. (1978). *J. Chem. Soc. Perkin Trans. I*, p. 1336.

Leigh, C., and Taylor, A. (1976). *In* "Advances in Chemistry Series" (J. V. Rodricks, ed.), No. 149, p. 228. Amer. Chem. Soc., Washington, D. C.

Lowe, G., Taylor, A., and Vining, L. C. (1966). *J. Chem. Soc. C*, p. 1799

MacDonald, J. C., and Slater, G. P. (1975). *Can. J. Biochem.* **53**, 475.

McInnes, A. G., Taylor, A., and Walter, J. A. (1976). *J. Am. Chem. Soc.* **98**, 6741.

Michel, K. H., Chaney, M. O., Jones, N. D., Hoehn, M. M., and Nagarajan, R. (1974). *J. Antibiot.* **27**, 57.

Minato, H., Matsumoto, M., and Katayama, T. (1973). *J. Chem. Soc. Perkin Trans. 1*, p. 1819.

Moncrief, J. W. (1968). *J. Am. Chem. Soc.* **90**, 6517.

Nagarajan, R., Huckstep, L. L., Lively, D. H., DeLong, D. C., March, M. M., and Neuss, N. (1968a). *J. Am. Chem. Soc.* **90**, 2980.

Nagarajan, R., Neuss, N., and Marsh, M. M. (1968b). *J. Am. Chem. Soc.* **90**, 6518.

Neuss, N., Boeck, L. D., Brannon, D. R., Cline, J. C., DeLong, D. C., Gorman, M., Huckstep, L. L., Lively, D. H., Mabe, J., Marsh, M. M., Molloy, B. B., Nagarajan, R., Nelson, J. D., and Stark, W. M. (1968a). *Antimicrob. Agents Chemother.* p. 213.

Neuss, N., Nagarajan, R., Molloy, B. B., and Huckstep, L. L. (1968b). *Tetrahedron Lett.*, p. 4467.

Przybylska, M., Gopalakrishna, E. M., Taylor, A., and Safe, S. (1973). *J. Chem. Soc. Chem. Commun.*, p. 554.

Rahman, R., Safe, S., and Taylor, A. (1969). *J. Chem. Soc. C*, p. 1665.

Ronaldson, J. W., Taylor, A., White, E. P., and Abraham, R. J. (1963). *J. Chem. Soc.*, p. 3172.

Sammes, P. G. (1975). *In* "Progress in the Chemistry of Organic Natural Products" (W. Herz, H. Grisebach, and G. W. Kirby, eds.), Vol. XXXII, p. 51. Springer-Verlag, Vienna and New York.

Siuda, J. F., and DeBernadis, J. F. (1973). *Lloydia* **36**, 107.

Slater, G. P., MacDonald, J. C., and Nakashima, R. (1970). *Biochemistry* **9**, 2886.

Strunz, G. M., Kakushima, M., Stillwell, M. A., and Heissner, C. J. (1973). *J. Chem. Soc. Perkin Trans. 1*, p. 2600.

Strunz, G. M., Kakushima, M., and Stillwell, M. A. (1975). *Can. J. Chem.* **53**, 295.

Suhadolnik, R. J., and Chenoweth, R. G. (1958). *J. Am. Chem. Soc.* **80**, 4391.

Taylor, A. (1967). *In* "Biochemistry of Some Foodborne Microbial Toxins" (R. I. Mateles and G. N. Wogan, eds.), p. 69. MIT Press, Cambridge, Massachusetts.

Taylor, A. (1971). *In* "Microbial Toxins" (S. Kadis and A. Ciegler, eds.), Vol. VII, p. 337. Academic Press, New York.

Towers, N. R., and Wright, D. E. (1969). *N. Z. J. Agric. Res.* **12**, 275.

Turner, W. B. (1971). "Fungal Metabolites." Academic Press, New York.

Weber, H. P. (1972). *Acta Crystallogr. Sect. B* **28**, 2945.

Winstead J. A., and Suhadolnik, R. J. (1960). *J. Am. Chem. Soc.* **82**, 1644.

10

The Biosynthesis of Cyclopiazonic Acid and Related Tetramic Acids

CEDRIC W. HOLZAPFEL

I. INTRODUCTION

The fungus *Penicillium cyclopium* Westling has been isolated from a variety of commodities in many parts of the world. Wilson *et al.* (1968) and Wilson (1971) reported two outbreaks of a disease which occurred after the ingestion of moldy feed contaminated with *P. cyclopium*. A similar

The Biosynthesis of Mycotoxins
Copyright © 1980 by Academic Press, Inc.
All rights of reproduction in any form reserved.
ISBN 0-12-670650-6.

outbreak of a disease in England was reported by Harrison (1971), who isolated *P. cyclopium* from crushed barley. Holzapfel (1968) was the first to report the isolation of a major toxic metabolite from *P. cyclopium*. The strain of *P. cyclopium* (C.S.I.R. 1082) used in this study was isolated from groundnuts and was toxic to ducklings and rats, when grown on sterilized moistened corn meal. The toxin, designated cyclopiazonic acid (CA), later designated α-cyclopiazonic acid (αCA), was extracted with chloroform–methanol and isolated by chromatography on formamide-impregnated cellulose powder followed by ion-exchange chromatography. This tetramic acid was subsequently isolated by Ohmomo *et al.* (1973) from surface and submerged cultures of *Aspergillus versicolor* (Vuill.) Tiraboschi and, more recently, by Luk *et al.* (1977) from *Aspergillus flavus* Link.

The toxicity of αCA was investigated by Purchase (1974). Histological investigations of organs in rats that died after oral and intraperitoneal administration revealed changes in liver, kidney, heart, pancreas, and spleen. Single-cell and focal necrosis of the hepatocytes and necrosis of the bile duct cells were observed in the liver.

Meronuck *et al.* (1972) showed that another tetramic acid, tenuazonic acid, was the major toxin from *Alternaria alternata*, while Umetsu *et al.* (1974a) isolated this compound from the broth of *Pyricularia oryzae* Cavara, the causal fungus of the rice blast disease. Holzapfel (1965, unpublished results) studied the toxigenicity of several South African isolates of *Alternaria tenuis* Auct. cultivated on corn and characterized tenuazonic acid as the causal mycotoxin. Tenuazonic acid exibits a conspicuous stunting effect on seedling growth of rice (Umetsu *et al.*, 1974b). Steyn and Rabie (1976) showed that the magnesium and calcium complexes of tenuazonic acid represent the toxicity of *Phoma sorghina* Sacc., the fungus implicated in the etiology of onyalai, a hematologic disorder. Tenuazonic acid was investigated by Gitterman (1965) and Kaczka *et al.* (1964) for its antineoplastic activity and by Miller *et al.* (1964) for its antiviral activity. The ability of tenuazonic acid to block peptide bond formation in protein synthesis was extensively investigated by Carrasco and Vazquez (1973).

Another tetramic acid, erythroskyrine, is one of three mycotoxins produced by *Penicillium islandicum* Sopp. The acute toxicity and pathological changes effected by this orange red metabolite were described by Ueno *et al.* (1975). It is a hepatotoxin, but its role in the carcinogenesis of mice and rats fed with *P. islandicum*-molded rice is still obscure.

As a result of the real and potential importance of the tetramic acids as mycotoxins, their chemistry and biochemistry have received considerable attention. In this chapter, studies on the biosynthesis of cyclopiazonic acid and related tetramic acids will be reviewed.

II. THE STRUCTURES OF NATURALLY OCCURRING TETRAMIC ACIDS

Stickings (1959) reported the first example of a naturally occurring tetramic acid, designated tenuazonic acid, isolated from a strain of *A. tenuis* Auct. It was formulated as an enolic tautomer of the acetyltetramic acid (**1**), formally derived from L-isoleucine, on the basis of chemical studies. A recent investigation (Dippenaar *et al.*, 1978) of copper bistenuazonate established that the chelate is formed between the enolic C(10)–O and the amide C(2)–O, as shown in **2**. The cations of the calcium and magnesium complexes of

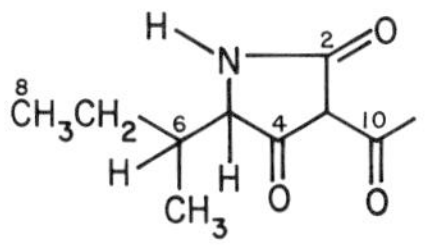

I	2

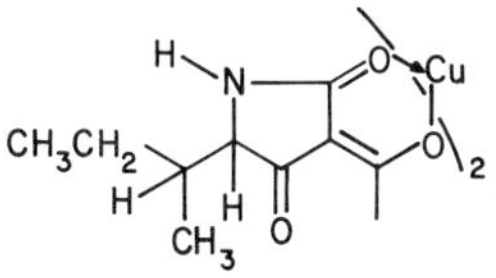

tenuazonic acid, isolated by Steyn and Rabie (1976), probably occupy the same position as the copper cation in **2**. The calcium and magnesium complexes contain the same absolute configuration as reported for tenuazonic acid. Gandhi *et al.* (1973) described the isolation of a magnesium complex in which the metal ion is bound to tetramic acid moieties. The compound, an antibiotic called magnesidin, was obtained from cultures of *Pseudomonas magnesiorubra*. The toxicity and other biological activities of the tetramic acids may, at least in part, be related to their ability to complex selectively *in vivo* with trace metals.

The nitrogen-containing pigment, named erythroskyrine, was first isolated by Howard and Raistrick (1954) from *P. islandicum* Sopp. Shoji *et al.* (1965) isolated this compound from another strain of the same fungus and elucidated its structure as **3**. The compound, which contains a polyene system, is an acyltetramic acid formally derived from *N*-methyl-L-valine.

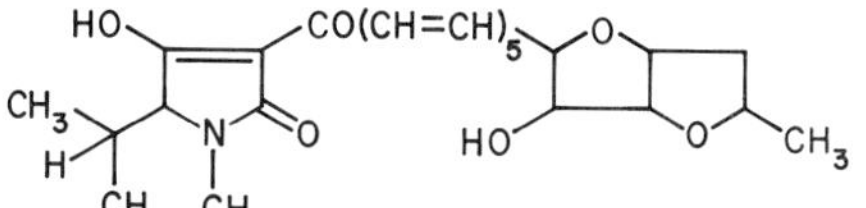

3

The structure of αCA was deduced by Holzapfel (1968) on the basis of chemical and physicochemical investigations. The compound was originally formulated as the enol tautomer (**5**) of the acyltetramic acid (**4**). A recent ^{13}C nuclear magnetic resonance (NMR) study (Steyn and Wessels, 1978) of cyclopiazonic acid indicated that it exists as a mixture of three tautomers,

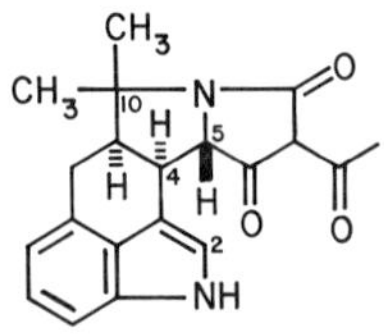

4

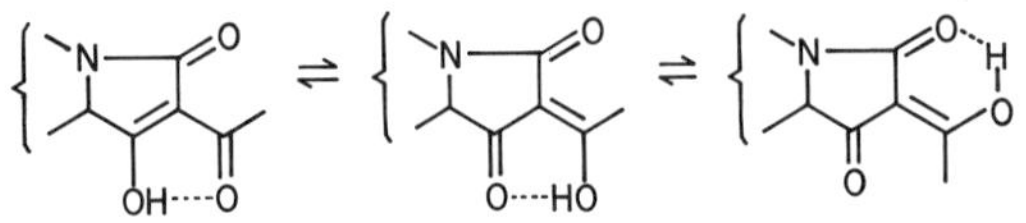

5   6   7

5, 6, and 7, in deuteriochloroform. However, the interconversion between tautomers 5 and 6 is so fast on the ^{13}C NMR time scale that these two tautomers give rise to a single line for the resonance of a specific carbon atom. A comparison of the peak intensities of those signals assigned to 7 with those of 5/6 showed that the ratio of 7 to 6 and 5 in deuterochloroform is ca. 6:1.

Holzapfel and Schabort (1977) recently presented evidence that position 5 of αCA has the L-configuration. Earlier, Holzapfel et al. (1970) isolated two metabolites chemically related to αCA from shake cultures of P. cyclopium. These compounds, cyclopiazonic acid imine and bissecodehydrocyclopiazonic acid [also designated β-cyclopiazonic acid (βCA)], have the structures 8 and 9, respectively.

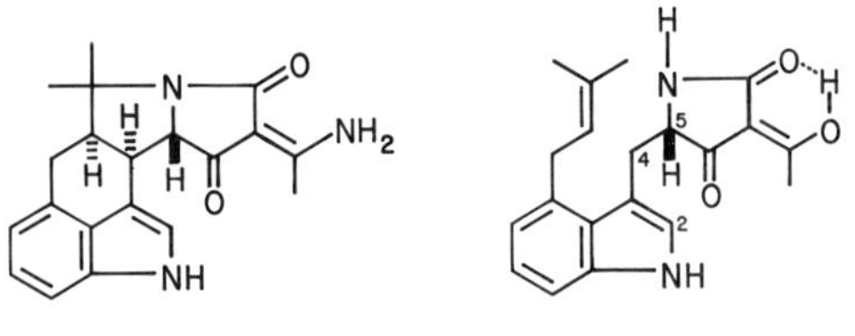

8   9

III. THE BIOSYNTHESIS OF TETRAMIC ACIDS

A. The Origin of the Carbon Skeletons of Tetramic Acids

1. Tenuazonic acid

Tenuazonic acid was the first tetramic acid whose biosynthesis received attention (Stickings and Townsend, 1961). A strain of A. tenuis Auct. growing on Czapek–Dox medium has been shown to incorporate more than 4% of the ^{14}C from added sodium [1-^{14}C]acetate into tenuazonic acid (1).

Hydrolysis of the labeled compound with 2 N sulfuric acid furnished 3-amino-4-methyl-2-hexanone which, on treatment with iodine in the presence of sodium hydroxide, furnished isoleucine and iodoform. The iodoform was oxidized to carbon dioxide, while treatment of isoleucine with ninhydrin furnished 2-methylbutanal, isolated as its 2,4-dinitrophenylhydrazone. Kuhn–Roth oxidation of the aldehyde gave acetic acid which was degraded by the Schmidt procedure to carbon dioxide and methylamine. The 2-methylbutanal was also degraded stepwise by the method of Strassman. Determination of the radioactivity of the various degradation products showed that 94% of the activity was equally shared between the lactam C(2) and side-chain C(10) carbonyl atoms. The remaining activity was shared between C(4) of the lactam ring and the ω carbon atom of the *sec*-butyl side chain. The results are consistent with derivation of tenuazonic acid from isoleucine and two molecules of acetic acid. However, the direct incorporation of isoleucine into tenuazonic acid was not investigated.

No information is available about the biochemical process which converts isoleucine and acetic acid (two units) into tenuazonic acid. By analogy with fatty acid and polyketide biosynthesis (cf. Turner, 1971), it is possible that an acetate (via acetyl coenzyme A) and a malonate unit (the monocoenzyme A derivative of malonic acid formed from acetyl-CoA and carbon dioxide) combine with the loss of a free carboxy group to give enzyme-bound acetoacetic acid. Condensation of this activated keto acid with isoleucine would give rise to tenuazonic acid. This suggested process is analogous to the laboratory synthesis of α-acetyltetramic acids (Lacey, 1954).

2. Erythroskyrin

The biosynthesis of erythroskyrin was investigated by Shibata *et al.* (1966), who established the distribution of ^{14}C in the molecule which was obtained by cultivation of the mold on Czapek–Dox media containing various ^{14}C-labeled substrates. The degradation reactions which were carried out on the labeled erythroskyrin are summarized in Fig. 1 (**10**–**12**). Erythroskyrin containing the label from added DL-$[1-^{14}C]$valine was decomposed into N-methylvaline (**10**) by ozonolysis. The product was converted into its N-(2,4-dinitrophenyl) derivative, which was decomposed photochemically into isobutanal (**11**). The 2,4-dinitrophenylhydrazone derivative of the aldehyde contained no radioactivity, while the N-(2,4-dinitrophenyl)-N-methylvaline contained 79% of the activity of the erythroskyrin. The result showed that $[1-^{14}C]$valine was incorporated (essentially) intact into the lactam portion of erythroskyrin, with the radioactivity located mainly at C(4).

Labeled erythroskyrin was also obtained from the mold fed separately with sodium $[1-^{14}C]$- and $[2-^{14}C]$acetates and with $[1-^{14}C]$- and $[2-^{14}C]$-diethyl malonates. Hydrogenation of this material furnished a decahydro

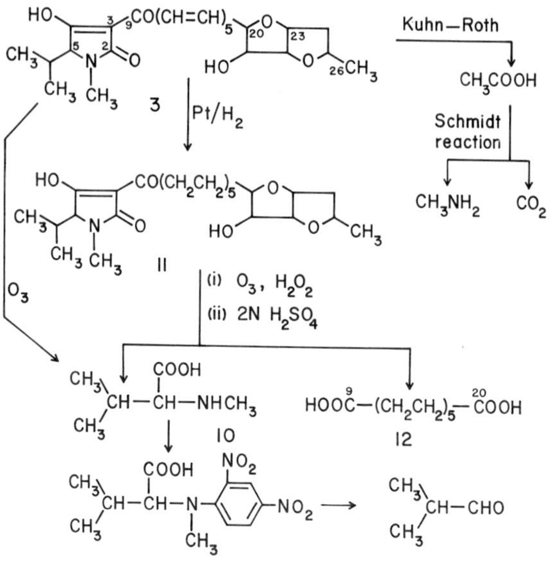

Fig. 1. Degradation of erythroskyrin.

derivative (11) which, on ozonolysis followed by hydrolysis, furnished
N-methylvaline and dodecanedioic acid (12). The diacid was isolated as its
dimethyl ester, while the amino acid was isolated as its N-(2,4-dinitrophenyl)
derivative. The erythroskyrin obtained from [1-^{14}C]acetate and from
[1-^{14}C]- and [2-^{14}C]malonates afforded dodecanedioic acid which contained 58% (6/10), 71% (6/9) and 63.5% (6/9), respectively of the total radioactivity. In each case, the corresponding N-methylvaline was essentially
inactive.

From these results it was deduced that any radioactivity in the acetic acid
obtained by Kuhn–Roth oxidation of [2-^{14}C]acetate-labeled erythroskyrin
must be derived from C(26). The acetic acid contained 4.45% of the total
activity, and this was shown by the Schmidt degradation procedure to be
located in the methyl group. The acetic acid obtained by Kuhn–Roth
oxidation of [1-^{14}C]- and [2-^{14}C]malonate-derived erythroskyrin was
inactive. These results proved that the biosynthesis of erythroskyrin involved the condensation of valine and a polyketide moiety. More specifically,
the results were taken as evidence that erythroskyrin is biosynthesized from
valine [N(1) and C(4) to C(8)], one acetate [C(25) and C(26)], and nine
malonate [C(2), C(3), C(9) to C(24)] units. This conclusion must, however,
be considered as tentative, particularly as no direct evidence was obtained
on the incorporation of ^{14}C from the various substrates into C(2) and

C(3). Two possibilities remain for the sequence in which the biogenetic units are joined together. The first involves condensation of valine with a C_{20}-polyketide. The other possibility involves the condensation of a C_{18}-polyketide with a five-membered ring formed from valine and one malonate unit. Similar possibilities, but with a C_4-dicarboxylic acid replacing valine, have been considered by Bentley *et al.* (1962) for tetronic acid biosynthesis in *Penicillium charlessi*.

3. α-Cyclopiazonic Acid

The origin of the carbon skeleton of a third tetramic acid, αCA, has been established. Structure analysis of the compound suggested that it is probably derived either from tryptophan, a C_5 unit formed from mevalonic acid and two molecules of acetic acid, or from tryptophan and two C_5 units formed from mevalonic acid. Holzapfel and Wilkins (1971) studied the biosynthesis of αCA in *P. cyclopium* grown in shake culture on a (basically) Czapek medium with sodium nitrate as nitrogen source and a trace element supplement. Labeled substrates were added on the sixth day after the start of the fermentation, and αCA was isolated 24 hr later. The following incorporations were obtained: 3.5, 7.1, and 24.7% from sodium $[1-^{14}C]$acetate, $[2-^{14}C]$mevalonic acid, and DL-tryptophan universally labeled in the benzene ring, respectively. The efficient incorporation of tryptophan was taken as evidence that it is a direct precursor. McGrath *et al.* (1976) carried out double-labeling experiments which showed that all the carbon atoms of tryptophan were incorporated directly into αCA.

αCA derived from either $[1-^{14}C]$acetate or $[2-^{14}C]$mevalonic acid was degraded (Holzapfel and Wilkins, 1971) by chemical methods. αCA suffered a retro-Claisen reaction when a dilute solution of the compound in 0.1 *M* sulfuric acid–methanol (1:1) was heated under reflux for 22 hr. One mole of acetic acid was obtained together with deacetylcyclopiazonic acid (**13**) and deacetylisocyclopiazonic acid. These deacetyl compounds were converted into the corresponding *O*-methyl derivatives by reaction with diazomethane and were crystallized to constant activity. Part of the acetic acid was converted into the *p*-bromophenacyl ester, whereas the remainder was degraded by the Schmidt procedure to give carbon dioxide collected as barium carbonate. The acetic acid obtained from $[2-^{14}C]$mevalonate-derived αCA was inactive, whereas the acetic acid obtained from αCA labeled with $[1-^{14}C]$acetic acid accounted for 35% of the total activity. The labeled acetic acid carried all its activity in the carboxy group.

Treatment of deacetyltenuazonic acid (**13**) with dilute sulfuric acid under drastic conditions effected a retro-Claisen reaction to give an *N*-acetylamino acid which was further hydrolyzed to acetic acid and the amino acid (**15**),

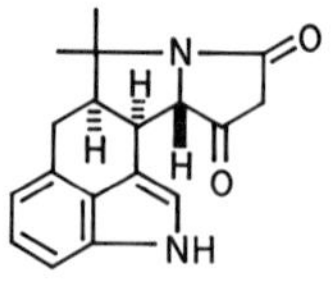

13 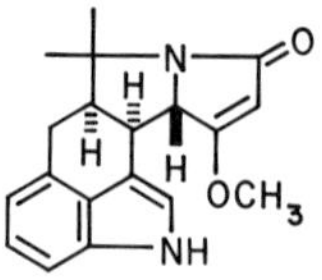   14

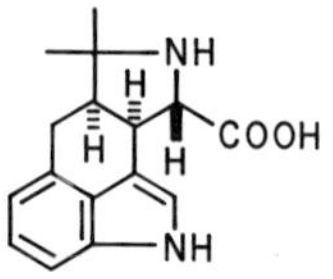

15

isolated as its methyl ester. A portion of the acetic acid obtained from labeled starting material was converted into its p-bromophenacyl ester, and the remainder was degraded by the Schmidt procedure which yielded carbon dioxide. The acetic acid obtained from [2-^{14}C]mevalonate-derived αCA was inactive, whereas the acetic acid obtained from [1-^{14}C]acetate-labeled αCA accounted for 33% of the total activity. This labeled acetic acid carried all its activity in the carboxy group.

Kuhn–Roth oxidation of O-methyldeacetylcyclopiazonic acid (14) yielded 0.34 mole of acetic acid, which was degraded by the Schmidt procedure to carbon dioxide, and methylamine, isolated as N-methylnitroaniline. The N-methylnitroaniline obtained in this way accounted for 96% of the total activity, while the carbon dioxide from [1-^{14}C]acetate-derived αCA contained 15% of the activity of the starting material.

From the above results, it follows that the atoms from [1-^{14}C]acetate and [2-^{14}C]mevalonate are incorporated into αCA as shown in Fig. 2. This distribution of labeled atoms is in agreement with the proposal that αCA is derived from tryptophan, an isoprene unit (formed from mevalonic acid), and two molecules of acetic acid.

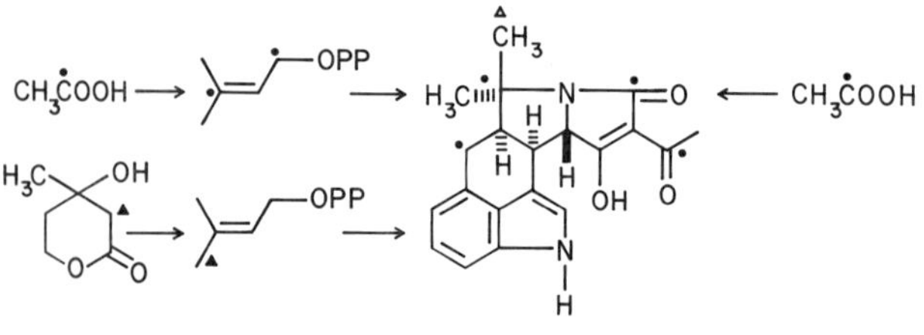

Fig. 2.   Incorporation of labeled acetate and mevalonate into cyclopiazonic acid. ● and ▲ designate ^{14}C.

B.   Intermediates in the Biosynthesis of α-Cyclopiazonic Acid

Several possibilities must be considered for the sequence in which the simple precursors of the tetramic acids are assembled. This problem has received attention only in the case of αCA. The possibility that γγ-dimethylallyltryptophan, the direct precursor of the ergot alkaloids, may be an early precursor was eliminated by the biosynthetic studies of McGrath *et al.* (1976). The possibility that β-cyclopiazonic acid (βCA) may be a precursor of cyclopiazonic acid was suggested by the following observations of Holzapfel and Wilkins (1971). βCA is already present in the mycelium at a stage when only trace amounts of αCA can be detected. Initially, its concentration increases; it then falls rapidly as soon as αCA formation is accelerated. To test the proposal that βCA is a direct precursor of αCA, [1-^{14}C]acetate-labeled βCA was distributed between two flasks containing 6 day old cultures of *P. cyclopium*. The αCA isolated 48 hr later contained 67% of the added label (Holzapfel and Wilkins, 1971). The labeled starting material which was recovered from the fermentation accounted for 18% of the added label, while cyclopiazonic acid imine accounted for 3.5%. The result was taken as evidence that βCA is a direct precursor of αCA. The enzyme responsible for the conversion of βCA into αCA was subsequently isolated by Schabort *et al.* (1971).

McGrath *et al.* (1973) prepared a cell-free extract (CFE) containing some of the enzymes involved in the biosynthesis of αCA. A mixture of L-[G^3H] tryptophan and [1-^{14}C]dimethylallyl pyrophosphate was incubated with this CFE at 30°C for 1 hr. αCA isolated from the reaction mixture contained no ^{3}H or ^{14}C, while βCA contained no ^{3}H but 19% of the added ^{14}C. It was clear that the CFE contained both an enzyme and a substrate which, along with dimethylallyl pyrophosphate (DMAPP), would produce βCA. This cosubstrate was a derivative of tryptophan (Trp), which was isolated and identified as α-acetyl-γ-(β-indolyl)methyltetramic acid (cycloacetoacetyl-L-tryptophanyl, cAATrp), **16**. It was also established that this indole, like

16

αCA, has the L-configuration at the asymmetric center. The CFE catalyzed the conversion of exogenous cAATrp and exogenous DMAPP into βCA in 1:1 stoichiometry. Further investigations (McGrath *et al.*, 1976) showed that cAATrp was present maximally 4 days after the start of the fermentation. It was found in the mycelium and in the culture filtrate in approximately equal concentration, which suggests that its distribution was due to a process of diffusion rather than active excretion.

The mechanism of the conversion of Trp into cAATrp remains to be investigated. The biochemical process in this case may be similar to that suggested earlier for the biosynthesis of tenuazonic acid. The mechanism of the isoprenylation at the least nucleophilic position of the indole ring system of cAATrp has not as yet been elucidated. The corresponding isoprenylation of Trp in ergot alkaloid biosynthesis has received considerable attention (cf. Bellatti *et al.*, 1977), but the mechanistic problem remains unsolved.

IV. ENZYMES IN THE BIOSYNTHESIS OF α-CYCLOPIAZONIC ACID

A. β-Cyclopiazonate Oxidocyclase

1. The Isolation and Physical Properties of Five Isoenzymes

Schabort *et al.* (1971) described the isolation of five isoenzymes, designated β-cyclopiazonate oxidocyclase, that could catalyze the conversion of βCA into αCA. The mycelium of *P. cyclopium* grown in shake culture under αCA production conditions was used as a source of these isoenzymes. All steps of the isolation procedure were carried out at $0°–5°C$. The mycelium, suspended in a $0.05\ M$ sodium maleate buffer (pH 6.6), was homogenized in a Sorvall Omnimix blender and then in a Edmund Bühler vibrator using glass beads. The suspension was centrifuged at $44,000\ g$ for 30 min. The supernatant solution which contained the isoenzymes was treated with increasing amounts of ammonium sulfate. The protein fraction that was precipitated between 25 and 94% saturation contained nearly all the enzyme activity. After dialysis, this fraction was chromatographed over DEAE-cellulose. The enzyme activity was located in one of the bands eluted from the column. This material was chromatographed over Sephadex-100. Enzyme activity was associated with only one of the protein peaks eluted with $0.05\ M$ sodium maleate. Final purification of the enzyme preparation was effected by chromatography on CM-Sephadex C-50. Five bands were obtained which showed β-cyclopiazonate oxidocyclase activity.

β-Cyclopiazonate oxidocyclase activity was determined after each step of the above isolation procedure. Dehydrogenating activity was determined by a spectrophotometric method employing 2,6-dichlorophenolindophenol (DCIP) as terminal electron acceptor. DCIP was found to be a very effective terminal acceptor of electrons in the dehydrogenation of βCA by β-cyclopiazonate oxidocyclase. The decrease in absorbance at 600 nm at $25°C$ and pH 6.82 was used to calculate the dehydrogenating activity which was expressed in nmole DCIP reduced per min, while specific activity was expressed in nmoles/min per mg protein. A colorimetric assay method was used for the conversion of βCA into αCA. This method was based on the finding that αCA gave a purple–blue Ehrlich color reaction, whereas the same reaction with βCA was negative. Enzyme activity determined by the colorimetric method was expressed as μmoles αCA formed per min, and specific activity as μmoles/min per mg protein. The reaction rates determined by the two methods were similar, and the specific activities for each of the five isoenzymes were in the range of 54.5–61.1 nmoles DCIP reduced/min per mg protein. The purification factors (ca. 130-fold) for the isoenzymes were also similar. The final total yield of enzyme activity was 64%, and the total amount of enzyme protein obtained from 350 gm mycelium (wet weight) was 33.7 mg.

The isoenzymes appeared to be homogenous, differing only slightly in their electrophoretic mobility toward the pH values employed in microzone (pH 4.85, 6.7, and 8.6) and polyacrylamide gel (pH 4.5 and 6.7) electrophoresis. It was evident that the isoenzymes were all positively charged, even at a pH value as high as 8.6. They differed only slightly in their positive charge and were numbered in increasing order of charge. The homogeneity of the isoenzymes was also illustrated by the sharpness of the single sedimentary boundaries obtained in sedimentation velocity experiments. The molecular weights, estimated by chromatographic behavior on columns of Sephadex G-200 for isoenzymes I–V, were 47,000, 50,000, 49,000, 48,000 and 48,000, respectively, at pH 6.6 as well as pH 7.5. Determination of molecular weights by analytical ultracentrifugation gave similar results. The five isoenzymes had essentially the same sedimentation coefficients ($s_{20,w}^0$ ca. 4.0×10^{-13} sec), diffusion coefficients ($d_{20,w}$ ca. 7.3×10^{-7} cm^{2}sec^{-1}), and partial specific volumes ($\bar{v}$, 0.73 cm^3 gm^{-1}).

The spectrophotometric methods described earlier were used to determine the optimum pH for the isoenzymes (Schabort et al., 1971). Cytochrome c [together with a small amount of phenazine methosulfate (PMS) as intermediate electron acceptor] was particularly useful for determinations below pH 6.4, because the absorbance of DCIP at 600 nm decreases rapidly below this value. The five isoenzymes showed the same optimum pH of 6.8 for both the dehydrogenation and the total conversion of βCA into αCA. The temperature stability of the five isoenzymes was essentially the same. They lost all their activity after heat treatment for 10 min at 75.5°C, but retained 70% of their activity after 10 min at 55°C.

2. The Chemical Composition of β-Cyclopiazonate Oxidocyclase

The amino acid composition of the β-cyclopiazonate oxidocyclases was determined (Schabort and Potgieter, 1971) after hydrolysis in vacuo in 6 M hydrochloric acid at 110°C for 24 hr. Eighteen different amino acids were detected in the hydrolysate. The most significant differences in amino acid content of the five isoenzymes were their basic and acidic amino acids content and the ammonia content. A gradual increase in basic amino acids [lysine, histidine, and arginine] of isoenzymes I–V of 41–53 residues and in ammonia content from 33 to 76 residues, with a concomitant decrease in acidic amino acids [aspartic and glutamic acids] from 81 to 74 residues, was found. These results are in agreement with the observed differences in the magnitude of the positive charge of the isoenzymes. The purified isoenzymes I and II contained, in addition to the pentose content of a flavin residue, small amounts of carbohydrate. The composition of the carbohydrates was not determined, and their function in terms of the catalytic activity of the isoenzymes is still obscure. Their presence may be ascribed to previous association of the isoenzymes with the cell walls. Emission spectroscopy (Schabort and Potgieter, 1971) showed that the isoenzymes did not contain significant quantities of metal ions. In this respect the isoenzymes correspond to the majority of flavoproteins and the flavodoxins (Mayhew and Schmid, 1969; Knight and Hardy, 1966). The fact that anions such as citrate, cyanide, and sulfide did not show any inhibitory effect provides additional support that the oxidocyclase did not contain any metal ion.

Schabort and Potgieter (1971) showed that each of the β-cyclopiazonate oxidocyclases contain one covalently linked molecule of flavin per molecule of enzyme. The purified enzymes had a yellow color, and their ultraviolet and visible spectra showed maxima at 276, 366, and 450 nm. The addition of sodium dithionite or of βCA caused the disappearance of the 450 nm peak because of the reduction of the flavin moiety. The flavin residues released from the protein molecules by proteolytic digestion with pronase showed absorption peaks at 262, 370, and 450 nm. The released flavin residues, separated by paper chromatography, were found to contain a covalently bound amino acid or small peptide. It was concluded that in the native enzyme, the flavin was bound by covalent linkage to the protein and that, during digestion with pronase, proteolysis stops at points determined by the specificity of the pronase or by structural or steric hindrance by the flavin. Pentose determination on the flavin residues showed that the flavins were dinucleosides.

In subsequent studies (Kenney et al., 1974a, 1976a) of the flavin prosthetic group of the β-cyclopiazonate oxidocyclases, the isoenzymes were digested with trypsin and chymotrypsin. A flavin mononucleotide peptide was isolated from the resultant mixture by chromatography on Florisil and diethylaminoethyl cellulose and by hydrolysis with nucleotide pyrophosphatase. Its amino acid composition was determined after hydrolysis in

6 M hydrochloric acid at 107°C for 18 hr. The hydrolysate contained tryptophan, valine, glycine, proline, threonine, aspartic acid, and histidine in the (nearest integer) ratio of 1:1:1:1:2:2:1. The amino-terminal residue of the flavin peptide was found to be aspartic acid by the subtractive Edman method, with glycine as the next residue. Hydrolysis of the flavin peptide with 6 M hydrochloric acid for 17 hr at 95°C gave a histidylflavin which was purified by thin layer chromatography. Histidine was liberated from this histidylflavin by incubation at 125°C in 6 M hydrochloric acid.

The corrected fluorescence and absorption spectra of the flavin peptide and of the corresponding histidylflavin showed a hypsochromic shift of the second absorption maximum relative to flavin mononucleotide (FMN) or riboflavin, which is characteristic of flavin peptides in which the peptide moiety is linked to the 8α position of the riboflavin moiety. Furthermore, the pK_a of fluorescence quenching of 5.05 of the histidylflavin was indicative of the presence of a tertiary nitrogen at the 8α position of the flavin. It remained only to establish whether the 8α substituent of the histidylflavin was linked via N^1 or N^3 of the imidazole ring. Its structure was established as 8α-(N^1-histidyl)-2′,5′-anhydroriboflavin by direct comparison with the unambiguously characterized compound obtained by synthesis. Proof that unmodified riboflavin is present in the enzyme itself was obtained by methylating the FMN peptide with methyl iodide, followed by reductive cleavage with Zn and dephosphorylation, which yielded riboflavin. Clearly, acid treatment of the flavin peptide resulted in an acid-modified histidylflavin. This property was also observed with synthetic 8α-(N^1-histidyl)riboflavin, which yielded the corresponding 2′,5′-anhydrocompound on treatment with acid. By summation of the results discussed above, it follows that the prosthetic group of β-cyclopiazonate oxidocyclase is 8α-(N^1-His)FAD (17).

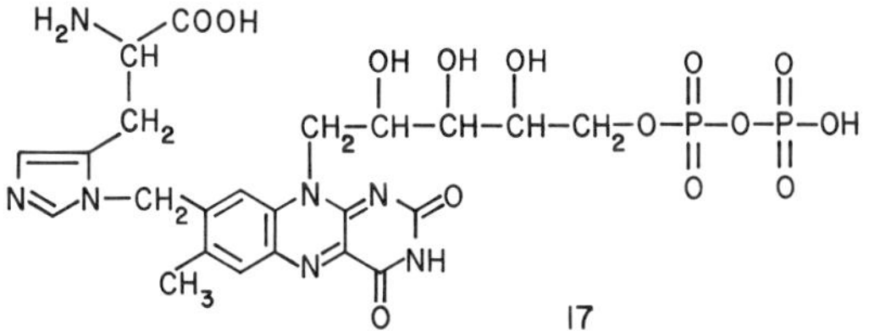

17

The same flavin occurs at the active center of bacterial thiamine dehydrogenase (Singer and Kenney, 1974, Kenney *et al.*, 1974b) and in L-gulono-γ-lactone oxidase from rat liver (Kenney *et al.*, 1976b).

In the course of the chemical studies of the FMN peptide from β-cyclopiazonate oxidocyclase, Kenney *et al.* (1974a, 1976a) observed that its fluorescence is extensively quenched even at acid pH values where quenching by the imidazole moiety is precluded. This quenching is abolished on oxidation of the tryptophan moiety with performic acid, and is not observed after degradation to the histidylriboflavin level. It was concluded that fluorescence quenching was due to interaction of the riboflavin moiety with the tryptophan moiety. Circular dichroism studies, however, indicated that the mutual quenching of flavin and tryptophan was the result of Förster energy transfer or of collisional transfer between the moieties rather than of direct molecular overlap of the aromatic ring systems.

3. The Catalytic Activity of β-Cyclopiazonate Oxidocyclase

Schabort and Potgieter (1971) carried out an extensive investigation of electron carriers, electron acceptors, and other cofactor requirements for the reaction catalyzed by the β-cyclopiazonate oxidocyclases. Ferricyanide, 2-methyl-1,4-naphthoquinone, methylene blue, coenzyme Q, NAD^+, $NADP^+$, FAD, and FMN did not act as electron acceptors or carriers for the oxidative cyclization of βCA under aerobic as well as anaerobic conditions. Cytochrome c and DCIP have been described previously as terminal electron acceptors in the dehydrogenation of βCA. The presence of oxygen had no effect on the dehydrogenating activity of the enzymes when these compounds were used as terminal electron acceptors. However, oxygen was an effective terminal electron acceptor in the presence of PMS as an intermediate electron carrier. The highest reaction rate obtained for the dehydrogenation reaction was observed when a combination of PMS and DCIP was used. This indicated that PMS was the most effective immediate acceptor of electrons and that the dehydrogenation reaction may be rate limiting in the conversion of βCA into αCA. It was subsequently shown (Steenkamp et al., 1974) that the reduction of the flavoenzyme was indeed the rate-limiting step when the (first-order) reaction is carried out in the presence of an excess of DCIP.

Essentially similar results for the five isoenzymes were obtained (Schabort and Potgieter, 1971) from kinetic studies on the effect of pH on the dehydrogenating activity. A pH optimum of 6.8 was obtained. The effect of substrate concentration on the dehydrogenating activity of the isoenzymes was studied (Schabort and Potgieter, 1971) by employing the spectrophotometric assay method with DCIP as terminal electron acceptor. The apparent Michaelis constants (K_m) for βCA varied considerably among the isoenzymes (e.g., 2.1 μM and 13.9 μM for isoenzymes I and III, respectively), while the K_m (DCIP) values (1.1–2.8 μM) showed less variation. The isoenzymes also differed in the order of the dehydrogenation reaction with respect to βCA (0.25–0.51), the half-periods of the dehydrogenation reaction (16–20 min), catalytic constants ($k_2 = 0.042$–$0.052 \sec^{-1}$), and the rate constants ($K = 1.2$–2.9

nmoles sec^{-1}) under conditions where the reaction was zero order with respect to DCIP.

The thermodynamic properties of the isoenzymes, however, were found to be similar. With respect to the dehydrogenation reaction, the following values were found: Activation energy (E_a ca. 7.2 kcal $mole^{-1}$), enthalpy change of activation (ΔH^* ca. 6.6 kcal $mole^{-1}$), entropy change of activation (ΔS^* ca. -42 cal $mole^{-1}$), and free energy change of activation (ΔG^* ca. 19.3 kcal $mole^{-1}$). The negative change in the entropy of activation, as also reported for most other enzyme-catalyzed reactions, suggests a structural change (folding) in the enzyme molecule during formation of the activated complex. The positive change in ΔG^* also falls within the range for many enzyme-catalyzed reactions.

The essential irreversibility of the oxidative cyclization of βCA was established by Steenkamp et al. (1973), who also determined the kinetics of the inhibition of the enzymatic reaction by αCA. The inhibition appears to be competitive with respect to βCA, and was explained in terms of the formation (supported by spectrophotometric studies) of a dead-end inhibitor complex between the oxidized enzyme and αCA.

Low-temperature studies (Steenkamp et al., 1973) showed that the reduction of the enzyme by βCA is at least biphasic. An initial fast (second-order) reaction may be interpreted as giving rise to the formation of an βCA-oxidized enzyme complex which is converted into the fully reduced enzyme by a slow process. Determination of the initial velocity of the reaction in the presence of DCIP, using variable concentrations of one substrate (βCA or DCIP) and changing fixed levels of the other, furnished results which indicated a "Ping-Pong-Bi-Bi" mechanism. Initial velocity studies in the presence of the competitive inhibitor 3-acetyl-5-skatyltetramic acid provided additional support (Steenkamp and Schabort, 1973) for enzyme catalysis by a Ping-Pong-Bi-Bi mechanism.

Extensive studies (Schabort et al., 1971) on the pH dependence of the velocity of the oxidocyclase reaction indicated that amino acid residues with pK_a and pK_b values of 7.8 and 5.3, respectively, were directly involved in the redox reaction of the enzyme-substrate complex. A pK_a value of 7.8 is consistent with the dissociation of an α-ammonium group, while a pK_b value of 5.3 falls nearly in the range of the ring nitrogen of the imidazole ring of histidine. The role of such groups was also suggested by the inhibitory effects of 2,6-dinitro-1-fluorobenzene (DNFB) and L-1-tosylamide-2-phenylethyl-chloromethyl ketone (TPCK).

A study of the pH dependence of the binding of various substrate analogues to β-cyclopiazonate oxidocyclase yielded results which were taken as indirect evidence for the presence of two histidyl residues (i.e., involvement of two groups with pK_a values of 6.0 and 7.0) in the active site of the enzyme (Steenkamp *et al.*, 1974). However, this interpretation was based on a model which allowed for binding of substrates with the enzyme in different states of protonation, but neglected different possible protonated species of the substrate analogues. Independent evidence (Steenkamp *et al.*, 1974) for the presence of histidyl residues in the active site was obtained by a study of the reaction of diethyl pyrocarbonate with the enzyme. This resulted in carbethoxylation of histidyl residues (as indicated by the change in absorbance at 242 nm) and inactivation of the enzyme. A complete loss of activity was obtained by the modification of approximately three histidyl residues per mole of enzyme. The enzyme was slowly reactivated on incubation with hydroxylamine at room temperature. Modification of the enzyme protein by carbethoxylation resulted in a marked decrease in affinity for indole derivatives, while the visible spectrum of the carbethoxylated enzyme–substrate complex was similar to that of the enzyme–substrate complex. It must be pointed out, however, that diethyl pyrocarbonate cannot be regarded as sufficiently specific to distinguish between essential and nonessential histidyl residues in enzymes.

The results of spectrophotometric titrations (Steenkamp *et al.*, 1973, 1974) of the oxidized enzyme with a number of substrate analogues [e.g., L-tryptophan, 3-acetyltryptophan tetramic acid, dihydro-βCA, 2-(indolyl-2)-propionic acid, and 3-acetyltrimethylenetetramic acid] indicated that the tetramic acid residue, and especially its NH group, is primarily responsible for binding at the active site. The effects of the substrate analogues on the visible spectrum of the enzyme-bound flavin, which were similar to that caused by the normal substrate βCA, were taken as evidence that all the compounds were bound at the active site. The possible importance of flavin–indole complexes in flavoenzyme catalysis has been pointed out be several workers, but, as in the present case, there is some uncertainty as to whether these are of the charge-transfer type. Studies on the effect of pH on the formation of flavin–indole complexes indicated that N(3) of the isoalloxazine ring is important (Wilson, 1966). This prompted a study (Steenkamp and Schabort, 1973) of the effect of the reduction at the N(3) position of the isoalloxazine on the binding of indole compounds by β-cyclopiazonate oxidocyclase. The reduction of the flavin coenzyme to the 3,4-dihydroflavin was achieved by consecutive cycles of reduction with sodium borohydride and reoxidation with atmospheric oxygen. The reduced enzyme showed a similar affinity for indole derivatives as does the native enzyme, but was inactive.

A number of divalent cations are reported to be strong inhibitors of certain flavoprotein enzymes, such as NADH dehydrogenases. Most divalent cations had a moderate to strong inhibitory effect (Schabort *et al.*, 1971) on β-

cyclopiazonate oxidocyclase, and the important role of Zn^{2+} and Fe^{2+} in the production of αCA is definitely not attributable to their action as cofactors or activators of the oxidocyclases.

B. β-Cyclopiazonic Acid Synthetase

The enzyme in the CFE of *P. cyclopium* Westling which catalyzes the conversion of cAATrp and DMAPP into βCA was designated (McGrath *et al.*, 1976) cycloacetoacetyltryptophanyl dimethylallyltransferase. It was also referred to as β-cyclopiazonate synthetase, or prenyl-aryl transferase, or secondary dimethylallyltransferase (S) in order to distinguish it from the transferase (T), important in primary metabolism, which catalyzes the formation of farnesylpyrophosphate (FPP) via geranylpyrophosphate (GPP) which is formed from one molecule of DMAPP and one molecule of isopentenyl-pyrophosphate (IPP). Preliminary investigations of the physical and catalytic properties of βCA synthetase were described (McGrath *et al.*, 1976, 1977).

The enzyme was purified by McGrath *et al.* (1977) in the following way. The CFE (obtained by breaking the cells of the mycelia by means of ice shear) was centrifuged at $110,000 g$ for 1 hr at $0°-5°C$, and the clear straw-colored supernatant was adjusted to contain Tris–chloride buffer (pH 7.9), $5 mM$ dithioerythritol (DTE), and $5 mM$ EDTA in order to maintain enzyme activity. The bulk of enzyme S was precipitated between 45% and 60% saturation with ammonium sulfate. This precipitate was fractionated on a BioGel A column in a Tris–chloride buffer (pH7.9). The purified enzyme (16-fold purification from the CFE) had an isoelectric point of 5.3 and a molecular weight (in the absence of divalent cations and in the presence of a thiol reductant) of ca. 95,000. It was stable for at least six months at $-20°C$ in a glycerol–water solution containing $10 mM$ EDTA.

Enzyme S was quite specific for DMAPP and cAATrp, neither IPP, GPP, Trp nor N-acetyltryptophan being used as substrates. In this connection it is of interest to note that another secondary transferase, 4-dimethylallyl-L-tryptophan synthetase, utilizes Trp as a cosubstrate with DMPP en route to the clavine alkaloids (Heinstein *et al.*, 1971; Lee, 1974), while in this case Trp did not even bind to the enzyme. The specificity of S for a cyclized Trp may be compared with that established by Allen (1972) for cyclo-L-alanyl-2-(1, 1-dimethylallyl)-L-tryptophanyl synthetase. In this case, however, the substrate, cyclo-L-alanyl-L-tryptophanyl, could be replaced by cyclo-L-prolyl-L-tryptophanyl (Deyrup and Allen, 1975).

The pH profile of βCA synthetase is broad, with an optimum value lying between 6.9 and 7.5 (McGrath *et al.*, 1976).

The enzyme exhibited Michaelis constants (K_m) for CAA Trp and DMAPP of 6.0 μM and 2.0 μM, respectively (McGrath *et al.*, 1977). The enzyme is

Cedric W. Holzapfel

not inhibited by EDTA which could mean either that the enzyme does not require a divalent cation or that, if it does, the cation is not removed from the enzyme by EDTA. The enzyme possesed a subunit structure. The addition of Mg^{2+} caused a diminution in size to ca. 75,000, whereas Mn^{2+} caused major disruptive changes and inhibition of the enzyme. These changes were, however, reversible, and removal of the Mn^{2+} by gel filtration or by chelation resulted in recovery of activity.

The appearance of βCA synthetase and soluble protein are coincident (McGrath et al., 1976, 1977), indicating that normal protein-synthesizing mechanisms, involved in primary metabolism, are likewise essential for secondary metabolism. The concentration of βCA synthetase (whose in vivo half-life is fairly short) reached a maximum ca. 60 hr after the start of the fermentation. The maximum pool of βCA and the highest rate of βCA synthesis occurred 12 hr after the maximum concentration of βCA synthetase was observed. A direct relationship between enzyme concentration and the rate of βCA production exists when both substrates are present in excess. However, a study of the level of enzyme activity throughout the growth period indicated that the enzyme concentration is not the rate-limiting factor in the production of αCA.

V. THE MECHANISM OF THE OXIDATIVE CYCLIZATION OF β-CYCLOPIAZONIC ACID

From a formal point of view, the conversion of βCA into αCA may be regarded as a didehydrogenation followed by cyclization. It has been suggested (Schabort et al., 1971) that the first step may involve the formation of a double bond in the 4,5-position. This possibility can, however, be excluded on the basis of a recent study (Holzapfel and Schabort, 1977) which showed that tritium in position 5 of βCA is retained during enzyme-catalyzed oxidative cyclization of αCA. In this experiment a mixture of DL-[5-^{3}H]βCA and DL-[4-^{14}C]βCA, both prepared by the reaction of π-dimethylallylnickel(I) bromide with suitable derivatives of 4-bromotryptophan (Holzapfel and Gildenhuys, 1977), was incubated with purified β-cyclopiazonate oxidocyclase in the presence of DCIP. The labeled αCA formed in the reaction contained 44% of the initially added label, while the ^{3}H:^{14}C ratio was essentially unchanged.

In a study of the steric course of proton removal during the cyclization of βCA, (3R)- and (3S)-[3-^{3}H,3-^{14}C]Trp were fed separately to cultures of P. cyclopium Westling (Steyn et al., 1975). Good incorporation (18–25%) into the cyclopiazonic acids was observed. Retention of the tritium from (3R)-[3-^{3}H]Trp [18, when H_R = T and H_S = H (see diagram)] during conversion into αCA was essentially complete for both the L- and DL-forms of

$$\text{18}$$

the amino acid. Conversely, $(3S)$-$[3\text{-}^3\text{H}]$Trp (**18**, $H_R = H$, $H_S = T$) lost almost all its tritium. All the tritiated tryptophans were incorporated into βCA with high retention of tritium. These results demonstrated the integrity of the methylene group of Trp during the early stages of the biosynthesis and that C–C bond formation at C(4) occurs from the opposite side of the molecule from proton removal. Furthermore, these results, taken together with the finding that C(5)–H is not directly involved in the oxidative cyclization of βCA, are consistent with cyclization via 1,4-didehydro-βCA.

Several examples of flavoprotein-catalyzed double-bond formation are known. The mechanism of the dehydrogenation reaction may be regarded as principally similar to that described for dehydrogenations, such as the conversion of succinic acid to fumaric acid. (England and Colowick, 1956; Tchen and van Milligan, 1960) and of 3-oxosteroids into $\Delta^{1,4}$-3-oxosteroids (Ringold *et al.*, 1963; Jerrussi and Ringold, 1965). This two-step mechanism involves the initial removal of a proton from the carbon atom adjacent to an electron-withdrawing group, followed by hydride transfer to a suitable oxidizing agent. It should be pointed out, however, that a dehydrogenation mechanism that does not involve hydride transfer or direct electron transfer has been proposed (Brown and Hamilton, 1970) for flavoenzyme-catalyzed reactions. In the case of βCA, proton removal followed by electron transfer (equivalent to hydride ion transfer) would result in the formation of an indolenine (3*H*-indolylidene) cation intermediate (see Fig. 3). Cyclization

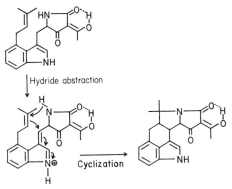

Fig. 3. Proposed mechanism of oxidative cyclization of β-cyclopiazonic acid.

could now occur by (a) nucleophilic attack by the π electrons of the double bond in the mevalonate-derived C_5 unit on the electron-deficient carbon at position 4, and (b) a concerted attack by the lone pair of electrons on N(9) on the developing carbonium ion at position 10. This cyclization may be activated by removal of a proton from N(9) of βCA which will enhance the nucleophilicity of this nitrogen atom. This proposed mechanism for the oxidative cyclization reaction involves two proton-removal steps. These steps may be catalyzed by one or two imidazole groups and the α- or ε-amino groups of lysine which, on the basis of the inhibition studies discussed earlier, appear to be directly involved in the enzymatic reaction.

No proof has been obtained that a $3H$-indolylidene (or the corresponding cation) is an intermediate in the oxidative cyclization, and it must be concluded that the substrate remains bound to the same site on the enzyme molecule throughout the whole process. It can be expected that a (reactive) compound similar in structure to the proposed intermediate will not be released from the enzyme after the dehydrogenation reaction. Further elucidation of the mechanism of the conversion of βCA into αCA requires more definite evidence that the cyclization step is also catalyzed by the enzyme. Efforts to obtain such evidence are complicated by the fact that the isoenzymes do not catalyze the reverse reaction; namely, the conversion of αCA into βCA (Schabort and Potgieter, 1971).

Irrespective of whether the oxidative cyclization of βCA is a concerted reaction or involves two (or more) steps, the reaction requires a single enzyme molecule. This conversion, therefore, differs from squalene oxidative cyclization, which requires an enzyme for the oxidative step and another enzyme (2,3-oxidosqualene lanosterol cyclase) for the cyclization (Singer *et al.*, 1956). The possibility that the oxidative cyclization of βCA may be a true concerted (one step) process cannot be ruled out at this stage. It may explain the specificity (Steenkamp *et al.*, 1974) of the enzyme for βCA as substrate and the observation that in all reaction mixtures αCA was formed at approximately the same rate as the rate of dehydrogenation of the electron acceptor.

VI. METABOLIC DEVELOPMENT OF *PENICILLIUM CYCLOPIUM* DURING α-CYCLOPIAZONIC ACID PRODUCTION

A. Nutrient Changes during α-Cyclopiazonic Acid Production

Neethling and McGrath (1977) studied the effect of a number of nitrogen sources (including most amino acids, urea, sodium, and ammonium nitrate) on αCA production in shake culture on synthetic liquid media (based on glucose as carbon source), and found that sodium nitrate gave the best specific yield of αCA; i.e., the activity of the primary pathways was minimized and that of the secondary maximized. In subsequent studies, nitrate (or other source of nitrogen), glucose, and phosphate in the medium were quantitated during the course of a standard growth of *P. cyclopium*. The results showed that at all times PO_4^{3-} was in excess while the glucose and NO_3^- (or NH_4^+) disappeared rapidly. However, at a time when NO_3^- was completely depleted, the glucose concentration was about 25% of its value at the start of the fermentation.

Although the biosynthesis of βCA and αCA occurs even in the trophophase (balanced growth), a rapid increase in secondary metabolite production begins when the nitrogen concentration (NO_3^- or NH_4^+) of the medium has reached a value of approximately 10 mmoles (see Fig. 4). Secondary metabolite production begins at an earlier time with NH_4^+, reflecting the faster growth and nitrogen uptake in this case. On complete depletion of nitrogen in the medium (around 72 hr in the case of NO_3^-), the secondary metabolite production begins to drop rapidly.

Neethling and McGrath (1977) measured the free amino acids during CA production, and showed that they are all present, with the exception of Trp, cysteine, asparagine and β-alanine, which were always absent, in quite substantial pools up to 84 hr, quite long after the depletion of nitrogen in the medium. These results suggest that nitrogen utilization controls CA production and that the message to cell metabolism is given by nutrient or extracellular levels of nitrogen. This is in keeping with suggestions (Bu'Lock, 1975; Righelato, 1975) that it is nutrient changes that terminate the balanced phase of growth. It might be, however, that external nitrogen levels are in a coarse control of the more finely controlled internal enzymatic, nitrogen-utilizing pathways. The external message occurring at nitrogen levels of 10 mmoles in the case of *P. cyclopium* suggests that it is at this level that the nitrogen-utilizing routes become imbalanced.

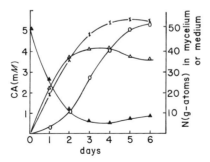

Fig. 4.   Production of αCA (O) and mycelium (×), showing the nitrogen content of the mycelium (△) during depletion of medium N (▲), calculated by N (supplied) – N(mycellium) – N(αCA). NaNO$_3$ was the N source.

348   Cedric W. Holzapfel

The dramatic change in cell metabolism coincident with increased CA production was further evidenced by a decline in the glucose uptake. Glucose utilization, measured by the release of $^{14}CO_2$ from $[U\text{-}^{14}C]$glucose, continued to decline rapidly during the period (around 75 hr) of maximum CA biosynthesis, which coincided with nitrogen depletion and the end of the growth phase of the fungus (Neethling and McGrath, 1977). It is of interest to note that total lipid content, excepting αCA and βCA, decreases rapidly at the time corresponding to the fall in glucose uptake and increased CA biosynthesis. Presumably the lipids are being mobilized, not to supply acetyl-CoA for energy requirements because the organism is entering the idiophase (stationary phase), but to meet the precursor requirements of CA production. Furthermore, disruption of the mitochondria (Neethling and McGrath, 1977), which contain 180–300 μg lipid/mg protein, started at a time of maximum CA production. However, it is not known whether mitochondrial disruption is the effect rather than the cause of the slow down in metabolism.

The relative importance of the Embden–Meyerhof (E.M.) pathway and the pentose cycle in the catabolism of glucose in *P. cyclopium* was determined by feeding $[1\text{-}^{14}C]$- and $[6\text{-}^{14}C]$glucose (Neethling and McGrath, 1977). The E.M. route creates two indistinguishable ^{14}C moieties from both $[^{14}C]$-glucose isotopes, whereas the pentose cycle expels $[1\text{-}^{14}C]$ as $^{14}CO_2$. It was found that during the early stage of growth all the glucose was utilized via the pentose cycle. By 46 hr a greater proportion was being metabolized by the alternative route. At 64 hr, near the time of maximum CA biosynthesis, a halt in the decline of the pentose cycle was seen. The maintenance of a minimum activity of the pentose cycle may be, to a large extent, associated with the production of Trp, an intermediate in CA production, which is derived from erythrose 4-phosphate, an intermediate in the pentose cycle. The relationship between Trp and CA biosynthesis has received considerable attention (McGrath et al., 1977).

Trp biosynthesis, together with protein production, decreased rapidly at the end of the growth phase which was coincident with the disappearance of medium nitrate. In fact, when the medium nitrogen was depleted, protein started to disappear, presumably to recycle amino acids and nitrogen. By 90 hr all the Trp synthesised was utilized for CA biosynthesis. This may suggest that Trp availability is important in the control of CA production.

B. Effect of Added Precursors, pH, and Trace Metals on α-Cyclopiazonic Acid Production

The effect of adding excess Trp on αCA production was investigated in some detail (Neethling and McGrath, 1977). It was found that exogenous Trp was rapidly taken up and depleted within 2 days after the start of the

fermentation. The addition of Trp caused a two-day delay in mycelium production and a three-day delay in both the rate of and total CA production.
Furthermore, the specific production of αCA was much lower in the Trp-
supplemented experiments than in the controls. These observations are in
sharp contrast with other results (McGrath *et al.*, 1976) which showed that
[^{14}C]-Trp was incorporated to the extent of 10–25% depending on the
duration of feeding. A possible explanation of these observations might be
in the existence of both feedback inhibition and repressing mechanisms
brought about by Trp on Trp synthetase, as found in *Neurospora crassa*
(Yanofksy, 1955; Lester, 1968) and in *Claviceps paspali* (Lingens *et al.*, 1967).
On day 2, when all exogenous Trp has been utilized by *P. cyclopium*, inhibition and repression would cease. Tryptophan production could now be a
rate-limiting step for CA and mycelium production if the kinetics of Trp
synthetase induction were slower than the utilization of Trp by routes which
have already been set up by the exogenous Trp. This may explain the delay
in the production of both αCA and mycelium caused by the presence of
exogenous Trp in the medium.

The effect of added DMAPP, another early precursor of CA, and its own
precursor, mevalonic acid, on CA production was studied by Neethling
and McGrath (1977). DMAPP and mevalonic acid were added separately
before inoculation. It was found that mevalonic acid was not rate limiting,
while its derivative DMAPP was rate limiting, at least from day 3 onward.
This suggests that the rate-limiting step lies somewhere between mevalonic
acid and DMAPP. The fact that DMAPP is rate limiting in all but the early
stages is in agreement with earlier experiments (McGrath *et al.*, 1976) which
demonstrated the presence of a pool of cAATrp (the cosubstrate of DMAPP
for βCA synthetase) from day 2 onward, and maximally on day 4.

When casein was used as the sole source of nitrogen, the pH dropped
rapidly from 5.5 to 3.5, and there was an accumulation of βCA. αCA was
produced normally if the pH decrease was prevented by the addition of
aqueous sodium hydroxide. The total CA production was, however, similar whether the pH was maintained at 5.5 or allowed to drop. This suggested
that βCA synthetase is not very sensitive to pH but that β-cyclopiazonate
oxidocyclase is not fully active at the lower pH.

Neethling and McGrath (1977) studied the effect of a number of trace
metals on growth and CA production. Of the trace metals examined, only
Zn^{2+} and Fe^{2+} were shown to be essential for growth. The specific yield of
αCA was constant over the concentration range 36–2.7 μM for Fe^{2+} and
24.5–1.2 μM for Zn^{2+}. Below these lower limits there was a rapid fall in
mycelial weight, αCA production, and specific yield. In both cases, the pH
of the medium fell to 3.6–3.8 and resulted in the accumulation of βCA.
Unfortunately, only αCA was measured in these experiments. It is likely

that had the total αCA and βCA been estimated, the actual changes in the specific yield would have been smaller than those recorded for αCA. Nevertheless, the change (ca. 50%) in specific yield of αCA resulting from a deficiency of Fe^{2+} or Zn^{2+} was negligible compared to the changes in growth and the total production of αCA. It may be concluded that αCA production in *P. cyclopium* is not dependent on the presence of common trace metals, in spite of the large mass of evidence accumulated that implies an important role for Mn^{2+}, Zn^{2+}, and Fe^{2+} in fungal secondary metabolism.

VII. LINKS BETWEEN PRIMARY METABOLISM AND THE SYNTHESIS OF α-CYCLOPIAZONIC ACID

The addition of cycloheximide, an inhibitor of protein synthesis, to cultures of *P. cyclopium* inhibited the growth of the fungus but had little effect on αCA production (Neethling and McGrath, 1977). This is in agreement with a conclusion based on the levels of βCA synthetase and β-cyclopiazonate oxidocyclase discussed earlier and suggests that the production of αCA is not directly related to the rate of synthesis or concentration of the enzymes involved in the synthesis of the compound, but rather to the competition of other growth-associated processes which restrict the activity of preformed enzymes.

The role of (catabolic) repression as a control mechanism for αCA production has received little attention. A significant finding (McGrath *et al.*, 1977) in this regard was that adenosine 5'-triphosphate (ATP) depressed the production of αCA and increased mycelial weight. However, cyclic adenosine 5'-phosphate (cAMP), which is known to have a number of regulatory effects in the cell, had no effect on αCA production.

The finding that DMAPP was rate limiting in the production of αCA was followed by studies (McGrath *et al.*, 1977) on the diversion of this metabolite from polyisoprenoid to CA biosynthesis in *P. cyclopium*. The enzymes S and T from *P. cyclopium* were separated in order to study the control at the branch point. The enzyme isopentylpyrophosphate isomerase (EC 5.3.3.2) (I) was also included in the study, because it is responsible for the production of DMAPP from IPP. The early control of the diversion of DMAPP away from polyisoprenoids to secondary metabolites must, of course, be the appearance of cAATrp. Both transferases are not utilized to their maximum capacity, and the production of their end products seem to bear no relationship to their concentrations. It is apparent, therefore, that simple enzyme concentrations alone do not control the branch point. As cAATrp and DMAPP pools become rate limiting, other enzyme regulatory mechanisms must become more important. In this regard it is probably significant that

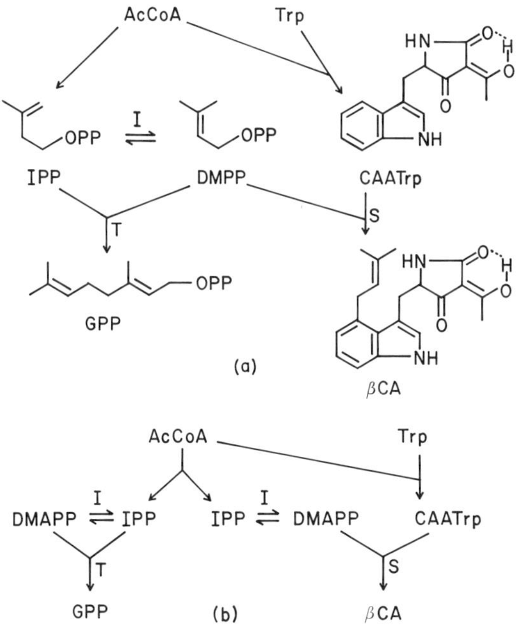

Fig. 5. Isoprenoid and α-cyclopiazonic acid branch points: (a) S and T competing for one pool of DMAPP; (b) compartmentation of DMAPP into two pools.

cAATrp inhibited T, the competitor with S for DMAPP, while at the same time it activated I. The product βCA was found to activate I in concentrations up to 0.5 mM after which it became strongly inhibiting. The level of βCA, however, never exceeded 0.5 mM in the fungus. The combined effect of cAATrp and βCA must, therefore, be to activate I and, in the case of direct competition (see Fig. 5), to favor secondary metabolism, particularly as cAATrp exists in the cell as a pool. The production of βCA will, therefore, depend largely on the DMAPP concentration (and its rate of production), while farnesylpyrophosphate production will depend not only on DMAPP, but more importantly on IPP (requiring 2 molecules). In compartmentation (see Fig. 5), this argument will only apply if isomerization of IPP was the rate-limiting step in the synthesis of βCA. Current knowledge of the pathway to polyisoprenoids suggests that the isomerization is not rate limiting. However, assuming that the rate-limiting step for CA production lies between the compartmented branch and I, the activation of I by cAATrp or βCA would not favor deflection. Control by direct competition is, therefore, considered the more likely of the two possible control systems.

Other possible controls on the direct competition of S and T for DMAPP were considered by McGrath *et al.* (1977). These included (a) the appearance of αCA, which inhibited T more effectively than S; (b) the removal of free Mn^{2+} and Mg^{2+} (by chelation with cAATrp, βCA, and αCA) both essential for I and T but not for S; and (c) the drop in the pH of the medium (with NO_3^- as nitrogen source) from 7.20 to 6.0 (between days 3 and 4). At pH 6.0 the activity of S was unaltered, I was at its highest, and T exhibited 50% of its maximum activity.

The question of the metabolic control of cAATrp production is also of interest, particularly because no pool of Trp, its direct precursor, was detected in the organism. A branch must occur between cAATrp and Trp–tRNA production. Whether this branch serves as a shunt which depends on Trp that is not required for protein synthesis, or whether it competes for Trp, is not known. McGrath et al. (1977) consider the first possibility to be more likely in view of the early appearance and nonutilization of the penultimate enzyme S. The early appearance and nonutilization of enzymes involved in αCA synthesis, like the early production of nonutilized secondary enzymes in Bacillus subtilis (Weinberg and Tonnis, 1967), raises a question as to the correctness of Bu'Lock and Powell's (1965) hypothesis of induced enzyme mechanisms in secondary metabolism. Furthermore, it suggests that the system for secondary metabolism exists before the primary pools become unbalanced—a built-in overflow mechanism. This view would be consistent with Woodruff's hypothesis (1966) that secondary metabolism serves to keep primary pools in balance.

A major control of secondary metabolite production would be the availability of substrates. At the end of primary growth, acetyl-CoA is likely to be in excess, because its main utilizer (the Kreb's cycle) will be slowing down. As primary growth ends, this acetyl-CoA is utilized along with Trp to yield cAATrp. This metabolite in turn deflects excess DMAPP (whose synthesis requires 3 molecules of acetyl-CoA) away from isoprenoid biosynthesis. Therefore, it appears that secondary metabolism is an interlock mechanism, linking in this case protein biosynthesis and energy metabolism, and perhaps polyisoprenoid biosynthesis, which is called into play when a restraint is placed on a specific area of primary metabolism.

VIII. SUMMARY

Investigations of the biosynthesis of three tetramic acids, namely, tenuazonic acid (1), erythroskyrin (3), and αCA (4), indicated that the primary step of tetramic acid biosynthesis involves the condensation of an amino acid (L-isoleucine, valine, and L-tryptophan, respectively) with an acetate-derived polyketide [(acetoacetic acid in the case of (1) and (4), a C_{20} polyketide in the case of (3)]. The details of the polyketide assembly and the final condensation leading to the tetramic acid ring system have yet to be established. The biosynthesis of erythroskyrin involves additional modifications (reduction and dehydration with the formation of double bonds and ether links) of the polyketide moiety as well as N-methylation of the tetramic acid system. No information is available on the sequence of these various modification steps.

αCA is the only tetramic acid whose biosynthesis has been elucidated in considerable detail. Isoprenylation takes place at the level of cAATrp (16) to furnish βCA (9), in contrast to ergot alkaloid biosynthesis, which involves isoprenylation of Trp at an early stage of the biosynthesis. Elucidation of the mechanism of the isoprenylation at the least nucleophilic position of the indole ring remains one of the most interesting problems of the CA biosynthesis.

The mechanism and stereochemistry of the unique oxidative cyclization of βCA to give αCA have been investigated in considerable detail, and the process appears to be concerted. The enzymes responsible for catalyzing the two final steps in the biosynthesis of αCA have been isolated, and the study of their physical properties and catalytic activity has received considerable attention. A study of the metabolic development of *P. cyclopium* during αCA production resulted in the establishment of links between primary metabolism and the synthesis of αCA as well as some of the factors involved in the control of αCA synthesis. The detailed investigations on the biosynthesis of αCA have contributed greatly to an increased understanding of the interlock mechanism linking primary and secondary metabolism.

REFERENCES

Allen, C. M., Jr. (1972). *Biochemistry* **11**, 2154.
Bellatti, M., Casnati, G., Palla, G., and Minghetti, A. (1977). *Tetrahedron* **33**, 1821.
Bentley, R., Bhate, D. S., and Keil, J. G. (1962). *J. Biol. Chem.* **237**, 859.
Brown, L. E., and Hamilton, G. A. (1970), *J. Am. Chem. Soc.* **92**, 7225.
Bu'Lock, J. D. (1975). *In* "The Filamentous Fungi" (J. F. Smith and D. R. Berry, eds.), Vol. I, pp. 33–58. Arnold, London.
Bu'Lock, J. D., and Powell, A. J. (1965). *Experientia* **21**, 55.
Carrasco, L. and Vazquez, D. (1973). *Biochim. Biophys. Acta* **319**, 209.
Deyrup, C. L. and Allen, C. M., Jr. (1975). *Phytochemistry* **14**, 971.
Dippenaar, A., Holzapfel, C. W., and Boeyens, J. C. A. (1977). *J. Cryst. Mol. Struct* **7**, 189.
Englard, S., and Colowick, S. P. (1956). *J. Biol. Chem.* **221**, 1019.
Gandhi, N. M., Nazareth, J., Divekar, P. V., Kohl, H., and De Souza, N. J. (1973). *J. Antibiot.* **26**, 797.
Gitterman, C. O. (1965). *J. Med. Chem.* **8**, 478.
Harrison, J. (1971). *Trop. Sci.* **13**, 57.
Heinstein, P. F., Lee, S. L., and Floss, H. G. (1971). *Biochem. Biophys. Res. Commun.* **44**, 1244.

Holzapfel, C. W. (1968). *Tetrahedron* **24**, 2101.

Holzapfel, C. W., and Gildenhuys, P. J. (1977). *S. Afr. J. Chem.* **30**, 125.

Holzapfel, C. W., Hutchison, R. D. and Wilkins, D. C. (1970). *Tetrahedron* **26**, 5239.

Holzapfel, C. W., and Schabort, J. C. (1977). *S. Afr. J. of Chem.* **30**, 233.

Holzapfel, C. W., and Wilkins, D. C. (1971). *Tetrahedron* **10**, 351.

Howard, B. H., and Raistrick, H. (1954). *Biochem. J.* **57**, 212.

Jerrussi, R., and Ringold, H. J. (1965). *Biochemistry* **4**, 2113.

Kaczka, A. E., Gitterman, C. O., Dulaney, E. H., Smith, M. C., Hendlin, G., Woodruff, H. B., and Folkers, K. (1964). *Biochem. Biophys. Res. Commun.* **14**, 54.

Kenney, W. C., Edmondson, D. E., Singer, T. P., Steenkamp, D. J., and Schabort, J. C. (1974a). *FEBS Lett.* **41**, 111.

Kenney, W. C., Edmondson, D. E., and Singer, T. P. (1974b). *Biochem. Biophys. Res. Commun.* **57**, 106.

Kenney, W. C., Edmondson, D. E., Singer, T. P., Steenkamp, D. J., and Schabort, J. C. (1976a). *Biochemistry* **15**, 4931.

Kenney, W. C., Edmondson, D. E., Singer, T. P., Nakagawa, H., Asano, A., and Sato, R. (1976b). *Biochem. Biophys. Res. Commun.* **71**, 1194.

Knight, E., and Hardy, R. W. F. (1966). *J. Biol. Chem.* **241**, 2752.

Lacey, R. N. (1954). *J. Chem. Soc.*, p. 850.

Lee, S. L. (1974). *Diss. Abstr. Int. B.* **35**, 2617.

Lester, G. (1968). *J. Bacteriol.* **96**, 1768.

Lingens, F., Goebel, W., and Vesseler, H. (1967). *Eur. J. Biochem.* **2**, 442.

Luk, K. C., Kobbe, B., and Townsend, J. M. (1977). *Appl. Environ. Microbiol.* **33**, 212.

McGrath, R. M., Steyn, P. S., and Ferreira, N. P. (1973). *J. Chem. Soc. Chem. Commun.*, p. 812.

McGrath, R. M., Steyn, P. S., Ferreira, N. P., and Neethling, D. C. (1976). *Biorg. Chem.* **4**, 11.

McGrath, R. M., Nourse, P. N., Neethling, D. C., and Ferreira, N. P. (1977). *Biorg. Chem.* **6**, 53.

Mayhew, S. G., and Schmid, K., (1969). *J. Biol. Chem.* **244**, 794.

Meronuck, R. A., Steele, J. A., Mirocha, C. J., and Christensen, C. M. (1972). *Appl. Microbiol.* **23**, 613.

Miller, F. A., Rightsel, W. A., Sloan, B. J., Ehrlich, J., French, J. C., and Bartz, Q. R. (1964). *Nature (London)* **200**, 1338.

Neethling, D. C., and McGrath, R. M. (1977). *Can. J. Microbiol.* **23**, 856.

Ohmomo, S., Sugita, M., and Abe, M. (1973). *J. Agric. Chem. Soc. (Japan)* **47**, 83.

Purchase, I. F. H. (1974). *In* "Mycotoxins" (I. F. H. Purchase, ed.), pp. 149–162. Elsevier, Amsterdam.

Righelato, R. C. (1975). *In* "The Filamentous Fungi" (J. F. Smith and D. R. Berry, eds.), pp. 79–103. Arnold, London.

Ringold, H. J., Hayano, M., and Stefanovic, V. (1963). *J. Biol. Chem.* **238**, 1960.

Schabort, J. C., and Potgieter, D. J. J. (1971). *Biochim. Biophys. Acta* **250**, 329.

Schabort, J. C., Wilkins, D. C., Holzapfel, C. W., Potgieter, D. J. J., and Nietz, A. W. (1971). *Biochim. Biophys. Acta* **250**, 311.

Shibata, S., Sankawa, U., Taguchi, H., and Yamasaki, K. (1966). *Chem. Pharm. Bull.* **14**, 474.

Shoji, J., Shibata, S., Sankawa, U., Taguchi, H., and Shibanuma, Y. (1965). *Chem. Pharm. Bull.* **13**, 1240.

Singer, T. P., and Kenney, W. C. (1974). *Vitam. Horm. (N.Y.)* **32**, 1.

Singer, T. P., Massey, V., and Kearney, E. B. (1956). *Biochim. Biophys. Acta* **19**, 200.

Steenkamp, D. J., and Schabort, J. C. (1973). *Eur. J. Biochem.* **40**, 163.

Steenkamp, D. J., Schabort, J. C., and Ferreira, N. P. (1973). *Biochim. Biophys. Acta* **309**, 440.

Steenkamp, D. J., Schabort, J. C., Holzapfel, C. W., and Ferreira, N. P. (1974). *Biochim. Biophys Acta* **358**, 126.

Steyn, P. S., and Rabie, C. J. (1976). *Phytochemistry* **15**, 1.

Steyn, P. S., Vleggaar, R., Ferreira, N. P., Kirby, G. W., and Varley, M. J. (1975). *J. Chem. Soc. Chem. Commun.*, p. 465.

Steyn, P. S., and Wessels, P. L. (1978). *Tetrahedron Lett.*, p. 4707.

Stickings, C. E. (1959). *Biochem. J.* **72**, 332.

Stickings, C. E. and Townsend, R. J. (1961). *Biochem. J.* **78**, 412.

Tchen, T. T., and van Milligan, H. (1960). *J. Am. Chem. Soc.* **82**, 4115.

Turner, W. B. (1971). "Fungal Metabolites," p. 79. Academic Press, New York.

Ueno, Y., Kato, Y., and Enomoto, M. (1975). *Jpn J. Exp. Med.* **45**, 525.

Umetsu, N., Kaji, J., Aoyma, K., and Tamari, K. (1974a). *Agric. Biol. Chem.* **38**, 1867.

Umetsu, N., Maramatsu, T., Honda, H., and Tamari, K. (1974b). *Agric. Biol. Chem.* **38**, 791.

Weinberg, E. D., and Tonnis, S. (1967). *Can. J. Microbiol.* **13**, 614.

Wilson, B. J. (1971). *In* "Mycotoxins in Human Health" (I. F. H. Purchase, ed.), pp. 223–229. Macmillan, New York.

Wilson, J. E. (1966). *Biochemistry* **5**, 1351.

Wilson, B. J., Wilson, C. H., and Hayes, A. W. (1968). *Nature* (*London*) **220**, 77.

Woodruff, H. B. (1966). Symposia of the Society for General *Microbiology* **16**, 22.

Yanofsky, C. (1955). *Methods Enzymol.* **2**, 233–238.

11

The Biosynthesis of Anthraquinonoid Mycotoxins from Penicillium islandicum Sopp and Related Fungi

U. SANKAWA

I. INTRODUCTION

Japan had an insufficient domestic rice crop after World War II. Large amounts of rice were, therefore, imported from Egypt, Spain, and the Southeast Asian countries. Government inspection of the imported rice established the presence of fungal-infected yellow rice grains. This discovery led to the so-called "Yellow Rice Event," which drew immediate attention

The Biosynthesis of Mycotoxins

ISBN 0-12-670650-6.

from Japanese mycologists and physiologists owing to their knowledge that rice contaminated by pigment-producing fungi might cause diseases. In 1918, the Japanese mycologist Miyake initiated pioneering research on the isolation of toxigenic fungi from stored rice. His approach was based on the idea that cardiac beriberi might be associated with the consumption of rice contaminated by toxigenic fungi. Cardiac beriberi had been prevalent in the big cities in Japan since the 17th Century. However, this disease disappeared after the introduction of a strict inspection system in all the districts of Japan. The work of Miyake was continued by the physiologist Uraguchi, who isolated a toxigenic fungus from moldy yellow rice. This fungus was identified as *Penicillium citreo-viride* Biourge (Uraguchi, 1971; Uraguchi and Saito, 1972). Uraguchi also found that a yellow pigment produced by this fungus caused in experimental animals symptoms similar to cardiac beriberi. This pigment was called citreoviridin, and structure elucidation established the polyene nature of the compound (Sakabe *et al.*, 1964).

These early studies led to general awareness that fungal-contaminated foodstuffs might cause diseases and to the establishment of a mycological inspection system in Japan. *Penicillium islandicum* Sopp was isolated in 1948 from imported rice (Tsunoda, 1951, 1952). It was subsequently established that rice contaminated by *P. islandicum*, the so-called "Islandia Yellow Rice," induced liver atrophies, cirrhosis, and carcinoma (Uraguchi *et al.*, 1961a,b). (−)-Luteoskyrin was soon isolated as a lipophilic toxin which caused liver damage in experimental animals, from cultures of *P. islandicum* (Shibata *et al.*, 1955b, 1956a; Uraguchi *et al.*, 1961a,b). (−)-Luteoskyrin caused liver damage in the experimental animals. Advanced toxicological and biochemical studies of (−)-luteoskyrin showed that it caused mitochondrial respiratory impairment in the rat liver (Ueno *et al.*, 1964a,b, 1966) and the formation of a complex with DNA and nucleohistone, resulting in the impairment of RNA synthesis (Ueno *et al.*, 1966; 1967a,b,c). In addition to (−)-luteoskyrin, two other mycotoxins belonging to different classes of metabolites have been isolated from *P. islandicum*. Cyclochloretine (islanditoxin) is a cyclic peptide (Uraguchi *et al.*, 1961a,b; Marumo, 1955, 1959; Yoshioka *et al.*, 1973), whereas erythroskyrin is a tetramic acid which contains a polyene side chain (Howard and Raistrick, 1954b; Shoji and Shibata, 1964, 1965; Ueno *et al.*, 1975) (see Chapter 10).

II. CHEMICAL STUDIES OF THE ANTHRAQUINONOID MYCOTOXINS

A. Earlier Investigations on the Metabolites of *Penicillium islandicum*

Penicillium islandicum Sopp was first isolated in 1912 from "Skyr," a kind of yogurt produced in Iceland (Sopp, 1912). Pigments which were subsequently isolated from this fungus were named after the domestic name of yogurt. Since 1940, Raistrick and his associates have studied the metabolites of *P. islandicum* NRRL 1036 and isolated two red pigments, islandicin and (−)-rubroskyrin (Howard and Raistrick, 1949, 1954a). In addition, yellow and orange pigments, namely, skyrin and (−)-flavoskyrin, were isolated from *P. islandicum* NRRL 1175 (Breen *et al.*, 1955; Howard and Raistrick, 1954 c). The structure of islandicin (**1**) was elucidated as a monomeric anthraquinone, whereas skyrin was proved to be the dimer of emodin (Howard and Raistrick, 1954a). Skyrin (**2**) was reductively cleaved by treatment with sodium dithionite into emodin (**3**) in a yield of more than 90% (see Scheme 1). The position of the C—C linkage involved in the connection of the two monomeric moieties was located by an unambiguous synthesis of the hexamethyl ether (Tanaka and Kaneko, 1955). In the early 1950's, Shibata and associates isolated both an orange and a yellow pigment from the wood rotting fungi, *Endothia parasitica* (Murr) P. J. et H. W. Ando, and *Endothia fluvens* (Sow) Ehear et Stevens, and named them endothianin and radicalisin (Shibata *et al.*, 1953). Raistrick's group isolated two pigments from *Penicillium rugulosum* Thom; the orange pigment was identified as skyrin (**2**). The other yellow pigment was named (+)-rugulosin (Breen *et al.*, 1955). Shibata *et al.* (1955a) showed that endothianin and radicalisin were identical to skyrin and (+)-rugulosin, respectively. (+)-Rugulosin is bacteriostatic against gram-positive and gram-negative bacteria and cytotoxic against Ehrlich cells. The hepatotoxicity of (+)-rugulosin was established by observing the change of GOT activity in mice (Sato *et al.*, 1977).

The close structural relationship between (−)-luteoskyrin and (+)-rugulosin was soon evident from experimental results (see Scheme 1). Both these substances gave bisanthraquinones on mild dehydration, whereas they furnished monomeric anthraquinones on pyrolysis (Shibata *et al.*, 1956a,b). (−)-Luteoskyrin yielded catenarin (**4**) and islandicin (**1**) in a 1:1 ratio on pyrolysis, whereas (+)-rugulosin gave emodin (**3**) and chrysophanol (**5**) in the same ratio. Dehydration of (+)-rugulosin gave dianhydrorugulosin (dichrysophanol) (**6**), and (−)-luteoskyrin gave iridoskyrin (diislandicin) (**7**). These findings indicated that the two compounds are dimers of partially hydrogenated anthraquinones and that luteoskyrin is in fact dihydroxyrugulosin. On the other hand, (−)-rubroskyrin, a quinonoidal pigment, was found to be converted into the nonquinonoidal (−)-luteoskyrin on treatment with pyridine. This observation was in agreement with the report of Zahn and Koch (1938) that a quinonoidal dihydroanthraquinone was easily converted into the corresponding nonquinonoidal enol tautomer by base treatment (Scheme 2). Thus, (−)-luteoskyrin and (−)-rubroskyrin were once formulated as a pair of tautomeric isomers represented by the structures of the dimeric anthraquinones, **8** and **9**, respectively. (+)-Rugulosin was formulated as **10**.

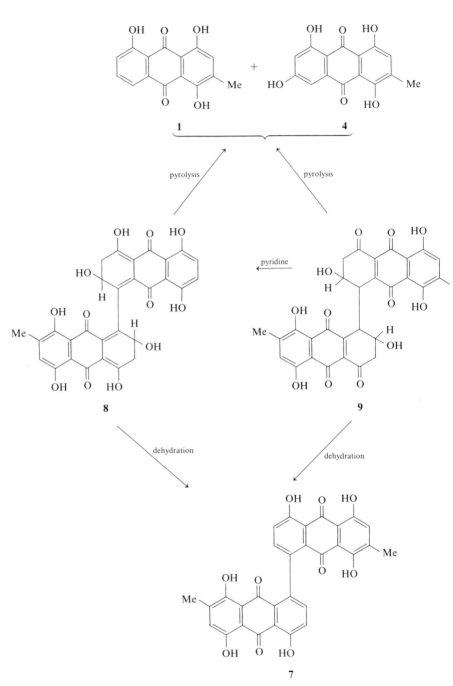

Scheme 1. Chemical reactions of skyrin (**2**), (−)-luteoskyrin, (−)-rubroskyrin, and (+)-rugulosin.

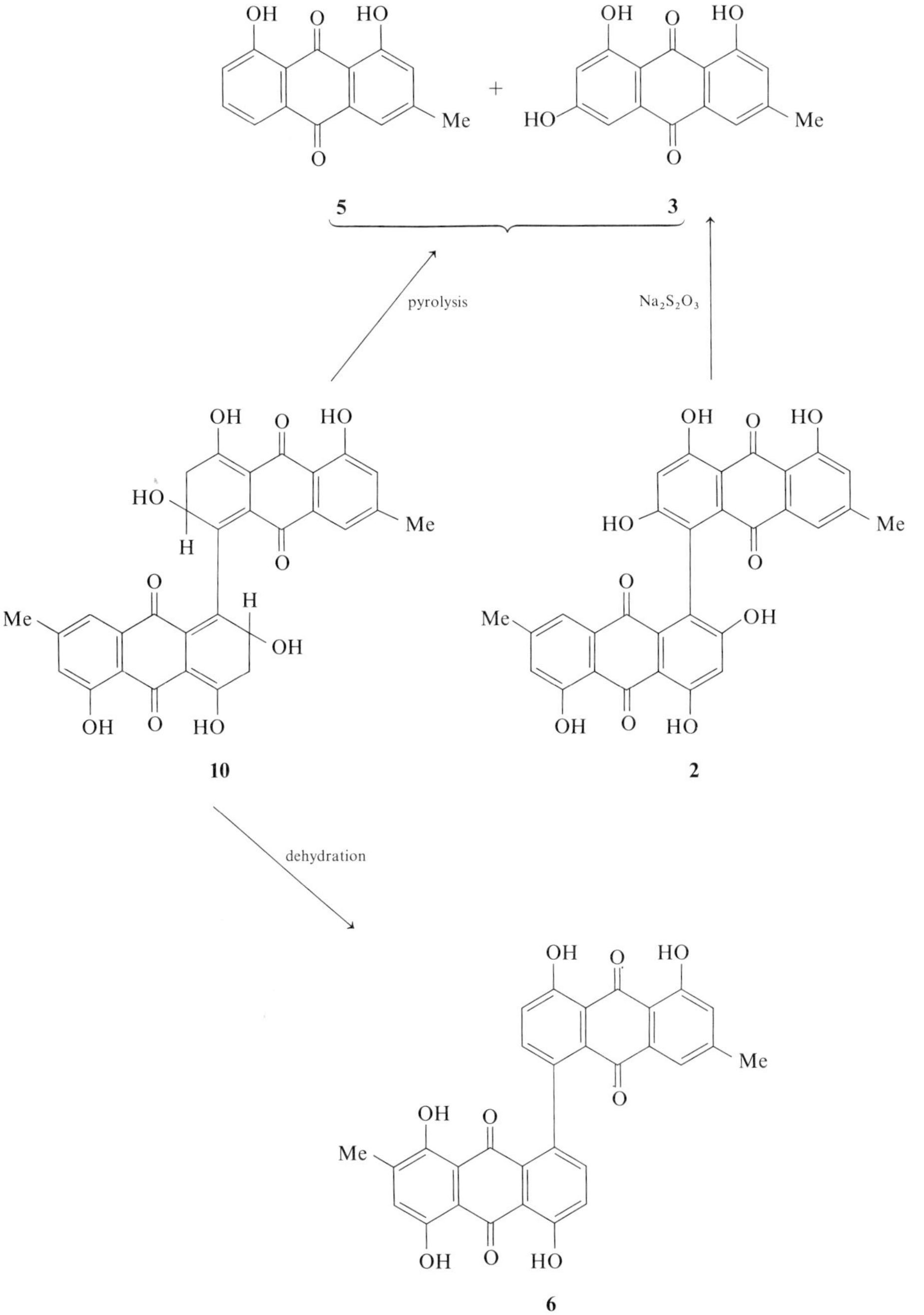

Scheme 1 (*continued*)

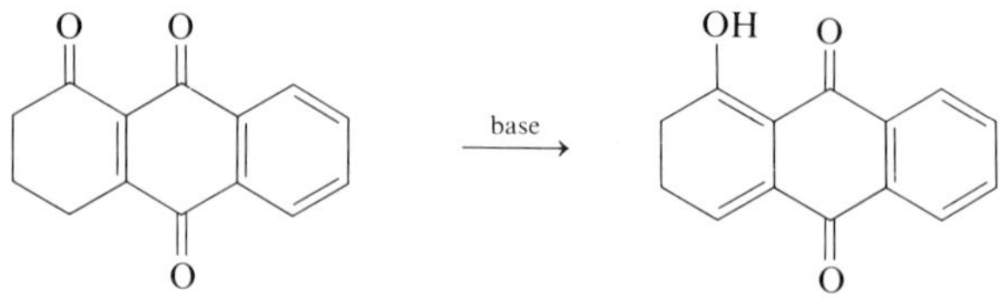

O   O   OH   O

$\xrightarrow{\text{base}}$

O   O

Quinonic dihydroanthraquinone   Enolic dihydroanthraquinone

Scheme 2. Keto–enol tautomerism of dihydroanthraquinone (Zahn and Koch, 1938).

B. Revised Structures of (−)-Luteoskyrin, (−)-Rubroskyrin, and (+)-Rugulosin

The renewed investigations of the structural chemistry of these anthraquinones were initiated by the advent of advanced NMR spectroscopic
techniques (Ogihara *et al.*, 1968). The NMR spectra of (−)-luteoskyrin and
(+)-rugulosin (Fig. 1) showed signals corresponding to the two halves of
these molecules and thereby established their symmetrical nature. Signals
attributable to the aromatic and methyl protons, as found in structures **8** and
10, were present. However, the expected ABX signals from the partially
hydrogenated rings were not observed; instead, three signals characteristic
of methine protons were observed in the aliphatic region.

One of the signals shifted downfield on acetylation and was assigned to a
proton on a carbon atom bearing a secondary hydroxy group. Decoupling
experiments proved that both of the remaining methine protons were located
in positions adjacent to the secondary hydroxy group. (−)-Tetrahydroluteo-
skyrin and (+)-tetrahydrorugulosin, obtained on catalytic reduction, showed

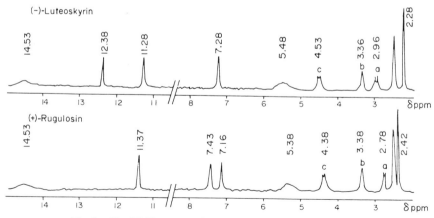

Fig. 1.   The NMR spectra of (−)-luteoskyrin and (+)-rugulosin.

additional signals attributable to the newly formed hydroxy groups. Infrared spectra indicated that nonchelated carbonyl groups of (+)-rugulosin had been reduced to hydroxy groups. The NMR spectrum of the acetate of (+)-tetrahydrorugulosin gave a sharp singlet signal attributable to the proton on the carbon atom bearing the newly formed acetoxy group; this established the quaternary nature of both carbon atoms adjacent to the carbonyl group. Therefore, partial structures for (+)-rugulosin (**11**) and (−)-luteoskyrin (**12**) were deduced from the spectral data. Arrows indicate the presence of C–C bonds in these formulas (Ogihara *et al.*, 1968).

At this stage, biogenetic considerations played an important role in formulating structures for the anthraquinonoid mycotoxins. If a hypothetical intermediate (**13**) possessing the structure of a partially hydrogenated bis-anthraquinone is postulated in the biosynthesis of anthraquinoids, then the formation of the additional C–C bonds which are required in the partial structures (**11** and **12**) can be explained reasonably by a Michael-type reaction between two monomeric moieties. Thus, (−)-luteoskyrin and (+)-rugulosin were formulated as **14** and **15**, respectively (Sankawa *et al.*, 1968). The validity of the structures was supported by the structural study of (−)-rubroskyrin. The NMR spectrum of (−)-rubroskyrin triacetate showed a broad AB quartet indicating the presence of a methylene group which is absent in (−)-luteoskyrin (**14**) and (+)-rugulosin (**15**) (Fig. 2). Successive

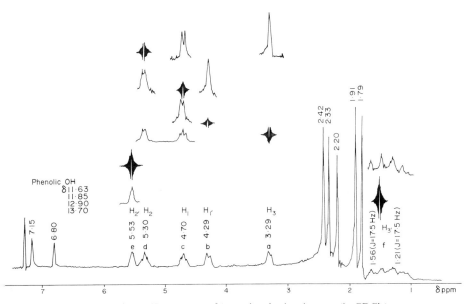

Fig. 2.   The NMR spectrum of (−)-rubroskyrin triacetate (in CDCl$_3$).

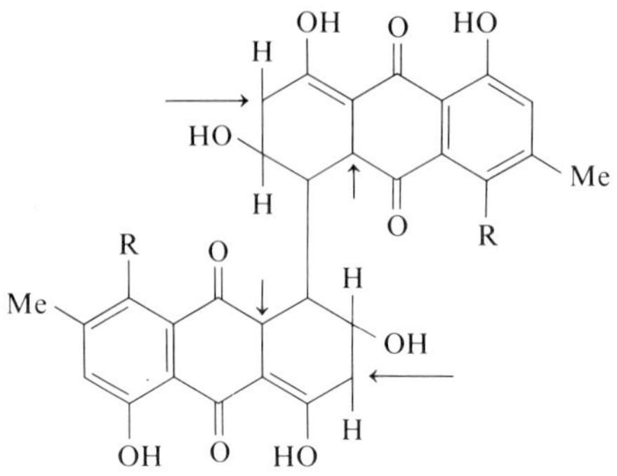

11 R = H
12 R = OH

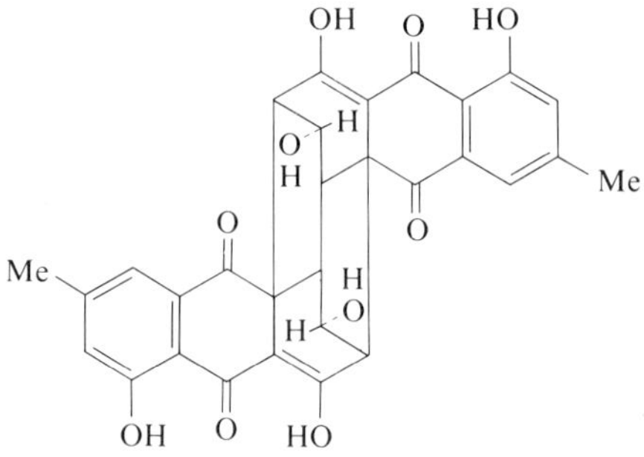

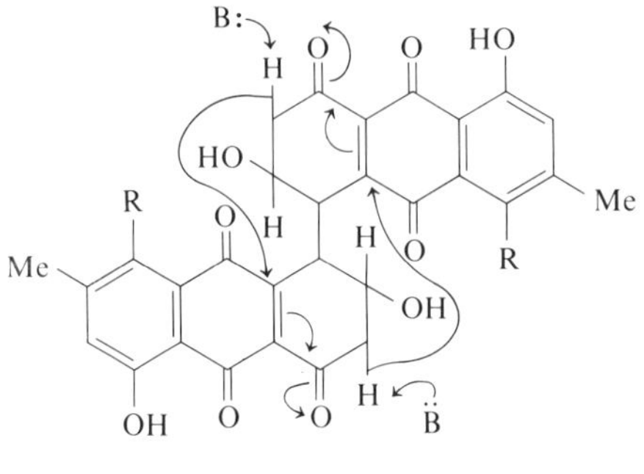

13

15

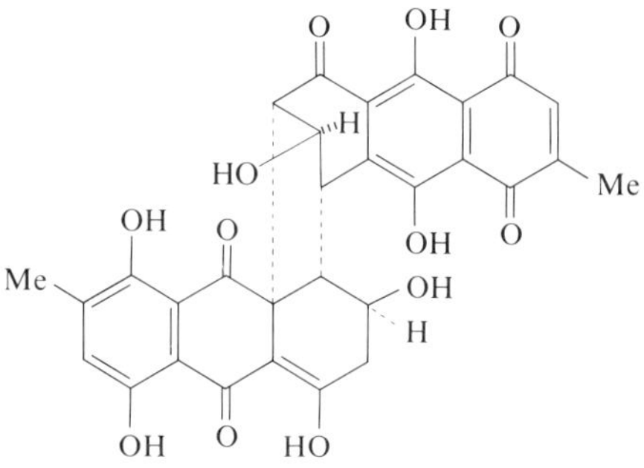

16

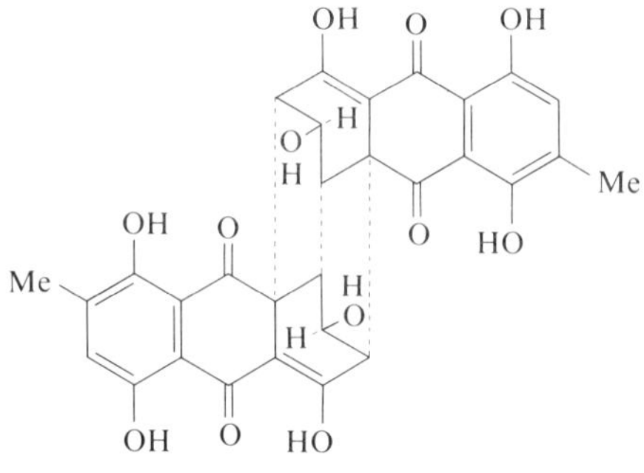

14

decoupling experiments revealed the following linkage in (–)-rubroskyrin

—C—CH—CH(OAc)—CH—CH · · · CH(OAc)—CH$_2$—C—

(–)-Rubroskyrin was again formulated as **16** by assuming a single Michael-type reaction in the hypothetical intermediate **13** instead of the double-Michael reaction in the biosynthesis of (–)-luteoskyrin (**14**). The established structure thus indicated that the conversion of (–)-rubroskyrin (**16**) into (–)-luteoskyrin (**14**) is not a simple keto–enol tautomerism, but the Michael-type reaction between two monomeric moieties. Anthraquinonoid mycotoxins can thus be regarded as the dimers of partially hydrogenated anthraquinones which are connected by three C–C bonds. Their unique structures were unambiguously established by the X-ray analysis of a bromination product of (+)-tetrahydrorugulosin (Kobayashi *et al.*, 1968,1970).

III. BIOSYNTHETIC ORIGIN OF ANTHRAQUINONOID MYCOTOXINS

The close biosynthetic relationship of (–)-luteoskyrin (**14**) and (+)-rugulosin (**15**) to the aromatic anthraquinones was indicated by the ready chemical conversion of these compounds to monomeric and dimeric anthraquinones by pyrolysis and dehydration. The anthraquinones produced by the fungi belonging to the genera *Aspergillus* and *Penicillium* possess an arrangement of oxygen atoms typical of polyketides derived from acetyl- and malonyl-CoA. Their polyketide nature was demonstrated relatively early by Gatenbeck (1958,1960b) by incorporation studies using [^{14}C]acetate and by successive degradation experiments. [^{14}C]Acetate-derived skyrin (**2**) and islandicin (**1**) obtained from a culture of *P. islandicum* were shown to be labeled at alternate carbon atoms, as expected from the "acetate theory" (Birch *et al.*, 1953; 1955). Noteworthy results were also obtained in the feeding experiment with [^{14}C,^{18}O]acetate. The polyketides are a class of compounds which are formed by the cyclization of polyketomethylene intermediates, in which carbonyl or its equivalent functions should be derived from (labeled) ^{18}O from [^{18}O]acetate. In cyclization processes, some of the oxygen atoms are lost as the result of aldol condensation reactions between carbonyl and active methylene groups, whereas the rest of the oxygen atoms are retained in the polyketide molecule as phenolic hydroxy groups or oxo or carboxy groups.

A preliminary experiment was carried out in *Chaetomium cochlioides* to study the potential of [^{14}C,^{18}O]acetate in the investigation of the origin of oxygen atoms. This fungus produces orsellinic acid (**17**), a typical tetraketide, which is derived from one molecule of acetyl-CoA and three molecules of malonyl-CoA without oxidation or reduction. The incorporation of ^{18}O into

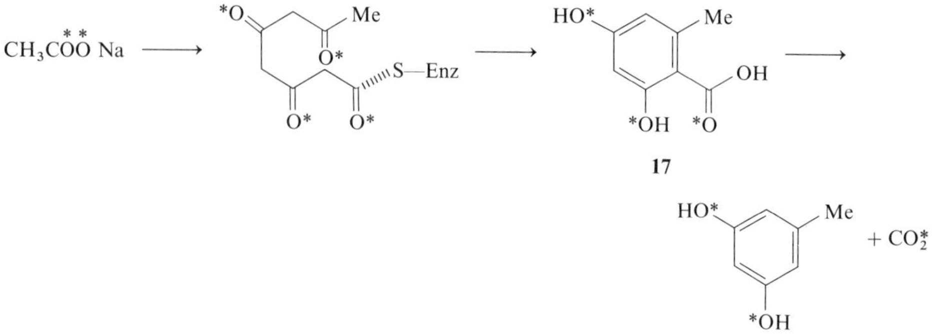

Scheme 3.   Incorporation of $[^{14}C,^{18}O]$acetate into orsellinic acid (17).

TABLE I

Ratio of ^{18}O to ^{14}C in Orsellinic Acid (17) Labeled by $[^{14}C,^{18}O]$Acetate

	Na Acetate	Carboxyl (CO_2)	Orcinol
$^{18}O:^{14}C$ Ratio	3.13	0.89	1.64
^{18}O Dilution in relation to ^{14}C	1	3.6	1.9

the carboxy group of orsellinic acid (17) (see Scheme 3, Table I) was half as much as that into the phenolic groups, indicating the exchange of one of the two oxygen atoms, presumably at the stage when orsellinic acid (17) was released from the enzyme template (Gatenbeck and Mosbach, 1959).

Analogous experiments in *P. islandicum* using $[^{14}C,^{18}O]$acetate proved the incorporation of ^{18}O into the anthraquinonoids (Scheme 4). The main metabolite of the fungus is skyrin (2). However, for the estimation of the ^{18}O incorporation data, it was necessary to convert labeled 2 into emodin by reductive cleavage. According to the polyketide theory, four of the five oxygen atoms of emodin (3) are derived from acetate and one from atmospheric oxygen, whereas in islandicin (1), three of the five oxygen atoms are derived from acetate and two from atmospheric oxygen.

Table II shows the results of the incorporation experiments (Gatenbeck, 1960a). The values of the ^{18}O dilution in relation to ^{14}C were calculated from the average ^{18}O content. The ^{18}O content in the labeled positions of emodin (3) and islandicin (1), for three hydroxy and one carbonyl groups, was 1.09 and 1.08, respectively. The results clearly demonstrated the validity of the polyketide theory and at the same time showed that there were negligible exchanges of ^{18}O during the biosynthesis of the anthraquinonoids. In the experiment with orsellinic acid (17), however, the dilution of ^{18}O vs. that of ^{14}C was 1.9 in the hydroxy group, indicating that about half the oxygen atoms

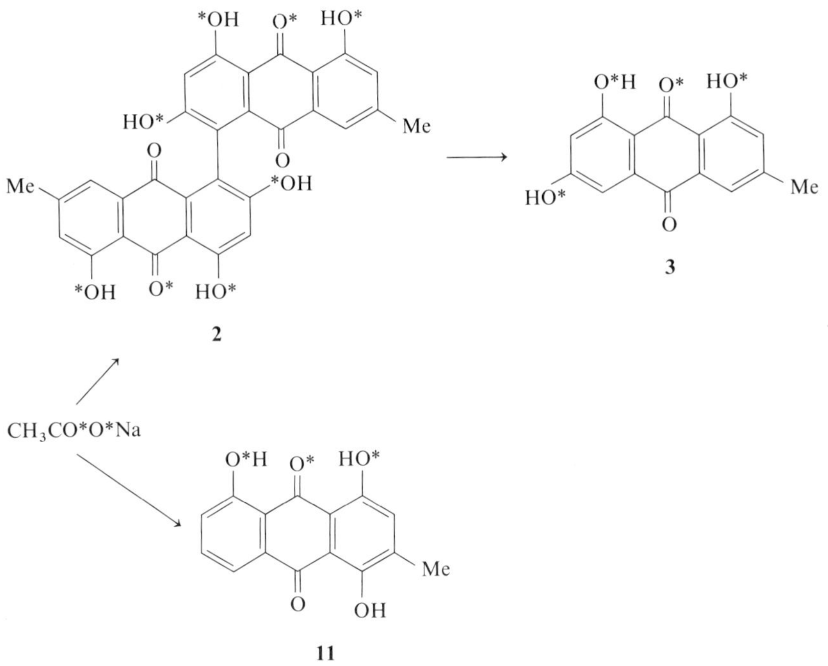

Scheme 4.   Incorporation of $[^{14}C,^{18}O]$acetate into anthraquinonoids.

TABLE II

Ratio ^{18}O to ^{14}C in Anthraquinones (1,3) Labeled by $[^{14}C,^{18}O]$Acetate

	Na Acetate	Islandicin	Emodin	(−)-Rubroskyrin
Average ^{18}O content	21.6	0.64	0.82	0.54(H_2O)
Calculated ^{18}O content in labeled positions	—	1.07	1.02	—
^{18}O dilution in relation to ^{14}C	1	1.08	1.09	—

originally present in $[^{14}C,^{18}O]$acetate had been exchanged during biosynthesis. These findings may indicate that the biosynthetic reaction is much faster in *P. islandicum* than that in *C. cochlioides*. The incorporation of ^{18}O into the secondary hydroxy groups of (−)-rubroskyrin (**16**) was also demonstrated in the same experiment, indicating that the secondary hydroxy group of the anthraquinonoid mycotoxins are formed by the reduction of polyketomethylene intermediates or an aromatic polyketide.

Shibata and Ikekawa (1962; 1963) studied the specific incorporation of $[^{14}C]$acetate and $[^{14}C]$malonate into (+)-rugulosin (**15**); the proven labeling patterns were as expected in a dimeric octaketide derived from two units of acetyl-CoA and 14 units of malonyl-CoA. Recently, the biosynthesis of (+)-rugulosin (15) was investigated by extensive use of ^{13}C NMR data obtained from (+)-rugulosin (15) derived from $[1\text{-}^{13}C]\text{-}$, $[2\text{-}^{13}C]\text{-}$, and $[1,2\text{-}^{13}C]$acetate labeling experiments. The $(^{13}C,^{13}C)$ coupling constants observed in $[1,2\text{-}^{13}C]$acetate-derived (+)-rugulosin (15) were particularly useful (Akiyama et al., 1978 unpublished work). Table III shows the values of the chemical shifts and the $(^{13}C,^{13}C)$ coupling constants. The incorporation patterns of the acetate units (18) unambiguously showed that (+)-rugulosin (15) is the dimer of an octaketide.

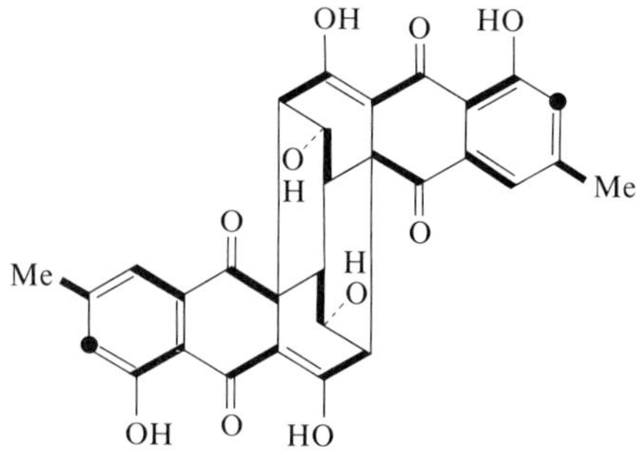

18

TABLE III

Chemical Shift and Coupling Constant Values of (+)-Rugulosin (15) Labeled by $[1,2\text{-}^{13}C_2]$Acetate

Carbon[a]	Chemical shift (ppm)	$(^{13}C,^{13}C)$ Coupling (Hz)
C(1)	47.7	37
C(2)	68.5	37
C(3)	58.2	47
C(4)	185.6	47
C(4a)	106.2	63
C(5)	160.2	65
C(6)	124.0	—
C(7)	147.5	43
C(8)	120.5	56
C(9)	193.9	43
C(9a)	55.6	43
C(10)	181.0	63
C(10a)	114.1	65
C(11)	21.4	43

[a] Numbering is shown in Figs. 3 and 4.

The fate of acetate hydrogen atoms in the biosynthesis of anthraquinones is particularly important in relation to the dimerization mechanism; this aspect is dealt with in the following section. A new method was applied for the tracing of hydrogen incorporation from acetate in the biosynthesis of (+)-rugulosin (15) (Sankawa *et al.*, 1978). The method is based on the use of [2-^{13}C,2-^{2}H$_3$]acetate as a tracer, and the incorporation of deuterium is detected by ^{13}C NMR spectroscopy. Because ^{2}H is directly attached to the ^{13}C, its incorporation was observed by ^{13}C signals showing ^{13}C–^{2}H coupling and isotopic shifts of 0.3 ppm per ^{2}H atom. The detection of the ^{13}C–^{2}H signal in methine and aromatic carbons is difficult under proton-noise-decoupled (PND) conditions because of the lack of the NOE effect and the longer T_1 attributable to the presence of ^{2}H. The incorporation of ^{2}H can be conveniently detected by comparison of the signal intensities between the ^{13}C NMR spectra of samples derived from [2-^{13}C]acetate and [2-^{13}C,2-^{2}H$_3$]acetate labeling experiments (Fig. 3). The signal intensities of carbon atoms labeled by ^{2}H are markedly suppressed, because the ^{13}C–^{2}H signals shift to higher field and signal intensities are then determined by ^{13}C which is not labeled by ^{2}H. The ^{13}C–^{2}H signals of methine and aromatic carbon atoms can be directly detected by recording the ^{13}C NMR spectrum under conditions of deuterium noise decoupling. The ^{13}C–^{2}H signals are observed as singlets between the coupled signals of the ^{13}C–^{1}H species.

The PND ^{13}C NMR spectra of (+)-rugulosin (15) labeled by [2-^{13}C]- and [2-^{13}C,2-^{2}H$_3$]acetates are shown in Fig.4. The signals of the ^{2}H-labeled carbon atoms [C(1), C(3), C(8), and C(11)], indicated by solid circles in Fig. 4, are markedly decreased in their intensities compared with the corresponding carbon atoms in undeuterated (+)-rugulosin (15). This conventional method for the detection of deuterium incorporation would be particularly useful when the deuterium noise decoupling is not available. Figure 4 shows the deuterium-noise-decoupled spectrum of (+)-rugulosin (15) labeled by [2-^{13}C,2-^{2}H$_3$]acetate. The ^{13}C–^{2}H signals of C(1) and C(3) appear as singlets between the corresponding doublet signals of the ^{13}C–^{1}H species. They show a shift of 0.3 ppm to high field compared with the ^{13}C–^{1}H signals. The C(11) methyl group gives rise to both a singlet and a doublet owing to the presence of ^{13}C–^{2}H$_3$ and ^{13}C–^{2}H$_2$ ^{1}H species. The two signals show isotope effects of 0.9 and 0.6 ppm, respectively. The presence of ^{13}C–^{2}H$_2$^{1}H in the methyl group indicates that interconversion took place in the organism between acetyl- and malonyl-CoA. The absence of ^{2}H at C(6) is in accordance with the fact that the carboxy group at C(6) is lost in the course of the biosynthesis, probably after skeletal formation. The incorporation of ^{2}H from acetate into C(1) is a particularly important finding, as it supports the reaction mechanism for the dimerization of the anthraquinonoids.

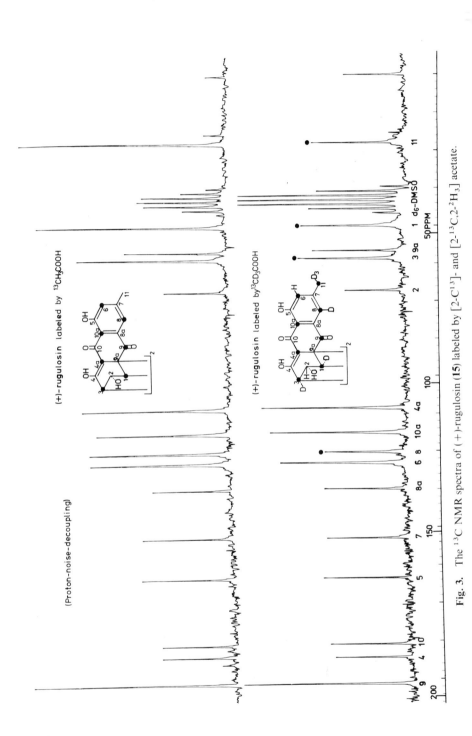

Fig. 3. The ^{13}C NMR spectra of (+)-rugulosin (15) labeled by [2-C^{13}]- and [2-^{13}C,2-$^2H_3$] acetate.

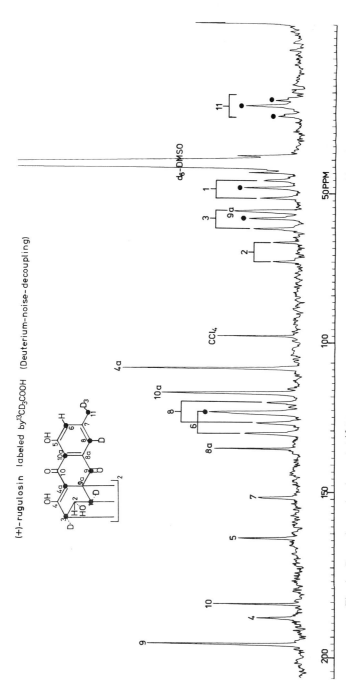

Fig. 4.   Deuterium noise decoupled ^{13}C NMR spectrum of (+)-rugulosin (15) labeled by [2-^{13}C,2-$^2H_3$]acetate.

371

IV. METABOLIC RELATIONSHIP
   OF THE ANTHRAQUINONOIDS PRODUCED
   BY *PENICILLIUM ISLANDICUM* AND RELATED FUNGI

A. Study by the Use of Mutants

The biosynthesis of anthraquinonoids in *P. islandicum* drew special attention from the point of their metabolic relationship. In an earlier stage of the investigation, before the structures of (−)-luteoskyrin (14) and (−)-rubroskyrin (16) were correctly established, the modified bisanthraquinones were regarded either as partially hydrogenated bisanthraquinones or as hydrated bisanthraquinones. On mild dehydration, they (14 and 16) yielded the bisanthraquinone iridoskyrin (7), which was further cleaved with alkaline dithionite into the monomeric anthraquinone islandicin (1). In living organisms the series of reactions might occur in this order or in reverse. Gatenbeck (1960a) studied the sequence of the production of the anthraquinonoids by investigating the metabolites at suitable time intervals. In this study, *P. islandicum* NRRL 1036 was grown on the normal Czapek–Dox medium. Skyrin (2) appeared considerably earlier than any of the other anthraquinonoids which were examined; in fact, no other pigment could be detected until 24 hr after the appearance of skyrin (2). It was not possible to determine the order of the appearance of (−)-luteoskyrin (14), (−)-rubroskyrin (16), or iridoskyrin (7). An intensive investigation of the appearance of these metabolites in *P. islandicum* NRRL 1175 by Hayashi *et al.* (1959) revealed that the first pigment which appeared was again skyrin (2), which was subsequently followed by oxyskyrin (19) and chrysophanol (5). Emodin (3) and (−)-flavoskyrin appeared last. However, the sequence of the appearance of the metabolites does not necessarily coincide with the metabolic sequence.

Time-course incorporation studies were carried out by Gatenbeck (1960a) to clarify the metabolic sequence among these pigments (Fig. 5). The specific activity of the mixture of islandicin (1) and iridoskyrin (7) was definitely higher than that of (−)-rubroskyrin (16). This finding ruled out the possibility that the former was derived from the latter. The time-course variation of the specific activities in the experiments where medium containing [^{14}C]-acetate was replaced by fresh medium after a very short incubation period clearly demonstrated that the specific activities of islandicin (1), iridoskyrin (7), and (−)-luteoskyrin (14) decreased continuously parallel to each other; this indicated that these anthraquinonoids are not formed in a sequential manner and that there is no product–precursor relationship among them. It is of interest to note that iridoskyrin (7) is not formed by the dimerization of the corresponding monomer, islandicin (1).

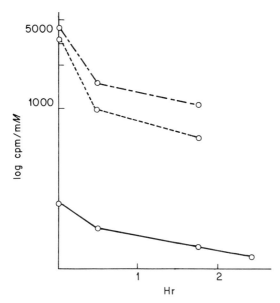

Fig. 5.   Time course changes of specific activities of (−)-luteoskyrin (**4**), — — ; iridoskyrin
(**7**), ‐‐‐ ‐‐‐; and islandicin (**1**), —‐ —‐ . (Gatenbeck, 1960a).

These observations were also supported by experiments using mutants.
The mutants of *P. islandicum* which were prepared by ultraviolet (UV)
irradiation were examined in a search for an intermediate that would
accumulate owing to the lack of a specific enzyme of the normal strain.
Chromatographic analysis of the metabolites formed by the mutants showed
that the UV mutation induced only a quantitative variation of the normal
metabolites (Gatenbeck and Barbesgard, 1960; Nakahara and Kikuchi,
1961). The stability of the metabolic pathway under conditions of successive
transplantation was studied by Kikuchi and Nakahara (1961) to identify
the group of metabolites belonging to the same metabolic pathway. Successive transplantations of the fungus on the Czapek–Dox agar medium
led to the gradual loss of the ability to produce certain of the metabolites
which are formed by an unstable metabolic pathway. The metabolic pathway
leading to skyrin (**2**), oxyskyrin (**19**) and skyrinol (**20**) was the most stable,
whereas (−)-luteoskyrin (**14**) disappeared fairly easily. The pathway of
islandicin (**1**) and iridoskyrin (**7**) was relatively stable, but this pathway
was lost faster than the skyrin pathway. The investigation of the metabolic
relationship among anthraquinonoids at an early stage gave only incon-
clusive results.

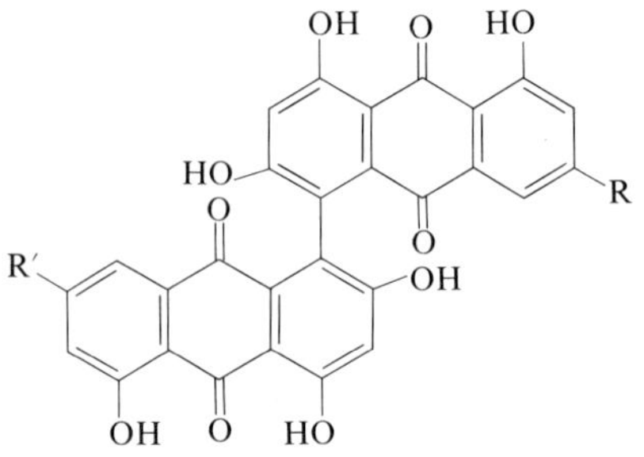

OH   O   HO

HO
O
                                    R
R′
          O
                          OH

OH   O   HO

19   R = Me, R′ = CH₂OH
20   R = R′ = CH₂OH

B. Biosynthetic Incorporation of Monomeric Anthraquinones into Anthraquinonoid Mycotoxins

Emodin (**3**) is an octaketide anthraquinone which is widely distributed among fungi such as *Penicillium* and *Aspergillus*. It has been known to play an important role as an intermediate in the biosynthesis of some fungal metabolites. Gröger *et al.* (1968) have shown that emodin (**3**) is a good precursor in the biosynthesis of the ergochromes, the pigments of *Claviceps purpurea* (ergot), possessing dimeric xanthone structures. The incorporation ratios of [¹⁴C]emodin into the ergochromes (secalonic acids) were 0.31–1.51% in *Claviceps* and *Penicillium oxalicum*. The biosynthetic pathway of the ergochromes from emodin (**3**) involves not only ring cleavage followed by the reaction which forms the xanthone skeleton, but the steps involved in the elimination of the hydroxy group and dimerization (see Chapter 5). The elimination of a hydroxy group of an anthraquinone during biosynthesis also occurs during the formation of sterigmatocystin and aflatoxin B_1; in this case, the β-hydroxy group of the anthraquinone precursor, averufin, was lost during the course of the biosynthesis (see Chapter 4). The potential of emodin (**3**) as a precursor of the anthraquinonoids was regarded as a subject worth investigation, because the elimination of the hydroxy group would require reduction and subsequent dehydration.

Significant incorporation ratios into (+)-rugulosin (**15**) were found with feeding experiments in *Penicillium brunneum* using [¹⁴C]emodin (**3**) and [¹⁴C]emodinanthrone (**21**) the [¹⁴C]emodinanthrone (**21**) was prepared from [¹⁴C]skyrin (**2**) obtained biosynthetically by feeding [¹⁴C]acetate to *P. islandicum*. However [¹⁴C]penicilliopsin (= diemodinanthrone) (**22**) prepared by feeding [¹⁴C]malonate to *Penicilliopsis calvariaeformis* showed no significant incorporation into (+)-rugulosin (**15**). [¹⁴C]Skyrin (**2**) was not converted into (+)-rugulosin (**15**), and a considerable amount of the radioactive skyrin (**2**) was recovered from the culture. The lack of incorporation of the dimeric anthraquinonoids does not necessarily mean that they are not involved in the biosynthesis of (+)-rugulosin (15); the negative results may be caused by a lack of permeability of the cell walls. However, the incorporation of ^{2}H from [2-^{13}C,2-^{2}H$_3$]acetate into C(1) of (+)-rugulosin (15), as mentioned previously, excludes the possibility that the aromatic bisanthraquinones or bisanthrones are involved in the biosynthesis of (+)-rugulosin (15) (Scheme 5). It was evident at the same time that the dimerization reaction does not take place at the anthrone or anthraquinone stages. (+)-[^{14}C]Rugulosin (15), labeled biosynthetically, showed no significant conversion into the other metabolites. The recovery of (+)-[^{14}C]-rugulosin (15) was low (4–5%), contrary to the experiment with [^{14}C]skyrin (2) (see above). A thin layer chromatography (TLC) scanning experiment revealed that the radioactivity in the medium was found mainly at the origin of the TLC plate, whereas work-up of the mycelium gave a radioactive peak at the spot of (+)-rugulosin (15). Therefore, the (+)-[^{14}C]rugulosin (15) absorbed on the mycelium seems to stay unaffected, whereas the (+)-rugulosin in the medium suffered extensive catabolism to yield highly polar compounds. Emodin (3) is a normal metabolite of *P. brunneum*; therefore, its biological conversion into (+)-rugulosin (15) substantiates its role in the actual biosynthesis (Sankawa *et al.*, 1973) (Table IV).

Similar results were also obtained using *Myrothecium verrucaria*, a fungus which produces (−)-rugulosin (23). Both [^{14}C]emodin (3) and [^{14}C]-emodinanthrone (21) were efficiently converted into (−)-rugulosin (23). [^{14}C]Emodin (3) was a better precursor in the specific strain used in this experiment (Sankawa *et al.*, 1973) (Table V).

In the feeding experiment using *P. islandicum* NRRL 1036, [^{14}C]emodin (3) and [^{14}C]emodinanthrone (21) showed incorporation into almost all of the anthraquinonoids which were produced by this fungus. However, the incorporation of [^{14}C]emodin (3) was less significant than that of [^{14}C]emodinanthrone (21). [^{14}C]-Labeled precursors for the feeding experiments were prepared as follows. (−)-[^{14}C]Rubroskyrin (16) and [^{14}C]-islandicin (1) were labeled biosynthetically by feeding [^{14}C]malonate to cultures of *P. islandicum* NRRL 1036. [^{14}C]Catenarin (4) was prepared by the pyrolysis of (−)-[^{14}C]rubroskyrin (16) and [^{14}C]chrysophanol (5) from (+)-[^{14}C]rugulosin (15) by dehydration followed by reductive cleavage with alkaline dithionite. It is evident from the data in Table VI that none of these labeled compounds showed significant incorporation into the other metabolites and that the compounds used in the feeding experiments were recovered intact from the culture medium and still contained considerable radioactivity (Sankawa *et al.*, 1973).

The exact role of emodin (3) and emodinanthrone (21) in the biosynthesis of the other anthraquinonoids of *Penicillium* and *Myrothecium* was not

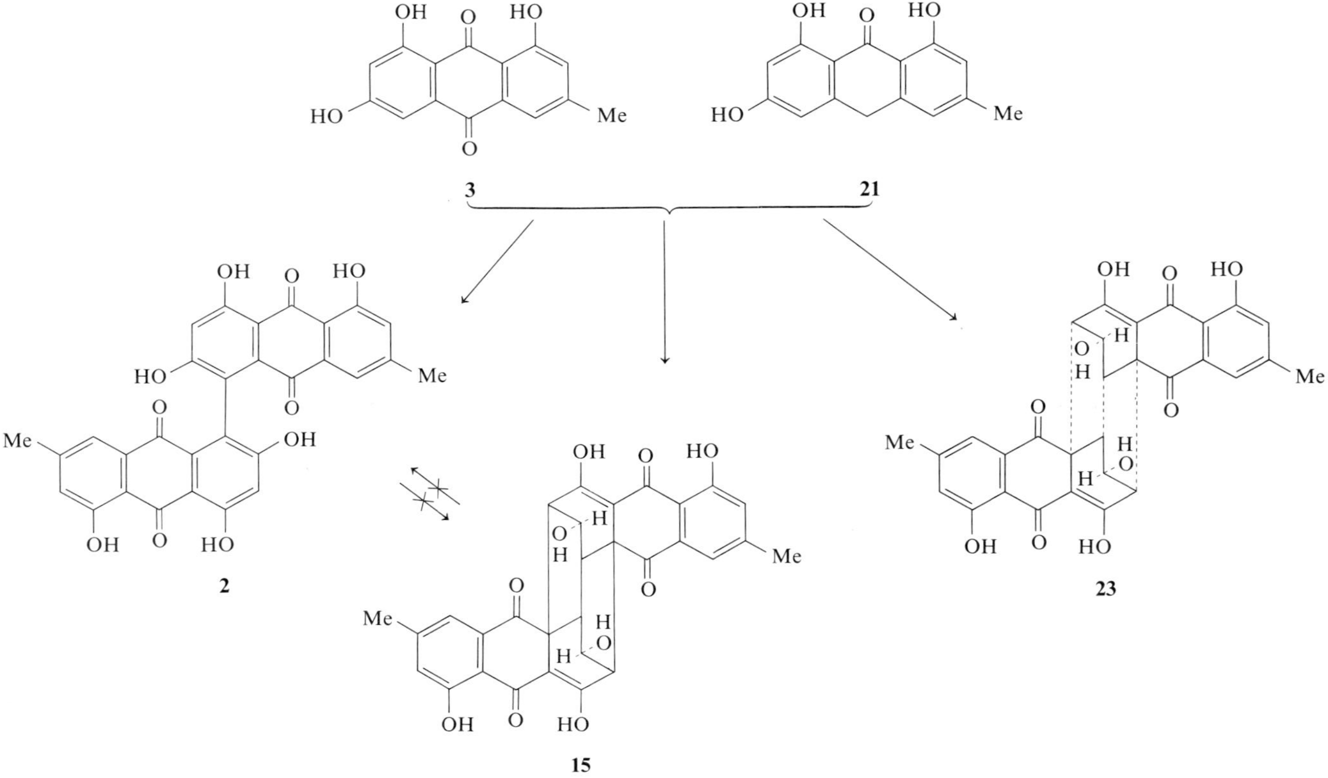

Myrothecium verrucaria

Penicillium brunneum

21

3

23

15

2

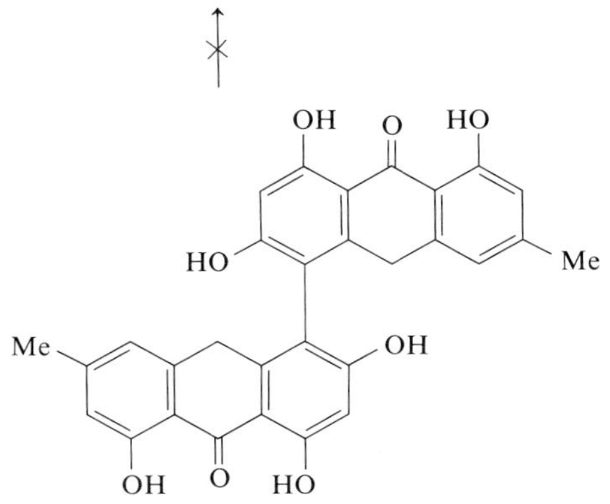

22

Scheme 5. Incorporation experiments with monomeric precursors in *Penicillium brunneum* and *Myrothecium verrucaria.*

TABLE IV

Feeding Experiments Using *Penicillium brunneum* Udagawa

	Incorporation (%) in isolated compounds (specific incorporation, %)		
Labeled compounds	Emodin (3)	Skyrin (2)	(+)-Rugulosin (15)
Emodinanthrone (21)	1.9 (4.7)	4.4 (12.5)	63.7 (14.0)
Emodin (3)	0.38 (−)	1.6 (12.5)	25.0 (13.6)
Penicilliopsin (22)	0(0)	3.8 (19.2)	0.7 (0.09)
Skyrin (2)	—	42. (45.8)	0.07 (0.12)
(+)-Rugulosin (15)	—	0.07 (0.21)	5.2 (2.7)

TABLE V

Feeding Experiment Using *Myrothecium verrucaria* (Alb. et Schw.) Ditmar ex Fr.

Labeled compounds	Incorporation (%) in (−)-rugulosin (23) (specific incorporation, %)
Emodinanthrone (21)	7.25 (5.81)
Emodin (3)	13.2 (8.25)

clear, although the efficient conversion of **3** and **21** into these anthra-quinonoids established them as precursors. Emodin (**3**) may be reduced to emodinanthrone (**21**) before it enters into the normal biosynthetic pathway, or else both emodin (**3**) and emodinanthrone (**21**) may be converted into the same intermediate, such as emodinhydroquinone, which does not exist in the free form. One of the possible intermediates beyond anthrone is hydroanthracene, which corresponds to dihydroemodinathrone (**24**). Recently, a yellow characteristic pigment of the seedlings of *Cassia torosa*, a plant belonging to the Leguminosae, was found to possess structure **24** (Takahashi *et al.*, 1976). Parietin glycoside (**25**), the main constituent of the seeds, disappears rapidly during the germination, and germichrysone (**24**) appears at the same time as the characteristic pigment in the seedlings. This finding seems to suggest that germichrysone (**24**) is formed from the anthraquinone glycoside **25**, for the appearance of **24** coincides with the disappearance of **25**. However, this possibility was ruled out by the observation that [^{14}C]malonate was incorporated efficiently into germichrysone (**24**). The *de novo* synthesis of germichrysone (**24**) from acetyl- and malonyl-CoA was also supported by the fact that a callus cell line derived from

TABLE VI

Feeding Experiments in *Penicillium islandicum* Sopp NRRL 1036

Labeled compounds	Incorporation (%) in isolated compounds (specific incorporation, %)				
	Islandicin (1)	Iridoskyrin (7)	Skyrin (2)	(−)-Rubroskyrin (16)	Others
Emodinanthrone (21)	20.3 (3.84)	0.35 (10.2)	5.25 (8.12)	2.2 (4.7)	
Emodin (3)	0.12 (1.2)	0.05 (1.6)	0.2 (12.0)	— (—)	
Islandicin (1)	58.6 (7.6)	0.07 (0.25)	0.06 (0.36)	— (—)	
Chrysophanol (5)	0.47 (0.10)	0.02 (0.02)	0.01 (0.36)	— (—)	Chrysophanol 28.6 (65.5)
Catenarin (4)	0.14 (0.018)	— (—)	1.3 (0.71)	0.18 (0.57)	Catenarin 13.8 (82.0)
Iridoskyrin (7)	0.11 (0.03)	45.7 (54.3)	0.8 (0.18)	0 (0)	
Skyrin (2)	0.14 (0.02)	— (—)	22.2 (6.2)	0 (0)	
(−)-Rubroskyrin (16)	0 (0)	— (—)	0 (0)	8.6 (22.2)	

the seedlings produces germichrysone (25) in high yield. Although [^{14}C]-emodin (3) and [^{14}C]emodinanthrone (21) showed no significant incorporation into germichrysone (24) in the seedlings and the callus culture, no definite conclusion can be drawn from these observations. It became possible to prepare [^{14}C]germichrysone (24) by using the callus culture. Feeding experiments in *M. verrucaria* using 24 gave significant incorporation into (−)-rugulosin (23) (Sankawa and Noguchi, 1979, unpublished work).

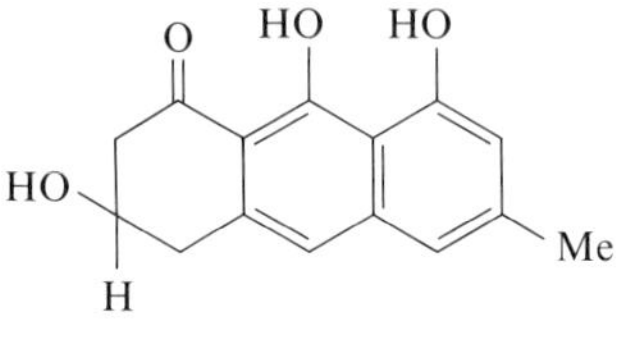

24 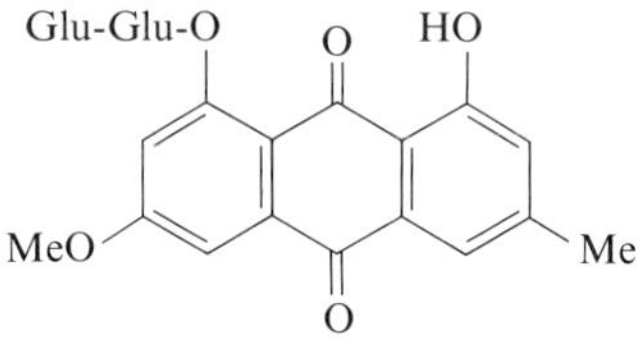   25

C. Structure of (−)-Flavoskyrin and Its Chemical Conversion into (−)-Rugulosin

(−)-Flavoskyrin is a nonquinonic yellow pigment which was first isolated by Howard and Raistrick (1954a,b) from cultures of *P. islandicum*. (−)-Flavoskyrin afforded chrysophanol (5) and water in quantitative yield on pyrolysis and emodin (3) on air oxidation in the presence of magnesium acetate; these findings are contrary to the reactions of (−)-luteoskyrin (14) and (+)-rugulosin (15) (Shibata *et al.*, 1960). However, a synthetic model compound, 29, prepared from chrysazine (26) via tetrahydroanthraquinone (27) and dihydroanthraquinone (28) according to the procedure of Zahn and Koch (1938), showed a UV spectrum almost superimposable on that of (−)-flavoskyrin. (−)-Flavoskyrin should, therefore, contain the same chromophore as model compound 29 (Shibata *et al.*, 1956a,1960). Furthermore, a characteristic infrared (IR) absorption of (−)-flavoskyrin at 1715 cm^{-1} was also observed in 29. The molecular formula given on the basis of elemental analysis, $C_{15}H_{12}O_5$, corresponded to dihydroemodin. On the basis of these observations, (−)-flavoskyrin was once formulated as (30) (Shibata *et al.*, 1956a, 1960).

In the course of renewed investigations of the anthraquinonoid mycotoxins, the conversion of (−)-rubroskyrin (16) into (−)-luteoskyrin (14) has been clarified as to involve a Michael-type condensation reaction between two monomeric moieties and not enolization of the keto tautomer. Because synthesis of model compound 29 involved the enolization of keto tautomer 28, it became necessary to reinvestigate the isomerization reaction as well as the structure of (−)-flavoskyrin (30); the structure of (−)-flavoskyrin was based on the model compound 29.

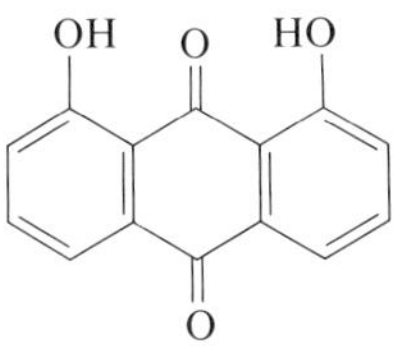

26 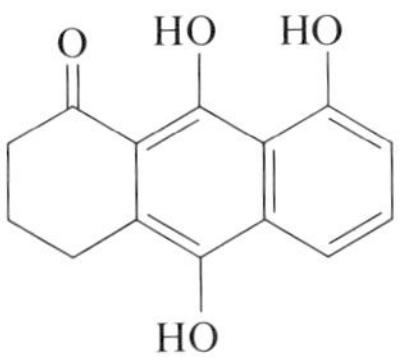   27 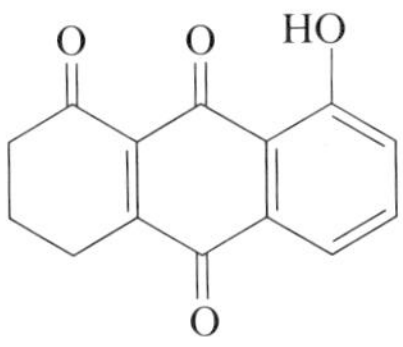   28 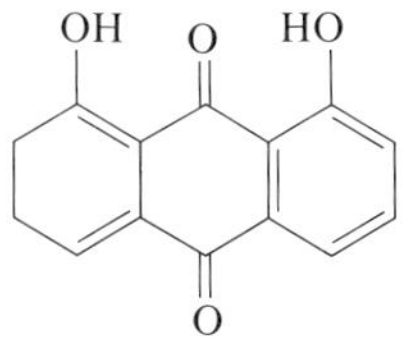   29

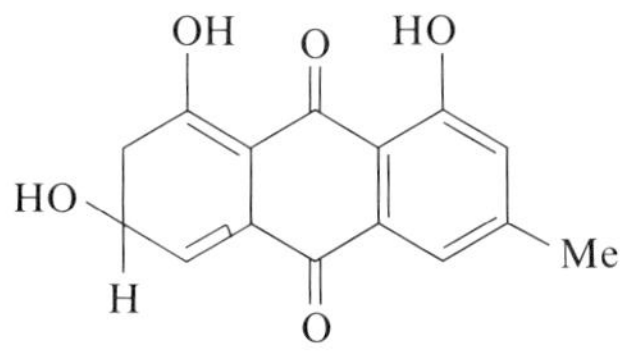

30

(−)-Flavoskyrin gave optically active (+)-dianhydrorugulosin (6) on mild dehydration, such as treatment with thionyl chloride–pyridine and auroskyrin (31) on chromic acid oxidation. Furthermore, it was inadvertently found that (−)-flavoskyrin was converted into (−)-rugulosin (23) on treatment with pyridine. Therefore, it is clear that (−)-flavoskyrin should be reformulated as a dimeric compound with the molecular formula $C_{30}H_{24}O_{10}$. The ^1H NMR spectrum of (−)-flavoskyrin showed signals arising from an unsymmetrical dimer, and revealed the presence of two aromatic methyl groups from aromatic protons, two secondary hydroxy groups, and four phenolic and enolic hydroxy groups (Scheme 6).

A new model compound was prepared from chrysophanol (5) as starting material for the comparison of spectral data. The IR and ^1H NMR spectra of the model compound and of (−)-flavoskyrin were very similar to each other. It was therefore concluded that the model compounds previously formulated as the enolic tautomers of monomeric dihydroanthraquinones are in fact unsymmetrical dimers. The model compound prepared from chrysophanol (5) as starting material is in fact identical to dideoxyflavoskyrin (34). Mass-spectral investigation of the model compound supported its dimeric nature, and simultaneously brought new evidence on the chemical properties of the partially hydrogenated anthraquinones. Tetrahydrochrysophanol (32) obtained by the catalytic reduction of chrysophanol (5) gives the molecular ion, M^+ (the highest mass ion), whereas dihydrochrysophanol (33), obtained by further oxidation with lead tetraacetate (Scheme 7), gives the peaks corresponding to (M^+ +2), M^+, and (M^+ −2). The appearance of such a strong (M^+ +2) peak was reported in some benzoquinones (Heiss et al., 1969). The synthetic model compounds also showed (M^+ +2), M^+, and (M^+ −2) peaks corresponding to the dimeric structure, indicating

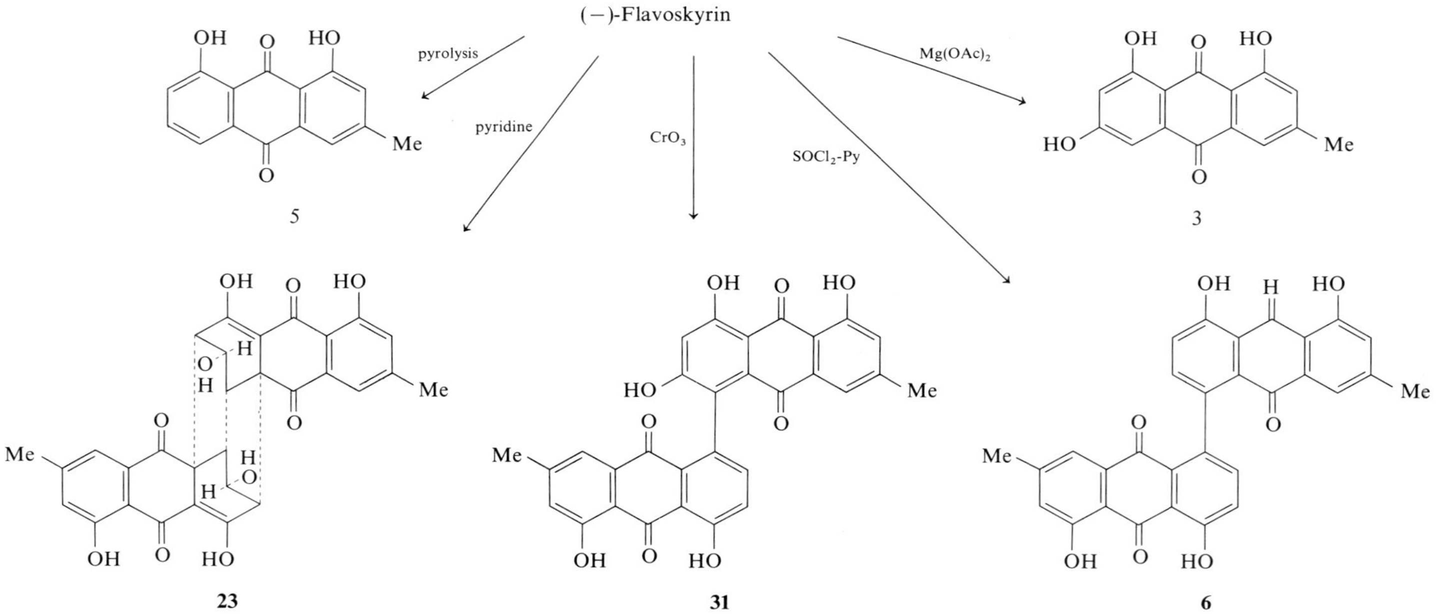

Scheme 6. Chemical reactions of (−)-flavoskyrin.

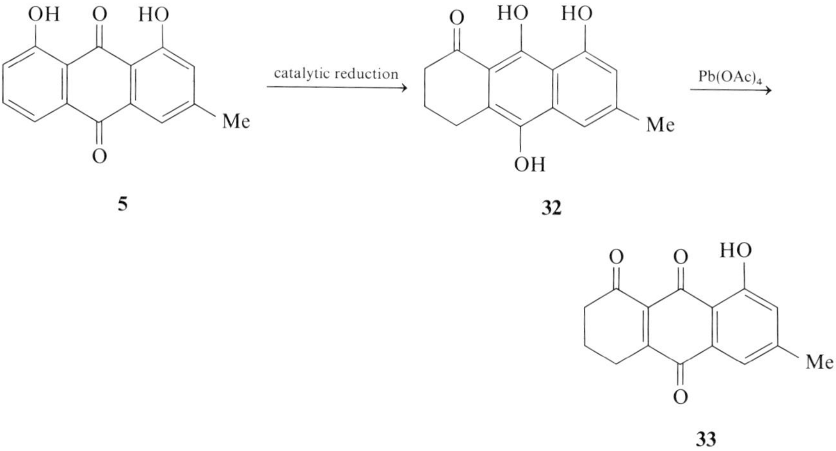

Scheme 7.   Synthesis of dihydrochrysophanol (**33**).

that the last step of the synthesis is in fact not the enolization of the keto tautomer but a dimerization reaction (Seo *et al.*, 1973) (Scheme 8).

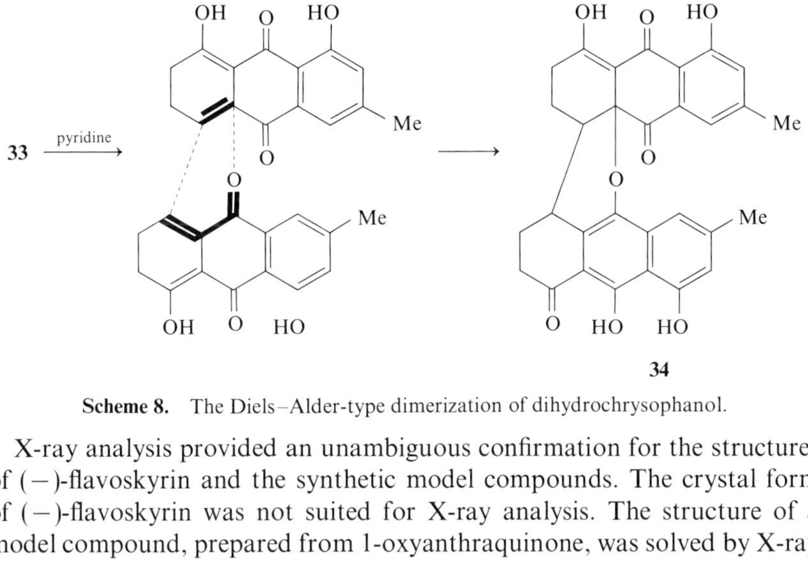

Scheme 8.   The Diels–Alder-type dimerization of dihydrochrysophanol.

X-ray analysis provided an unambiguous confirmation for the structures of (−)-flavoskyrin and the synthetic model compounds. The crystal form of (−)-flavoskyrin was not suited for X-ray analysis. The structure of a model compound, prepared from 1-oxyanthraquinone, was solved by X-ray crystallography using the direct method (Fig. 6). The structure (**35**) given by the X-ray analysis consists of two monomeric moieties bonded by C–C and C–O linkages, and the dimerization reaction is suggested to be a Diels–Alder-type cycloaddition reaction between two monomeric molecules represented by the structure formerly given to the model compound (Zahn and Koch, 1938) (Scheme 9).

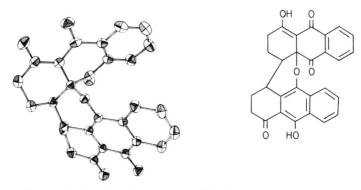

Fig. 6. Perspective drawing of the structure of the dimerization product prepared from 1-oxyanthraquinone.

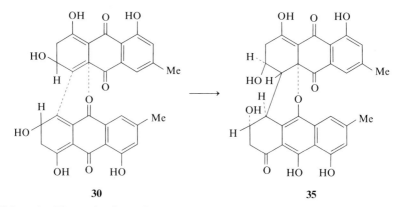

30   35

Scheme 9. Biogenesis of (−)-flavoskyrin (**35**) from enolic form of dihydroemodin (**30**).

The reaction mechanism of the dimerization is supported by mass spectroscopy. The dimeric compounds showed strong peaks corresponding to $[(M^+/2)+2]$, $(M^+/2)$, and $[(M^+/2)-2]$, which are identical to the peaks observed in the mass spectra of the corresponding dihydroanthraquinones. The series of peaks should arise from the dihydroanthraquinones formed by the retro-Diels–Alder reaction of monomeric compounds (Seo *et al.*, 1973).

Biogenetic considerations are at this stage again valuable in the formulation of the structure of (−)-flavoskyrin. If the enol form of dihydroemodin (**30**) [former structure of (−)-flavoskyrin] is assumed as the substrate of the dimerization in the biosynthesis, then a Diels–Alder-type cycloaddition reaction between two molecules of (**30**) should lead to the structure (**35**) of (−)-flavoskyrin.

D. Possible Role of (−)-Flavoskyrin in the Biosynthesis of Anthraquinonoid Mycotoxins

The characteristic chemical reactions of (−)-flavoskyrin (35) which yield various anthraquinonoids are summarized in Scheme 6. Its conversion into (−)-rugulosin (23) and the facile dimerization to analogues of flavoskyrin strongly suggested that flavoskyrin was derived from a Diels–Alder-type dimerization of dihydroemodin (30) and that it acts as a key intermediate in the biosynthesis of some anthraquinonoids (Seo *et al.*, 1973).

Several problems were anticipated in the feeding experiments to establish the biosynthetic conversion of (−)-flavoskyrin (35) into (−)-rugulosin (23) (Table VII). (−)-Flavoskyrin (35) is a rather unstable compound which easily decomposes into chrysophanol (5) by a retro-Diels–Alder reaction followed by dehydration. In an incubation experiment it was found that (−)-flavoskyrin (35) changed completely in distilled water at 28°C into chrysophanol (5). The low permeability of (−)-flavoskyrin (35) and the difficulty in distinguishing between biological conversion from a nonbiological conversion during feeding experiments could cause other problems. Because the preparation of (−)-[^{14}C]flavoskyrin (35) by biosynthetic approaches is difficult, (−)-[^{3}H]flavoskyrin (35) was prepared by the Wilzbach method and used in the feeding experiments.

The incorporation of (−)-[^{3}H]flavoskyrin (35) into (−)-rugulosin (23) in *M. verrucaria* was 5.2%; the labeling in (−)-rugulosin (23) was confirmed by dilution experiments. In an incubation experiment of labeled 35 with sterilized mycelium, no significant incorporation was observed in (−)-rugulosin (23). Experimental proof was obtained for the biosynthetic conversion of (−)-flavoskyrin (35) into (−)-rugulosin (23). The results do not necessarily imply that (−)-flavoskyrin (35), as absorbed by the fungus, was directly converted into (−)-rugulosin (23), because 35 undergoes a retro-Diels–Alder reaction (see above), and the compound which is absorbed by the fungus and therefore enters the biosynthetic pathway might be dihydroemodin.

In *P. brunneum* the incorporation of (−)-[^{3}H]flavoskyrin (35) into rugulosin (15) was 0.34%, and the specific incorporation was 0.008%.

TABLE VII

Incorporation of (−)[^{3}H] Flavoskyrin (35) into Anthraquinonoids

Fungi	Incorporation, (%) (specific incorporation, %)	
Penicillium islandicum	Chrysphanol (5) 2.11 (26.4)	(−)-Rubroskyrin (16) 1.01 (4.47)
Penicillium brunneum	Skyrin (2) 1.35 (0.47)	(+)-Rugulosin (15) 0.34 (0.008)
Myrothecium verrucaria	(−)-Rugulosin (23) 5.24 (0.49)	

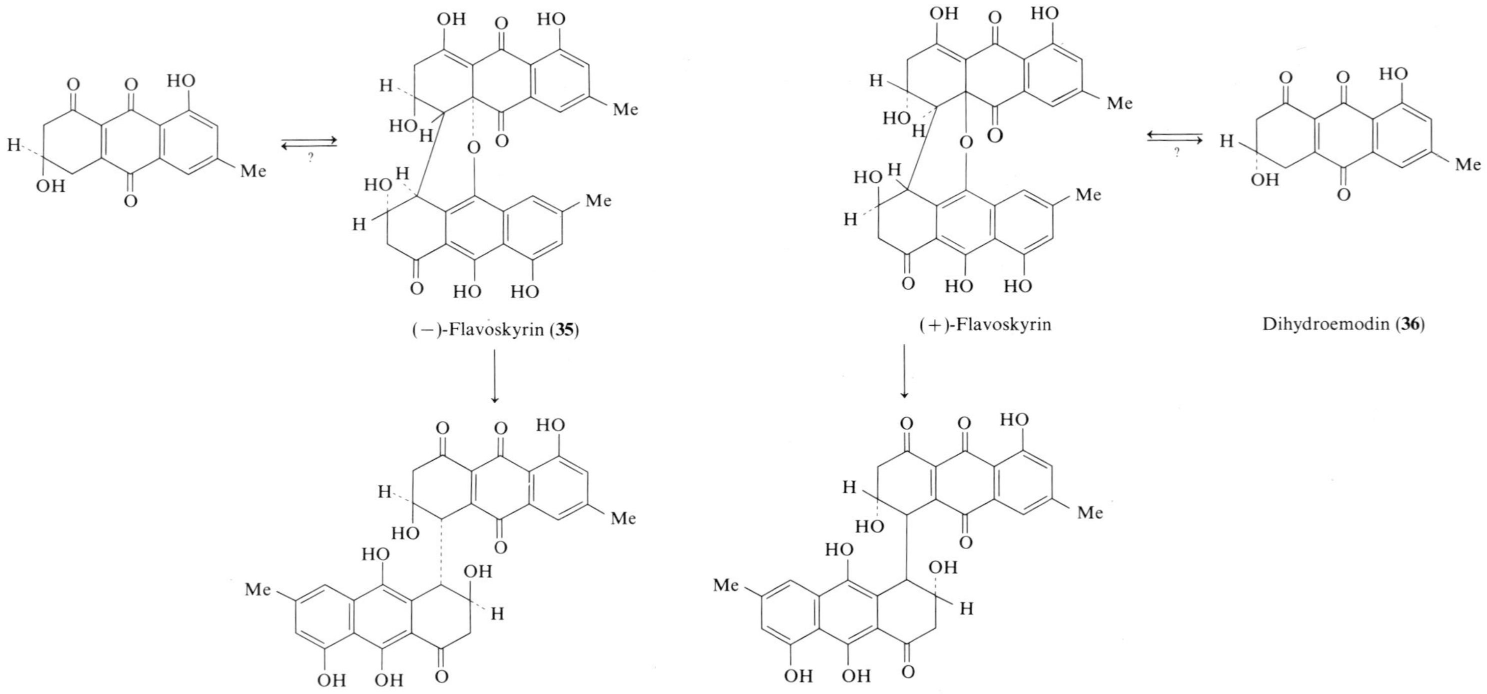

Dihydroemodin (36)

(+)-Flavoskyrin

37b

(−)-Flavoskyrin (35)

37a

386

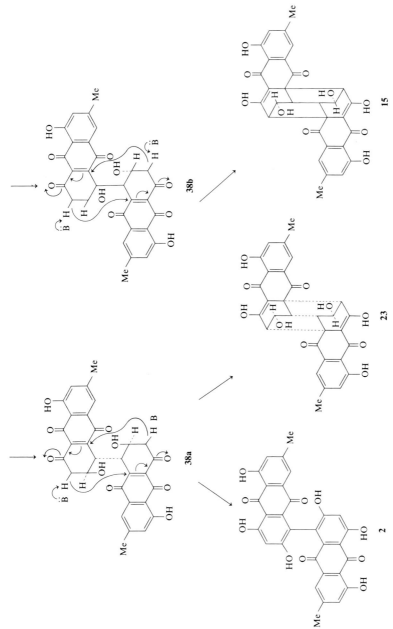

Scheme 10. Biosynthesis of anthraquinonoids in *Penicillium brunneum* and *Myrothecium verrucaria*.

387

(−)-Flavoskyrin (**35**) cannot act as a precursor of (+)-rugulosin (**15**), for its absolute configuration is opposite to that required for the specific precursor. The results of the feeding experiments in *P. brunneum* supported this view. The incorporation ratio of (−)-[³H]flavoskyrin (**35**) into skyrin (**2**) seemed to be significant. Skyrin (**2**) as isolated from the fungi showed optical activity. A comparative optical rotatory dispersion (ORD) study revealed that all the dimeric bisanthraquinones showed positive optical rotations and strong positive Cotton effects (Ogihara *et al.*, 1968). On the other hand, dianhydrorugulosin (**6**) derived from (+)-rugulosin (**15**) showed a negative Cotton effect in the ORD, whereas (−)-flavoskyrin (**35**) displayed a positive Cotton effect. The absolute configuration around the C–C bond [C(1) and C(1')] in the aromatic bisanthraquinones is the same as that of (−)-flavoskyrin (**35**) and (−)-rugulosin and opposite to that of (+)-rugulosin (**15**). (−)-Flavoskyrin (**35**), therefore, possesses the required absolute configuration concerning the C–C bond for an intermediate leading to skyrin (**2**). If the dimerization reaction in the biosynthesis of skyrin (**2**) is different from the Diels–Alder type, for instance, phenol oxidative coupling, then two completely different reactions would occur in the same organism. However, if all the dimeric anthraquinonoids are formed via the Diels–Alder dimerization step, then both the enantiomeric forms of flavoskyrin should be formed in *P. brunneum*. The last route, as illustrated in Scheme 10, seems more probable.

The C–O bond cleavage of flavoskyrin gives the dimeric intermediate (**37a** and **37b**) consisting of tetrahydro- and dihydroemodins. Successive oxidation of the tetrahydro moiety affords the key intermediate (**38a** and **38b**) which had been assumed in the structural study of modified bisanthraquinonoids (Section II,B). Both (+)- and (−)-rugulosin (**14** and **23**) would then be formed by the double Michael condensation between two monomeric moieties. The formation of skyrin (**2**) is explained in terms of the oxidation of secondary alcoholic groups of intermediate **38a**.

(−)-[³H]Flavoskyrin (**35**) showed, according to Ebizuka *et al.* (1977, unpublished work), considerable incorporation into (−)-rubroskyrin (**16**) in *P. brunneum*. As discussed above, dihydroemodin (**36**) may be the true precursor that enters the biosynthetic pathway during the biosynthesis of (−)-rugulosin (**23**) from (−)-flavoskyrin (**35**). Although the exact role of (−)-flavoskyrin (**35**) in the biosynthesis of (−)-luteoskyrin (**14**) and (−)-rubroskyrin (**16**) has not been fully clarified, possible biosynthetic pathways are shown in Scheme 11. There are two possible pathways leading to the key intermediate, **39**, which is the substrate of the Michael reaction yielding (−)-rubroskyrin (**16**) and (−)-luteoskyrin (**14**). One route involves the oxidation of (−)-flavoskyrin (**35**); the other route is by dimerization of the quinone B (**40**), which was isolated by Bu'Lock and Smith (1968) (Scheme II).

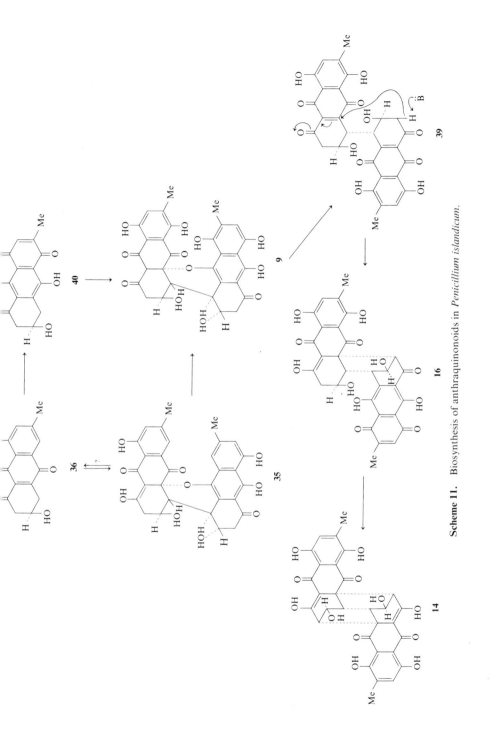

Scheme 11. Biosynthesis of anthraquinonoids in *Penicillium islandicum*.

The Diels–Alder-type dimerization is the characteristic reaction involved in the biosynthesis of anthraquinonoid mycotoxins. The biological Diels–Alder reaction is not limited to the biosynthesis of anthraquinonoids only, but there are in fact a few other examples. Flavonolignans are a new class of compounds isolated from a higher plant, *Sylibum marianum*. These compounds also possess structures which consist of flavonoid and phenylpropanoid units. The Diels–Alder reaction between taxifolinquinone (**41**) and coniferyl alcohol (**42**) has been suggested for possible biosynthesis by Abraham *et al.* (1970). A Diels–Alder reaction involving the dione of taxifolinquinone (**41**) would give silymarin (**43**), whereas the involvement of the dione would afford silidianin (**44**) (Scheme 12). The proposed name "flavonolignans" has been based on this biogenesis.

Thamnosin (**45**) is a dimeric coumarin which was isolated by Kutney *et al.* (1972) from a Rutaceous plant, *Thamnosa montata*, along with the corresponding monomer, thamnosmin (**46**). The biosynthesis of **45** is explained

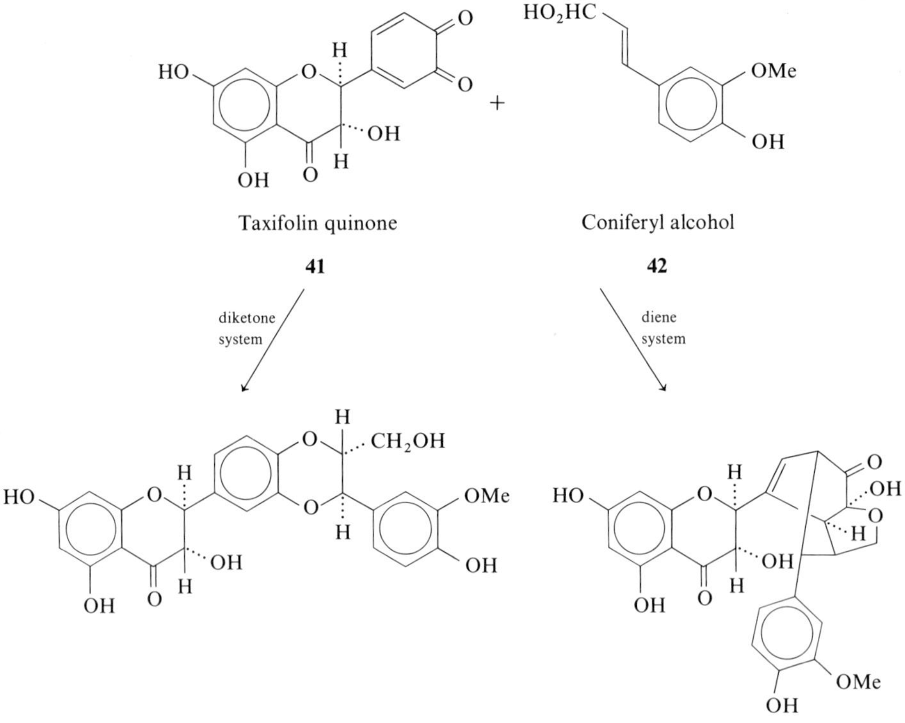

Taxifolin quinone

41

Coniferyl alcohol

42

Silymarin

43

Silydianin

44

Scheme 12. Biosynthesis of flavonolignans.

in terms of a Diels–Alder reaction between two molecules of thamnosmin (**46**) (Scheme 13).

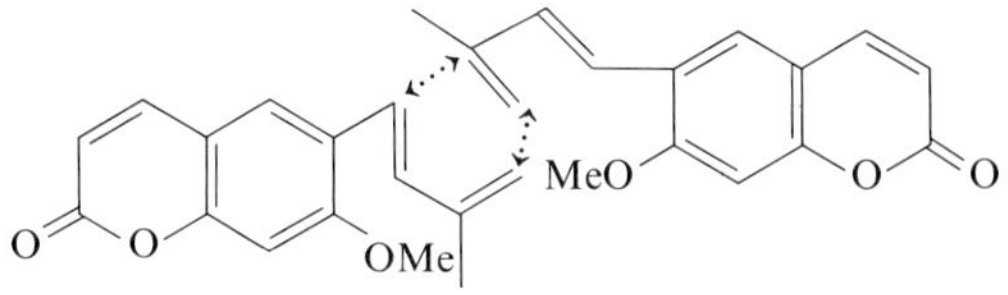

Thamnosmin

46

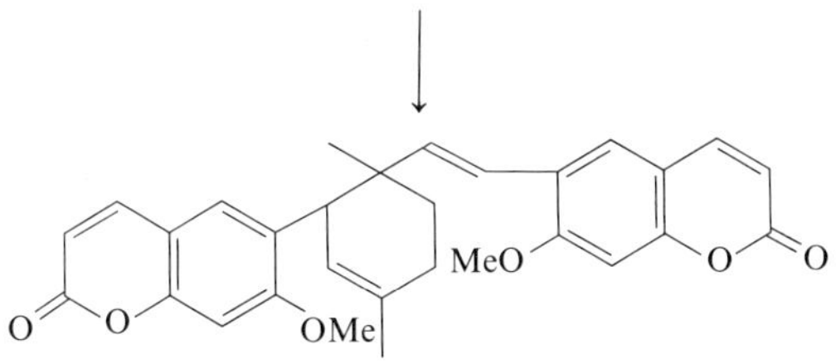

Thamnosin

45

Scheme 13. Biosynthesis of thamnosin.

V. BIOMIMETIC SYNTHESIS OF ANTHRAQUINONOIDS

Because the biomimetic synthesis of bisdeoxyflavoskyrin (**34**) had been achieved in the course of a chemical study on (−)-flavoskyrin (**35**) and its synthetic model compounds, only its conversion into bisdeoxyrugulosin (**47**) was necessary to complete the biogenetic-type synthesis of a rugulosin analogue. (−)-Flavoskyrin (**35**) can be converted into (−)-rugulosin (**23**) on treatment with pyridine. This unique reaction was recognized when a solution of (−)-flavoskyrin (**35**) in [^{2}H$_5$]pyridine exhibited three methine signals in the NMR region characteristic of rugulosin and (−)-luteoskyrin. Subsequent investigations revealed that (−)-flavoskyrin (**35**) yielded (−)-rugulosin (**23**) and dianhydrorugulosin (**6**) on base treatment (Seo *et al.*, 1973).

Bisdeoxyflavoskyrin (**34**), obtained by the Diels–Alder-type dimerization reaction of dihydrochrysophanol (**46**), was subjected to base treatment by keeping it in pyridine for three weeks with occasional warming. The solution turned yellow and showed a pale yellow fluorescence. Bisdeoxyrugulosin (**47**) was obtained in low yield (less than 10%). This conversion involves C–O bond cleavage followed by oxidation of the hydroquinone moiety and then Michael-type condensation between two monomeric moieties. The partially hydrogenated bisanthraquinone **48** is the direct substrate of the

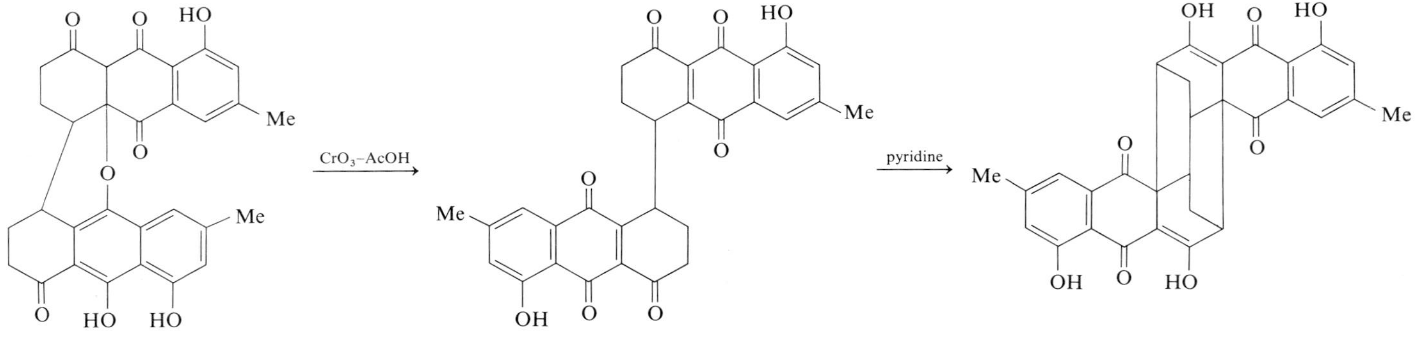

Scheme 14. Biomimetic synthesis of bisdeoxyrugulosin (**47**).

double Michael reaction, and its synthesis was the next subject of study. Oxidation of bisdeoxyflavoskyrin (34) with chromic oxide in acetic acid yielded 48. On treatment with pyridine, 48 afforded bisdeoxyrugulosin (47) along with dianhydrorugulosin (6).

The Diels–Alder-type dimerization of dihydroanthraquinone, successive oxidation, and Michael-type condensation exactly reproduced the reactions involved in the biosynthesis. The biomimetic synthesis of bisdeoxyrugulosin (47) has been accomplished by Yang et al. (1976) (Scheme 14).

REFERENCES

Abraham, D. J., Takagi, S., Rosenstein, R. D., Shiono, R., Wagner, H., Hörhammer, L., Seligmann, O., and Farnsworth, N. (1970). Tetrahedron Lett., p. 2675.
Birch, A. J., and Donovan, E. W. (1953). Aust. J. Chem. 6, 360.
Birch, A. J., Massy-Westropp, R. A., and Meye, C. J. (1955). Aust. J. Chem. 8, 539.
Breen. J., Dacre, J. C., Raistrick, H., and Smith, G. (1955). Biochem. J. 60, 618.
Bu'Lock, J. D., and Smith, J. R. (1968). J. Chem. Soc. C, p. 1941.
Gatenbeck, S. (1958). Acta Chem. Scand. 12, 1211.
Gatenbeck, S. (1960a). Acta Chem. Scand. 14, 102.
Gatenbeck, S. (1960b). Acta Chem. Scand. 14, 296.
Gatenbeck, S., and Barbesgard, P. (1960). Acta Chem. Scand. 14, 230.
Gatenbeck, S., and Mosbach, K. (1959). Acta Chem. Scand. 13, 1561
Gröger, D., Erge, D., Frank, B., Ohnsorg, U., Flasch, H., and Hüper, T. (1968). Chem. Ber. 101, 1970
Hayashi, K, Kikuchi, M., and Okamoto, Y. (1959). Shokubutsugaku Zasshi 72, 220.
Heiss, J., Zeller, K. P., and Rieder, A. (1969). In "Organic Mass Spectroscopy," Vol. II, pp. 1325–1334. Heyden, North Ireland.
Howard, G. H., and Raistrick, H. (1949). Biochem. J. 44, 227.
Howard, B. H., and Raistrick, H. (1954a). Biochem. J. 56, 56.
Howard, B. H., and Raistrick, H. (1954b). Biochem. J. 56, 216.
Howard, B. H., and Raistrick, H. (1954c). Biochem. J. 57, 212.
Kikuchi, M., and Nakahara, M. (1961). Shokubutsugaku Zasshi 74, 42
Kitagawa, I., and Shibata, S. (1960a), Chem. Ind. 1054.
Kitagawa, I., and Shibata, S. (1960b). Chem. Pharm. Bull. 8, 884.
Kobayashi, N., Iitaka, Y., Sankawa, U., Ogihara, Y., and Shibata, S. (1968). Tetrahedron Lett., p. 6135.
Kobayashi, N. Iitaka, Y., and Shibata, S. (1970). Acta. Cryst. B26 188.
Kutney, J. P., Verma, A. K., and Young, R. N. (1972). Tetrahedron 28, 5091.
Marumo, S. (1955). Bull. Agric. Chem. Soc. (Japan) 19, 258.
Marumo, S. (1959). Bull. Agric. Chem. Soc. (Japan) 23, 428.
Nakahara, M., and Kikuchi, M. (1961). Shokubutsugaku Zasshi 74, 463.
Ogihara, Y., Kobayashi, N., and Shibata, S. (1968). Tetrahedron Lett., p. 1881.
Sakabe, N., Goto, T., and Hirata, Y. (1964). Tetrahedron Lett., p. 1825.
Sankawa, U., Seo, S, Kobayashi, N., Ogihara, Y., and Shibata, S. (1968). Tetrahedron Lett., p. 5557.
Sankawa, U., Ebizuka, Y., and Shibata, S. (1973). Tetrahedron Lett., p. 2125.
Sankawa, U., Shimada, H., and Yamasaki, K. (1978). Tetrahedron Lett., p. 3375.

Sato, N, Ueno, Y., and Ueno, I. (1977). *J. Toxic Sci.* **2**, 261.

Seo, S., Sankawa, U., Ogihara, Y., Iitaka, Y., and Shibata, S. (1973). *Tetrahedron* **29**, 3721.

Shibata, S., and Ikekawa, T. (1962). *Chem. Ind.*, p. 360.

Shibata, S., and Ikekawa, T., (1963). *Chem. Pharm. Bull.* **11**, 368.

Shibata, S., and Kitagawa, I. (1956). *Chem. Pharm. Bull.* **4**, 309.

Shibata, S., and Tanaka, O, Chihara, T., and Mitsuhashi, H. (1953). *Pharm. Bull.* **1**, 302.

Shibata, S., Tanaka, O., Murakami, T., Chihara, G., and Sumimoto, M. (1955a). *Pharm. Bull.* **3**, 274.

Shibata, S., Takido, M., and Nkajima, T. (1955b). *Pharm. Bull.* **3**, 286.

Shibata, S., Ikekawa, T., and Takido, M. (1956a). *Pharm. Bull.* **4**, 303.

Shibata, S., Murakami, T., Kitagawa, I., and Kishi, T. (1956b). *Pharm Bull.* **4**, 111.

Shibata, S., Ikekawa, T and Kishi, T. (1960). *Chem. Pharm. Bull.* **8**, 889.

Shibata, S., Ogihara, Y., Kobayashi, N., Seo, S., and Kitagawa, I. (1968). *Tetrahedron Lett.*, p. 3179.

Shoji, J., and Shibata, S. (1964). *Chem. Ind.*, p. 19

Shoji, J., Shibata, S., Sankawa, U., Taguchi, H., and Shibanuma, Y. (1965) *Chem. Pharm. Bull.* **4**, 309.

Sopp, O. J. O. (1912). *Skr. Nor. Vidensk. Selk, Christ.* **161**.

Takahashi, S., Takido, M., Sankawa, U., and Shibata, S. (1976). *Phytochemistry* **15**, 1295.

Takeda, N., Seo, S., Ogihara, Y., Sankawa, U., Iitaka, Y., Kitagawa, I., and Shibata, S. (1973). *Tetrahedron* **29**, 3703.

Tanaka, O., and Kaneko, C. (1955). *Pharm. Bull.* **3**, 284.

Tshunoda, H. (1951). *Jpn J. Nutr.* **8**, 186.

Tshunoda, H. (1952). *Jpn J. Nutr.* **9**, 1.

Ueno, I. (1966). *Seikagaku* **38**, 741.

Ueno, I., Ueno, Y., Tatsuno, T., and Uraguchi, K. (1964a). *Jpn. J. Exp. Med.* **34**, 135.

Ueno, Y., Ueno, I., Tatsuno, T., and Uraguchi, K. (1964b). *Jpn. J. Exp. Med.* **34**, 197.

Ueno, Y., Ueno, I., Ito, K., and Tatsuno, T. (1966) *Seikagaku* **38**, 687.

Ueno, Y., Ueno, I. and Mizunoto, K. (1965). *Jpn. J. Exp. Med.* **38**, 47.

Ueno, Y., Platel, A and Fromgeot, P. (1967a). *Biochem. Biophys. Acta* **134**, 27.

Ueno, Y., Ueno, I., Ito, K and Tatsuno, T. (1967b). *Experientia* **23**, 1001.

Ueno, Y., Yeno. I., Mizumoto, K., and Tatsuno, T. (1967c). *J. Biochem.* **63**, 395.

Ueno, Y., Kato, Y., and Enomoto, M. (1975). *Jpn. J. Exp. Med.* **45**, 525.

Uraguchi, K. (1971). *In* "The Encyclopedia of Pharmacological and Therapeutic," Sect. 71 Vol II, p. 143. Pergamon Press, Oxford.

Uraguchi, K., and Saito, M. (1972). *Food Cosmet. Toxicol.* **10**, 193.

Uraguchi, K., Tatsuno, T., Tukioka, M., Sakai, Y., Sakai, F., Kobayashi, Y., Saito, M., Enomoto, M., and Miyake, M. (1961a). *Jpn. J. Exp. Med.* **31**, 1.

Uraguchi, K., Tatsuno, T., Skai, F., Tsukioka, M., Sakai, Y., Ynemitsu, O., Ita, H., Miyake, M., Saito, M., Enomoto, M., Shibata, T., and Ishiko, T., (1961b). *Jpn. J. Exp. Med.* **31**, 19.

Yang, D-M., Sanakwa, U., Ebizuka, Y., and Shibata, S. (1976). *Tetrahedron* **32**, 333.

Yoshioka, H., Nakatsu, K., Sato, M., and Tatsuno, T. (1973). *Chem. Lett.*, p. 1319.

Zahn, K., and Koch, H. (1938). *Chem. Ber.* **71**, 172.

12

The Biosynthesis
of Some Miscellaneous Mycotoxins

ROBERT VLEGGAAR AND PIETER S. STEYN

I. INTRODUCTION

The proliferation in the number of new and diverse fungal metabolites in recent years complicates a comprehensive survey of their biogenetic origin. The biosynthesis of many metabolites appears to be trivial, because a cursory chemical inspection of the structure allows the formulation of a plausible biosynthetic pathway. For many new metabolites, no toxicological data are available and only the structural elucidation together with a biosynthetic postulate is reported. Thus the biosynthetic origin of viridicatumtoxin (**1**), a toxic metabolite from *Penicillium viridicatum* (Kabuto *et al.*, 1976), has not been studied, but is most probably closely modeled on that of the tetracyclines (McGormick, 1967). Similarly, verruculotoxin (**2**), isolated from cultures of *Penicillium verruculosum*, is most probably derived from two L-amino acids, phenylalanine and pipecolic acid (Macmillan *et al.*, 1976).

395

The Biosynthesis of Mycotoxins
Copyright © 1980 by Academic Press, Inc.
All rights of reproduction in any form reserved.
ISBN 0-12-670650-6.

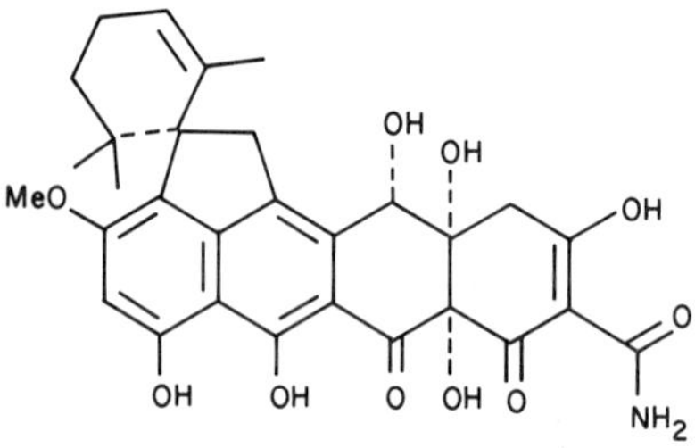

I

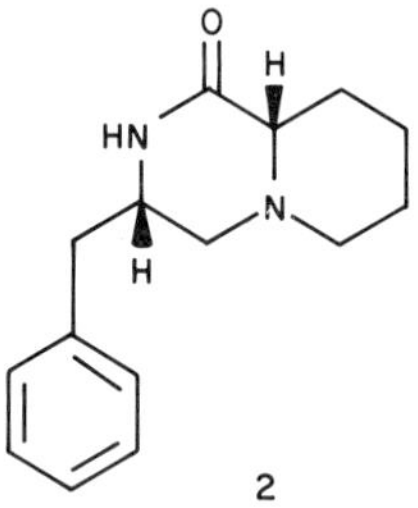

2

The malformins (A_1, A_2, B_1, B_2, and C) are a group of cyclic pentapeptides isolated from *Aspergillus niger*. Anderegg *et al.* (1976) characterized mal-formin C as the disulfide of cyclo-D-cysteinyl-D-cysteinyl-L-valyl-D-leucyl-L-leucyl. Austin (**3**), a mycotoxin from *Aspergillus ustus*, is probably derived from a polyisoprenoid precursor (Chexal *et al.*, 1976). The structure and synthesis of moniliformin (**4**), a toxigenic product of *Fusarium moniliforme*, has been reported (Springer *et al.*, 1974), but the biosynthesis remains an unsolved challenge.

In this final chapter we would like to discuss the biosynthesis of some unrelated fungal metabolites for which toxicological data have been reported.

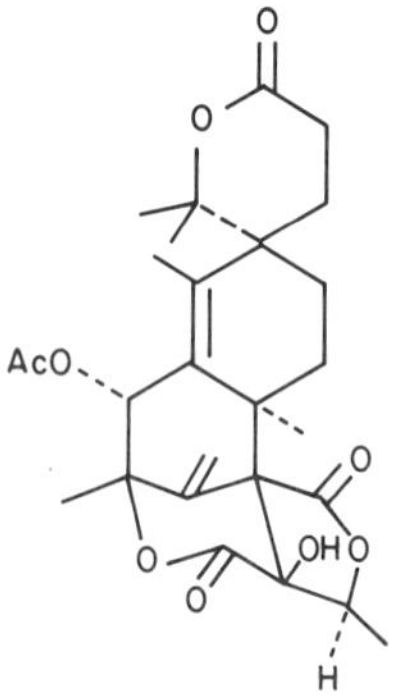

3

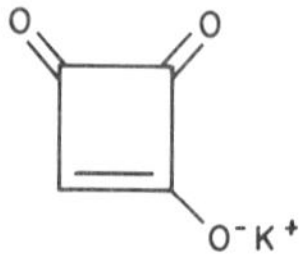

4

II. OCHRATOXIN AND RELATED DIHYDROISOCOUMARINS

A. Ochratoxin A

The discovery of toxigenic strains of the fungus *Aspergillus ochraceus* Wilh. (Scott, 1965) led to the isolation and structure elucidation of ochratoxin A (**5**) and ochratoxin B (**6**) (Van der Merwe *et al.*, 1965a,b); the structures were subsequently proved by synthesis (Steyn and Holzapfel, 1967; Roberts and Woolven, 1970). The ochratoxins are naturally occurring nephrotoxic and hepatotoxic metabolites elaborated by several species within the *Aspergillus* and *Penicillium* genera (Lai *et al.*, 1968; Hesseltine *et al.*, 1972; Van Walbeek *et al.*, 1969; Scott *et al.*, 1972; Ciegler *et al.*, 1972). Their biological activity has been well documented (Steyn, 1971; Chu, 1974; Harwig, 1974).

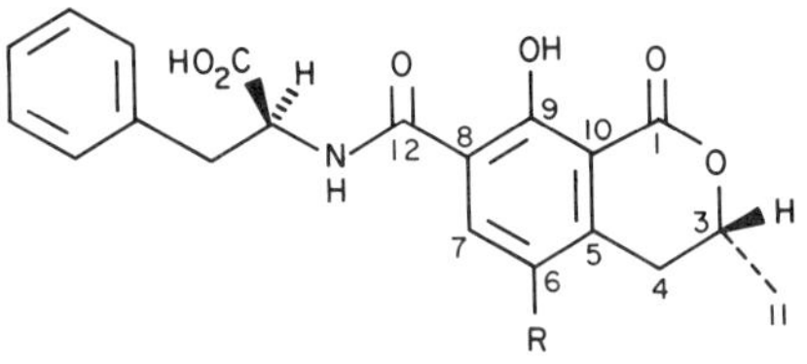

```
5   R = Cl

6   R = H
```

The toxins comprise a 3,4-dihydro-3-methylisocoumarin moiety which is linked to L-β-phenylalanine through a carboxy group at C(8). Cell-free extracts of *A. ochraceus* capable of effecting this amide bond formation were reported by Ferreira and Pitout (1969).

The biosynthesis of ochratoxin A has been studied using both ^{14}C- and ^{13}C-labeled precursors. In preliminary studies, Ferreira and Pitout (1969) showed that DL-$[1-^{14}C]$-β-phenylalanine was incorporated into ochratoxin A by cultures of *A. ochraceus*. Hydrolysis of the labeled ochratoxin A with 6 *N* hydrochloric acid gave the isocoumarin acid **7** and L-β-phenylalanine. The amino acid was found to contain all the activity. These results were confirmed by Steyn *et al.* (1970) and Maebayashi *et al.* (1972) using L-$[U-^{14}C]$-β-phenylalanine, as well as by Searcy *et al.* (1969) using $[1-^{14}C]$-β-phenylalanine.

The biosynthesis of ochratoxin A was, therefore, reduced to a study of the origin of the isocoumarin acid, **7**; this investigation was carried out by Steyn *et al.* (1970). Sodium $[1-^{14}C]$acetate was added to resting cultures of *A. ochraceus*. On acid hydrolysis of the labeled ochratoxin A, the isocoumarin acid **7** was found to contain all the activity. Kuhn–Roth oxidation of compound **7** gave acetic acid which contained 20% of the total activity. Schmidt

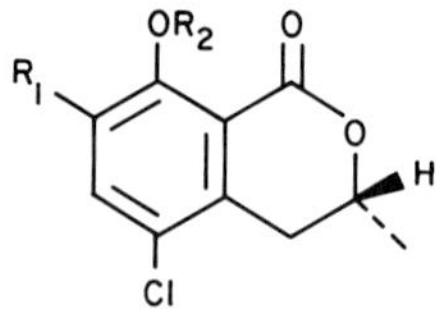

7 R_1 = CO_2H, R_2 = H

8 R_1 = CO_2Me, R_2 = Me

9 R_1 = CO_2H, R_2 = Me

10 R_1 = CON_3, R_2 = Me

11 R_1 = NH_2, R_2 = Me

degradation of the labeled acetic acid showed that all its activity was contained in the carboxy group. Treatment of the $[1\text{-}^{14}C]$acetate-derived isocoumarin acid (7) with diazomethane gave 8 which, on alkaline hydrolysis, yielded the acid 9. Treatment of the corresponding azide (10) with sulfuric acid gave inactive carbon dioxide and the amine 11, which had the same specific activity as the starting material.

Unequivocal evidence for the acetate origin of the isocoumarin moiety in ochratoxin A was obtained by Steyn et al. (1978 unpublished results). The complete assignment of the signals in the natural abundance ^{13}C NMR spectrum of ochratoxin A allowed a study of its biosynthesis using ^{13}C-labeled precursors. The proton noise decoupled (PND) ^{13}C NMR spectrum of $[1\text{-}^{13}C]$acetate-derived ochratoxin A, obtained from cultures of P. viridicatum, showed that only C(1), C(3), C(5), C(7), and C(9) were enriched. The arrangement of intact acetate units in the dihydroisocoumarin moiety as shown in Fig. 1 was proved by Steyn et al. (1978, unpublished results). A culture of Aspergillus sulphureus was supplemented with sodium $[1,2\text{-}^{13}C]$-acetate. The PND ^{13}C NMR spectrum of the derived ochratoxin A showed that the signals arising from the following carbon atoms exhibited directly bonded ($^{13}C,^{13}C$) couplings: C(11)–C(3), C(4)–C(5), C(6)–C(7), C(8)–C(9), and C(10)–C(1).

The origin of the carboxy group at C(8) was established by Steyn et al. (1970) through addition of DL-[methyl-^{14}C]methionine to a resting culture of A. ochraceus. The resulting radioactive ochratoxin A was hydrolyzed and the isocoumarin acid, 7, was converted into the acid azide, 10. Schmidt decarboxylation of 10 yielded active carbon dioxide, whereas the amine (11) contained no activity.

The participation of a C_1 unit in the formation of the carboxy group at C(8) was verified by Maebayashi et al. (1972), who showed that increasing concentrations of ethionine inhibited the formation of ochratoxin A. The

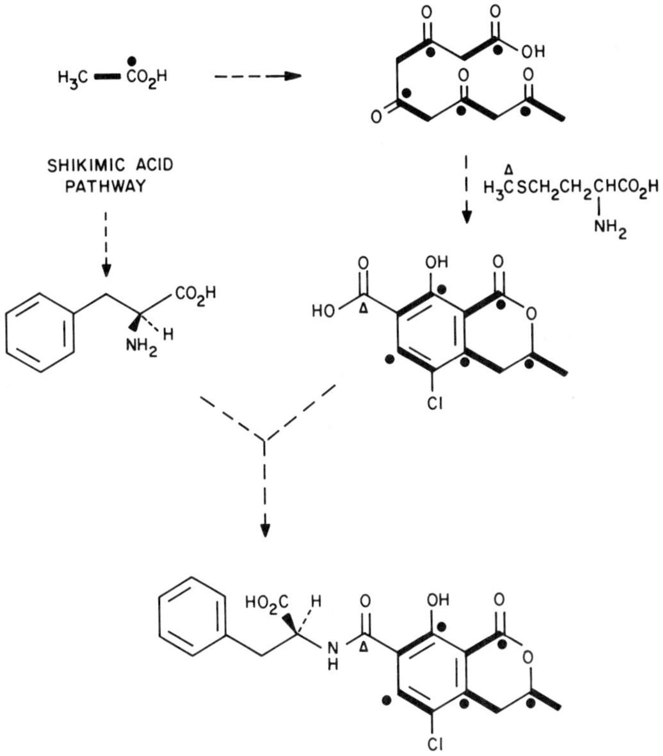

Fig. 1.   Biosynthesis of ochratoxin A (5).

involvement of sodium [^{13}C]formate (65% ^{13}C) was established by feeding this precursor to a culture of *A. ochraceus*. The ^{13}C-enriched ochratoxin was hydrolyzed to the isocoumarin acid 7 which was converted into ester 8 using diazomethane. The PND ^{13}C NMR spectrum of 8 indicated that only the signal at δ165.1 (relative to tetramethylsilane), which had been assigned to C(12), was enhanced.

The results showed that the isocoumarin moiety of ochratoxin A is formed via the acetate–polymalonate pathway from one acetate and four malonate units, whereas the carbonyl carbon atom C(12) is derived from the C_1 pool.

Incubation of *A. ochraceus* in a medium containing sodium [^{36}Cl]chloride resulted in the incorporation (0.75%) of ^{36}Cl into ochratoxin A (Wei *et al.*, 1971). It has not been established at what point in the biosynthesis of ochratoxin A the chlorine atom is introduced.

Biosynthetic data on a number of other dihydroisocoumarins will also be reported, although no toxicity data are available for these compounds.

B. Biosynthesis of Related Dihydroisocoumarins

1. *Dihydroisocoumarin from Periconia macrospinosa*

In a study of the biosynthesis of the cyclopentene derivative (12) by *Periconia macrospinosa*, Holker and Young (1975) showed by using ^{13}C-labeled precursors and ^{13}C NMR spectroscopy that the compound is derived from the structurally related cometabolite 13 by ring contraction involving fission of the C(8)–C(9) bond.

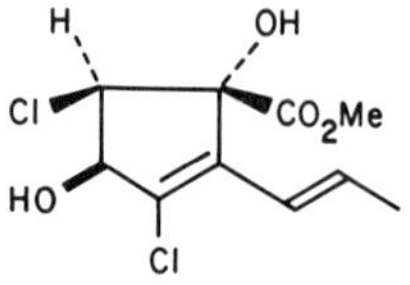

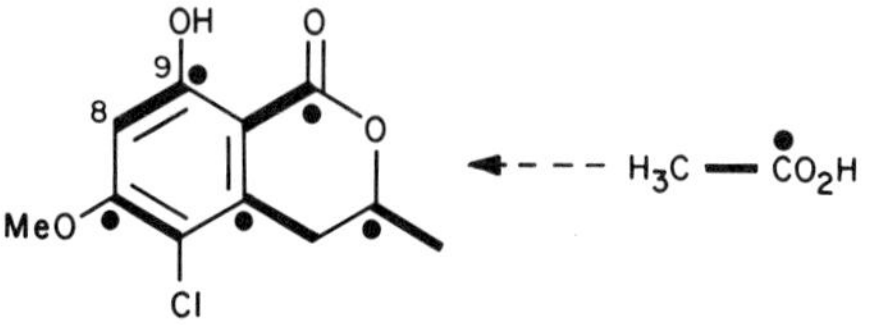

The penta-β-ketide origin of the dihydroisocoumarin (13) was established by the PND ^{13}C NMR spectrum of the [1,2-^{13}C]acetate-enriched 13, which showed five pairs of coupled ^{13}C satellites superimposed on the natural abundance spectrum. The spectra of the [1-^{13}C]- and [2-^{13}C]acetate-derived samples of 13 showed enhancements of individual carbon signals as required by structure 13.

2. Terrein

Hill *et al.* (1975) have proved that terrein (14), a metabolite of *Aspergillus terreus*, is derived from the cometabolite 3,4-dihydro-7,9-dihydroxy-3-methylisocoumarin (15).

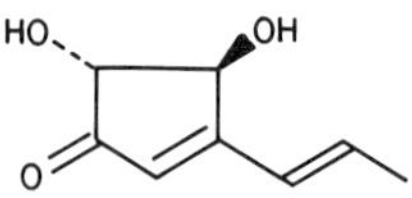

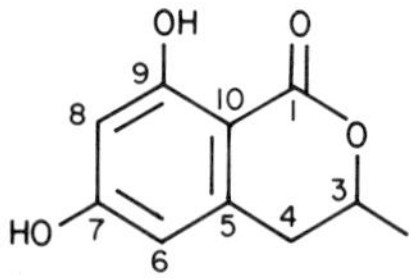

3. *Asperentin*

Cattel *et al.* (1973) showed that incorporation of sodium [1-^{13}C]acetate by an entomogenous strain of *Aspergillus flavus* into the dihydroisocoumarin asperentin 16 gave a labeling pattern consistent with its formation via the acetate–polymalonate pathway from one acetate and seven malonate-derived two-carbon units. The acetate-derived chain-initiating unit was distinguished by the addition of [2-^{14}C]malonate to the cultures of *A. flavus*. The C(6')–C(7') unit was significantly less radioactive than the malonate-derived two-

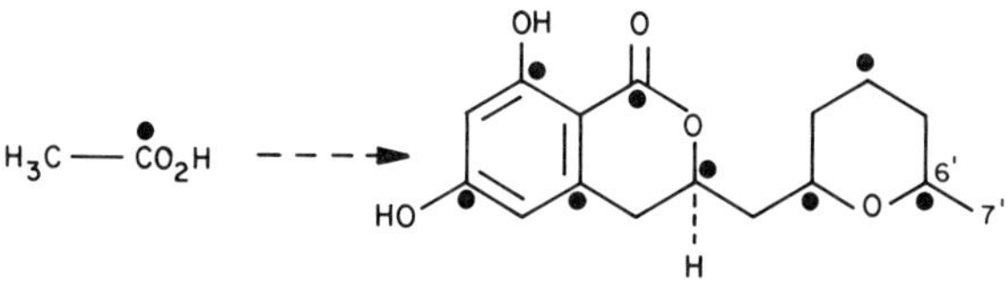

$$H_3C-\overset{\bullet}{C}O_2H \dashrightarrow$$

16

carbon units. This result is to be expected if reconversion of malonate into acetate occurs only to a limited extent.

4. Oospolactone and Oosponol

Nitta *et al.* (1966) studied the biosynthesis of oospolactone (**17**) and oosponol (**18**), two metabolites from *Oospora astringenes*. The results from the addition of $[1-^{14}C]$- and $[6-^{14}C]$glucoses and of $[2-^{14}C]$malonate were comparable, and showed that activity was located at carbon atoms C(11), C(4), C(6), C(8), and C(10) of oospolactone and at C(12), C(4), C(6), C(8), and C(10) of oosponol. The origin of C(12) of oospolactone and C(3) of oosponol from a C_1 pool was confirmed by addition of $[^{14}C]$formate to the medium: in each case, 98% of the activity was located at these carbon atoms, respectively.

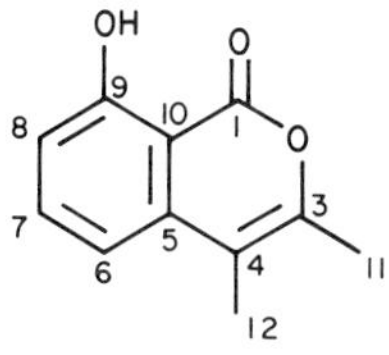

17

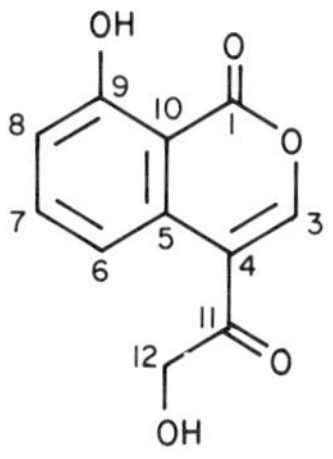

18

The results indicate that these metabolites are derived from five C_2 units, via the acetate–malonate pathway, and one C_1 unit.

5. Xanthomegnin and Related Metabolites

The isolation of the fungal pigments xanthomegnin (**19**), viomellein (**20**), rubrosulphin (**21**), and viopurpurin (**22**) from the mycelium of *Aspergillus sulphureus* and *Aspergillus melleus* was described by Durley *et al.* (1975). Xanthomegnin (**19**) had previously been isolated from *Trichophyton* species and assigned structure **19** (Just *et al.*, 1963). The four metabolites have also been isolated from toxigenic cultures of *P. viridicatum* (Carlton and Tuite, 1977). Carlton *et al.* (1976) reported that xanthomegnin and viomellein produced hepatic lesions in mice.

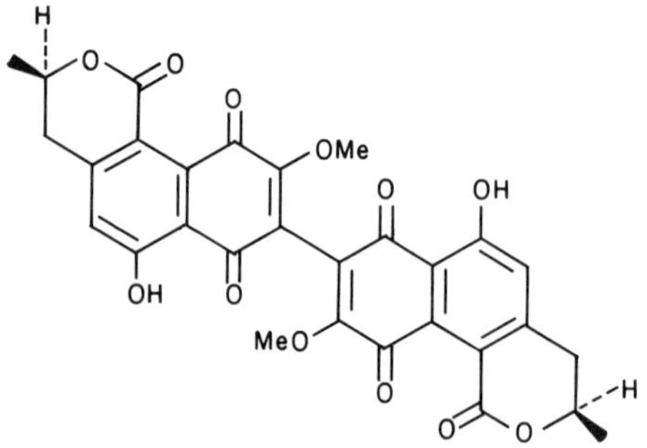

19

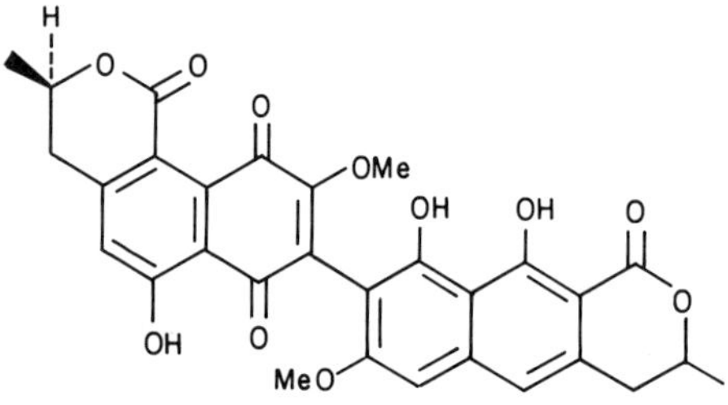

20

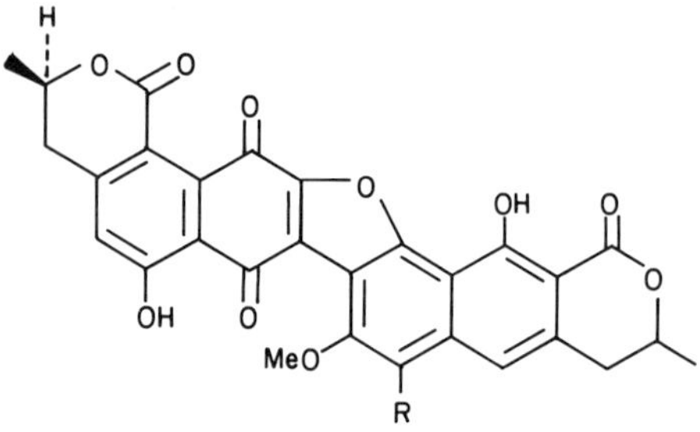

21 R = H
22 R = OH

Simpson (1977) assigned the ^{13}C NMR spectra of these metabolites and proved their origin via the acetate–malonate route by adding [1-^{13}C]- and [1,2-^{13}C]acetates to cultures of *A. melleus*.

The structures **19, 10, 21**, and **22** assigned to the metabolites are based on chemical and spectroscopic evidence. The alternative and more probable linear structures for these metabolites, e.g., **23** for xanthomegnin, were reported in a communication by Höfle and Röser (1978). Their findings are based on a study of the long-range (C,H) coupling constants in the proton-coupled ^{13}C NMR spectrum of xanthomegnin. The biosynthetic conclusions are, however, not affected by the structural change.

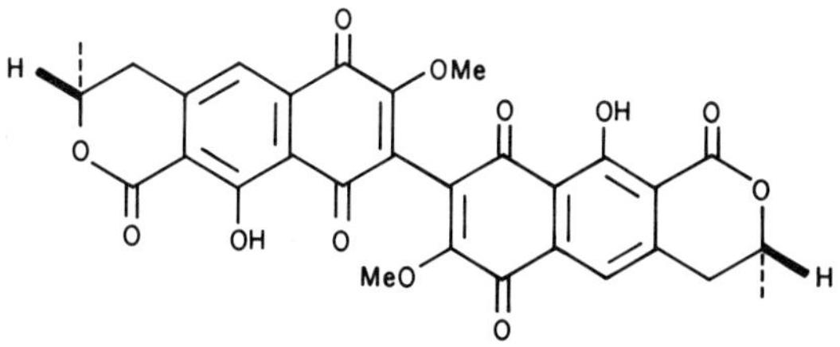

23

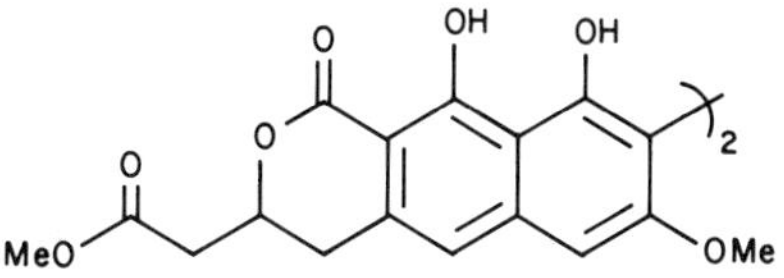

24

A related toxic metabolite, viriditoxin (**24**), was isolated from the mycelia of *Aspergillus viridinutans* (Weisleder and Lillehoj, 1971).

III. CITRININ

Citrinin (**25**), first isolated from *Penicillium citrinum* (Hetherington and Raistrick, 1931), is produced by numerous *Penicillium* and *Aspergillus* species. The compound exhibited marked antibiotic activity *in vitro* (Raistrick and Smith, 1941), but its toxic properties prevented therapeutic application; it has assumed importance as a nephrotoxin (Krogh *et al.*, 1973).

The biosynthetic origin of citrinin was determined initially by Birch *et al.* (1958a). Addition of sodium $[1\text{-}^{14}C]$acetate to cultures of *Aspergillus candidus* gave $[^{14}C]$citrinin. Acid hydrolysis of the labeled citrinin resulted in the formation of three products: (a) inactive carbon dioxide, derived from C(11); (b) formic acid, derived from C(1) and representing 20% of the total radioactivity; and (c) the phenol **26**, carrying 78% of the radioactivity. The C_1 methyl donors formate (Birch *et al.*, 1958a) and methionine (Schwenk

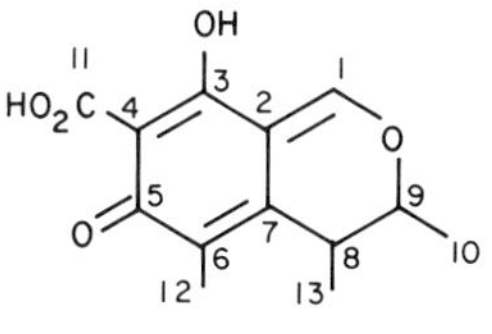

25

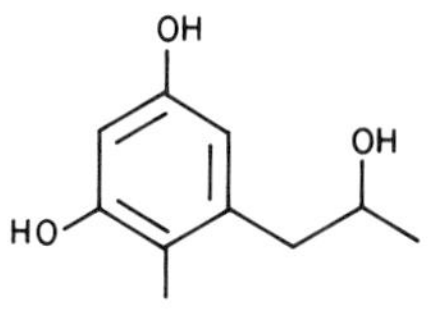

26

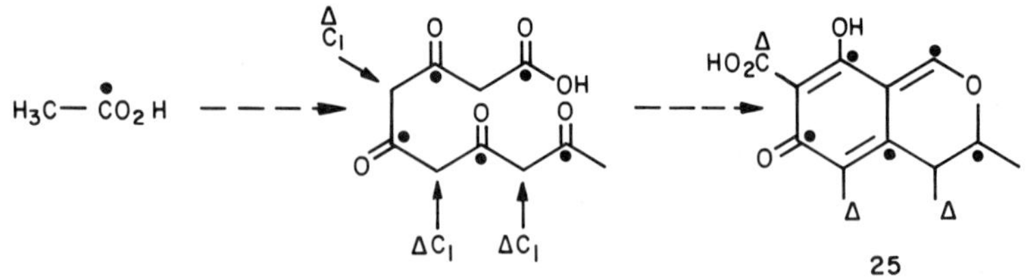

Fig. 2. Biosynthesis of citrinin (**25**).

et al., 1958) were demonstrated to give rise to the extraskeletal groups C(11), C(12), and C(13) in citrinin (see Fig. 2). The inequality in the labeling of C(12), C(13) (determined together as the phenol, **26**), and C(11) in citrinin derived from sodium $[^{14}C]$formate suggested to Birch *et al.* (1958a) a sequential rather than a simultaneous attachment of these groups. However, from their studies with $[methyl-^{14}C]$methionine and cultures of *P. citrinum*, Schwenk *et al.* (1958) reported that C(11), C(12), and C(13) had essentially the same activity. The problem was reexamined by Rodig *et al.* (1966) using $[1-^{14}C]$- and $[6-^{14}C]$glucoses. Their results confirmed the acetate origin of citrinin,

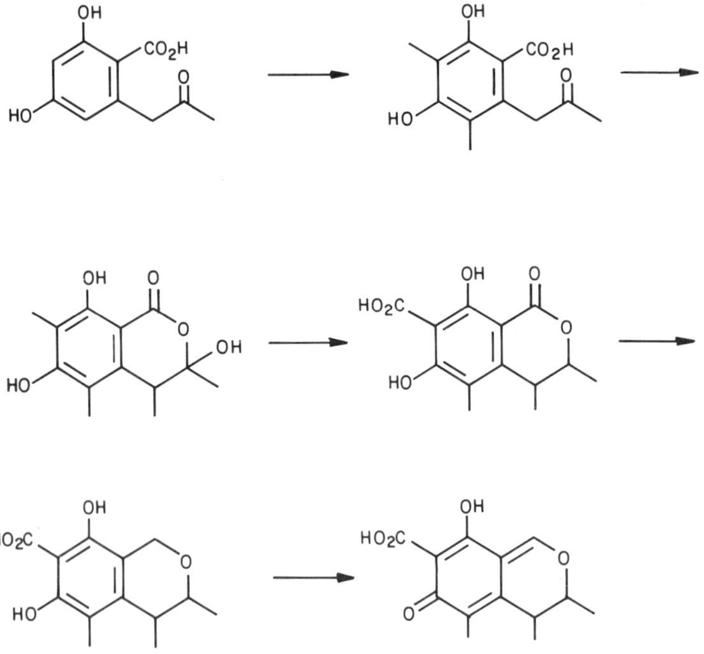

Fig. 3. Postulated intermediates in the biosynthesis of citrinin (**25**).

and the relative activities of the C_1 groups suggest that they are introduced in the order C(11), C(12), C(13); no evidence was obtained for the timing of the oxidation of C(11) or of the cyclizations. In an attempt to answer these questions, Curtis *et al.* (1968) examined the metabolites from mutants of *P. citrinum*. They suggest the biosynthetic sequence as shown in Fig. 3, but in the absence of experiments with labeled precursors this idea must be regarded as speculative.

IV. CITROMYCETIN

On the basis of experiments with sodium [1-^{14}C]acetate as precursor, Birch *et al.* (1958a) proposed that citromycetin (**27**) is derived from seven acetate units. Unfortunately, relatively few degradations are known for citromycetin, so the location of radioactive label was determined by direct measurement only for C(6) and certain carbon atoms located in the pyrone ring. For the remainder of the molecule, only minimal support was obtained for the proposed labeling pattern.

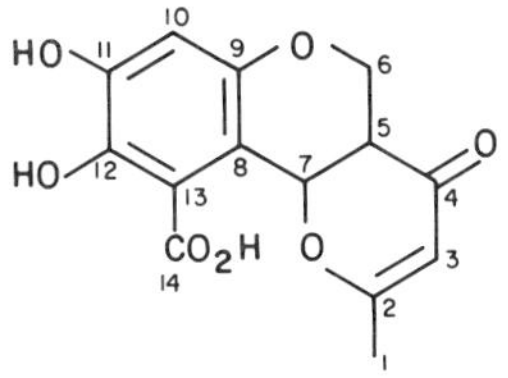

27

In further experiments by Gatenbeck and Mosbach (1963) and Birch *et al.* (1964), it was found that addition of [2-^{14}C]malonate to cultures of *Penicillium frequentans* Westling gave labeled citromycetin with a nonuniform distribution of activity, in which C(11) and C(14) each carried less activity than the average of the remaining labeled carbons. On this basis it was proposed that two initial polyketide chains are involved in the biosynthesis of citromycetin.

In view of the above results, Evans and Staunton (1976) reexamined the pattern of incorporation using ^{13}C-labeled precursors. The assignment of the signals in the natural-abundance PND ^{13}C NMR spectrum of citromycetin was based on calculated values of chemical shifts and was supported by off-resonance techniques, pulse relaxation techniques (Wehrli, 1973), and the observed (^{13}C,^{13}C) couplings in the spectrum of citromycetin derived from sodium [1,2-^{13}C]acetate. The experiments with sodium [1-^{13}C]- and [2-^{13}C]acetates established rigorously the complete pattern of incorporation, as shown in Fig. 4. The experiment with sodium [1,2-^{13}C]acetate

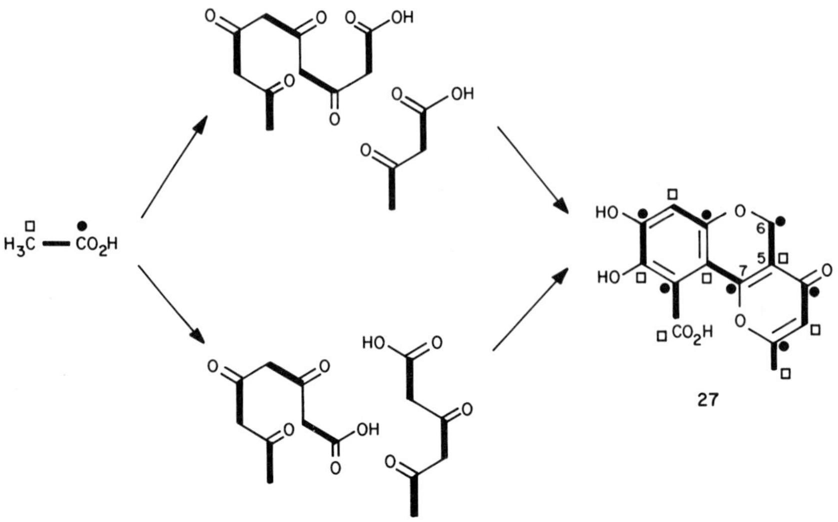

Fig. 4. Biosynthesis of citromycetin (**27**) from [1,2-^{13}C]acetate.

showed that all the C_2 units are intact and that the direction of the polyketide chain at the key branching point at C(5) is as shown in Fig. 4; thus
this carbon forms an intact C_2 unit with C(6) rather than C(7). The above
results point to a biosynthesis of citromycetin from two separate polyketide
chains along one of the two pathways shown in outline in Fig. 4.

V. ZEARALENONE AND RELATED METABOLITES

Zearalenone (**28**), a naturally occurring mycotoxin and a secondary metabolite of *Fusarium* species, is notable because of its estrogenic and anabolic
activity in animals (Pathre and Mirocha, 1976; Mirocha and Christensen,
1974). The structure of zearalenone indicates a biosynthetic pathway involving nine acetate units.

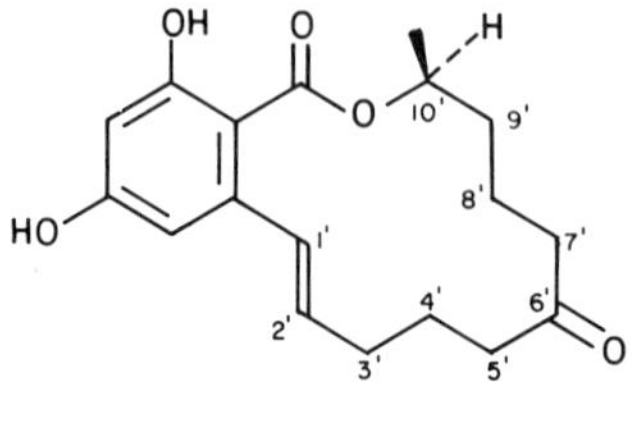

28

In the study of the biosynthesis of zearalenone, Steele *et al.* (1974) found that sodium [1-^{14}C]acetate and [2-^{14}C]malonate were efficiently incorporated. Chemical degradation of zearalenone obtained from [1-^{14}C]acetate followed by decarboxylation yielded $^{14}CO_2$ derived from the lactone carbonyl carbon atom. Oxidation of labeled zearalenone with nitric acid gave glutaric, succinic, and oxalic acids. The relative molar activities suggested a nonuniform ^{14}C distribution and alternative labeling of the carbon skeleton which is consistent with the acetate–malonate pathway.

Compounds structurally related to zearalenone but of dissimilar biological activity have been isolated from different fungi. Radicicol (**29**), an antibiotic, was first isolated from *Monosporium bonorden*. The structure was independently elucidated by McCapra *et al.* (1964) and Mirrington *et al.* (1964).

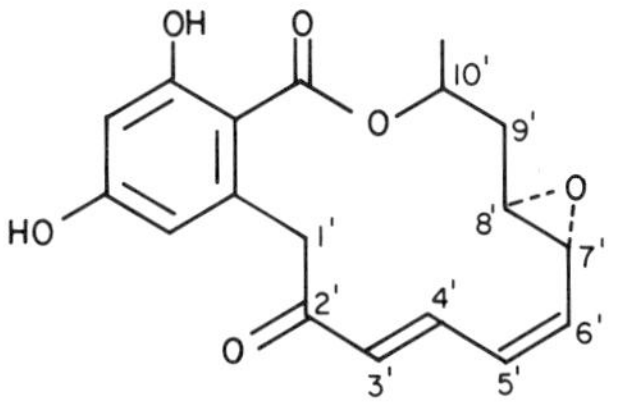

29

Musgrave (1956) isolated two related metabolites from species of *Curvularia*. The structure of the major metabolite curvularin (**30**) was deduced by Birch *et al.* (1959) and Musgrave (1956, 1957); the minor metabolite was 2′,3′-dehydrocurvularin (Munro *et al.*, 1967). Birch *et al.* (1959) found that sodium [1-^{14}C]acetate was efficiently incorporated (ca. 4%) into curvularin. Kuhn–Roth oxidation of the labeled product gave acetic acid containing approximately one-eighth the total activity, all of it in the carboxy carbon atom. Hydrobromic acid fission of the [^{14}C]curvularin gave octanoic acid and 3,5-dihydroxyphenylacetic acid, each containing 50% of the total activity. On the basis of these results, it was inferred that the C_{16} metabolite is derived from eight acetate units via the acetate–malonate pathway.

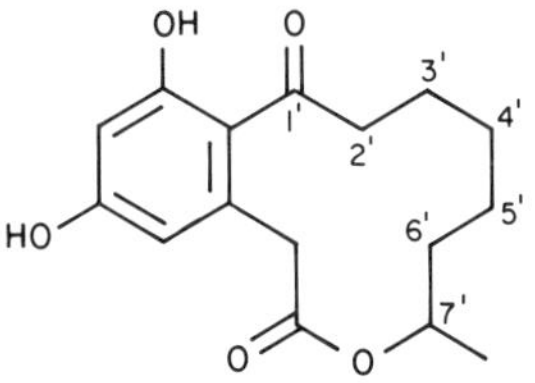

30

VI. RUBRATOXINS AND RELATED METABOLITES

Rubratoxin B is one of at least two toxins produced by certain strains of *Penicillium rubrum* isolated from feeds. The biological activity of both the rubratoxins and *P. rubrum* have been extensively reviewed (Moss, 1971; Newberne, 1974; Hayes, 1977). Rubratoxin B was shown by Moss *et al.* (1968) to be a bisanhydride (**31**); rubratoxin A was shown to possess essentially the same structure, with one of the anhydride groups reduced to the lactol (**32**) (Moss *et al.*, 1969).

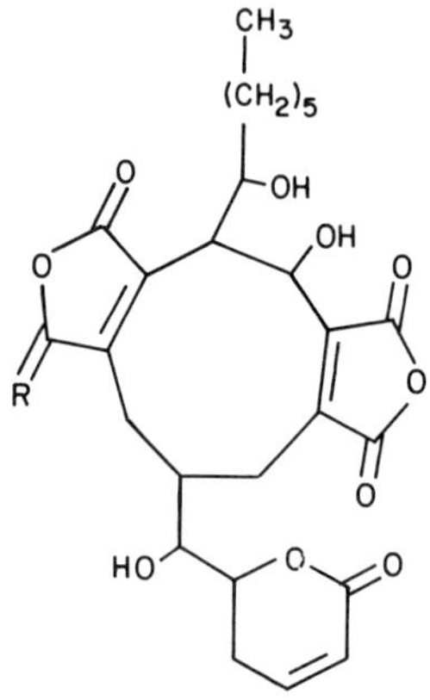

31 R = O
32 R = H,OH

The rubratoxins are unusual compounds in possessing relatively stable anhydride functions. They share this structural feature with the nonadrides, glaucanic acid (**33**) and glauconic acid (**34**), metabolites from *Penicillium purpurogenum*, as well as byssochlamic acid (**35**), produced by the ascomycete *Byssochlamys fulva*. The rubratoxins can be viewed as substituted higher homologues of byssochlamic acid (**35**).

Baldwin *et al.* (1962) described the constitution of glaucanic, glauconic, and byssochlamic acids and indicated how all three compounds could be derived by the coupling of two C_9 units of the form **36**. Moppet and Sutherland (1966) and Bloomer *et al.* (1968) presented sound evidence that such a C_9 compound, formed from the condensation of a β-polyketide-derived hexanoate residue with a C_3 fragment generated from the C_4 Krebs' cycle intermediate oxaloacetate, is indeed a precursor of glauconic acid (**34**). Addition of $[7\text{-}^3\text{H}]$ (**36**) to cultures of *P. purpurogenum* gave labeled glauconic acid (51.5% incorporation), with 97.5% of the activity located at C(7) and C(16). In feeding experiments with $[1\text{-}^{14}\text{C}]$- and $[2\text{-}^{14}\text{C}]$acetates, $[1\text{-}^{14}\text{C}]$-

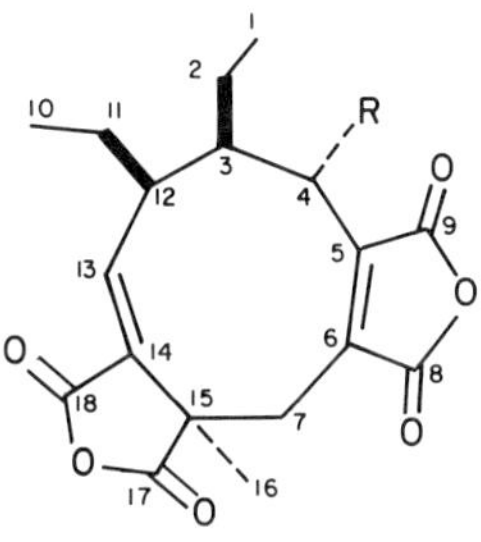

33   R = H
34   R = OH

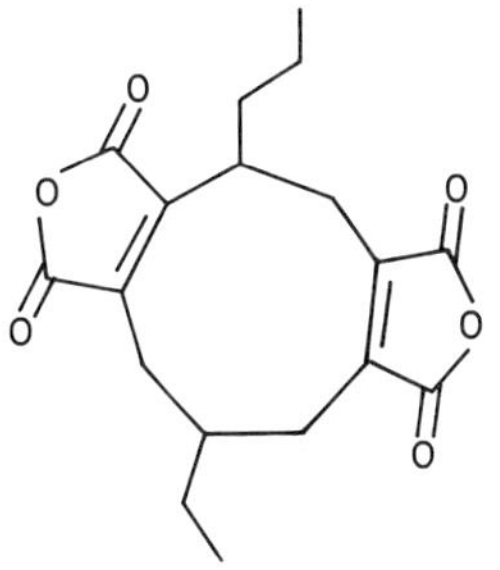

35

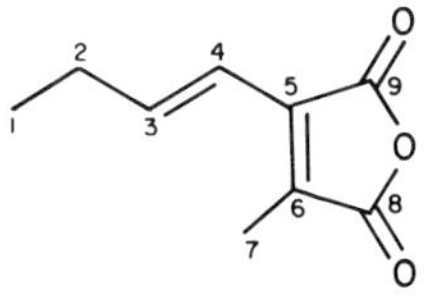

36

and [2-^{14}C]glucoses, [2-^{14}C]pyruvate, and [2,3-^{14}C]succinate, activity was found in both the β-ketide and the oxaloacetate-derived portions of the molecule. It was only by comparison of differential incorporations of individual precursors that firm conclusions could be derived. The problem of randomization of labels via the Krebs' tricarboxylate cycle tends to complicate all biosynthetic studies involving feedings with succinate and related precursors.

A more direct approach to glauconic acid biosynthesis was adopted by Cox and Holker (1976). Direct incorporation of the precursor [2,3-^{13}C]-succinate into the C$_3$ residue would be demonstrated by the appropriate (^{13}C,^{13}C) couplings observed in the ^{13}C NMR spectrum of the enriched metabolite, whereas any randomization that occurred via [1,2-^{13}C]oxaloacetate and [2,3-^{13}C]pyruvate into [1,2-^{13}C]acetate would be shown by (^{13}C,^{13}C) couplings in the hexanoate residue. The PND ^{13}C NMR spectrum of [2,3-^{13}C]succinate-derived glauconic acid showed (^{13}C,^{13}C) couplings for C(15)–C(16) and C(6)–C(7). The absence of couplings elsewhere in the spectrum indicated that there was negligible randomization of label into the hexanoate residue via [1,2-^{13}C]acetate.

By analogy, the biosynthesis of the rubratoxins can be postulated as the coupling of two C$_{13}$ units, each of which is derived from an acetate-derived decanoic acid derivative and oxaloacetic acid (see Fig. 5).

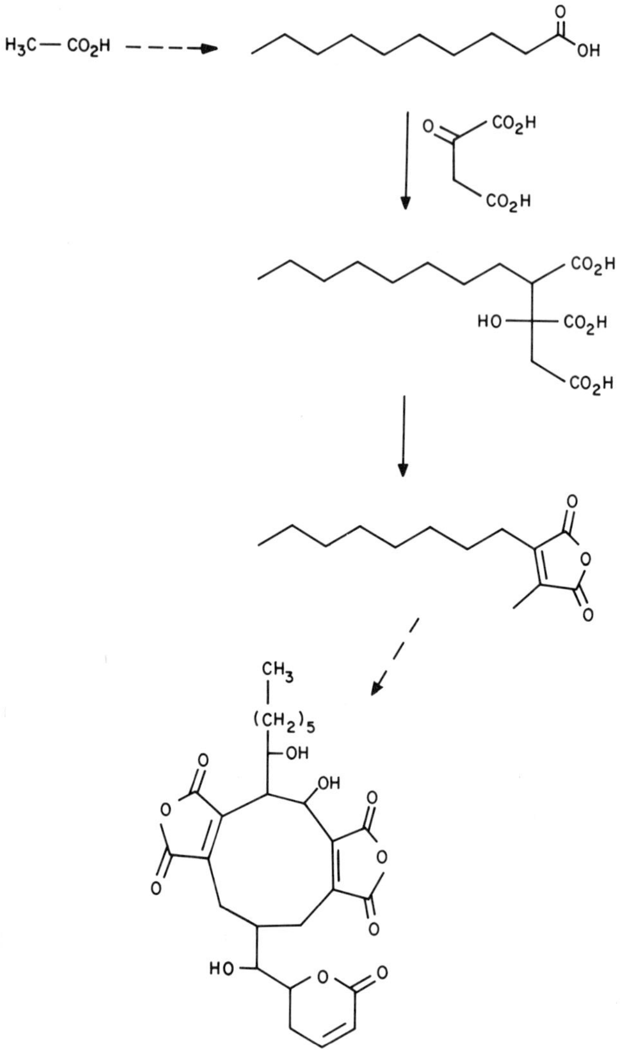

Fig. 5. Postulated biosynthesis of rubratoxin A (**31**).

VII. XANTHOCILLINS

The antibiotic xanthocillin X, first isolated from *Penicillium notatum* by Rothe (1950), was shown to be 1,4-di-(*p*-hydroxyphenyl)-2,3-diisonitrilo-1,3-butadiene (**37**) by Hagedorn and Tönjes (1957). Achenbach and Grisebach (1965) and Achenbach and König (1971) studied the biosynthesis of this unusual metabolite. DL-[2-^{14}C]Tyrosine was efficiently incorporated (18–25%) into xanthocillin X, whereas no activity from DL-[1-^{14}C]tyrosine was found in the metabolite. The origin of the isonitrile carbon atom remains unknown, for neither [1-^{14}C]-acetate, [2-^{14}C]acetate, [^{14}C]formate, or [*methyl*-^{14}C]methionine was incorporated to any extent into the carbon atom of the isonitrile group.

Achenbach and König (1972) also studied the biogenetic equivalence of the two C$_6$–C$_2$–N parts in the xanthocillin X molecule. The results from feeding experiments with DL-[^{15}N]tyrosine showed that only one nitrogen atom in the symmetric xanthocillin molecule originates directly from tyrosine. The presence of *p*-hydroxyphenylpyruvic acid in the medium in the above experiments caused a significant increase in ^{15}N enrichment in the formed xanthocillin and a simultaneous decrease of formation of dilabeled species. On the basis of these results, it was concluded that one molecule each of tyrosine and *p*-hydroxyphenylpyruvic acid is involved in the biosynthesis of xanthocillin X.

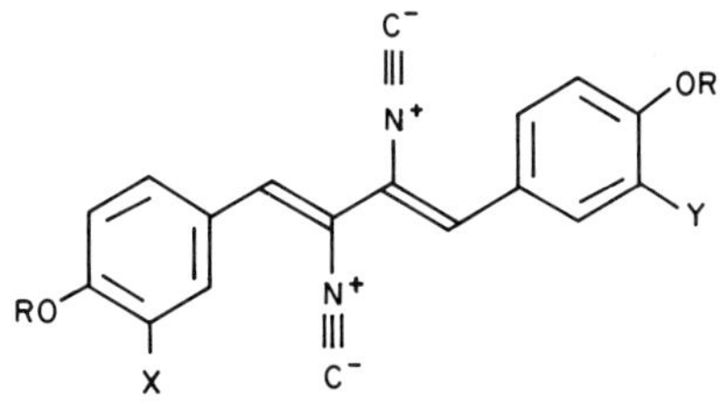

37	R = X = Y = H
39	R = Y = H , X = OH
40	R = H, X = Y = OH
41	R = X = Y = H ; – NH·CHO INSTEAD OF – $\overset{+}{N}\equiv\overset{-}{C}$
42	R = Me, X = Y = H
43	R = Me, X = OMe, Y = H

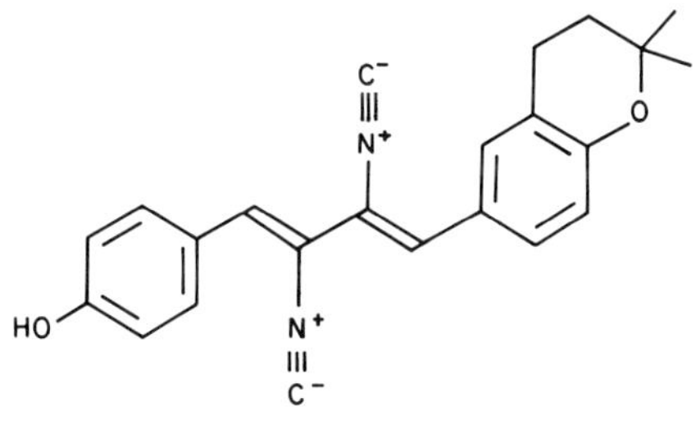

38

A xanthocillin analogue, xanthoascin (**38**), isolated from *Aspergillus candidus* by Takahashi *et al.* (1976), exhibited both hepato- and cardiotoxic properties in experimental animals. Some of the xanthocillin analogues (**39–43**) isolated from *P. notatum* (Hagedorn and Tönjes, 1957; Achenbach *et al.*, 1972; Pfeifer *et al.*, 1972), *Dichtomomyces albus* (Ando *et al.*, 1968) and *Aspergillus chevalieri* (Takatsuki *et al.*, 1968) exhibit cytotoxic activity to HeLa cells (Takahashi *et al.*, 1976).

VIII. TOXIC FURANOSESQUITERPENOIDS

Fungal contamination of sweet potatoes (*Ipomoea batatas*) or stress conditions (e.g., treatment with heavy metal salts) often results in the production of stress metabolites, including the well-known hepatotoxin ipomeamarone (**44**). In addition, the potent lung toxins 4-ipomeanol (**45**), 1-ipomeanol (**46**), ipomeanine (**47**), and 1,4-ipomeadiol (**48**) are sometimes produced (Burka and Wilson, 1976; Wilson and Boyd, 1974).

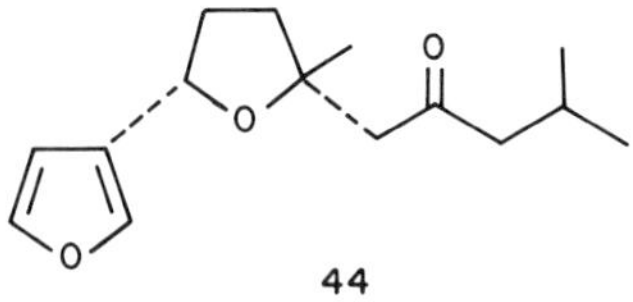

44

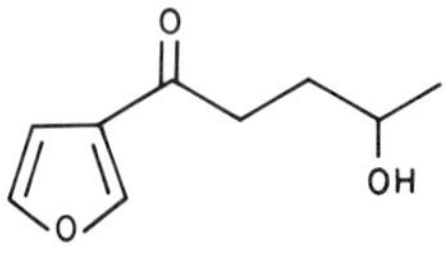

45 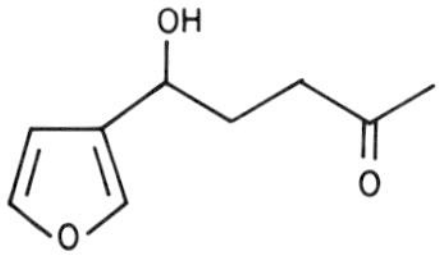   **46**

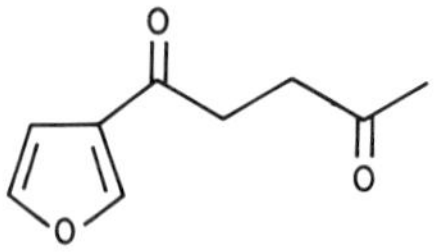

47 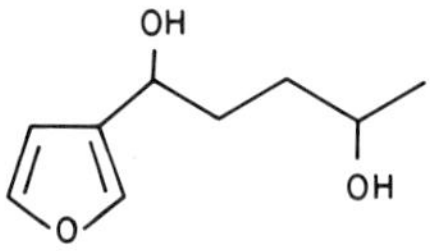   **48**

Available evidence suggests that ipomeamarone (**44**) arises from alterations of the tricarboxylic acid cycle and fatty acid synthesis. A postulated biosynthetic pathway is as follows:

Acetate ⟶ acetyl-CoA ⟶ acetoacetyl-CoA ⟶ β-hydroxy-β-methylglutaryl-CoA ⟶ mevalonate ·····▶ isopentenyl pyrophosphate ·····▶ farnesyl pyrophosphate ·····▶ ipomeamarone

(Oguni *et al.*, 1969). The incorporation of acetate, mevalonate, citrate, ethanol, leucine, and farnesol into ipomeamarone has been demonstrated.

Burka and Kuhnert (1977) showed that [¹⁴C]ipomeamarone, prepared by treating sweet potato slices with mercury(II) chloride in the presence of [2-¹⁴C]acetate, is a precursor of 4-hydroxymyoporone (**49**). Incubation of

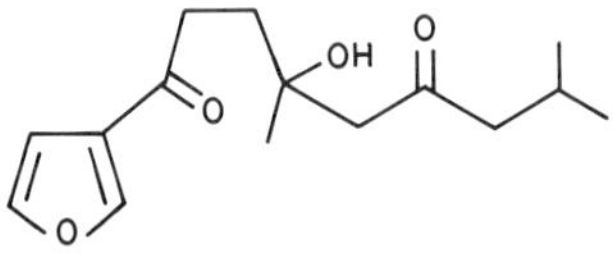

49

[¹⁴C]-4-hydroxymyoporone with the fungus, *Fusarium solani*, a common fungal contaminant of sweet potatoes, demonstrated that **49** can serve as a precursor to the lung toxins (Burka *et al.*, 1977). A retroaldol reaction would convert 4-hydroxymyoporone (**49**) into ipomeanine (**47**). Reduction of **47** would then lead to the other lung toxins, **45**, **46**, and **48**.

IX. DIPLOSPORIN

A novel mycotoxin, diplosporin, is produced by a toxigenic strain of *Diplodia macrospora* Earle, a fungus isolated from Zambian corn (Chalmers *et al.*, 1978). The structure **50** [(5S,6X)-6-ethyl-5-hydroxy-3-hydroxymethyl-5,6,7,8-tetrahydrobenzo[*b*]pyran-4-one] was assigned to this metabolite on the basis of physicochemical data and especially ¹H and ¹³C NMR data.

The biosynthesis of diplosporin was studied utilizing both ¹⁴C- and ¹³C-labeled precursors (Chalmers *et al.*, 1979). Initial experiments showed that sodium [1-¹⁴C]acetate was efficiently incorporated (2.5%) into diplosporin by growing cultures of *D. macrospora*. Feeding experiments with ¹³C-labeled acetate showed that carbon atoms C(4), C(7), C(9), C(11), and C(13) were derived from [1-¹³C]acetate. In a complementary experiment, the [2-¹³C]-acetate origin of carbon atoms C(3), C(6), C(8), C(10), and C(12) was confirmed. In the PND ¹³C NMR spectrum of the [1,2-¹³C]acetate-derived diplosporin, all the signals, with the exception of those for C(2) and C(5), exhibited (¹³C,¹³C) couplings and proved the presence of the following intact acetate units: C(13)–C(3), C(4)–C(10), C(9)–C(8), C(7)–C(6), and C(11)–C(12). These results established the folding of the original polyketide chain to be as shown in Fig. 6.

The origin of C(2) and C(5) from a C_1 pool was confirmed by addition of L-[*methyl*-¹⁴C]- (11% incorporation) and L-[methyl-¹³C]methionines. The ¹³C NMR spectrum of diplosporin derived from the latter precursor showed two enhanced signals caused by C(2) and C(5), thus confirming their origin.

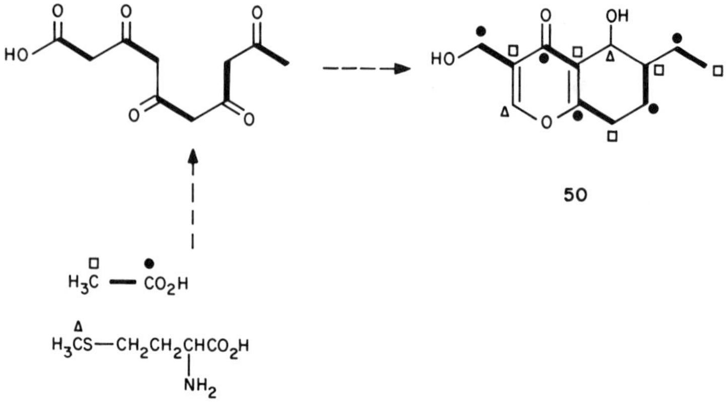

Fig. 6.   Biosynthesis of diplosporin (38).

Both C- and O-methylation of precursors in a biosynthetic pathway occur via S-adenosylmethionine, and are common occurrences. The introduction of a methionine-derived carbon atom into a heterocyclic ring is much less common but has been observed in, e.g., the biosynthesis of the rotenoids (Crombie et al., 1970, 1971a,b). The presence of a methionine-derived carbon atom in a carbocyclic ring has been demonstrated in two cases, namely, the biogenesis of the tropolones via a rearrangement of 3-methylorsellinic acid (Scott et al., 1971; McInnes et al., 1971; Scott and Wiesner, 1972) and the production of the cyclopropane ring in lactobacillic acid by C-methylation of a cis-vaccenic acid (Lederer, 1969).

The incorporation of a methionine-derived carbon atom into the carbocyclic ring of diplosporin is thus a highly unusual event. The mechanism probably proceeds by methylation of the C_{10}-polyketide progenitor chain at either the C(10) or the C(6) methylene group, followed by oxidative activation of the newly formed C-methyl group to facilitate ring closure.

A related metabolite, 5-deoxydiplosporin (51), was isolated from the culture medium of D. macrospora (Chalmers et al., 1979).

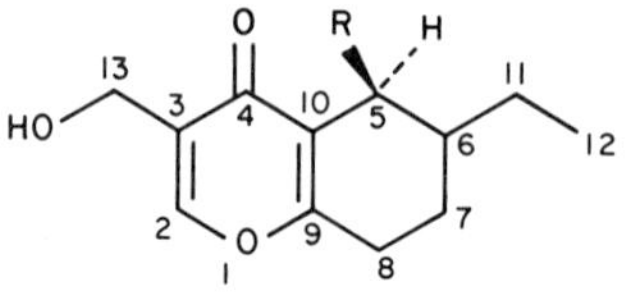

50   R = OH

51   R = H

X. GRISEOFULVIN

Griseofulvin (**52**), a chlorine-containing metabolite elaborated by *Penicillium griseofulvum* and related strains of *Penicillium*, has unique value as an antifungal antibiotic. Although it is apparently hepatotoxic and carcinogenic for experimental animals and may produce less serious toxic effects in humans, it continues to be used owing to its effectiveness (Wilson, 1971).

The polyketide origin of griseofulvin was demonstrated by incorporation studies with sodium[1-^{14}C]acetate by Birch *et al.* (1958b). On the basis of extensive degradations of the resultant labeled griseofulvin, a single polyketide chain formed from seven acetate units was formulated as a precursor. Tanabe and Detre (1966) studied the biosynthesis of griseofulvin using [2-^{13}C]acetate as a precursor. The detection and location of excess ^{13}C-label was performed by a study of the ^{13}C satellite signals in the ^{1}H NMR spectrum of the ^{13}C-enriched metabolite. In this manner, the presence of excess ^{13}C at C(7'), C(3'), and C(5) could be demonstrated.

In a communication, Sato *et al.* (1976b) reported the complete assignment of the signals in the ^{13}C NMR spectrum of griseofulvin. The alternate labeling pattern associated with the polyketide origin of the metabolite was verified by feeding experiments with *Penicillium urticae* using [1-^{13}C]- and [2-^{13}C]acetates. Furthermore, it was noted that incorporation of [2-^{13}C]acetate resulted in a substantial enrichment of the three methoxy groups of griseofulvin. These results were confirmed by Simpson and Holker (1977), who also reported that the apparent enrichment of labeled sites was very much lower with [2-^{13}C]acetate than with [1-^{13}C]acetate. However, mass spectrometry indicated that the total incorporation of the two precursors was comparable. This apparent discrepancy was explained by the fact that the label of [2-^{13}C]acetate becomes randomized into the 1 position via operation of the Krebs' cycle.

An acetate chain-initiating effect was also observed in the ^{13}C NMR spectra: the degree of enrichment at C(7') and C(6') was significantly higher than in the remaining acetate-derived carbon atoms. This observation was confirmed by addition of [2-^{14}C]malonate to cultures of *Penicillium patulum*. Kuhn–Roth oxidation of the [^{14}C]griseofulvin gave acetic acid with only 9.8% of the total activity of griseofulvin (even labeling requires 14.3%).

The enrichment of the methoxy groups by [2-^{13}C]acetate reported by Sato *et al.* (1976b) was confirmed and explained by Simpson and Holker (1977). Conversion of [2-^{13}C]acetate via the Krebs' cycle and pyruvate into [2,3-^{13}C]serine would lead to the specific enrichment of the methoxy groups in griseofulvin. The origin of the C(2) and C(3) carbon atoms of serine from C(2) of acetate has been noted (Ehrensvard *et al.*, 1950). Subsequent dehydroxymethylation of [2,3-^{13}C]serine would give [2-^{13}C]glycine and a

^{13}C-enriched C_1 pool (N^5,N^{10}-methylenetetrahydrofolate). The methyl carbons of the methoxy groups in griseofulvin have previously been shown to originate from the usual C_1 donors (Hockenhull and Faulds, 1955).

Administration of [1,2-^{13}C]acetate to *P. urticae* by Sato *et al.* (1976b) gave griseofulvin which showed characteristic satellite resonances in the PND ^{13}C NMR spectrum. Ten pairs of directly bonded (^{13}C,^{13}C) couplings were identified by matching coupling constants, and these indicated that

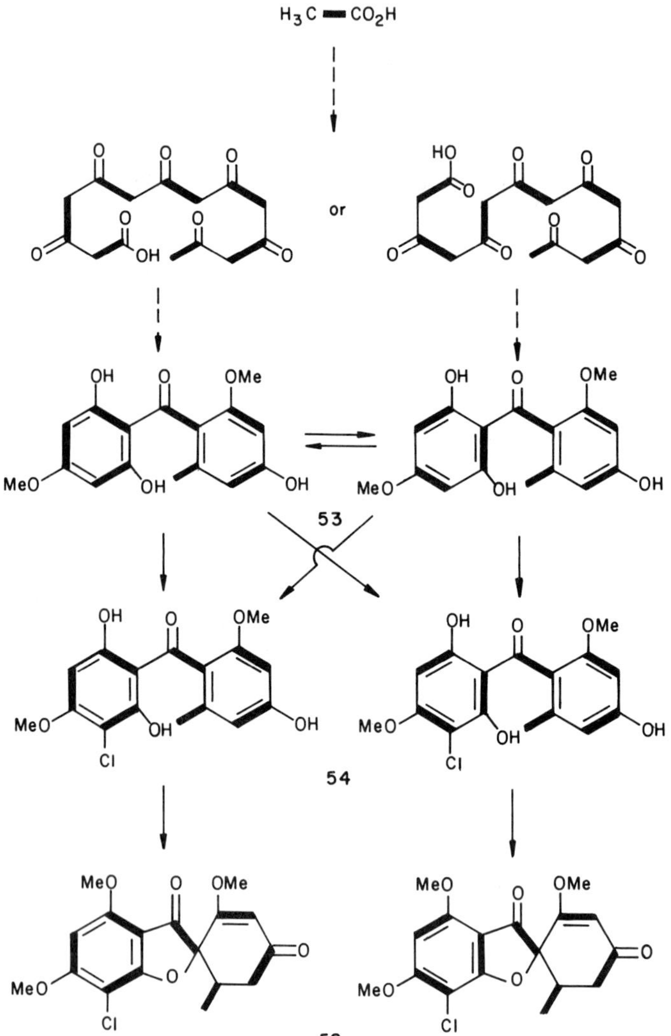

Fig. 7.   Biosynthesis of griseofulvin (52).

C(7′)–C(6′), C(5′)–C(4′), C(3′)–C(2′), C(1′)–C(3), C(3a)–C(4), C(5)–C(6), C(7)–C(7a), C(3a)–C(7a), C(7)–C(6), and C(5)–C(4) originated from intact C_2 units. It is noteworthy that C(7) was (^{13}C, ^{13}C) coupled to both C(6) and C(7a), C(5) to C(4) and C(6), and C(3a) to C(4) and C(7a). The above distribution of C_2 units arises from rotation about the twofold axis of symmetry in ring A of the precursor, griseophenone C (**53**). This rotation interchanges carbon atoms on opposite sides of the axis, and must occur when the precursor is not rigidly bound to an enzyme surface. Chlorination at either of the two equivalent positions C(7) or C(5), followed by ring closure using the hydroxy group *ortho* to the chlorine atom, would result finally in the formation of two differently labeled griseofulvin molecules (see Fig. 7). It is only by introducing cryptic asymmetry through ^{13}C-labeling with [1,2-^{13}C]acetate that this type of rotation can be observed. Similar results have been reported in the biosynthesis of ravenelin (Birch *et al.*, 1976) and secalonic acid A (Kurobane *et al.*, 1978).

Cometabolites of griseofulvin (**52**), which include the benzophenones griseophenone C (**53**), griseophenone B (**54**), and griseophenone A (**55**) as well

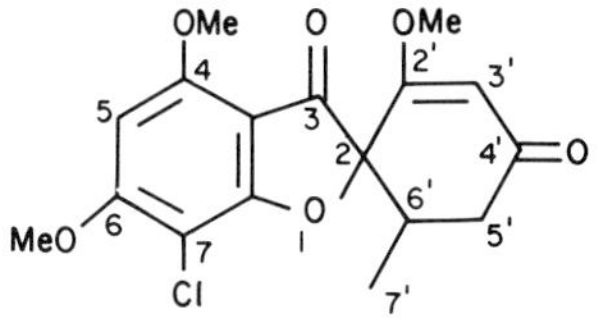

52

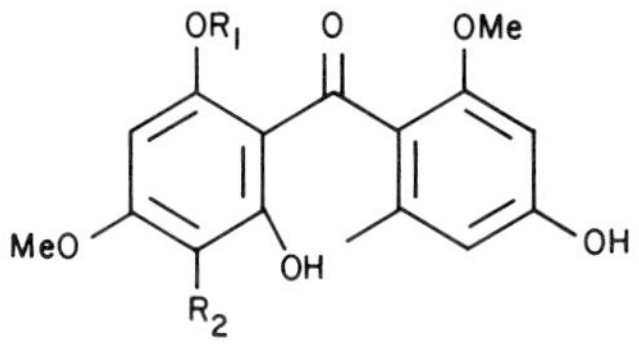

53 R$_1$ = R$_2$ = H

54 R$_1$ = H, R$_2$ = Cl

55 R$_1$ = Me, R$_2$ = Cl

as 5′,6′-didehydrogriseofulvin (**56**), have provided considerable insight into its biosynthesis. Rhodes *et al.* (1963) demonstrated the efficient incorporation of both griseophenone C (**53**) (21%) and griseophenone B (**54**) (71%) into griseofulvin. Griseophenone A (**55**), however, was not incorporated. The benzophenone **57** was shown by Harris *et al.* (1976) to be a precursor of griseofulvin by a feeding experiment in which **57** labeled with tritium in the

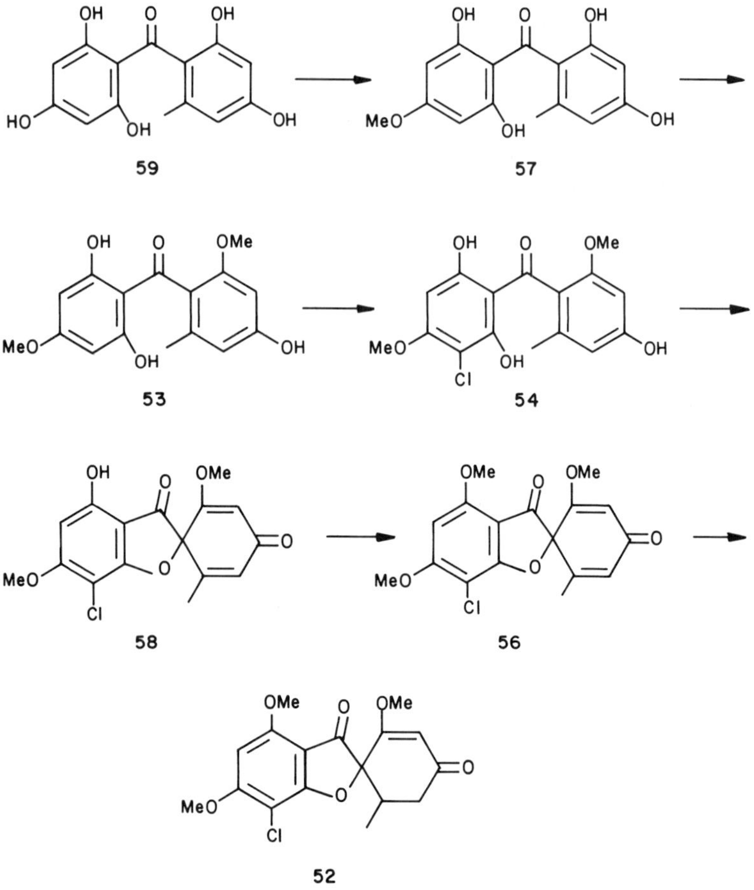

Fig. 8. Aromatic precursors in the biosynthesis of griseofulvin (**52**).

O-methyl group was incorporated (14%) into griseofulvin. Normethyldi-
dehydrogriseofulvin (**58**) proved to be an highly efficient (44%) precursor.
Indirect evidence for the precursor role of the benzophenone **59** was also
obtained by Harris et al. (1976). The findings of Harris et al. (1976), in conjunction with those of previous studies, support the biosynthetic sequence
as outlined in Fig. 8.

^{2}H NMR spectroscopy provides an excellent tool to study the fate of
hydrogen atoms in biosynthetic pathways. As ^{2}H NMR chemical shifts are
essentially the same as those of the ^{1}H isotope, assignments are greatly
simplified. Sato et al. (1975) studied the extent of incorporation of ^{3}H into
griseofulvin by feeding [2-^{3}H,2-^{14}C]acetate with a ^{3}H:^{14}C ratio of 6.27 to
cultures of P. urticae. The isolated griseofulvin had a ^{3}H:^{14}C ratio of 1.77,

which corresponds to the incorporation of six tritium atoms. The location of the hydrogen isotope labels was determined from feeding experiments using $[2\text{-}^2H_3]$acetate as precursor (Sato et al., 1976a). The ^2H NMR spectrum of the enriched griseofulvin indicated the presence of ^2H at the following positions: C(7'), 44%; C(5'α), 23%; C(3') and C(5), 24%. The presence of ^2H in the methoxy groups [C(2'), 3%; C(4) and C(6), 6%] is in agreement with the results obtained from $[2\text{-}^{13}C]$acetate incorporation studies (Sato et al., 1976b; Simpson and Holker, 1977). Analysis of the signal caused by the deuteriums at C(7') as well as mass spectrometric analysis of the labeled griseofulvin suggested that the deuteriated 6'-methyl group consisted of 75–89% CHD_2 and 14–22% CD_3. The mass spectral data of griseofulvin obtained from short-time incubation with $[2\text{-}^2H_3]$acetate suggested that the 6'-methyl group consisted only of CD_3.

^2H NMR spectroscopy was also used to establish that in *P. urticae*, the precursors $[5'\text{-}^2H]$griseophenone B (**54**) and 4-demethyl-5',6'-$[5'\text{-}^2H]$didehydrogriseofulvin (**58**) led to the formation of griseofulvin (**52**) with ^2H in the 5'α position (Sato et al., 1978). The stereochemical course of the 5'-hydrogen atoms is the same as that in the microbial hydrogenation of didehydrogriseofulvin (**56**) to griseofulvin (Sato et al., 1977).

REFERENCES

Achenbach, H., and Grisebach, H. (1965). *Z. Naturforsch* **20B**. 137.
Achenbach, H., and König, F. (1971). *Experientia* **27**, 1250.
Achenbach, H., and König, F. (1972). *Chem. Ber.* **105**, 784.
Achenbach, H., Strittmatter, H., and Kohl, W. (1972). *Chem. Ber.*, **105**, 3061.
Anderegg, R. J., Bieman, K., Büchi, G., and Cushman, M. (1976). *J. Am. Chem. Soc.* **98**, 3365.
Ando, K., Tamura, G., and Arima, K. (1968). J. Antibiot. **21**, 587.
Baldwin, J. E., Barton, D. H. R., Bloomer, J. L., Jackman, L. M., Rodriques-Hahn, L., and Sutherland, J. K. (1962). *Experientia* **18**, 345.
Birch, A. J., Fitton, P., Pride, E., Ryan, A. J., Smith, H., and Whalley, W. B. (1958a). *J. Chem. Soc.*, p. 4576.
Birch, A. J., Massey-Westropp, R. A., Rickards, R. W., and Smith, H. (1958b). *J. Chem. Soc.*, p. 360.
Birch, A. J., Musgrave, O. C., Rickards, R. W., and Smith, H. (1959). *J. Chem. Soc.*, p. 3146.
Birch, A. J., Hussain, S. F., and Rickards, R. W. (1964). *J. Chem. Soc.*, p. 3494.
Birch, A. J., Baldas, J., Hlubucek, J. R., Simpson, T. J., and Westerman, P. W. (1976). *J. Chem. Soc., Perkin Trans. 1*, p. 898.
Bloomer, J. L., Moppet, C. E., and Sutherland, J. K. (1968). *J. Chem. Soc. C.*, p. 588.
Burka, L. T., and Kuhnert, L. (1977). *Phytochemistry* **16**, 2022.
Burka, L. T., and Wilson, B. J. (1976). *Adv. Chem. Ser.* **149**, 387.
Burka, L. T., Kuhnert, L., Wilson, B. J., and Harris, T. M. (1977). *J. Am. Chem. Soc.* **99**, 2302.
Carlton, W. W., and Tuite, J. (1977). *In* "Mycotoxins in Human and Animal Health" (J. V. Rodricks, C. W. Hesseltine, and M. A. Mehlman, eds.), p. 525. Pathotox Publishers, Park Forest South, Illinois.

Carlton, W. W., Stack, M. E., and Eppley, R. M. (1976). *Toxicol. Appl. Pharmacol.* **38**, 455.

Cattel, L., Grove, J. F., and Shaw, D. (1973). *J. Chem. Soc. Perkin Trans. 1*, p. 2626.

Chalmers, A. A., Gorst-Allman, C. P., Kriek, N. P. J., Marasas, W. F. O., Steyn, P. S., and Vleggaar, R. (1978). *S. Afr. J. Chem.* **31**, 111.

Chalmers, A. A., Gorst-Allman, C. P., Steyn, P. S., Vleggaar, R., and Scott, D. B. (1979). *J. Chem. Soc., Perkin Trans. 1*, p. 1481

Chexal, K. K., Springer, J. P., Clardy, J., Cole, R. J., Kirksey, J. W., Dorner, J. W., Cutler, H. G., and Strawter, B. J. (1976). *J. Am. Chem. Soc.* **98**, 6748.

Chu, F. S. (1974). *C. R. C. Crit. Rev. Toxicol.*, p. 499.

Ciegler, A., Fennell, D. I., Mintzlaff, H-J, and Leistner, L. (1972). *Naturwissenschaften* **59**, 365.

Cox, R. E., and Holker, J. S. E. (1976). *J. Chem. Soc., Chem. Commun.*, p. 583.

Crombie, L., Dewich, P. M., and Whiting, D. A. (1970). *J. Chem. Soc. Chem. Commun.*, p. 1469.

Crombie, L., Dewich, P. M., and Whiting, D. A. (1971a). *J. Chem. Soc., Chem. Commun.*, p. 1182.

Crombie, L., Dewich, P. M., and Whiting, D. A. (1971b). *J. Chem. Soc. Chem. Commun.*, p. 1183.

Curtis, R. F., Hassal, C. H., and Nazar, M. (1968). *J. Chem. Soc. C.*, p. 85.

Durley, R. C., MacMillan, J., Simpson, T. J., Glen, A. T., and Turner, W. B. (1975). *J. Chem. Soc. Perkin Trans. 1*, p. 163.

Ehrensvard, G., Reio, L., Saluste, E., and Stjernholm, R. (1950). *J. Biol. Chem.* **183**, 93.

Evans, G. E., and Staunton, J. (1976). *J. Chem. Soc. Chem. Commun.*, p. 760.

Ferreira, N. P., and Pitout, M. J. (1969). *J. S. Afr. Chem. Inst.* **22**, S1.

Gatenbeck, S., and Mosbach, K. (1963). *Biochem. Biophys. Res. Commun.* **11**, 166.

Hagedorn, I., and Tönjes, H. (1957). *Pharmazie* **12**, 567.

Harris, C. M., Roberson, J. S., and Harris, T. M. (1976). *J. Am. Chem. Soc.* **98**, 5380.

Harwig, J. (1974). *In* "Mycotoxins" (I. F. H. Purchase, ed.), p. 344. Elsevier, Amsterdam.

Hayes, A. W. (1977). *In* "Mycotoxins in Human and Animal Health" (J. V. Rodricks, C. W. Hesseltine, and M. A. Mehlman, eds.), p. 507. Pathotox Publishers, Park Forest South, Illinois.

Hesseltine, C. W., Vandegraft, E. E., Fennel, D. I., Smith, M. L., and Shotwell, O. L. (1972). *Mycologia* **64**, 539.

Hetherington, A. C., and Raistrick, H. (1931). *Phil. Trans. R. Soc. London, Ser. B.* **220**, 269.

Hill, R. A., Carter, R. H., and Staunton, J. (1975). *J. Chem. Soc., Chem. Commun.*, p. 380.

Hockenhull, D. J. D., and Faulds, W. F. (1955). *Chem. Ind. (London)*, p. 1390.

Höfle, G. and Röser, K. (1978). *J. Chem. Soc., Chem. Commun.*, p. 611.

Holker, J. S. E., and Young, K. (1975). *J. Chem. Soc. Chem. Commun.*, p. 525.

Just, G., Day, W. C., and Blank, F. (1963). *Can. J. Chem.* **41**, 74.

Kabuto, C., Silverton, J. V., Akiyama, T., Sankawa, U., Hutchison, R. D., Steyn, P. S., and Vleggaar, R. (1976). *J. Chem. Soc., Chem. Commun.*, p. 728.

Krogh, P., Hald, B., and Pedersen, E. J. (1973). *Acta Pathol. Microbiol. Scand. Sect. B.* **81**, 689.

Kurobane, I., Vining, L. C., McInnes, A. G., Walter, J. A., and Wright, J. L. C., (1978). *Tetrahedron Lett.*, p. 1379.

Lai, M., Semeniuk, G., and Hesseltine, C. W. (1968). *Phytopathology* **58**, 1056.

Lederer, E. (1969). *Chem. Soc. Rev.* **4**, 453.

McCapra, F., Scott, A. I., Delmotte, P., Delmotte-Plaquee, J., and Bhacca, N. S. (1964). *Tetrahedron Lett.*, p. 869.

McGormick, J. R. D., (1967). *In* "Antibiotics Vol. II. Biosynthesis" (D. Gottlieb and P. D. Shaw, eds.), p. 113. Springer-Verlag, Berlin and New York.

McInnes, A. G., Smith, D. G., Vining, L. C., and Johnson, L. (1971). *J. Chem. Soc., Chem. Commun.*, p. 325.

Macmillan, J. G., Springer, J. P., Clardy, J., Cole, R. J., and Kirksey, J. W. (1976). *J. Am. Chem. Soc.* **98**, 246.

Maebayashi, Y., Miyaki, K., and Yamazaki, M. (1972). *Chem. Pharm. Bull.* **20**, 2172.

Mirocha, C. J., and Christensen, C. M. (1974). *In* "Mycotoxins" (I. F. H. Purchase, ed.), p. 129. Elsevier, Amsterdam.

Mirrington, R. N., Ritchie, E. Shoppee, C. W., Taylor, W. C., and Sternhell, S. (1964). *Tetrahedron Lett.*, p. 365.

Moppet, C. E. and Sutherland, J. K. (1966). *J. Chem. Soc. Chem. Commun.*, p. 772.

Moss, M. O. (1971). *In* "Microbial Toxins" (A. Ciegler, S. Kadis, and S. J. Ajl, eds.), Vol. VI, p. 381. Academic Press, New York.

Moss, M. O., Robinson, F. V., Wood, A. B., Paisley, H. M., and Feeney, J. (1968). *Nature (London)* **220**, 767.

Moss, M. O., Wood, A. B., and Robinson, F. V. (1969). *Tetrahedron Lett.*, p. 367.

Munro, H. D., Musgrave, O. C., and Templeton, R. (1967). *J. Chem. Soc. C.*, p. 947.

Musgrave, O. C. (1956). *J. Chem. Soc.*, p. 4301.

Musgrave, O. C. (1957). *J. Chem. Soc.*, p. 1104.

Newberne, P. M. (1974). *In* "Mycotoxins" (I. F. H. Purchase, ed.), p. 163. Elsevier, Amsterdam.

Nitta, K., Yamamoto, Y. Inoue, T., and Hyodo, T. (1966). *Chem. Pharm. Bull.* **14**, 363.

Oguni, I., Oshima, K., Imaseki, H., and Uritani, I. (1969). *Agric. Biol. Chem.* **33**, 50.

Pathre, S. V., and Mirocha, C. J. (1976). *Adv. Chem. Ser.* **149**, 178.

Pfeifer, S., Bär, H., and Zarnach, J. (1972). *Pharmazie* **27**, 536.

Raistrick, H., and Smith, G. (1941). *Chem. Ind. (London)* **160**, 331.

Rhodes, A., Somerfield, G. A., and McGonagle, M. P. (1963). *Biochem. J.* **88**, 349.

Roberts, J. C., and Woolven, P. (1970). *J. Chem. Soc. C.*, p. 278.

Rodig, O. R., Ellis, L. C., and Glover, I. T. (1966). *Biochemistry* **5**, 2458.

Rothe, W. (1950). *Pharmazie* **5**, 190.

Sato, Y., Machida, T., and Oda, T. (1975). *Tetrahedron Lett.*, p. 4571.

Sato, Y., Oda, T., and Saitô, H. (1976a). *Tetrahedron Lett.*, p. 2695.

Sato, Y., Oda, T., and Urano, S. (1976b). *Tetrahedron Lett.*, p. 3971.

Sato, Y., Oda, T., and Saitô, H. (1977). *J. Chem. Soc., Chem. Commun.*, p. 415.

Sato, Y., Oda, T., and Saitô, H. (1978). *J. Chem. Soc., Chem. Commun.*, p. 135.

Schwenk, E., Alexander, G. J., Gold, A. M., and Stevens, D. F. (1958). *J. Biol. Chem.* **233**, 1211.

Scott, D. B. (1965). *Mycopathol. Mycol. Appl.* **25**, 213.

Scott, A. I., and Wiesner, K. J. (1972). *J. Chem. Soc., Chem. Commun.*, p. 1075.

Scott, A. I., Guilford, H., and Lee, E. (1971). *J. Am. Chem. Soc.* **93**, 3534.

Scott, P. M., van Walbeek, W., Kennedy, B., and Anyeti, D. (1972). *J. Agric. Food. Chem.* **20**, 1103.

Searcy, J. W., Davis, N. D., and Diener, U. L. (1969). *Appl. Microbiol.* **18**, 622.

Simpson, T. J. (1977), *J. Chem. Soc. Perkin Trans. 1*, p. 592.

Simpson, T. J., and Holker, J. S. E. (1977). *Phytochemistry* **16**, 229.

Springer, J. P., Clardy, J., Cole, R. J., Kirksey, J. W., Hill, R. K., Carlson, R. M., and Isidor, J. L. (1974). *J. Am. Chem. Soc.* **96**, 2267.

Steele, J. A., Lieberman, J. R., and Mirocha, C. J. (1974). *Can. J. Microbiol.* **20**, 531.

Steyn, P. S. (1971). *In* "Microbial Toxins" (A. Ciegler, S. Kadis, and S. J. Ajl, eds.), Vol. VI, p. 179. Academic Press, New York.

Steyn, P. S., and Holzapfel, C. W. (1967). *Tetrahedron* **23**, 4449.

Steyn, P. S., Holzapfel, C. W., and Ferreira, N. P. (1970). *Phytochemistry* **9**, 1977.

Takahashi, C., Sekita, S., Yoshihira, K., and Natori, S. (1976). *Chem. Pharm. Bull.* **24**, 2317.

Takatsuki, A., Suzuki, S., Ando, K., Tamura, G., and Arima, K. (1968). *J. Antibiol.* **21**, 671.

Tanabe, M., and Detre, G. (1966). *J. Am. Chem. Soc.* **88**, 4515.

Van der Merwe, K. J., Steyn, P. S., Fourie, L., Scott, D. B., and Theron, J. J. (1965a). *Nature (London)* **205**, 1112.

Van der Merwe, K. J., Steyn, P. S., and Fourie, L. (1965b). *J. Chem. Soc.*, p. 7083.

Van Walbeek, W., Scott, P. M., Harwig, J., and Lawrence, J. W. (1969). *Can. J. Microbiol.* **15**, 1281.

Wehrli, F. W. (1973). *J. Chem. Soc., Chem. Commun.*, p. 379.

Wei, R-D., Strong, R. M., and Smalley, E. B. (1971). *Appl. Microbiol.* **22**, 276.

Weisleder, D., and Lillehoj, E. B. (1971). *Tetrahedron Lett.*, p. 4705.

Wilson, B. J. (1971). *In* "Microbial Toxins" (A. Ciegler, S. Kadis, and S. J. Ajl, eds.), Vol. VI, p. 459. Academic Press, New York.

Wilson, B. J., and Boyd, M. R. (1974). *In* "Mycotoxins" (I. F. H. Purchase, ed.), p. 327. Elsevier, Amsterdam.

INDEX

A